praise for the first edition of
The Unofficial LEGO® Technic Builder's Guide

"This is one of those books that just amazes me—complex ideas made easier to follow with what are basically toy pieces of plastic."
—JAMES FLOYD KELLY, *GeekDad*

"This book boggles the mind! Even if you're an accomplished builder, some of the techniques that Sariel shares are sure to expand your repertoire."
—KRIS BORDESSA, *WIRED*

"I would recommend this book for any adult builder who is interested in becoming more familiar with Technic and using Technic in their own creations. It is definitely an asset that deserves a place on the shelf."
—JOSH WEDIN, *THE BROTHERS BRICK*

"A very well-organized and clear guide to getting the most out of your hobby. Start at the beginning, work towards the end, and you'll be an expert modeler and maker of things LEGO Technic."
—GREG LADEN, NATIONAL GEOGRAPHIC'S *SCIENCEBLOGS*

"Sariel is a legend in the LEGO world. . . . His machines are fantastic."
—JESUS DIAZ, *GIZMODO*

"This book is a gem."
—RYAN MCNAUGHT, LEGO CERTIFIED PROFESSIONAL

THE UNOFFICIAL LEGO® TECHNIC BUILDER'S GUIDE, 2ND EDITION

Paweł "Sariel" **Kmieć**

THE UNOFFICIAL LEGO® TECHNIC BUILDER'S GUIDE, 2ND EDITION. Copyright © 2017 by Paweł "Sariel" Kmieć.

Printed in USA

First printing

20 19 18 17 16   1 2 3 4 5 6 7 8 9

ISBN-10: 1-59327-760-1
ISBN-13: 978-1-59327-760-4

Publisher: William Pollock
Production Editor: Serena Yang
Cover Illustration: Eric "Blakbird" Albrecht
Interior Design: Octopod Studios
Developmental Editor: Tyler Ortman
Technical Reviewer: Eric "Blakbird" Albrecht
Copyeditor: Anne Marie Walker
Compositor: Serena Yang
Proofreader: Paula L. Fleming
Indexer: BIM Creatives, LLC

Figures 3-17, 3-18, 3-19, 3-20, 3-21, 3-22, 3-23, 3-24, 3-44, 4-6, 7-11, 11-24, 12-29, 12-37, 16-16, 18-4, 23-3, 23-4, 23-8, 23-14, and 23-15 by Eric "Blakbird" Albrecht

Figure 5-11 courtesy of Michał Skorupka. Figure 5-12 courtesy of SevenStuds. Figure 17-13 by Jano Gallo, used under Creative Commons Attribution-ShareAlike 3.0 Unported.

Blueprint images (Figures 23-2, 23-5, 23-6, 23-18, 23-19, 23-20, 24-1, 24-6, 24-7, 24-8, and 24-9) are royalty-free images purchased from The-Blueprints.com.

Author's photo by Magda Andrzejewska

The following software has been used for illustrations: MLCAD by Michael Lachmann, LDView by Travis Cobbs and Peter Bartfai, and LPub by Kevin Clague.

For information on distribution, translations, or bulk sales, please contact No Starch Press, Inc. directly:
No Starch Press, Inc.
245 8th Street, San Francisco, CA 94103
phone: 1.415.863.9900; info@nostarch.com; www.nostarch.com

The Library of Congress has cataloged the first edition as follows:

Kmiec, Pawel.
   The unofficial LEGO Technic builder's guide / Pawel "Sariel" Kmiec.
       pages cm
   ISBN-13: 978-1-59327-434-4
   ISBN-10: 1-59327-434-3
   1. Machinery--Models. 2. LEGO toys. I. Title. II. Title: LEGO Technic builder's guide.
   TJ248.K57 2012
   621.8022'8--dc23

                              2012029840

about the author

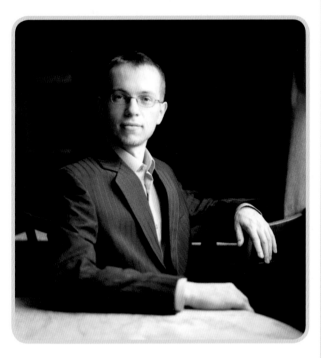

Paweł "Sariel" Kmieć is a LEGO Technic enthusiast based in Warsaw, Poland. A prolific blogger and model builder, Sariel's LEGO creations have been featured in many magazines and the world's most popular LEGO blogs, and even prompted the LEGO Group to ask for his help in developing some of its products. Sariel is an acting LEGO Ambassador and an official reviewer of LEGO sets, which he showcases on his popular YouTube channel (which has more than 40 million views) along with his own creations. His models have been praised by historians and military experts, and his articles are used as references by the University of Cambridge's engineering department. Check out his models and more at *http://sariel.pl/*.

about the tech reviewer

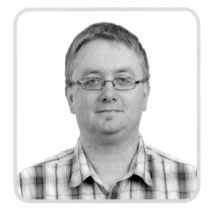

Eric "Blakbird" Albrecht is an aerospace engineer living in the northwest United States. He maintains the globally known Technicopedia, in which he documents the history of every Technic model beginning in 1977, all of which are on display on his shelves. Eric is also an avid user of LEGO CAD tools and has generated over 1,000 photo-realistic renders of official models and MOCs (My Own Creations). He has created dozens of sets of instructions for some of the best Technic MOCs from around the world, averaging 1,500 parts each. Check out his site at *http://www.technicopedia.com/*.

brief contents

contents in detail

PART I   BASICS

1

2

PART IV   ADVANCED MECHANICS

preface

The first edition of *The Unofficial LEGO Technic Builder's Guide* was written with one simple goal: to share everything I've learned about building with LEGO Technic during the past 20 years. This plan inevitably met with some limitations, not least of which were the page count and the vast amount of work involved. It was also an unprecedented book in LEGO Technic field, and we were sailing in uncharted waters, so to speak.

Fortunately, thanks to the warm welcome and great feedback of many great builders who found the original guide useful, you are now holding the second edition, which I was able to expand and update substantially. By necessity, it still does not cover *everything* you can build, and it never will, considering that just six basic 2×4 LEGO bricks can be combined in more than 915 million ways. The original guide consisted of 21 chapters. In this second edition, 13 of these chapters are updated and 4 brand-new chapters are added. The updates include introducing the new pieces the LEGO Group has released, as well as corrections, improvements, and newly developed mechanical solutions—for example, the best transmission design I've ever created (page 321). Many sections of the original text are revised or rewritten to make them easier to understand and more accurate; with the same goal in mind, many original figures and diagrams are newly created.

The new chapters cover a variety of topics, from the deceptively simple subject of LEGO wheels to the more obviously advanced, like planetary gearing and custom 3D-printed pieces. I also discuss the legendary LEGO RC system—a system that, although only available secondhand, in many respects still outperforms the solutions LEGO relies on today.

My goal in this new edition remains the same: to equip you for your own adventure in designing and building your own models with LEGO Technic. LEGO sets usually include complete building instructions but no explanations about how things work. I decided to take the opposite approach by introducing the principles that make LEGO constructions work and by showing you component mechanisms, such as transmissions or suspension systems, which you can then incorporate into your creations. It is my intent to offer you a choice: You can not only build LEGO sets, but you can also create new designs on your own. You can also try combining the two approaches by customizing LEGO sets, each of which can be changed in countless ways.

Any construction you find in this book should not be considered a definitive design. There's always room for tinkering and improvements. In fact, some of the constructions shown in this guide deliberately use basic LEGO pieces to help builders with limited LEGO resources. If you're fortunate to have newer, more sophisticated pieces at hand, don't hesitate to experiment with upgrades. If your collection is modest, keep in mind that creative thinking can overcome nearly any limitation.

As explained in "Where to Buy LEGO Pieces?" on page xix, this book intentionally relies on many earlier LEGO pieces and on the BrickLink's catalog for their numbers and names. BrickLink (*http://www.bricklink.com/*) offers a vast secondhand market right at your fingertips; you'll be able to find and purchase pretty much any kind of LEGO piece ever made.

Playing with LEGO is a fantastic hobby that comes in many flavors, from collecting pieces to customizing existing sets to creating models on your own. I strongly believe that the last one is the most satisfying—it's a unique experience to build something you've invented and see it work as you intended. I hope this book will help you to have this experience, too.

Have Fun!
Sariel

acknowledgments

Thanks to the many amazing and supportive readers of the first edition for making this new edition happen. Even though it's impossible to list all of you here, you are first and foremost when it comes to expressing my gratitude. Thank you all sincerely.

Thanks also to my publisher, who appreciated the potential of the first edition and allowed me to build upon it. The No Starch Press crew, and especially the lead editor of this book, Tyler Ortman, didn't hesitate for a moment when I presented him with this monster of a book requiring months of heavy work. The same can be said about Eric "Blakbird" Albrecht, whose expert engineering knowledge and unending patience in correcting me allowed many blunders to be avoided.

Many thanks go to the amazing, talented, and supportive people at No Starch Press, including but not limited to Bill Pollock, Serena Yang, Pam Watts, and Julia Borden.

Special thanks go to many amazing creators whose help made this book better: Philippe "Philo" Hurbain, Fernando "Conchas" Correia, and Paul "Crowkillers" Boratko, as well as to Michael Efferman and Micha Koren with their crazy and bold 3D-printing designs.

A very important thanks goes to Michael Lachmann, Travis Cobbs, and Kevin Clague for their talent and generosity in freely sharing their software, which was essential for creating figures and building instructions in this book.

I also owe thanks to the many amazing people from the LEGO Group, including Jan Beyer, Kim E. Thomsen, Ana Albouy, Gaute Munch, Monica Pedersen, and the entire Technic team.

There are no words that could sufficiently thank my friends and family for putting up with a fellow whose hobbies include filming hamsters in LEGO cars, even though he hasn't been a kid for a while.

Last but not least, I want to thank the many people who have been following my work for years, showing their support and interest through conversation, suggestions, and challenges. I hope that reading this book will be as rewarding to you as interacting with you is to me.

```
        #230   05-16-2018 12:02PM
    Item(s) checked out to p41983518.

TITLE: The amazing book of LEGO Star War
BRCD: 30653516595642
DUE DATE: 06-06-18

TITLE: 365 things to do with LEGO bricks
BRCD: 30632003573114
DUE DATE: 06-06-18

TITLE: The unofficial LEGO Technic build
BRCD: 31800003257173
DUE DATE: 06-06-18
```

where to buy LEGO pieces?

You may soon notice that several pieces used in this book are hard to find in the latest LEGO sets. That's natural—most LEGO sets are discontinued after two or three years of production, so many individual pieces go out of production as well. Some elements get replaced by something better; others are gone forever.

Luckily, finding these older pieces isn't an issue thanks to the secondhand market. Countless international sellers have all sorts of LEGO pieces available for purchase. The best place to look is, of course, online. Other than obvious websites, such as eBay (*http://www.ebay.com/*), there are specialized online LEGO markets, most notably BrickLink (*http://www.bricklink.com/*). It's Bricklink I am referring to when discussing availability and pricing of various pieces throughout this book, and it's Bricklink's vast and up-to-date catalog that the piece ID numbers in the book come from.

Bricklink has been operating since 2000, and over the years it has become the essential source of cheap pieces for the worldwide community of LEGO builders. It has a ratings system for each seller so you can check whether you're buying from someone trustworthy, and the prices can be quite good, often beating all alternatives. In short, it's safe, it's cheap, and it will let you find the pieces you need. Shopping at BrickLink is a daily routine for many builders. I've personally made more than 600 orders myself, and only 2 of these orders went missing (most likely because of the post office); in both cases, the sellers happily compensated the loss.

The key to using BrickLink effectively is understanding that it's not a single online shop but an immense collection of individual shops located all over the world. Almost all shopping starts by following these two steps: (1) Simply find the item you're interested in and (2) select your desired color, quality, and condition (new or used). BrickLink will

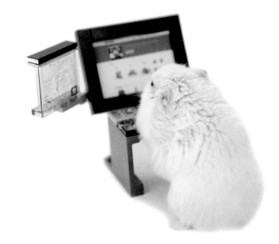

then provide you with a list of shops that have the desired item (or items) for sale, and you can narrow that list down by selecting the region you want to shop from (nobody wants to pay for shipping from across the world if they don't have to). From there, all that remains is to click the desired shop and add the items to your basket. (You can also browse what else this particular shop has to offer, which may end badly for your wallet.) Once you're happy with your basket, check out and wait for the seller to send you an invoice, which will also tell you how to pay for your order.

You pay individual sellers, not BrickLink itself, and there are many payment options available, from onsite PayPal payment to money transfers. When in doubt, refer to Brick-Link's extensive Help section.

PART I

basics

1

basic concepts

This chapter explains the basic concepts we'll be exploring as we build. Note that it aims for strictly practical knowledge. Its goal is to get you acquainted with the laws of physics involved in building working LEGO mechanisms, not to cover everything a practicing engineer or physicist needs to know. So let's get started with the basics.

speed

Speed describes how fast an object moves. When you think of speed, you likely think about the distance a vehicle can travel within a certain unit of time. We call this *linear speed*, and we will be measuring it in kilometers per hour (kph).

But there's another type of speed, called *rotational speed*, which tells us how fast an object rotates. We'll need to understand rotational speed, as most LEGO mechanisms are powered by spinning axles, whose rotary motion is transformed into a vehicle's linear speed using wheels or tank treads. Rotational speed is measured in rotations per minute (RPM). Various types of LEGO motors deliver different RPM, from less than 20 RPM to more than 1,000 RPM.

torque

Torque describes the turning force applied to an object. For example, when a LEGO motor drives an axle, it's applying torque to that axle. The more torque a motor applies, the stronger the rotation and the more resistance it takes to stop the motor. A motor that has enough torque to drive a 1 kg vehicle, for instance, might be stopped when trying to drive a 2 kg vehicle.

In LEGO Technic, the torque of LEGO motors can be measured in units called *Newton centimeters* (N•cm). The torque available from a motor is constant for a given power source: For example, the weakest LEGO motors provide 0.5 N•cm of torque, while the strongest ones provide 16.7 N•cm. The situation is different when you drive a mechanism manually—the amount of torque is variable and depends on how much physical strength you apply.

Understanding torque is crucial to understanding the capability of motors and the mechanisms they drive, as well as the limits of LEGO pieces. High torque creates stress that can damage and destroy LEGO pieces. We will learn how to prevent such damage in Chapter 12. Even more importantly, we'll explore the relationship between torque and rotational speed.

power

In this book, *power* refers to *mechanical power*, which is the product of torque and rotational speed. So torque multiplied by speed gives mechanical power, which is normally measured in watts (W). LEGO motors provide various degrees of power depending on their type, from 0.021 W to 2.38 W. While the concept of power is fairly complex, we will be using it mainly as a faster way to say "speed and torque together."

The power of a particular LEGO motor is affected by the *voltage* of its power source (that is, its battery). Most modern LEGO motors are meant to be powered at 9V. Although they can run at a lower voltage with lower power, a higher voltage can damage them.

friction

When two or more surfaces make contact and slide against each other, *friction* is a force that resists their movement. You'll see friction whenever two LEGO pieces are in contact and moving at different speeds. This means that every LEGO mechanism is affected by friction, which we have to overcome when we drive a mechanism. Friction dissipates some of the input force we've applied to the system, thus reducing both torque and speed.

The amount of friction increases as parts press against each other harder, and it also depends on the type of surface: Smooth, firm surfaces generate less friction than rough, soft ones. Friction can be decreased by separating the surfaces with a lubricating medium, such as a grease.

When building LEGO mechanisms, some notable points of friction are between two meshed gears, between a rotating axle and a piece with a pin hole that houses it, and between wheels and a surface they're rolling on. Large amounts of friction, resulting from a large number of moving parts, can render a mechanism useless and wear down or even damage LEGO pieces. (Of course, frictional forces are also present in static, nonmoving connections between LEGO pieces, which is why they stick together.)

traction

Traction, also called *grip*, describes the maximum frictional force that can be generated between two surfaces before they slip. We will be using the term when discussing tires—tires with good traction don't slip over a surface as easily as tires with poor traction.

Traction depends primarily on the hardness and shape of the tires as well as the material that the tires are made of. For example, rubber tires always have better traction than solid plastic wheels because rubber is soft and sticky compared to hard plastic. The differences in shape come down to the profile and tread of the tires. Traction is better when a tire contacts a large area of the road's surface, and a tire's profile and tread determine how much of a given type of surface the tire contacts.

As Figure 1-1 shows, tires that have a flat profile and a small, shallow tread have a larger area of contact on flat, smooth surfaces than tires that have a round profile and a large, deep tread. On the other hand, tires with a round profile and a large, deep tread have better contact with irregular, loose, or muddy surfaces. This is why the first

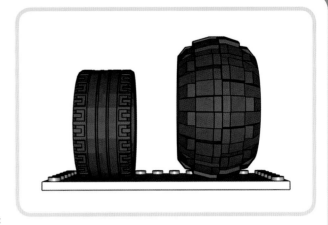

Figure 1-1: A tire with a flat profile and small tread (left) has better contact with a flat surface than a tire with a round profile and large tread (right).

type of tire is typical of sports cars designed for roads, while the second type of tire is typical of off-road cars designed for rough terrain.

Finally, the width of the tires also matters simply because wider tires will come into contact with a larger area of the road's surface.

In most cases, you want your tires to provide as much traction as possible. One exception is when you want your tires to slip—for example, to make your vehicle drift. The 8366 Supersonic RC set comes with two sets of rear tires: one with rubber tires for regular driving and one with solid plastic tires for drifting.

rolling resistance

Rolling resistance describes the resistance generated by rolling an object on a surface, and it is particularly important for wheels. All solid wheels have similar rolling resistance, but for wheels with tires, resistance varies a lot depending on the tires' characteristics.

Tires that are soft and wide, such as the one shown in Figure 1-2, generate more rolling resistance than tires that are hard and narrow. The resistance also depends on the vehicle's weight because weight deforms the tires, increasing their rolling resistance. Finally, the type of surface the wheels are in contact with affects the resistance. Smooth, flat, firm surfaces—such as asphalt or glass—lower the rolling resistance, while loose, boggy, soft, and sticky surfaces—such as sand, mud, or grass—increase it.

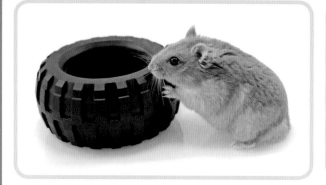

Figure 1-2: Typical off-road tires, which are soft and bulging, have particularly high rolling resistance. Apparently, they make up for it with their flavor.

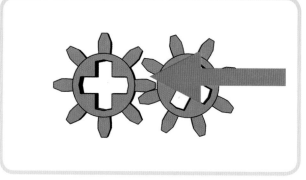

Figure 1-3: Backlash, in the form of a gap between the teeth of two mating gears, is particularly large for 8-tooth gears.

Rolling resistance is an important factor when choosing wheels and tires, but it is usually less important than traction. There are only a few types of LEGO tires whose rolling resistance is a serious concern, so in most cases you will find improved traction worth a little more resistance. Good traction almost always comes at the cost of extra rolling resistance.

backlash

Backlash describes the gaps between mating components, such as two gears, as shown in Figure 1-3. Practically every LEGO Technic connection has some backlash, and too much backlash is highly undesirable. When you start, stop, or reverse a mechanism, backlash will create a delay in the motion between its input and output. High backlash results in a longer delay, making the whole mechanism inaccurate and sluggish.

While building, remember that the backlash of many moving parts sums up, meaning that it accumulates over the entire mechanism. So a mechanism with four gears will have more backlash than a mechanism with two gears. One way to reduce backlash is to make your mechanism as simple as possible, and another is to replace high-backlash components, such as gears, with low-backlash ones, such as pneumatic cylinders (see Chapter 10) or linear actuators (see Chapter 14).

efficiency

Efficiency describes how much of the power we apply to a mechanism is actually used and how much is dissipated as friction. It is usually expressed as a percentage: For example,

a 50 percent efficiency means that a mechanism effectively uses half of the power delivered to it and the other half is lost.

In LEGO mechanisms, efficiency is generally low because LEGO pieces are simple and lack sophisticated mechanical solutions designed to lower friction, such as ball bearings. It is difficult to accurately measure the efficiency of any LEGO mechanism. Instead, we should focus simply on keeping the friction as low as possible.

The only way to improve efficiency is to reduce friction in our mechanism, and the simplest way to do reduce friction is to limit the number of moving parts. Weight is also an important factor because heavy moving parts generate more friction than light ones; size is a factor, too, as larger parts are heavier. In general, the simpler and lighter the mechanism, the more efficient it is.

vehicular concepts

At this point, we should have a good understanding of the basic physics and engineering concepts that apply to various constructions. Next we'll focus on issues related to vehicles. Since vehicles form the vast majority of both LEGO Technic sets and custom builds, we will be referring to these concepts throughout this book.

driveshaft

A *driveshaft* is a mechanical component, usually an axle, that transmits power from the motor to a mechanism. It connects—sometimes not directly—two components: one that *generates* power and a second that *receives* it. A typical

car, for example, has a single driveshaft that connects its gearbox to one or both of its axles. In other words, the driveshaft connects the engine indirectly, through a gearbox, to a *receiving mechanism*, which in this case is the wheels.

Driveshafts can also incorporate universal joints or extendable sections, as shown in Figure 1-4. These incorporated pieces allow for variations in the alignment of and distance between the power input and the receiving mechanism.

drivetrain

The *drivetrain*, also called a *powertrain*, is a group of components that generate power and deliver it in a vehicle. This group typically includes the motor, transmission (also known as a *gearbox*), driveshaft, axles, and final drive (the wheels, tracks, or propellers). While components in the middle of a drivetrain may vary—for example, there may be no transmission—the ends of the drivetrain remain the same: One is the propulsion motor (or motors), and the other is the final drive.

driveline

The *driveline* refers to the three final components: the driveshaft, axle, and final drive. In other words, the driveline is the drivetrain minus the motor and gearbox. If you consider a regular bicycle, the drivetrain would include the bicyclist (acting as a motor), the pedals, the gears, the chain, and the rear wheel as the final drive. The driveline, on the other hand, would include just the chain and the rear wheel.

turning radius

The *turning radius*, also called the *turning circle*, is the radius of the smallest U-turn the vehicle can make. Note that a vehicle's bodywork often overhangs the wheels, and the turning radius can be measured including its frame (a *wall-to-wall* turning radius) or without the frame, taking only the wheels into consideration (a *curb-to-curb* turning radius).

The turning radius is affected by several factors, including the maximum steering angle, the wheelbase, and the number of steered axles. The smaller this radius is, the better it is for the vehicle, as it can maneuver within tighter spaces. Note that certain vehicles, like tanks and other tracked vehicles, can turn in place, meaning they have a turning radius of zero.

FWD, RWD, 4×4, 4WD, and AWD

FWD, RWD, 4×4, 4WD, and AWD are abbreviations referring to the arrangement of driven axles in a vehicle. For example, a car with only the front axle driven has *FWD*, or *front-wheel drive*, while a car with only the rear axle driven has *RWD*, or *rear-wheel drive*.

A 4×4 vehicle is an automobile whose four wheels are all driven. With LEGO 4×4 vehicles, we are dealing with *4WD*, or *four-wheel drive*, where the motor's power is split equally among all wheels. Real 4×4 vehicles can also have something called *AWD*, or *all-wheel drive*, where the power distribution is constantly adjusted to driving conditions by electronic components—something that is extremely difficult to achieve with LEGO pieces.

Note that a third number can be added to the 4×4 description. For example, an SUV or Jeep is 4×4×2, which means four wheels total with four wheels driven and two wheels steered. Such descriptions are particularly important for multi-axle vehicles, such as mobile cranes and armored personnel carriers, which have many axles driven and steered. For instance, many small armored personnel carriers are 6×6×4, which stands for six wheels, all of which are driven and four of which are steered.

steering lock

When we talk about the steering lock in this book, we aren't referring to a physical lock you put on your steering wheel to prevent theft. The *steering lock* is the maximum steering angle—that is, the maximum angle to which wheels

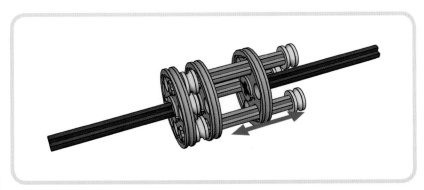

Figure 1-4: An extendable driveshaft section, consisting of two axles with three wedge belt wheels (the thin grey discs) and another three axles inside them. The three axles transmit rotation to all the discs, and these axles are able to slide through the single disc shown on the right, effectively changing the driveshaft's length even as it spins.

on a steered axle can be turned. Usually the greater the steering lock, the better, as it allows the vehicle to make tighter turns. However, a very large steering lock can be undesirable because it enables the vehicle's direction to change very rapidly, making the vehicle less stable and exerting significant stress on parts of the steering system. See Figure 1-5 for a model with a large steering lock.

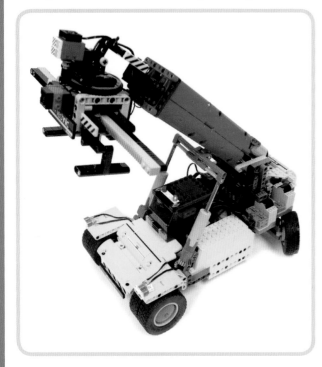

Figure 1-5: My reach stacker model had a rear axle (right) with a particularly large steering lock, just like that of a real vehicle. Designed to stack containers in ports' loading areas, reach stackers need to be able to maneuver in limited space.

ground clearance

Ground clearance, also called *ride height* or simply *clearance*, is the distance between the underside of the chassis and a flat, level surface the vehicle is standing on, as shown in Figure 1-6. It determines the height of obstacles the vehicle can drive over without scraping them with the chassis. Ground clearance depends primarily on the suspension system.

High ground clearance allows a vehicle to negotiate bigger obstacles but makes it taller and less stable due to a higher center of gravity. Low ground clearance improves stability but reduces the ability to drive over rough terrain. High ground clearance is therefore typical of off-road vehicles, whereas low ground clearance is common in sports

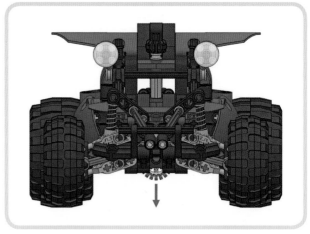

Figure 1-6: The green arrow indicates this simple buggy's ground clearance. Note that the ground clearance is usually measured in the center of the vehicle as seen from front or rear, because this part is most likely to contact obstacles.

cars because they are designed for flat roads and benefit from good stability, which allows them to make turns at higher speeds.

suspension travel

Suspension travel is the maximum length of a suspension's up-and-down movement. Consider a simple suspension system where an axle is connected to the chassis by a vertical shock absorber, as shown in Figure 1-7. In this case, the suspension travel is the difference between the chassis height when the shock absorber is fully compressed and when the shock absorber is unloaded (that is, the vehicle is standing on a level surface and only its weight is acting on the absorber). Usually, suspension travel is expressed in units of length: In Figure 1-7, it appears to be two studs.

Any suspension system has some travel, regardless of whether it uses shock absorbers or it's sprung or unsprung (see Chapter 17 for details). If the suspension allows the wheels to go up or down relative to the chassis, the maximum range of that up-and-down movement is suspension travel. A large suspension travel is valuable in off-road cars because it enables them to negotiate large obstacles while keeping all the wheels on the ground.

However, large suspension travel comes at a cost. The larger the suspension travel, the farther a wheel can go up or down and the more space is needed to prevent the wheel from hitting the chassis or the body of the car. This is obvious in off-road cars where there is plenty of room between the fender and the wheel. The result is that the whole car is taller, making it less stable.

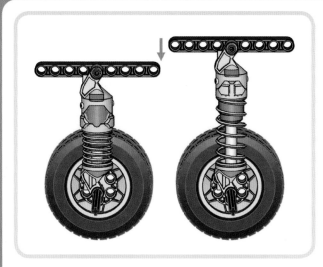

Figure 1-7: The suspension travel is the difference in height between a fully compressed (left) and unloaded (right) shock absorber.

camber angle

The *camber angle* is the angle between the centerline of a wheel and the surface the wheel rolls on. It determines whether the wheel is tilted inward or outward, or not tilted at all (see Figure 1-8). A wheel that's perfectly vertical has a neutral camber angle. A wheel tilted inward so its top is closer to the center of the vehicle than its bottom has a negative camber angle. A wheel tilted outward so its top is farther from the center of the vehicle than its bottom has a positive camber angle.

A negative camber angle improves car handling by increasing traction when the car is turning. In a turn, the car's outer wheel bears most of the weight. The tire is slightly deformed by the vehicle's weight, and a negative camber angle

helps to apply load to the tire evenly, increasing the tire's surface contact with the road. A negative camber angle is most common in cars built for drifting because they need to handle well in the many turns they make.

On the other hand, a negative camber angle doesn't work as well when driving straight because it puts more load on the tire's inner edge. With a neutral camber angle, the load is applied mostly to the tire's outer edge. A neutral angle is best while driving in a straight line because it balances the load on the tire evenly.

A positive camber angle is generally avoided because it impairs a vehicle's handling. Vehicles with Tatra-type suspension are an exception. These have a positive camber angle if there isn't much weight acting on their suspension (see Chapter 17 for details). With LEGO models, the camber angle usually has little effect because the tires are relatively hard and less prone to deformation than real tires.

caster angle

The *caster angle* is the angle of a wheel's pivot in the longitudinal direction (see Figure 1-9). *Pivot* refers to the line around which the wheel turns when you steer left or right—in other words, the wheel's *steering axis*. If the pivot is perfectly vertical, the wheel has a neutral caster angle. If the pivot is inclined so it "precedes" the wheel, the wheel has a positive caster angle. If the pivot is inclined so it "follows" the wheel, the wheel has a negative caster angle.

A car with a positive caster angle has better stability while traveling in a straight line and steers better, but it requires a greater force for steering. Positive caster angles are common in fast sport cars: Stability and steering are crucial, and steering is power assisted. A positive caster angle is also ubiquitous in motorbikes and bicycles because it dramatically improves their stability (see Figure 1-10).

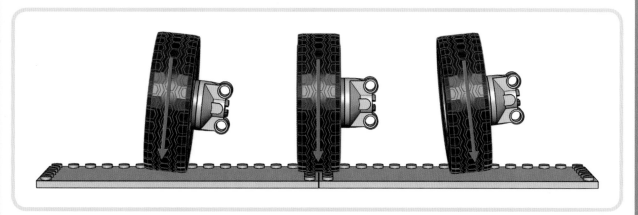

Figure 1-8: Assuming the car is on the right side of the wheel, the angles shown are a negative camber angle (left), a neutral camber angle (center), and a positive camber angle (right).

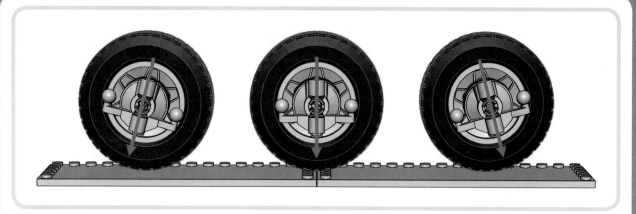

Figure 1-9: Assuming that the wheel shown is a front wheel of a vehicle moving from right to left, the angles shown are a negative caster angle (left), a neutral caster angle (center), and a positive caster angle (right).

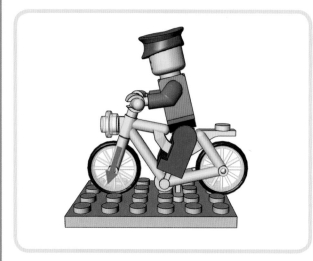

Figure 1-10: A typical bicycle has a positive caster angle on the front wheel. It's achieved by inclining the fork away from the vertical position (a red arrow indicates the fork's angle), and it improves the bicycle's stability.

A car with a negative caster angle behaves in the opposite way: The amount of force needed to steer is reduced, but the steering is less efficient and the car is more likely to wander off the straight line. Wheels with a negative caster are found mostly in old, obsolete vehicles without power-assisted steering. Most shopping carts come with a steep negative caster on all wheels because it makes changing their direction easier: As you push the cart, the wheels simply trail behind it.

toe angle

A *toe angle* is the angle between the left and right wheel on the same axle as viewed from above (see Figure 1-11). The wheels can be parallel or facing inward or outward (relative to the front of the car). Toe angle has a different significance for steered and for non-steered axles.

Wheels that are perfectly parallel have a *neutral toe* angle. Wheels that are facing inward have a *toe-in* angle. A toe-in angle makes a car more stable when driving in a straight line but less responsive to steering (understeer). For non-steered axles that aren't driven, a toe-in angle may be desirable because these axles are pushed or pulled by other axles, and backlash in the wheel hubs can make the wheels face outward. The correct amount of toe-in angle neutralizes that effect.

Wheels that face outward have a *toe-out* angle. It makes a car more responsive to steering (oversteer), but it also makes keeping the car going in a straight line more difficult. For non-steered axles that are driven, toe-out angles may be desirable because both wheels pull or push the rest of the vehicle and backlash in the wheel hubs can make the wheels face inward. The right amount of toe-out angle neutralizes that effect. However, it will only work in a vehicle that has just one driven axle. With multiple driven axles and with AWD vehicles, it's safest to use a neutral toe angle because no single axle is ever pulling the whole vehicle.

Note that both toe-in and toe-out angles result in heavy tire wear and considerable additional friction, which may slow down the vehicle. Too much of a toe-out angle can also cause a wheel to separate from the axle. For that reason, the vast majority of real cars use a neutral toe angle, and the

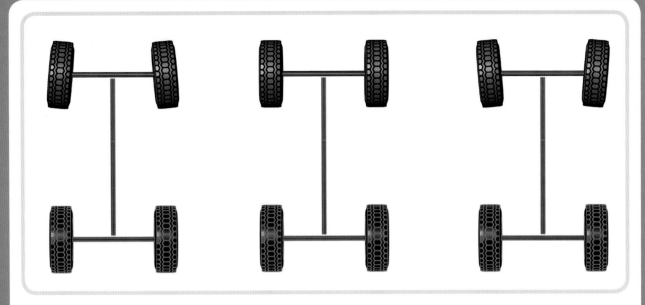

Figure 1-11: Assuming the blue axle is the front axle, the angles shown are toe-in (left), neutral toe (center), and toe-out (right).

other alignments are typical for specialized track-going cars. In LEGO models, however, there is more backlash between the wheel and the chassis than in real cars, so toe angle is something to consider.

weight distribution

Weight distribution, and in particular whether a vehicle is front heavy or rear heavy, can greatly affect the performance of a vehicle.

Weight distribution primarily affects traction and thus handling. Imagine a car with two axles: one steered in front and one driven in rear. If this car is front heavy, it will have better steering traction because its front wheels will have more weight on them. If this car is rear heavy, it will have better acceleration because its rear wheels will have better traction with more weight on them.

In four-wheeled vehicles, weight distribution is described as a ratio. For example, a 40:60 weight distribution means that 40 percent of the vehicle's weight rests on the front axle and 60 percent on the rear one. In off-road cars with 4WD, 50:50 weight distribution is considered ideal, while high-performance race cars with central engines often have more weight in the back.

Weight distribution is also important for tracked vehicles. Since tracks have poor traction on smooth surfaces, weight distribution significantly affects how a tracked vehicle turns and how it climbs obstacles. For example, a front-heavy tracked vehicle won't be able to turn in place because its center of rotation will be moved forward. But this type of vehicle will be good at climbing up hills because its front end will have better traction.

center of gravity

The *center of gravity* is the central point of an object's weight distribution. It can be located in the actual center of the object—in the case of a solid ball, for example—or elsewhere. The location of the center of gravity determines the object's likelihood of falling over, which is greater for objects with a high center of gravity than for ones with a low center of gravity. In other words, a low center of gravity makes objects more stable.

With LEGO vehicles, the center of gravity is greatly affected by the location of a vehicle's heaviest components, such as battery boxes, and it should always be as low as possible. This is why, for example, builders of off-road vehicles, which need to be very stable, always try to locate battery boxes low in the chassis.

Now that you have these basics down, let's start putting them into practice!

2

basic units and pieces

LEGO models and bricks are measured in a fanciful unit called the *stud* rather than in inches or centimeters. One stud equals the width of the smallest brick, which is 8 mm wide. We'll even use the stud to measure LEGO pieces that aren't bricks, like shock absorbers and axles.

When the unit of measurement for a LEGO piece is omitted, you can safely assume that it is the stud—for example, a *1×1 brick*, a *2×2 tile*, and so on. This is how we'll refer to pieces in this book.

NOTE You might also see the stud referred to by other names, such as *module*, *dot*, or *fundamental LEGO unit (FLU)*. The letter *L* is used to indicate length in studs. For example, a 6.5L shock absorber is 6.5 studs long.

LEGO builders generally measure the *height* of their creations, however, in terms of the height of a brick or plate. For example, we say that something is *1 brick tall* or *1 plate tall*. Note that 1 brick tall is equal to 9.6 mm, just a bit more than 1 stud (see Figure 2-1).

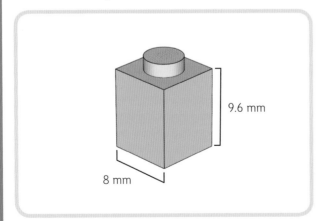

Figure 2-1: A 1×1 brick is 8 mm wide and 9.6 mm tall.

As illustrated in Figure 2-2, LEGO *plates* are only one-third as tall as a brick, meaning that three stacked plates are the same height as one brick.

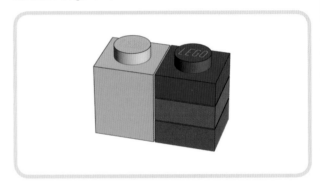

Figure 2-2: A LEGO brick (left) is the same height as three stacked LEGO plates (right).

NOTE The size of the round peg or stud at the top of a brick is not included in its height because the peg is completely hidden inside the brick on top of it. Instead, we measure the height of a brick only from corner to corner.

the Technic brick

As in the classic LEGO system, the basic building block in the Technic system is the *brick*: that easy-to-connect piece that we all know and love. But, as shown in Figure 2-3, Technic bricks are a little different. They have hollow studs, which make them harder to separate and better suited for heavy-duty use. Most Technic bricks also have pin holes centered

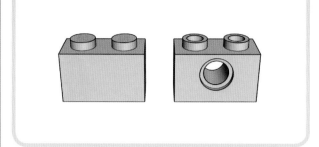

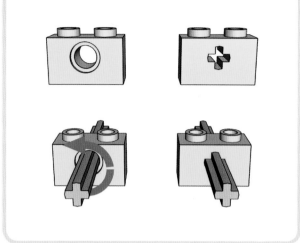

Figure 2-3: A regular 1×2 brick (left) has solid studs and sides, while a Technic 1×2 brick (right) has hollow studs and a center hole.

between the studs: A 1×2 brick has one hole, a 1×4 brick has three holes, and so on. The holes in Technic pieces are vital to the LEGO Technic building system, as they allow you to connect pieces with pins or run axles through them.

Although the holes in most Technic bricks are centered between the studs, you will find variants of 1×1 and 1×2 Technic bricks that have holes aligned with the studs—for example, see Figure 2-4. When the studs are aligned with the holes, the number of holes and studs is equal. Such an arrangement is useful for compact building with densely packed pins and axles, and these pieces can also be used to align pieces by half of a stud.

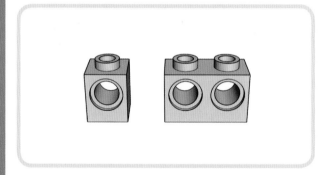

Figure 2-4: Some Technic bricks have holes aligned with the studs.

There are two types of holes in Technic bricks: round *pin holes* and X-shaped *axle holes*. Examine the shape of any LEGO axle, and the purpose of these holes should be obvious: Axles inserted in pin holes can rotate, but axles in axle holes cannot (see Figure 2-5). (Note that only 1×2 Technic bricks have an axle hole.)

Figure 2-5: Pin holes (left) allow axles to rotate, while axle holes (right) keep axles from turning.

pins, for joining and rotating

A pin is a small connector that you insert into pin holes or axle holes to connect two or more adjacent pieces. As shown in Figure 2-6, pins vary in length and shape. Although they are simple, pins are indispensable for holding together Technic constructions. The largest Technic sets can include hundreds of pins. They're just that important!

Like axles, you can put pins in either pin holes or axle holes. But unlike axles, each pin has a collar that makes it impossible to push it completely through a hole. For example, the most basic pin is 2 studs long, and you can push each of its ends 1 stud deep into a hole but no farther. The long pin, which is 3 studs long, has one end that you can push 1 stud deep and another that you can push 2 studs deep. The collars stay between the pieces you connect this way, and all pin holes are shaped to accommodate the collars (see Figure 2-7).

Many pins come in two variants: without friction (the pin can rotate freely inside a pin hole) and with friction (the pin requires some force to rotate inside a pin hole). Rotating

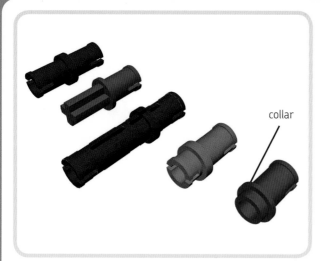

Figure 2-6: The most common Technic pins (from left to right: pin, axle pin, long pin, three-quarter pin, and half pin)

collar

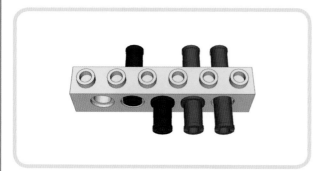

Figure 2-7: Pin holes (from left to right: empty pin hole, two pin holes with pins inserted from opposite sides, and two pin holes with long pins inserted from opposite sides)

anything inside an axle hole is of course not possible. You can identify the variants easily because those with friction are ridged and come in different colors than those without friction. When in doubt, insert the pin into a pin hole and give it a spin.

Table 2-1 lists all existing pins and their variations. As the table shows, some pins have only one variant, whereas others have two, which are always differentiated by their color (for example, a regular pin without friction is light grey, and a regular pin with friction is black). Some variants come in more than one color because LEGO changed its color coding at some point (for example, half pins come in light grey and blue, both without friction).

table 2-1: a list of all pins and variations in their most common colors

pin name	without friction	with friction
half pin		
three-quarter pin		
regular pin		
axle pin		
long pin		
long pin with 1L axle		
long pin with 2L axle		
pin with pin hole		
axle pin with pin hole		
axle pin with pin hole and 2 axles		

(continued)

table 2-1 (continued)

pin name	without friction	with friction
axle pin with axle hole and 3 axles		
long pin with pin hole		
half pin with 2L bar		
pin with towball		
axle pin with towball		
long pin with stop bush		

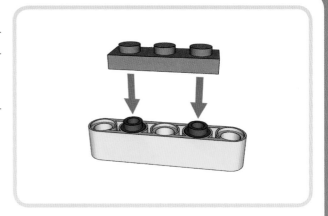

Figure 2-8: In half pins, tops act like studs and connect to studded pieces.

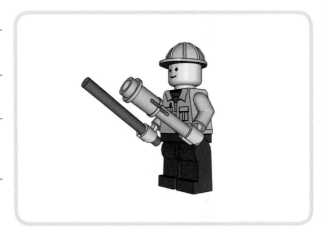

Figure 2-9: A LEGO minifigure holds a regular bar (red) and half-pin with 2L bar (light grey) in its hands.

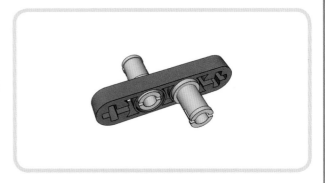

Figure 2-10: The three-quarter pins make strong connections with half-stud-wide beams because their tops are exactly half a stud long.

Certain pins have special properties:

half pin Its shorter side connects to studs. It acts like a single round stud (Figure 2-8) with a hole inside that you can insert a bar into (Figure 2-9).

three-quarter pin Its shorter side connects to half-stud-wide beams (Figure 2-10).

half pin with 2L bar The pin and bar are a single piece. The bar is as thick as a regular bar and is 2 studs long (Figure 2-9).

pin with towball and axle pin with towball These pins are commonly used as mounting points for steering links (Figure 2-11).

long pin with stop bush This pin comes in more than a dozen colors, all with friction. It is commonly used in LEGO sets as a push-in/pull-out piece when two modules of a construction need to be connected in a way that can easily be undone (Figure 2-12).

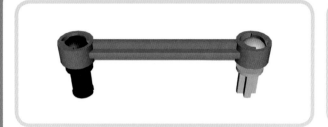

Figure 2-11: Two pins with towballs can be connected with a link if, for example, you need to connect suspension parts that move relative to each other.

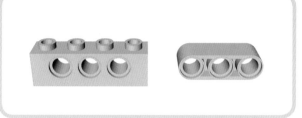

Figure 2-13: A 1×4 Technic brick (left) and a 1×3 Technic beam (right)

Because they lack regular LEGO studs on top, beams are called *studless*, while bricks and plates are called *studfull* (or *studded*) pieces. The same names—studless and studfull—are also applied to constructions that use mainly one type of piece. For example, you can build a car with a studfull body on a studless chassis. (Chapter 3 describes the differences between studfull and studless pieces in detail; we'll take only a brief look here.)

Many studless pieces come in complex shapes that have no counterpart among the studfull pieces, as you can see in Figure 2-14.

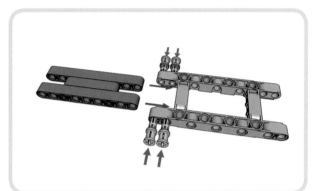

Figure 2-12: Long pins with bushes have a very specific role in LEGO sets. Large LEGO sets are often built as several separate modules, and these pins are used to connect the modules. The pins are usually half inserted into one module until the other module is in place. Then they are pushed in all the way. Unlike other pins, they can be easily pulled out due to the bush.

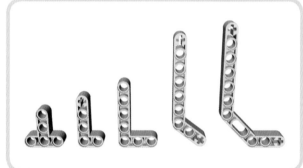

Figure 2-14: Complex studless shapes

beams, the studless alternative

In addition to bricks, the Technic system contains pieces called *beams* or *liftarms*. As shown in Figure 2-13, beams are like bricks reduced to mere pin holes. They come in many sizes and shapes, and some beams even include axle holes.

While bricks have a 6:5 height-to-width ratio, beams maintain a 7:8 ratio. A simple beam can be up to 15 studs long, but it is always 1 stud (8 mm) wide and 7 mm tall. For example, notice the slight height difference between the 9.6 mm tall brick and the 7 mm tall beam in Figure 2-15.

Note that the studfull pieces can be connected to the studless ones using pin holes.

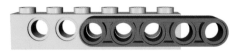

Figure 2-15: A brick (left) and a beam (right) are not the same height.

Studless pieces are symmetrical: Their tops and bottoms are identical, which makes them much more versatile than bricks, as shown in Figure 2-16. When building with bricks, the orientation of the brick and its studs is important; with beams, it's not.

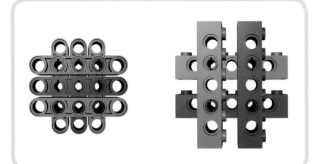

Figure 2-16: A comparison between a construction using beams (left) and one using bricks (right)

Consider that a block of six 1×5 beams connected with pins is symmetrical: It looks the same whether you rotate it 90, 180, or 270 degrees. In comparison, a block of four 1×6 bricks connected with pins is asymmetrical. Rotating it changes the orientation of the bricks and their studs, affecting how you can build onto it.

Studless pieces have nearly ousted studfull ones from LEGO Technic sets, making the use of bricks and plates as measurements of height obsolete. When it comes to measurements, studless pieces offer an advantage because they are orientation independent; therefore, it doesn't matter whether you place them vertically or horizontally.

When speaking in Technic terms, it is common to express height in studs and to measure height using the distance between holes in Technic bricks and beams. Note that these two distances can be aligned using plates. As shown in Figure 2-17, two bricks spaced apart by two plates have exactly 3 studs of distance between their pin holes.

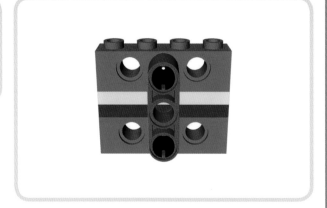

Figure 2-17: The basic rule of alignment for studless and studded pieces: Holes in two bricks separated by two plates are exactly 3 studs apart.

This trick shows how bricks with plates can be repeated at regular intervals to align with beams. For example, in order to have a 5-stud-long space between their pin holes, two bricks need to be spaced apart by seven plates, by a brick and four plates, or by two bricks and one plate, as 1 brick is 3 plates tall. Figure 2-18 provides more examples of studless and studfull pieces in alignment.

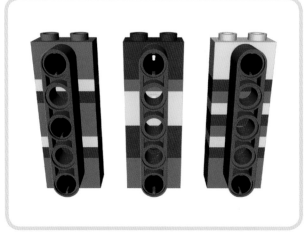

Figure 2-18: More examples of studless and studfull pieces in alignment

The difference between the height of a single stud and the height of a single brick makes 6 stacked bricks exactly 7 studs tall, as shown in Figure 2-19. This relationship is repetitive: 11 stacked bricks are 13 studs tall, and so on.

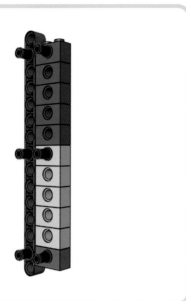

Figure 2-19: Once you connect a brick to a vertical beam, the next connections can be made every five stacked bricks.

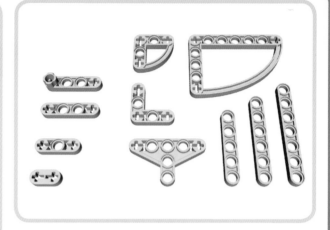

Figure 2-20: Various half-stud-thick pieces

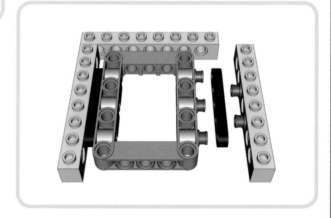

Figure 2-21: Of all Technic pins, the three-quarter pins are best suited to hold half-stud-thick pieces.

the half stud as the minimum building unit

While the basic building unit in the world of LEGO is a single stud, some pieces are smaller. For example, plates are one-third of a stud tall, and some beams are one-half of a stud thick. As shown in Figure 2-20, studless pieces that are half a stud thick typically include a lot of axle holes, which makes them useful for creating rigid structures with complex shapes.

With these pieces, it is possible to use a half stud as the minimum unit, which comes in handy when combining studless structures (normally with odd dimensions) with studfull ones (normally with even dimensions). The pin holes in half-stud-thick pieces won't really fit a regular pin, but a three-quarter pin fits perfectly. Figure 2-21 shows

how three-quarter pins can be used to combine half-stud-thick pieces with 1-stud-thick pieces. One end of the three-quarter pin fits perfectly into a half-stud-deep pin hole, while the other end fits perfectly into a 1-stud-deep pin hole.

Because half pins enter beams only partially, they can easily fall out. On the other hand, three-quarter pins enter the beam completely, securing it firmly in place, and fit inside it entirely with no parts protruding. Regular pins secure beams firmly, too, but they protrude by another half stud, which allows the beam to slide on the protruding part. Figure 2-22 illustrates these three types of pins as they are used to hold a half-stud-thick beam.

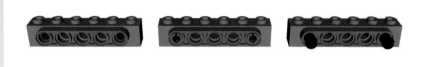

Figure 2-22: From left to right: a half pin, a three-quarter pin, and a regular pin used to hold a half-stud-thick beam

tricks with bricks

There are many unusual ways to connect bricks. One of the more popular ways is to place bricks half a stud off, which you can do by using jumper plates (see Figure 2-23) or Technic bricks (see Figure 2-24). You can also combine the two techniques. For example, if you want to create a tall "off" section, it's best to secure its bottom in place using jumper plates and its top using Technic bricks for the strongest connection.

Another effective technique that you can use for a variety of aesthetic effects is to connect bricks bottom to bottom. The key to this technique is to use brackets and bricks with studs on two sides, as shown in Figure 2-25.

You can use the same technique to cover the bottoms of bricks. This is useful, for example, if you want to make a smooth, seamless surface, as shown in Figure 2-26. It's also an easy way to join two smooth surfaces at a right angle (see Figure 2-27).

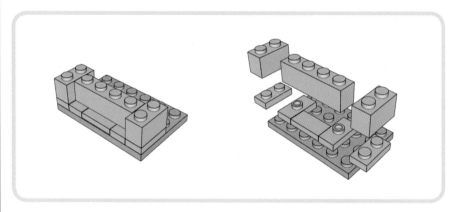

Figure 2-23: Using jumper plates to place a brick half a stud off (normal and exploded view)

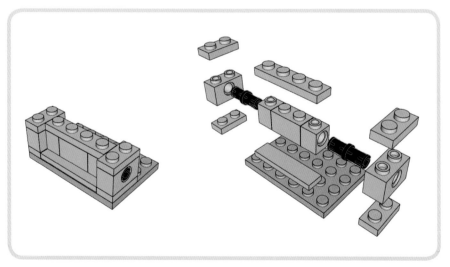

Figure 2-24: Using Technic bricks to place a brick half a stud off (normal and exploded view)

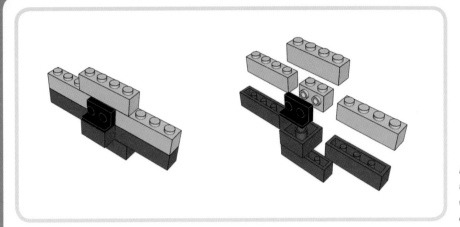

Figure 2-25: Connecting bricks bottom to bottom using a bracket and a brick with studs on two sides (normal and exploded view)

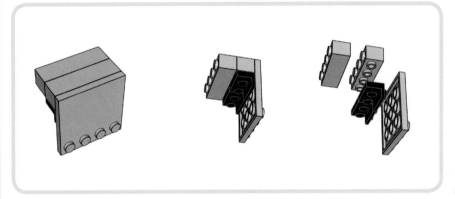

Figure 2-26: The bottom-to-bottom technique covers the bottom of a brick with a smooth surface. Shown from above (left), below (middle), and exploded (right).

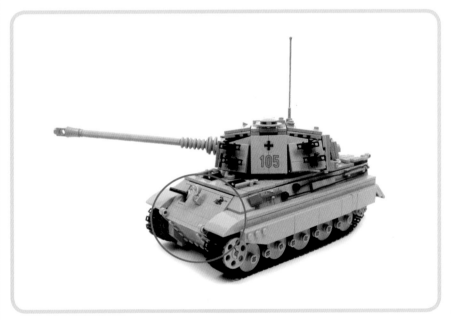

Figure 2-27: My model of a Tiger 2 tank. The front armor is made of an upper and lower plate connected using the technique in Figure 2-26.

3

studless or studfull?

In Chapter 2, we took a peek at the difference between two styles of building with LEGO pieces: studless (using beams) and studfull (using bricks and plates). The two styles are significantly different, and each offers advantages. The styles can also be combined in order to use the best qualities of each technique in a single construction. As a matter of fact, most of today's LEGO Technic sets and *MOCs* (*My Own Creations*, a term builders use for their custom models) use a combination of the two approaches rather than a purely studless or studfull building technique.

The successful builder knows which combination works best for a given construction, which style should serve as its basis, and to what extent the other style should be incorporated. We'll address these issues in this chapter.

First, we'll discuss the pros and cons of each technique and compare one to the other. Then we'll focus on how the two techniques can be combined to bring out the best from both, using official LEGO sets and amateur builders' MOCs (like my Monster Truck, shown in Figure 3-1) as examples.

LEGO evolving

The entire LEGO building system was originally 100 percent studfull. The first studless pieces appeared when the LEGO Technic line was already well developed and initially only complemented the studfull style rather than forming a new one. But as the Technic sets evolved, studless pieces grew very popular, and the studfull pieces were nearly entirely phased out.

Today, most Technic sets are studless, with studfull pieces used to add certain minor details to already mechanically functional and sound constructions. And when you consider the fact that most of the new specialized elements, such as electric motors, pneumatic switches, turntables, and

actuators, are designed specifically to fit the studless style rather than the studfull one, it becomes obvious that studless pieces are of primary importance to Technic today. Learning to build with studless pieces, which is usually more challenging than with studfull ones, is crucial to keeping up with new additions to the Technic system.

But we shouldn't abandon studfull pieces completely. Many amateur Technic builders don't follow the LEGO Group's doctrine, and they continue to publish primarily studfull MOCs that are both very functional and good-looking (like my Kenworth truck, shown in Figure 3-2).

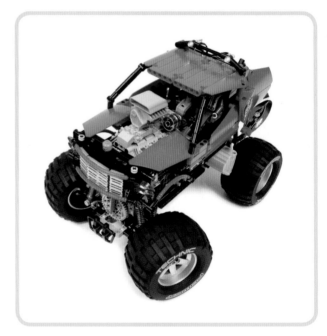

Figure 3-1: My Monster Truck model took the approach of modern LEGO Technic sets: It was almost entirely studless, with studfull pieces used only for minor details, like the grille.

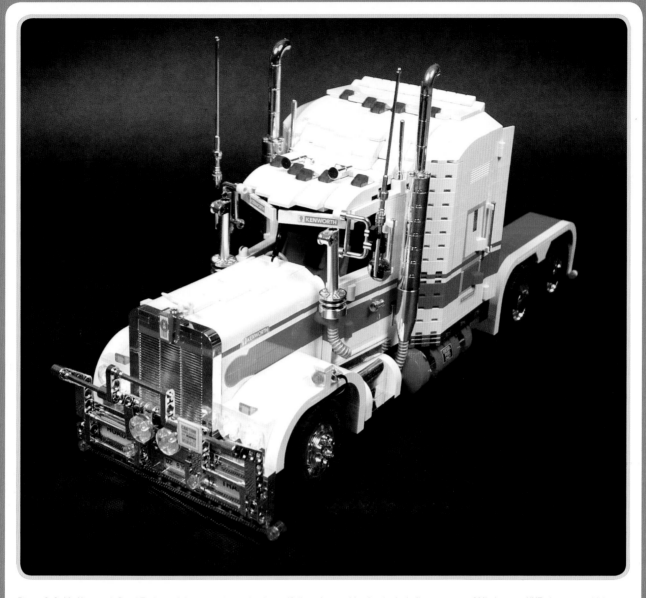

Figure 3-2: My Kenworth Road Train model appeared completely studfull on the outside, despite including an array of Mindstorms NXT elements, which are best suited for studless structures.

studfull building

Technic bricks and regular plates are the basis of the studfull style. Technic bricks differ from regular LEGO bricks (as shown in Figure 3-3) in that they have hollow studs on top and slightly thicker rods inside them.

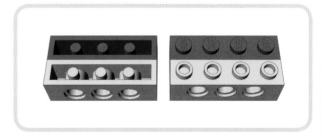

Figure 3-3: Side-by-side comparison of a regular LEGO brick (red) and a LEGO Technic brick (yellow)

Thanks to their altered design, Technic bricks are less likely to come apart when subjected to lateral pressure. (They are still easy to tug apart on purpose.) To make your designs resistant to high torque, you'll need to lock your studfull bricks using pins and other pieces. Studless beams are more space efficient than studfull Technic bricks, as shown in Figure 3-4.

reinforcing studfull constructions

When you add extra pieces to a combination of LEGO pieces to keep them together, you're *reinforcing* them. Technic bricks are usually combined with plates to allow vertical reinforcement. A *brick–two plates–brick* combination is used to ensure proper vertical spacing of the bricks and their pin holes to allow reinforcement with a vertical piece (shown in Figure 3-5). The corner and hinge plates allow for perpendicular connections, as shown in Figure 3-6, or angled connections, as shown in Figure 3-7.

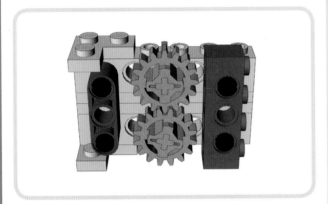

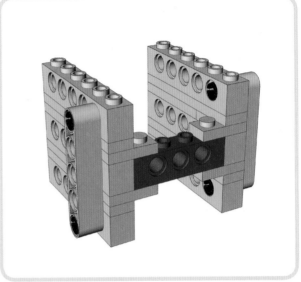

Figure 3-4: Two 1×6 Technic bricks are locked vertically to prevent them from coming apart when high torque is applied to the gears. The little space used by the studless locking piece (left) compared to the studfull one (right) leaves space for plates on the top and bottom of the two bricks and allows the use of bigger gears.

Figure 3-6: Even though the red brick is not reinforced directly, it is kept firmly in place by L-shaped corner plates that are locked with reinforced bricks.

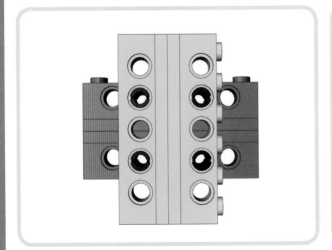

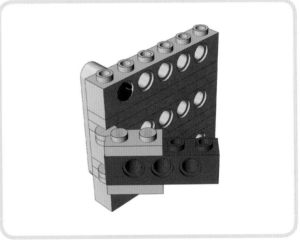

Figure 3-5: The brick–two plates–brick combination makes sure the spacing between bricks allows vertical connection. The addition of plates keeps the pin holes in the bricks exactly 1 stud apart.

Figure 3-7: Two reinforced hinge plates secure the red Technic brick while allowing it to be set at any angle.

The use of plates as spacers, however, has a disadvantage: It reduces the number of pin holes as compared to an entirely studless structure of the same size, as shown in Figure 3-8. Therefore, studfull structures can house fewer axles and other elements that require pin holes.

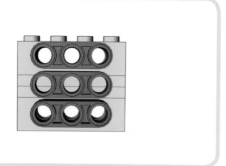

Figure 3-8: As these superimposed images show, the combination of bricks and plates (yellow) not only allows for fewer pin holes than the combination of studless beams (red)—six as compared to nine—but also takes up significantly more space.

In general, studfull constructions are bigger and heavier than studless ones, with a less dense internal structure. They often need to be reinforced, but the resulting structures are very rigid. They are also orientation dependent because of their asymmetry, meaning that the direction their studs face affects the number of possible combinations between pieces.

Additionally, studfull constructions don't work as well with vertical elements; for example, vertical axles are difficult to secure firmly in studfull structures.

studfull advantages

In general, studfull constructions are

* Easy to combine horizontally
* Easy to combine with non-Technic pieces and thus better suited to creative design
* Able to form very rigid constructions with firm horizontal connections
* Able to use a variety of plates for connections at many angles
* Able to create a rigid connection that maintains the relative orientation of the pieces

studfull disadvantages

In general, the disadvantages of studfull connections are that they

* Require reinforcements to prevent vertical separation under torque
* Have pin holes that are distributed less densely, making for bigger constructions
* Are not symmetrical, meaning that their orientation affects how easy they are to combine
* Do not easily fit most of the modern specialized pieces, such as motors and actuators
* Are a poor fit for vertical elements, such as axles and gear wheels
* Are bigger and heavier than studless pieces

studless building

The studless style consists of beams connected with pins, as well as a variety of specialized connectors. Beams are symmetrical, so they can be combined in any orientation, allowing for real three-dimensional building, as shown in Figure 3-9. In most cases, beams are connected with regular Technic pins, but some studless connectors come with integrated pins, as shown in Figure 3-10.

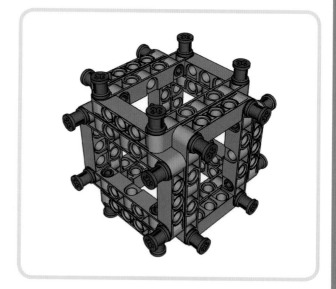

Figure 3-9: This structure, comprised of studless frames connected with pins and bushings, is symmetrical, meaning that it has no definite top or bottom. Unlike studfull structures, it can have axles inserted from any direction.

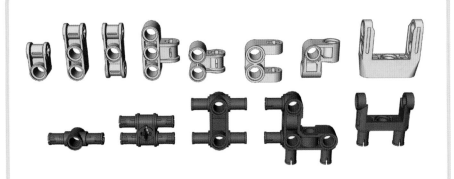

Figure 3-10: While most studless connectors have just pin and axle holes (yellow), some come with integrated pins (red).

creating rigid studless connections

Once connected, studless pieces are much more difficult to separate than bricks and plates, but that doesn't necessarily mean that they are rigid. Since pins are round, any two studless pieces connected with a single pin can oscillate relative to each other. Using pins with friction can make this oscillation a little less likely to occur, but using two or more pins for each connection ensures a truly rigid and static connection.

Figure 3-11 shows the difference between a rigid and nonrigid connection. The advantage of using rigid connections is that a rigid studless structure usually doesn't need additional reinforcement when axles and gears are added, because its pieces remain in place under torque (see Figure 3-12). The axle holes can be used to easily create a rigid connection, as shown in Figure 3-13.

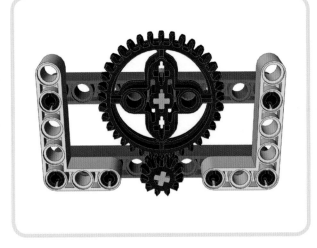

Figure 3-12: Pieces kept together by a rigid connection usually don't need extra reinforcement in order to stay together when torque is applied. These four pieces act as one due to their rigid connections.

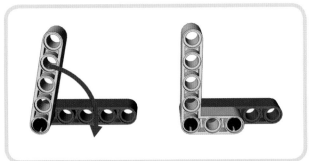

Figure 3-11: A comparison of nonrigid (left) and rigid (right) connections between studless pieces. In a nonrigid connection, pieces stay together, but their orientation can change—the yellow beam can be rotated left or right, regardless of the type of pin used for the connection. In a rigid connection, pieces are connected and fixed to each other so that their orientation does not change.

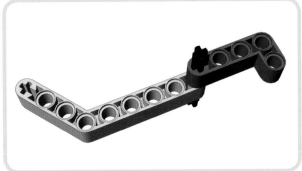

Figure 3-13: When two studless pieces have axle holes, a single axle is enough to create a rigid connection between them. However, such a connection won't be as strong as one made with two or more pins.

Beams are smaller and lighter than bricks, but they are also more elastic. Long beams are therefore more likely to bend or even buckle under a load than long bricks, making it more difficult to create large, rigid studless structures and requiring more complex connections using smaller pieces. Another difficulty comes when you want to create a perpendicular connection between beams without putting one beam on top of the other. It's possible to do so only with a right-angle connector or with a 5×7 studless frame (see Figure 3-14). These frames are quite popular and can also be used as a means of reinforcing builds.

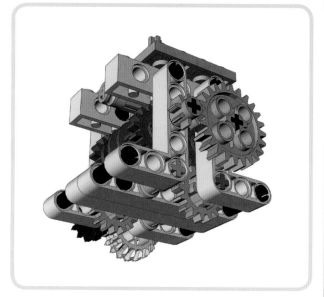

Figure 3-15: I used studless pieces to connect this gearbox. Thus, this build required me to plan which pin holes would be filled with axles and which with pins, to figure out how many connections would be needed to keep the structure rigid, and to carefully select pieces best suited in shape and size.

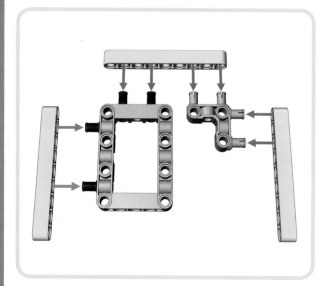

Figure 3-14: Only two types of pieces (light grey) allow you to easily create rigid connections between perpendicular beams on the same level.

The presence of both pin and axle holes means that studless pieces and connectors can also be connected with axles to create bigger, sturdier structures. These sorts of connections require advance planning because of the complexities of the studless technique (see Figure 3-15). When making a structural axle connection, you should have a good idea of the size of your structure and know which pin holes can be used for pins and which have to be reserved for axles. All of these considerations make it more challenging to build with studless pieces. There is even a popular saying that doing so resembles playing chess: The builder needs to plan a couple of steps ahead.

Learning to build primarily with studless pieces allows you to build stronger, sturdier, and more compact structures; hence, studless MOCs are usually more functional, smaller, and lighter than studfull ones. They can give your model a fairly skeletal or "hollow" appearance, though. To avoid this and to create a good-looking studless model (like the Ford GT40 in Figure 3-16), you can add panels and flexible axles, or you can combine a studless interior structure with a studfull body, an idea fully explored later in this chapter.

studless advantages

In general, the advantages of studfull connections are that they

* Are easy to combine in any direction, allowing for three-dimensional building
* Are easy to combine with most modern Technic pieces, such as motors and actuators
* Have more pin holes, making compact construction elements possible
* Rarely need extra reinforcement (if using rigid connections)
* Are smaller and lighter than studfull pieces

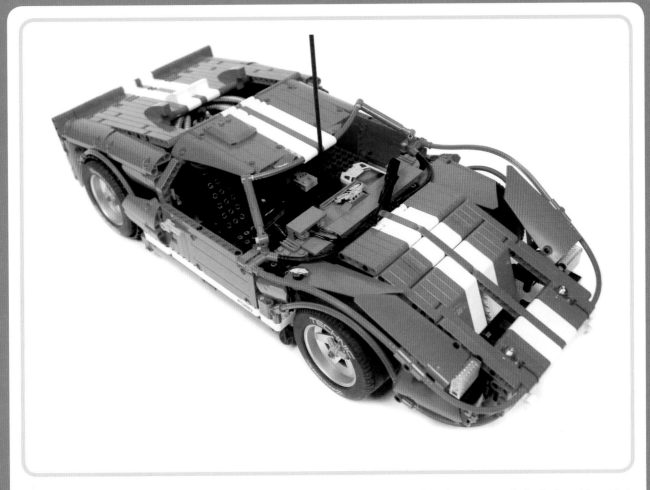

Figure 3-16: My Ford GT40 model had a completely studless body. It combined beams, panels, and flexible axles to re-create the flowing lines of the original car. Studless pieces can create shapes that are impossible to model with bricks, at the cost of certain conventions—in this case, panels approximated the shape of the hood in a way not possible with studfull pieces, but there were gaps between them.

studless disadvantages

In general, the disadvantages of studfull connections are that they

* Are less rigid; the largest studless structures have to be complex (or reinforced) to maintain rigidity
* Are harder to combine with non-Technic pieces
* Require at least two pins to create a rigid connection; extra pieces with complex shapes are often needed for rigidity
* Don't always look as good as bricks

combining the styles

Combining the two styles in a clever way can be a key to creating a good-looking, highly functional MOC.

With vehicular models, the chassis and the body are often independent, and we can take advantage of that independence. For example, adding a studless body to a studfull chassis results in a very sturdy but light model, and it's a popular combination when building in large scale, when weight is a serious concern. Adding a studfull body to a studless chassis, on the other hand, results in compact, good-looking models with many functions.

get inspired by Technic sets

Classic LEGO sets ingeniously mixed the two styles before the Technic line evolved into its primarily studless stage. Figures 3-17 through 3-27 provide examples of different styles of building, just to inspire your own creations.

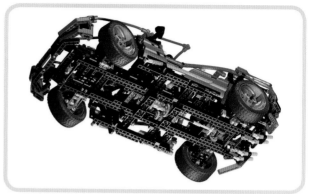

Figure 3-19: The 8448 Super Street Sensation set features a large supercar with a studfull chassis under a studless body. The model combines the rigidity of the studfull pieces, crucial at this size, with the lightness of studless ones.

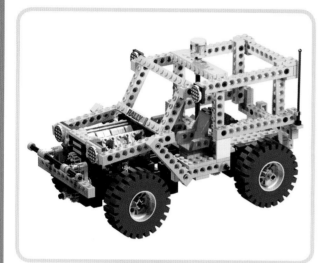

Figure 3-17: The 8850 Jeep is one of the last completely studfull LEGO Technic sets. Note that while the silhouette of the Jeep is modeled quite well, the bricks facing various directions look somewhat chaotic.

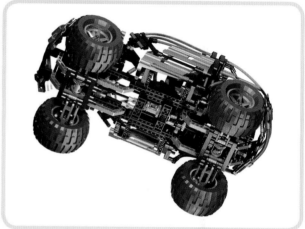

Figure 3-20: The 8466 4×4 Off-Roader set features another large car model, but this time only the center of the chassis remains studfull. This center provides the rigidity needed by the car's impressive suspension system, but the set itself is mainly studless.

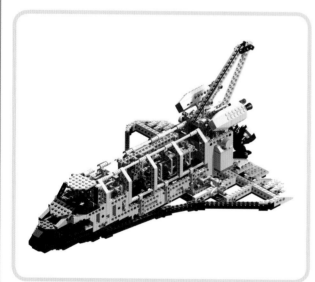

Figure 3-18: The 8480 Space Shuttle set does an excellent job of modeling the complex shape of the real vessel with bricks and hinge plates. Studless pieces are present, but they don't dominate yet.

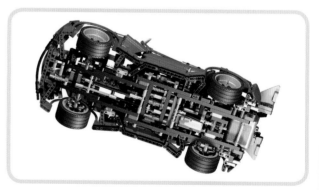

Figure 3-21: The 8070 Super Car set can be considered a direct descendant of the 8448 set. It's completely studless, with a very rigid, although shorter, chassis.

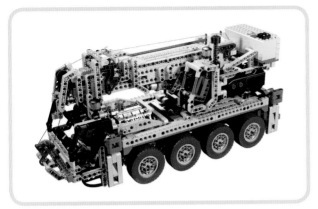

Figure 3-22: The acclaimed 8421 Mobile Crane set is primarily studless, but it uses a combination of bricks and plates for the most heavily loaded part of the boom.

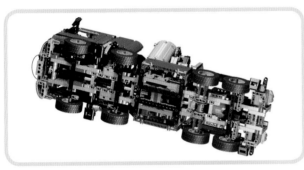

Figure 3-23: The 8285 Crane Truck set is an outstanding achievement in creating a rigid, sturdy studless chassis for a heavy vehicle. Studfull pieces are still there—note the clever use of a Technic brick to attach the license plate under the front bumper.

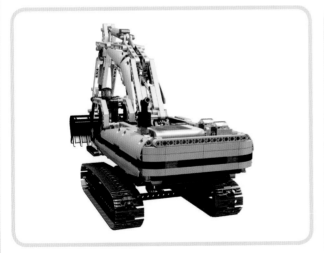

Figure 3-24: The 8043 Motorized Excavator set has a realistic silhouette created with studless panels, but it also uses studfull ones, mainly tiles and curved slopes, to model its rear end.

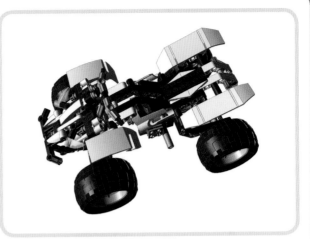

Figure 3-25: Some LEGO panels come in surprising shapes. The 8262 Quad-Bike set proves these panels can be used to excellent aesthetic effect.

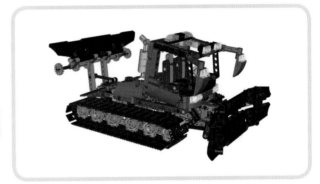

Figure 3-26: The 8263 Snow Groomer set uses a number of studfull pieces as cabin details, which are too small to be modeled with studless pieces.

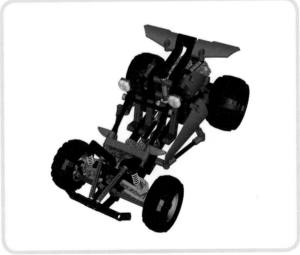

Figure 3-27: The 8048 Buggy set is a great example of creating a small, authentic-looking vehicle using studless pieces only.

While modern LEGO Technic sets use studfull bricks only when necessary, making the distinction between chassis and body quite subtle, MOCs can do something much more dramatic. You can create splendid-looking models by building a studfull body around a studless chassis and then incorporating large numbers of classic LEGO bricks. Many accomplished builders abandon the Technic aesthetic completely and instead aim to make their models look as authentic as possible using any LEGO pieces that suit their needs. This is often called the *Model Team approach*, in reference to the discontinued LEGO Model Team line of large-scale vehicular models. These are Technic models that really "work"—that steer, drive, shift gears, and so on—but don't resemble Technic models. This building technique, possible usually only at medium and large scale, involves covering the Technic structure with bricks and tiles, thus concealing any pin holes, axles, wires, and motors. Figures 3-28 through 3-30 show examples of the Model Team approach, while Figure 3-31 shows a build using studless pieces, panels, and flexible axles as a counterexample.

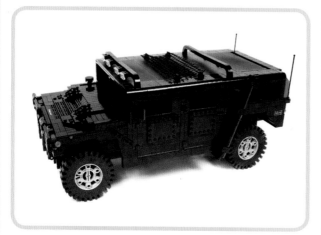

Figure 3-28: My Humvee model used a studfull body on a mixed chassis. The central bearing structure of the chassis was studfull, and the areas between wheels, where compactness was crucial, were studless. The resulting model was very rigid and compact for its functionality but also very heavy.

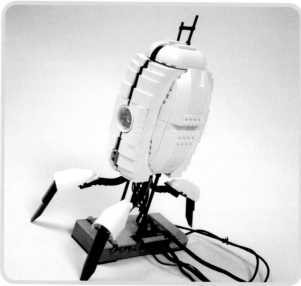

Figure 3-30: My model of a sentry turret from the Portal game used a complex combination of pieces to create an egg-shaped body. The body consisted of five separate studfull parts—front, rear, left, right, and top—attached around a studless skeleton. No existing studless pieces could achieve that body shape.

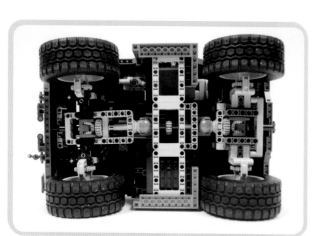

Figure 3-29: My model of the RG-35 4×4 MRAP vehicle (an armored personnel carrier) combined a completely studless chassis with a fully studfull body. The realistic model was extremely compact, but its densely built body made it top-heavy.

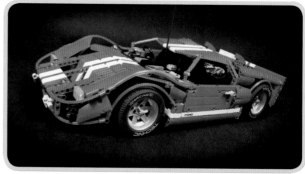

Figure 3-31: My Ford GT40 model used studfull pieces only for minor details of the body and cabin interior. It lacked some rigidity, but it weighed only 2.35 kg while being over 0.5 m long. It's the counterexample to Model Team builds.

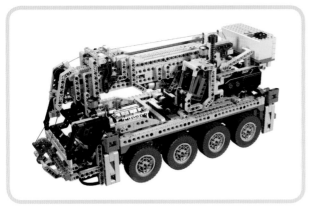

Figure 3-22: The acclaimed 8421 Mobile Crane set is primarily studless, but it uses a combination of bricks and plates for the most heavily loaded part of the boom.

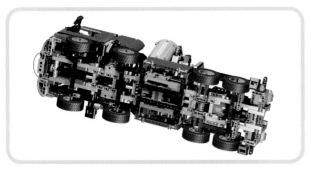

Figure 3-23: The 8285 Crane Truck set is an outstanding achievement in creating a rigid, sturdy studless chassis for a heavy vehicle. Studfull pieces are still there—note the clever use of a Technic brick to attach the license plate under the front bumper.

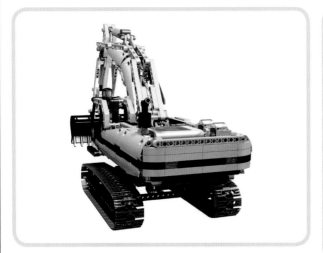

Figure 3-24: The 8043 Motorized Excavator set has a realistic silhouette created with studless panels, but it also uses studfull ones, mainly tiles and curved slopes, to model its rear end.

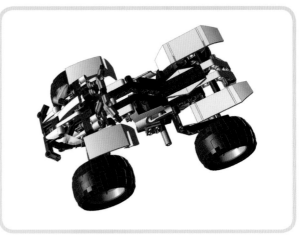

Figure 3-25: Some LEGO panels come in surprising shapes. The 8262 Quad-Bike set proves these panels can be used to excellent aesthetic effect.

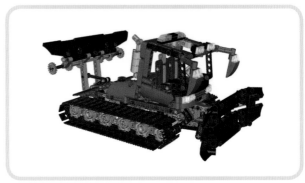

Figure 3-26: The 8263 Snow Groomer set uses a number of studfull pieces as cabin details, which are too small to be modeled with studless pieces.

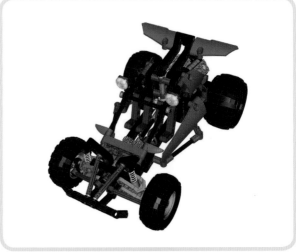

Figure 3-27: The 8048 Buggy set is a great example of creating a small, authentic-looking vehicle using studless pieces only.

While modern LEGO Technic sets use studfull bricks only when necessary, making the distinction between chassis and body quite subtle, MOCs can do something much more dramatic. You can create splendid-looking models by building a studfull body around a studless chassis and then incorporating large numbers of classic LEGO bricks. Many accomplished builders abandon the Technic aesthetic completely and instead aim to make their models look as authentic as possible using any LEGO pieces that suit their needs. This is often called the *Model Team approach*, in reference to the discontinued LEGO Model Team line of large-scale vehicular models. These are Technic models that really "work"—that steer, drive, shift gears, and so on—but don't resemble Technic models. This building technique, possible usually only at medium and large scale, involves covering the Technic structure with bricks and tiles, thus concealing any pin holes, axles, wires, and motors. Figures 3-28 through 3-30 show examples of the Model Team approach, while Figure 3-31 shows a build using studless pieces, panels, and flexible axles as a counterexample.

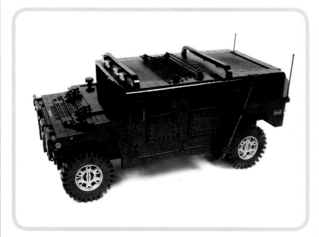

Figure 3-28: My Humvee model used a studfull body on a mixed chassis. The central bearing structure of the chassis was studfull, and the areas between wheels, where compactness was crucial, were studless. The resulting model was very rigid and compact for its functionality but also very heavy.

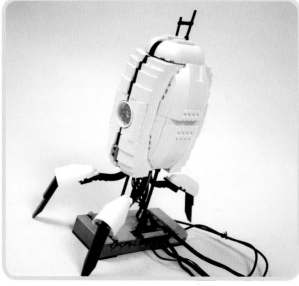

Figure 3-30: My model of a sentry turret from the Portal game used a complex combination of pieces to create an egg-shaped body. The body consisted of five separate studfull parts—front, rear, left, right, and top—attached around a studless skeleton. No existing studless pieces could achieve that body shape.

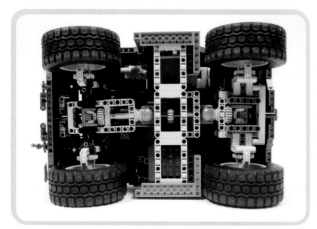

Figure 3-29: My model of the RG-35 4×4 MRAP vehicle (an armored personnel carrier) combined a completely studless chassis with a fully studfull body. The realistic model was extremely compact, but its densely built body made it top-heavy.

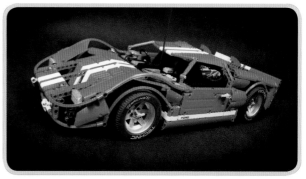

Figure 3-31: My Ford GT40 model used studfull pieces only for minor details of the body and cabin interior. It lacked some rigidity, but it weighed only 2.35 kg while being over 0.5 m long. It's the counterexample to Model Team builds.

methods for connecting bricks and beams

Now that you've been inspired by models that successfully combine studless and studfull pieces, let's consider the practical aspects of actually connecting the two. In addition to using pins to connect pieces, as shown in Figure 3-32, we can use half pins to work like regular studs, as shown in Figures 3-33 and 3-34.

Some connections are considered incorrect because they align pieces in a manner not equal to a full number of studs, as shown in Figure 3-35. While sturdy, these misaligned pieces will make finishing your model extremely difficult, as the relative spacing of the pieces is no longer 1 full stud.

Electric components are usually designed to fit with either studless or studfull constructions, so incorporating them into mixed models can be challenging. You'll need to think

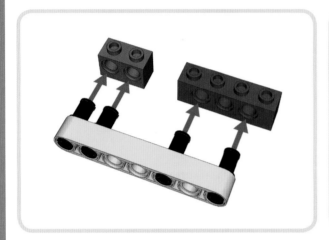

Figure 3-32: Beams can be easily connected with bricks using pins. Note that we can choose regular Technic bricks (blue) or bricks with centered pin holes (green) to adjust the alignment.

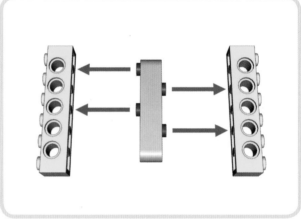

Figure 3-34: The symmetry of the studless pieces allows for complex connections that can grow in several directions.

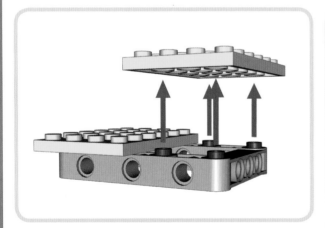

Figure 3-33: When half pins are inserted into pin holes, their tops work just like studs. Bricks or plates can be firmly attached to them, and we can select their exact alignment by carefully choosing the positions of our half pins.

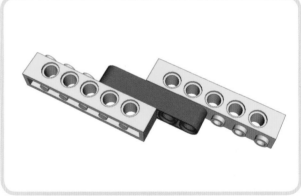

Figure 3-35: This connection, with studs inserted into the beam's pin holes, is sturdy but considered incorrect. This is because—unlike in the previous examples—the spacing between the bricks' pin holes is not equal to a full number of studs. In terms of LEGO units, the bricks are misaligned.

creatively to secure these mismatched elements into your constructions. The Power Functions IR receiver (Figure 3-36), Medium motor (Figure 3-37), and switch (Figure 3-38) are the most common examples. You'll learn more about the Power Functions system in Chapter 14.

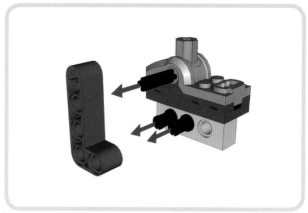

Figure 3-38: The Power Functions switch is easily connected to studfull pieces, but creating a rigid connection with a studless piece is more challenging.

even vs. odd

The final challenge is matching the two styles' widths. Studfull pieces are designed for even-numbered spacings of 2 or 4 or 6 studs, and so on. Studless pieces are designed for odd spacings, 3 or 5 or 7 studs. This difference raises difficulties when combining the two styles—for example, a studless chassis is in most cases an odd width, but a studfull body around it is easier to build at an even width. Of course, length and height often also require matching, but in practice width is usually the primary challenge, because the left and right sides of most models are symmetrical. In other words, making a model wider or narrower requires changing its central part, while length and height can be adjusted by adding pieces at the top or back of the model.

A pair of half-stud-wide liftarms (shown in blue in Figure 3-39) are well suited for matching a single-stud difference in width. Other pieces and connectors designed to overcome this spacing problem are shown in Figures 3-40 to 3-44.

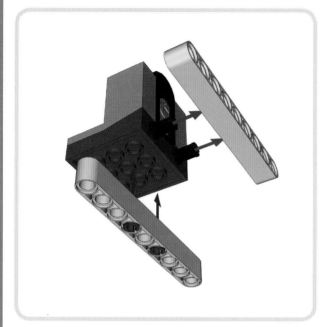

Figure 3-36: With its plate base, the Power Functions IR receiver is easily connected to studfull pieces. For studless connections, we have the option of using pins or half pins (as studs), shown above.

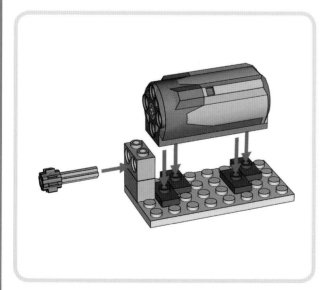

Figure 3-37: Jumper plates (blue) can be used to align the Power Functions Medium motor to studfull pieces.

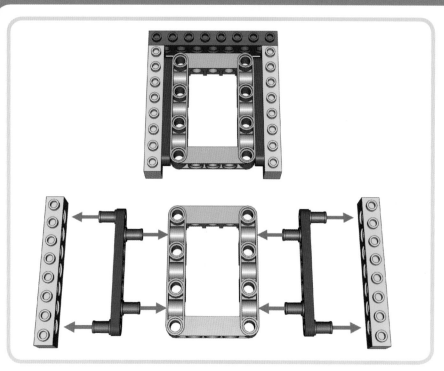

Figure 3-39: Half-stud-wide beams (blue) and three-quarter pins (dark grey) can be used to create a very firm connection between pieces of even and odd width.

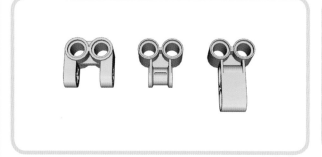

Figure 3-40: Three types of studless connectors created specifically to handle a half-stud difference

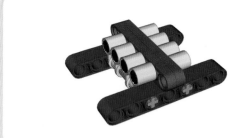

Figure 3-42: Connectors (yellow) used to align a 6-stud-long piece (red) to the center of a 5-stud-long structure (blue)

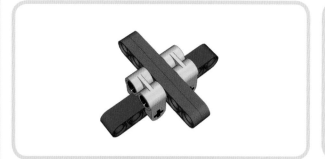

Figure 3-41: Connectors (yellow) used to align a 6-stud-long piece (red) to the center of a 7-stud-long piece (blue)

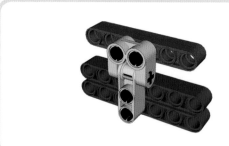

Figure 3-43: A combination of two connectors (yellow) used to align a 6-stud-long piece (red) to the center of a 7-stud-long structure (blue)

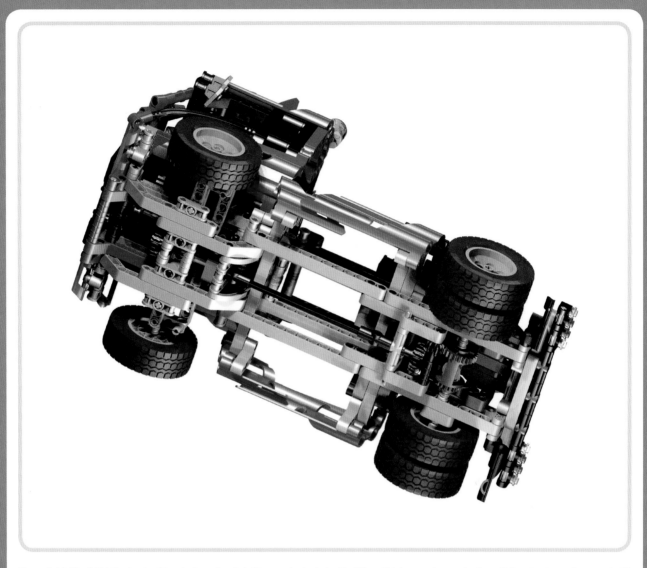

Figure 3-44: The 8436 Truck set, with a studless chassis built around a 4-stud-wide differential, is a great example of combining structures of even and odd width. The use of the adjusting connectors in this set creates a very rigid yet light structure.

Depending on where and when your adventure with LEGO Technic started, you may be unfamiliar with one building style or the other. The best way to understand how an unfamiliar style works is by playing with a LEGO set that uses it extensively. If this proves difficult, remember that there is nothing wrong with sticking to the system you know and like. After all, innovation is quite often driven by our creative constraints!

4

axles, bushes, and joints

We've already covered most of the basic LEGO Technic pieces. In this chapter, we discuss three other popular pieces: axles, bushes, and universal joints. While all of these elements can be used to transmit drive, they can also be used as structural elements in your builds. Let's take a look.

axles

Axles are one of the most basic and crucial pieces in LEGO Technic. They have a very special property: Depending on the shape of the hole they're put through, axles can either rotate inside other pieces or remain fixed to them (at the same time locking them together), as Figure 4-1 shows.

Axles have two essential tasks: transferring drive and structural reinforcement. The first task requires axles to rotate freely and to be connected to a motor, either directly or through gears, axle joiners, or other pieces.

The task of reinforcing requires axles to remain fixed relative to other pieces, which necessitates an axle hole. It is not uncommon to use an axle exclusively for holding together pieces at fixed angles, as shown in Figure 4-2.

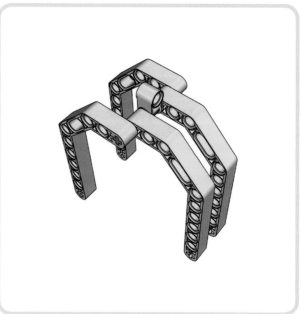

Figure 4-2: A 5-stud-long axle connecting five other pieces. All the pieces are fixed to the axle, and the axle alone keeps them at fixed angles.

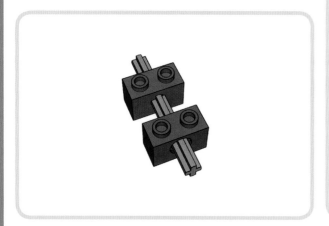

Figure 4-1: A regular axle put through two Technic bricks: The red brick has an X-shaped axle hole that locks the axle, while the green brick has a pin hole that allows the axle to rotate freely.

It is also possible to use an axle for both tasks at once—the axle can transfer drive through pieces while at the same time keeping other pieces locked to it. Such a combination is shown in Figure 4-3. Note that any axle that holds pieces together is subjected to structural stress, which adds friction to it. This will matter when you use the axle to transfer drive.

There are three categories of axles, each suitable for a different purpose. They are standard axles, modified axles, and flexible axles.

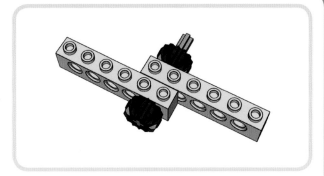

Figure 4-3: A 5-stud-long axle used to keep two bricks (yellow) together between two gears (black). The axle can rotate inside the bricks, and the gears' rotation can be used to transfer drive.

standard axles

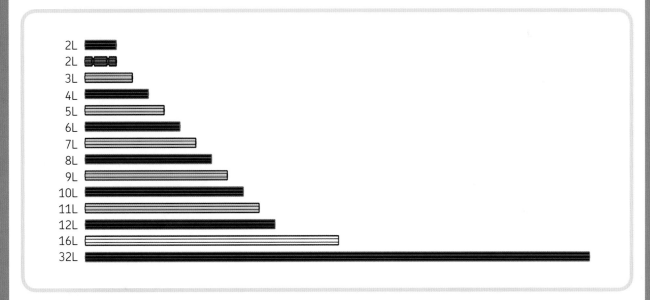

Standard axles come in 14 variants, which are shown above in their most recent colors. Historically, LEGO has changed the colors of the axles several times, as I'll explain here.

Originally, only axles of even length existed, and they were all black. Odd-length axles were introduced later; initially, these axles were also black, but they were later changed to light grey to provide a simple distinction between odd and even lengths. Then in 2016, LEGO started to make certain odd-length axles in yellow and certain even-length axles in red, but in an inconsistent manner (they appear in only some 2016 sets), suggesting a transition period between the old and new standards.

Other than their lengths, all axles are alike with three notable exceptions:

2L Has two variants: One is smooth (black) and the other is notched, which makes pulling it out easier (red and, rarely, black). The notch makes pulling the axle out easier. The smooth variant is obsolete, and the notched axle has replaced it.

11L Introduced in late 2016, this is the rarest of all axle variants.

16L In its usual white variant, this axle is noticeably more elastic than standard axles; it can easily bend and unbend. A rare black variant also exists that has a standard stiffness.

modified axles

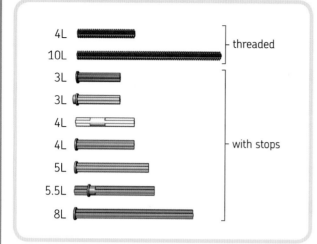

4L — threaded
10L — threaded

3L — with stops
3L —
4L —
4L —
5L —
5.5L —
8L —

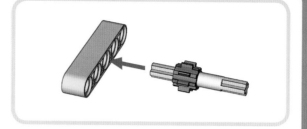

Figure 4-4: *A popular use of the 4L axle with center stop. By placing a gear wheel on it, you can prevent the axle from going deeper than 1 stud into the yellow beam because its center stop can't go through the gear wheel.*

Modified axles belong in two groups: threaded axles and axles with stops. Threaded axles are black, come in 4L and 10L variants (top two axles above), and were eliminated in LEGO Technic sets circa 1990. Along with threaded nuts to hold their ends, threaded axles work as bolts to hold parts together. They have a very thin cross section and will break if they're used to transmit torque. Given how rare and expensive they are, builders should be careful not to misuse them.

Axles with stops, on the other hand, are newer and have many practical applications. With the exception of the 4L axle with a center stop, these axles have stops that can't go through a pin hole, and none of them can go through an axle hole. Thus, these axles are commonly used when sliding of the axle is not desired. The modified axle variants are shown in the preceding figure in their most common colors, and each is described in the following list:

3L axle with stop   Has a standard, smooth stop that fits entirely inside a pin hole.

3L axle with stud   Has a special kind of stop that ends with a hollow stud, which actually makes the axle a little longer than 3 studs and allows you to connect studded pieces to its end. The end with the stud can also be inserted into a pin hole, making the axle rotate with extra friction.

4L axle with center stop   A unique axle that has a 1-stud-long smooth section 2 studs away from one end and 1 stud away from the other. The stop can go through a pin hole but not through an axle hole, so you can put pieces with axle holes (like gear wheels) on the axle to prevent it from sliding, as shown in Figure 4-4.

4L axle with stop   Has a standard, smooth stop that fits entirely inside a pin hole.

5L axle with stop   Has a standard, smooth stop that fits entirely inside a pin hole.

5.5L axle with stop   Has a midpoint stop located 1 stud away from one end (and therefore 4.5 studs away from the other); has a half-stud-long smooth section adjacent to the stop on the longer side. The stop can be used to prevent the axle from sliding through the beam, and the axle can be used to drive something on the other side of the beam safely. For this reason, and despite its odd length, this axle has several useful applications, such as the one shown in Figure 4-5. Also note that two 5.5L axles connected with an axle joiner can form a substitute 11L axle.

8L axle with stop   Has a standard, smooth stop that fits entirely inside a pin hole.

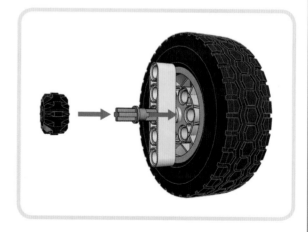

Figure 4-5: *Using the 5.5L axle with stop to keep the axle from being pulled out by the wheel, for example, while cornering*

flexible axles

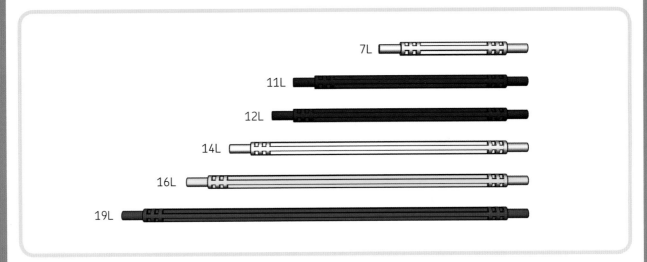

7L
11L
12L
14L
16L
19L

Flexible axles, also called *soft axles*, are made of soft material and are easily bent without incurring damage. While they can be put through a pin hole, their ends prevent them from being put through an axle hole. Each end has a 1-stud-long protrusion that is less thick than a full stud. The protrusions are most often inserted into half pins, which are then inserted into pin holes to anchor the axle. The axles come in many colors and six variants that vary only by length: 7L, 11L, 12L, 14L, 16L, and 19L.

Flexible axles have few practical or structural uses. It's extremely difficult to use them to transfer drive or to hold anything together. They are also too soft to act as springs, although they can be used instead of shock absorbers to stabilize pendular suspensions. They are most often used as decorative elements, bent to form various arches. Their flexibility makes them popular in LEGO Technic supercars (as Figure 4-6 shows), where they form mudguards, windshield edges, bumpers, hoods, and other curvy elements whose shapes are difficult to model with other LEGO pieces.

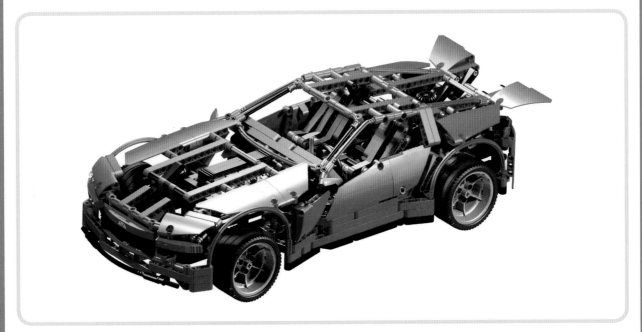

Figure 4-6: The 8070 Super Car set relies on flexible axles to model parts of the body such as the mudguards and the edges of the front bumper.

bushes

LEGO bushes, also called *bushings*, are small elements put on axles in order to maintain spacing between two or more other elements. They can also prevent pieces from sliding off of axles or keep axles in place. They come in three versions: a half bush (half stud long), a bush (1 stud long), and a bush with a long pin (3 studs long, including a 2-stud-long pin), all of which are shown in Figure 4-7.

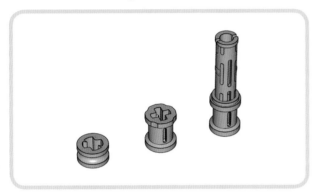

Figure 4-7: From left to right: a half bush, a bush, and a bush with a long pin

half bush

The half bush is the only piece from this group that comes in variants (as shown in Figure 4-8). Its variants include a toothed half bush, a toothed half bush with a cut-out axle hole, and the currently produced smooth half bush with a cut-out axle hole.

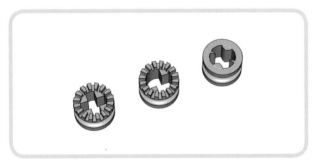

Figure 4-8: From left to right: a toothed half bush, a toothed half bush with a cut-out axle hole, and a smooth half bush with a cut-out axle hole

toothed half bush

The first variant, the toothed half bush, comes with a complete axle hole and 16 small teeth on one side. The other side is completely smooth. The rim of the half bush has a groove that allows it to act as a pulley for rubber bands, as shown in Figure 4-9. In fact, all half bushes have the ability to act as a pulley. For more information on pulleys, check out Chapter 7.

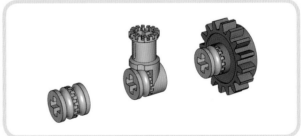

Figure 4-9: A half bush and a wedge belt wheel both have grooves for LEGO rubber bands and can be used as pulleys.

The toothed side of the half bush can be meshed with a number of other LEGO pieces: another toothed half bush, a toothed axle connector, or a toothed 16-tooth gear with clutch (as shown in Figure 4-10). It's important to keep in mind that when these pieces are meshed, they come roughly 1 mm closer to each other, which means that there is 1 mm of backlash behind them.

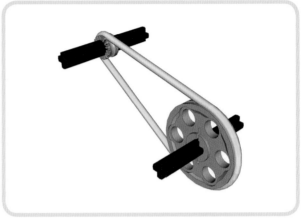

Figure 4-10: Several LEGO pieces can be meshed with a toothed half bush.

It's also useful to remember that the pieces can be meshed at various angles of rotation. Since there are 16 teeth on the side of the half bush, each tooth corresponds to 22.5 degrees; this is the minimum value by which we can change the angle of two meshed pieces. This arrangement creates some useful possibilities. For example, you can use two half bushes to couple two switches in such a way that turning one switch on turns the other one off (see Figure 4-11).

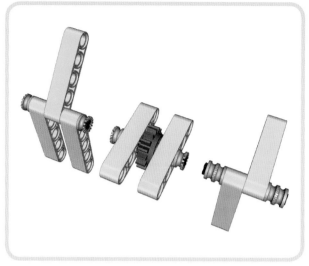

Figure 4-12: Several examples of securing an axle in place using toothed half bushes

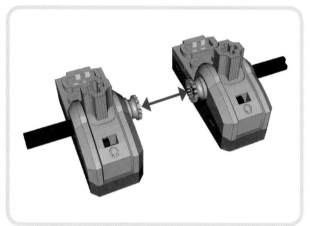

Figure 4-11: When these two half bushes are meshed at the same angle, the two switches will be coupled and work as one. But if the bushes are meshed with one rotated by just one tooth relative to the other, the two switches will be coupled so that only one of them can be on at a time; turning off one turns the other one on.

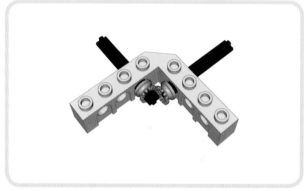

Figure 4-13: Toothed half bushes working as bevel gears. Note the quarter-stud spacings between the half bushes and the adjacent brick. Meshed this way, the half bushes can actually work very smoothly, provided high torque is not applied.

The toothed half bush is still popular today because it takes a lot of force to make it move on the axle. This makes it useful in high-load applications: Two toothed half bushes are preferable to one regular bush because they are less likely to slip along the axle when a load is applied (see Figure 4-12).

Finally, toothed half bushes can be used as bevel gears (as shown in Figure 4-13), but they must be shifted by a quarter stud each to mesh, and their teeth generate high friction and easily disengage under torque.

toothed half bush with a cutout

The second variant, the toothed half bush with a cutout, is exactly what its name implies: a copy of the previous version with part of the axle hole cut out, making the axle hole larger (see Figure 4-14). This modification was introduced

to make it easier for children to take half bushes on and off the axles, and that's exactly what makes it much less popular with builders: These bushes are more likely to shift when stressed than the first variant. Other than that, this bush has every quality of the original toothed half bush except that, having been introduced a few years later, it's newer and thus made of stronger material.

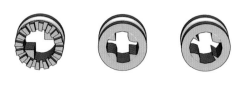

Figure 4-14: Half bushes with semireduced axle holes: the toothed half bush and two forms of the smooth half bush

smooth half bush with a cutout

The third and final variant, the smooth half bush with a cutout, is an exact copy of the previous variant minus teeth. More specifically, the teeth haven't been removed but rather have been filled in order to create a smooth side; thus, both sides of this variant are identical. This variant is also identical to the previous variant in terms of how much stress it can take before shifting along the axle. There are two forms of this variant, with the newer piece having a slightly expanded axle hole. The difference is barely noticeable and does not affect the properties of this piece. This half bush variant was introduced 13 years after the first version and is still in use today; therefore, it is always available in better condition than previous variants and is made of stronger material.

regular bush

The regular bush is a far less complex piece, with only one variant available. It can be used for securing axles or maintaining 1-stud spacings. One of its sides is smooth, and the other has four small notches in it. The notches fit LEGO studs and enable the bush to be placed in the middle of 4 studs, as shown in Figure 4-15. That means the bush can be connected to bricks and plates sized 2×2 studs or larger.

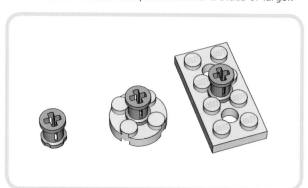

Figure 4-15: A regular bush and two examples of a regular bush connected to studded pieces

bush with a long pin

The bush with a long pin is a combination of two pieces: the long pin and a regular bush. One of its sides is just like a bush, except that its axle hole is only 1 stud deep and it has smooth rims. Its other side is identical to that of a long pin with friction, as shown in Figure 4-16.

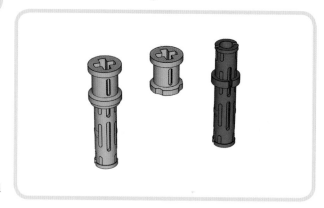

Figure 4-16: From left to right: a bush with a long pin, a regular bush, and a regular long pin

This combination was developed as a convenience for the official LEGO Technic sets. Large and complex sets are very often divided into several modules that are built separately and then connected. The bush with a long pin is well suited for this task because it can be pushed in and pulled out more easily than regular pins (see Figure 4-17).

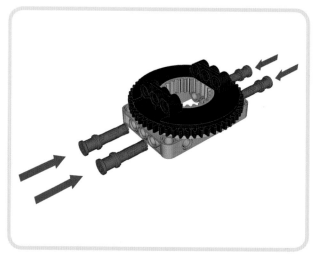

Figure 4-17: An example of the intended use of a bush with a long pin. Let's assume that we want to connect the turntable to a 5×7 frame so that they can be easily disconnected. We can do this by pushing the bushes in to lock the turntable into place and then pulling them out to free the turntable.

LEGO uses this piece for temporarily locking some modules together as well: For example, the bush with a long pin enables a truck's cabin to be lifted up, lowered back, and then locked in that position (as shown in Figure 4-18).

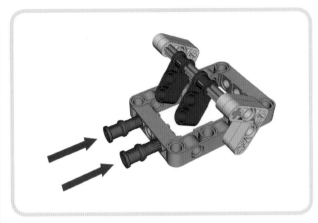

Figure 4-18: Another example of the intended use of a bush with a long pin. Let's assume that the 5×7 frame is part of the chassis and the yellow beams are part of the cabin of a truck. We can lower the cabin by rotating the yellow beams and then lock it in that position by pushing the red pieces in. Then we can pull them out and lift the cabin up again.

universal joints

LEGO universal joints, also called *u-joints* or *Cardan joints*, are used to transfer rotary motion from one axle to another at an angle. They consist of a central disc with four pegs, located between two hinges with two pegs per hinge, as shown in Figure 4-19.

The main advantage of universal joints is that they can transfer motion along a line, acting like a bent shaft.

Additionally, their angle can be changed at any moment without affecting the speed or torque they are transferring. Their only flaw is that if they are bent at more than 45 degrees, they generate fluctuations in transmitting the motion. These fluctuations increase as the angle increases, resulting in vibration, until the joint becomes completely locked at 90 degrees (see Figure 4-20).

Universal joints can be damaged by very high torque in one of two ways: The yoke (the part that embraces the axle) can crack, or the pegs on the cruciform (the disc in the center) can snap. The first type of damage can be prevented by using 2×2 round bricks or round plates, as shown in Figure 4-21. The latter type has no countermeasurebeyond building your own style of universal joint (see Chapter 9).

Universal joints were originally 4 studs long. Then in 2008, a new 3-stud-long version was introduced (shown in Figure 4-22). The new version fits well into studless structures thanks to its odd length (shown in Figure 4-23), and it is produced using stronger material than the old one. Additionally, its central disc is solid rather than hollow, and its pegs are less likely to snap; these features have made it much more popular and useful than the old version. Like the old version, though, it can be secured with round plates.

When dealing with high amounts of torque, we can also use a ball joint, which combines two studless pieces to create a sturdy, tight housing for the 3-stud-long universal joint (as shown in Figures 4-24 and 4-25). The universal joint can rotate inside the housing without being stressed or pulled. As a result, a ball joint can be used for connecting structures that exert some load on the universal joint between them. This method holds these structures together firmly while allowing a universal joint to pass through, while also giving these structures a large degree of free movement. The ball joint handles structural loads, leaving the universal joint with only the torsion of its shaft to handle. LEGO first used this method to connect suspended axles to a chassis while transferring drive from the chassis to the axles.

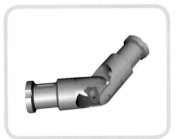

Figure 4-19: A universal joint

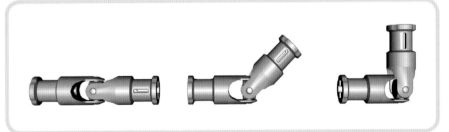

Figure 4-20: From left to right: a universal joint when it's straight, a universal joint bent at 45 degrees, and a universal joint bent at 90 degrees (unable to rotate)

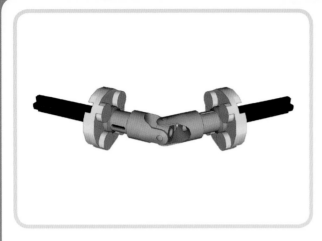

Figure 4-21: A universal joint secured against cracking with two round plates

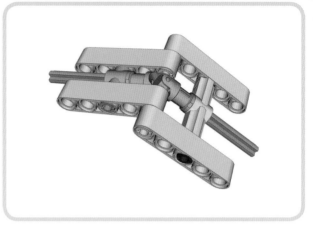

Figure 4-23: A 3-stud-long universal joint used to transfer drive through an articulation point

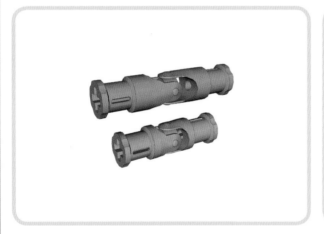

Figure 4-22: A 4-stud-long universal joint (top) and the newer 3-stud-long variant (bottom)

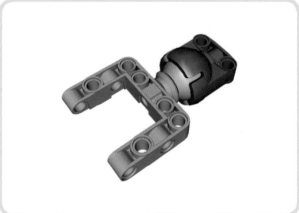

Figure 4-24: A complete ball joint includes two pieces, one inserted into the other. Note that the light grey part on the left comes with a frame large enough to house a differential; it can therefore be used directly as a basis for an axle.

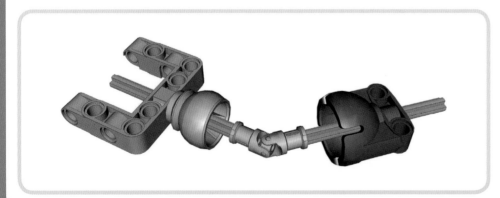

Figure 4-25: An open ball joint with a universal joint visible inside. A universal joint becomes more effective inside a ball joint because it's protected from structural stress; as a result, less friction is generated in it.

5

wheels

Simple as they are, wheels are vital pieces for any Technic vehicle builder. They're difficult to replace with other elements, their selection is limited, and they have a huge impact on the aesthetics and function of a model. In this chapter, I'll discuss how to choose the right wheels for the job and how to get the most out of them.

what makes a wheel

Most LEGO wheels are a combination of two pieces: a plastic rim and a rubber tire (see Figure 5-1). Many rim and tire combinations are unique, but some rims fit a number of tires (see Figure 5-2) and vice versa. You can find a list of popular LEGO rim and tire combinations at *http://www.wheels.sariel.pl/*.

The rare exception to the "rim + tire = wheel" rule is the tireless rim. Consider the 54 mm × 30 mm wheel shown in Figure 5-3. It's made so its outer rim replaces the tire. For this to work, the wheel must be solid plastic. I'll discuss the functional pros and cons of plastic wheels in "Material" on page 48, but one of their benefits is that they can serve as decorative elements. For instance, they can be part of a jet engine nozzle in LEGO spaceships.

In addition to rims and tires, some wheels have wheel covers or hubcaps. These elements are purely decorative. They connect to the front or back of the rim, typically with an axle, effectively hiding the rim and becoming the most visible part of the wheel. They're usually made to fit a specific rim, and they're a simple way to re-create the look of specific car's wheels. Often, they're a simple solution to the problem of having an inappropriate rim for the model. The wheels in the 8145 Ferrari 599 GTB Fiorano set, shown in Figure 5-4, are a typical example of this approach.

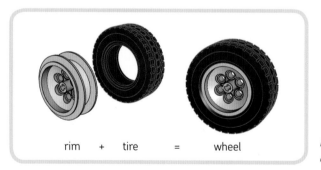

rim   +   tire   =   wheel

Figure 5-1: The popular 62.4 mm × 20 mm wheel (right) combines two elements: a plastic rim and a rubber tire.

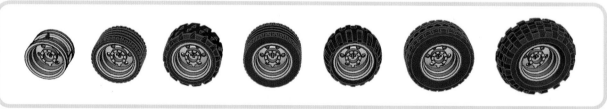

Figure 5-2: The 30.4 mm × 20 mm rim (leftmost) is one of the most versatile LEGO rims, fitting six different tires and effectively creating six different wheels.

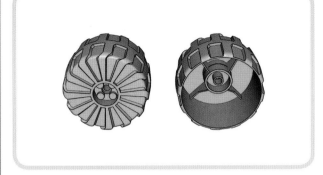

Figure 5-3: The 54 mm × 30 mm wheel (front and back) is actually just a rim that acts as complete wheel. It doesn't need a tire, and it's often used as a decorative element.

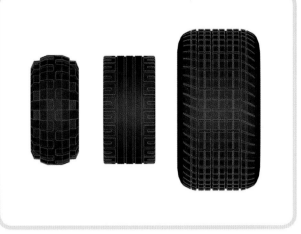

Figure 5-5: A balloon tire (left) and a regular tire (middle). Although these two tires are identical in diameter, their shapes are very different: the balloon tire is oval and the regular one is rectangular. The tire on the right combines both characteristics but performs like a regular tire.

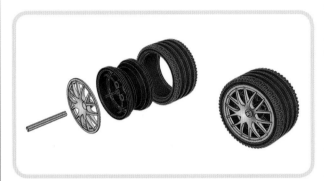

Figure 5-4: The wheel on the right is a combination of the four elements shown on the left: an axle, a wheel cover, a rim, and a tire. Note that the axle is required to connect the cover to the rim.

tires

Tires are an important wheel component. They're the only part that is supposed to come in contact with the ground, so they have a major impact on a wheel's performance. Tires can be grouped into a few categories based on their shape, their filling, and the material they're made of.

shape

Shape refers to a tire's form when it's viewed in profile, as shown in Figure 5-5. LEGO tires come in two basic shapes: balloon tires, which are oval-shaped, and regular tires, which are rectangular. The left tire in Figure 5-5 is an example of a balloon tire; the middle is a regular tire. Although these two tires are the same size, their shapes result in very different strengths and weaknesses.

Some tires, such as the tire on the right in Figure 5-5, combine characteristics of the two shapes. Because a tire's center has the most contact with the ground, these hybrids function largely like regular tires.

Tire shape affects a vehicle's functionality in many ways. The biggest difference is that balloon tires work better off-road, because their shape ensures better contact with uneven surfaces. Regular tires, on the other hand, work better on road surfaces that are generally smooth and flat. Tire shape also affects rolling resistance (see Chapter 1). Balloon tires are more deformed than regular tires when they come in contact with surfaces, which gives them better traction but also requires higher torque to make the wheel roll.

Regular tires are the opposite: They provide less traction, but they also have lower rolling resistance and require less torque. In real life, you see the difference all the time. Balloon tires are common in off-road cars, whereas sport cars meant only for roads have regular tires. Traction is crucial for off-road vehicles, so it makes sense for them to take on the extra rolling resistance, even if it requires a more powerful engine. In contrast, road cars drive on optimized road surfaces, and tires that provide less traction free up more of the engine's power for speed. And when road cars require increased traction, you can substitute wider tires or tires made of grippier material and still maintain the regular tire shape.

solid vs. hollow

After choosing the tire profile, you need to consider whether to choose a tire that is solid rubber or hollow with air inside. Solid tires have a smooth inner surface that wraps around the rim tightly, leaving nothing in between. These are rare in the LEGO world. Hollow tires, which are more widespread, have sidewalls that separate their inner surface from the rim, creating a gap inside that is filled with air. Hollow tires can be shallow or deep depending on the depth of the sidewalls (see Figures 5-6 and 5-7). With hollow tires, the sidewalls also hold the rim in place by overlapping the flanges on either side of the rim (see Figure 5-8). Solid tires, on the other hand, depend on friction between the rim and the tire inside for the same purpose; generally, this approach is less efficient. Note that if friction between the rim and tire is too low, the rim may start rotating inside the tire: This often occurs in off-road vehicles while negotiating obstacles.

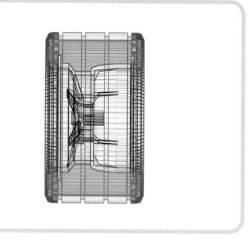

Figure 5-8: A see-through view of a hollow tire with the rim inside. The red marks the gap inside the tire, which is filled with air. Note the flanges on either side of the rim that overlap with the tire's sidewalls, helping to keep the rim inside the tire.

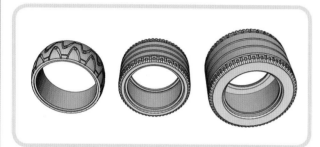

Figure 5-6: A solid tire (left), a shallow hollow tire (middle), and a deep hollow tire (right). The tires are colored yellow to highlight their inner shape.

Solid and hollow tires also differ in rolling resistance and cushioning. Solid tires have practically no rolling resistance because there is no air to be compressed inside, making it difficult to deform a solid tire. But hollow tires are still quite hard, and they only become significantly deformed under large loads. The difference between the two is only noticeable with heavy vehicles. In addition, solid tires transfer significantly more vibration to the rims and then the chassis than hollow tires, because there is no air-filled gap to act as a cushion between the tire and the rim. The vehicle's suspension system can absorb some of this vibration, but as a rule of thumb, solid tires are best suited for smooth, flat surfaces.

Note that LEGO's hollow tires are pneumatic, meaning the air inside them is not pressurized. Real cars use pressurized tires because their walls are proportionally thinner and the wheels carry proportionally heavier loads. LEGO tires are pretty thick and LEGO cars are relatively light, so pneumatic tires are a better solution they provide better cushioning and they're puncture proof. Pressurizing a LEGO tire is technically possible under certain conditions (for example, by sealing the tire and rim in an airtight connection and finding a way to feed air into the tire afterward), but there is no practical gain from doing so.

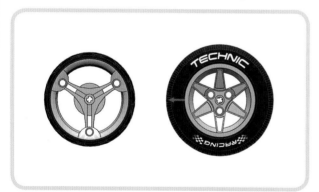

Figure 5-7: A solid tire (left) and a hollow tire (right). The red arrow shows the distance between the rim and the inner surface of the hollow tire, which is equal to the depth of the tire's sidewalls.

material

Another consideration is the material of the tires, but this choice is very simple. All modern LEGO tires are made of a complex compound of ingredients, which I'll call "rubber" for simplicity. LEGO has undoubtedly experimented with its rubber composition and quite possibly improved it over the years, but the rubber retains its essential characteristics. Some early tires were made of a different material resembling compressed foam. This foam was lighter than rubber but provided inferior traction, and for some reason all tires of this kind were solid. They also had poor contact with the rim and were likely to start rotating inside it.

Then there are solid plastic wheels, mentioned earlier, that are made of the same material as regular LEGO pieces. These wheels have advantages and disadvantages. Plastic wheels have much worse traction than wheels with rubber tires, but they offer the advantages of reduced weight (rubber tires are usually heavy), zero ground resistance (the plastic is not deformed as easily as rubber), increased resistance to wear (plastic is more durable than rubber), and color consistency (unlike rubber tires, plastic wheels can be made in any regular LEGO color).

Figure 5-9 compares the three essential tire types: rubber, foam, and plastic. Note that rubber tires are subject to aging. This process takes years, but brand-new rubber tires are clearly softer and grippier than the older ones—a result of the gradual evaporation of the compound's softening agent.

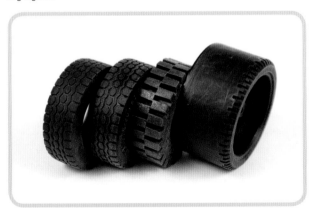

Figure 5-9: From left to right, the tires shown are a 10-year-old LEGO rubber tire, a brand-new rubber tire, a foam tire, and a solid plastic wheel.

size matters

The final critical consideration is a wheel's size or its total diameter, which is measured from one outer edge to the other. Wheel size affects speed, acceleration, and several other properties of a vehicle. Table 5-1 summarizes some of the key differences between big and small wheels.

table 5-1: functional differences between tire sizes

	small wheels	big wheels
top speed	low	high*
acceleration	high*	low
drivetrain stress	low*	high
torque required	low*	high
ground clearance	small	large*
off-road performance	poor	good*

* These properties are more desirable.

To understand how size affects speed and acceleration, it's useful to think about the wheel's circumference, which is the total distance around the wheel and thus the distance a wheel travels by making one full rotation. The circumference (C) equals π multiplied by the wheel's diameter, so a wheel's travel distance is always a little more than three times its diameter. A wheel with a diameter of 3 studs has a circumference of $C = 3.14 \times 3 = 9.42$ studs, meaning that a single revolution of that wheel lets it travel 9.42 studs. A wheel with a diameter of 9 studs has $C = 3.14 \times 9 = 28.26$ studs.

Circumference is directly proportional to the wheel's diameter: A three times larger wheel travels three times farther in a single revolution. This, in turn, means that a wheel's diameter affects the top speed of a vehicle. If you drive your wheels with a motor that rotates them 10 times per minute, the 3-stud wheel will travel 94.2 studs, whereas the 9-stud wheel will travel 282.6 studs a minute. So, the bigger wheel, in theory, will move a vehicle at three times the speed of the smaller wheel. Of course, this assumes that the wheels have perfect traction and never slip.

However, there is no free lunch in physics. Everything comes at a cost, and this applies to the big wheels' top speed as well. Bigger wheels allow for higher speeds, but they also require more torque to rotate. Compare a wheel to a lever. When a wheel rotates, it pushes itself against the surface at a pivot point just as a lever does (see Figure 5-10). The lever "pushes" a load, which is the surface in this case. I discuss levers in more detail in Chapter 8 when I talk about solutions for moving heavy loads. For now, you just need to know that the longer the lever, the harder it is to move something with it. The lever goes from the wheel axle to the ground, so in other words, the lever is equal to the length of the wheel's radius, or half the diameter. Thus, the bigger the wheel, the more power is required to move it. In real life, you might have experienced this if you've ridden bicycles with big and small wheels. In motorized LEGO vehicles, this difference translates into a sluggish acceleration with bigger wheels because the motor must work harder to get the vehicle up to speed. This also means that a bigger wheel generates more stress in the vehicle's drivetrain.

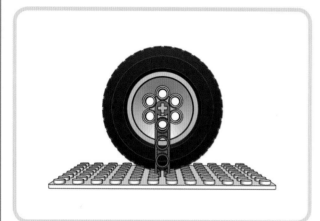

Figure 5-10: The way a wheel behaves on a surface can be compared to the action of a lever (shown in red) whose length is equal to the wheel's radius. Imagine the lever rotating and applying force to move the surface.

Wheel size also determines ground clearance and off-road performance. In general, the bigger the wheel, the greater the ground clearance. This principle can be mitigated somewhat by using portal axles, which I'll discuss in Chapter 17. Off-road performance, or how well a wheel handles obstacles, is also directly related to size: Bigger wheels have less chance of getting stuck in a hole, they can climb bigger obstacles, and they perform well on uneven terrain because they have more contact with the ground.

With the preceding characteristics in mind, it should be easier to choose the right wheels for your model. Choosing the biggest wheels possible—a natural temptation because big wheels look cool and usually mean bigger models—isn't always the best decision. In many cases, you'll do better with wheels that balance speed and performance over rough terrain against torque requirements.

beyond the basics

Sometimes the perfect wheel won't be available. Many builders have found the selection of LEGO wheels lacking. If this is your situation, you have a few options. One is to 3D print your own wheels, but this is expensive and subject to limitations, which I'll discuss in Chapter 22. Other options are to experiment with pairing different tires and rims that are not designed to work with each other or to look to other manufacturers for tires. The following sections discuss both options.

experimenting with rim and tire size

Although most LEGO tires are made to fit specific rims, you can still experiment. By doing so, you can change the shape of a LEGO tire and make it harder or heavier. This, in turn, can lower the vehicle's center of gravity. Here are some ways you can experiment with the LEGO wheels:

* You can squeeze a tire between dishes or turntables that replace the rim, making the tire taller and narrower (see Figure 5-11).
* You can build a custom rim. One method for doing this is to build a ring of angle joiners that goes inside the tire, changing its shape and making it harder.
* You can wrap a bigger tire around a smaller tire on the same rim, making the resulting tire harder and heavier.
* You can stuff a tire with small tires or other LEGO pieces that will make it harder and heavier; if you're not a purist, consider stuffing the tire with other materials, such as plasticine (modeling clay).
* You can submerge the tire in water as you put the rim inside. This will create a wheel with a water-filled tire, which will be harder and heavier than an air-filled tire. Some leaking will occur between the rim and tire, but it can be minimized depending on the type of rim and tire and the load applied to the wheel.

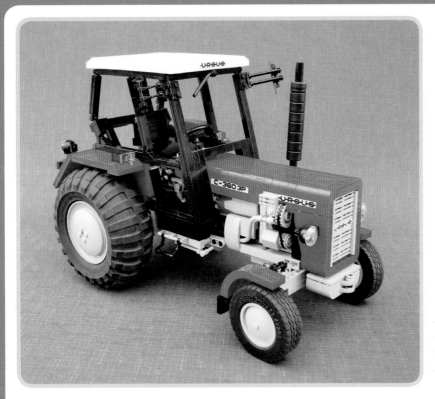

Figure 5-11: This model of the Ursus C360 3P tractor by Eric Trax has realistic-looking rear wheels that were created by squeezing LEGO Power Puller tires between two sets of dishes to make them taller and narrower.

when LEGO tires are not enough

Besides 3D printing a tire, another practical solution is to put third-party tires on LEGO rims. Some popular LEGO/RC combinations are shown in Figure 5-12. The best source of high-quality third-party tires are vendors of parts for RC models, such as Tamiya USA (*http://www.tamiyausa.com/product/category.php?sub-id=71200*) and US-based Pro-Line (*http://www.prolineracing.com/*) and RC4WD (*http://www.store.rc4wd.com/*), which sell a wide selection of tires in 1.55-inch, 1.7-inch, 1.9-inch, and 2.2-inch standards. The standard describes the inner diameter of a tire, and a popular standard with LEGO builders is the 1.9-inch standard, which fits the LEGO Technic Racing Medium rim. It's a well-tried combination, so when you're looking for 1.9-inch tires, you just need to pay attention to their width: The Technic Racing Medium rim is 34 mm wide, so you should look for tires that fall within a few millimeters of that width (RC tires are softer than LEGO tires and thus have a greater size tolerance). As shown in Figure 5-13, fitting 38.9 mm wide ROCK CRUSHER X/T 1.9-inch tires on the 34 mm wide

Technic Racing Medium rim isn't a problem. You'll find a list of many popular LEGO rims and their widths at *http://www.wheels.sariel.pl/*.

Here's how RC tires generally compare to LEGO tires:

* RC tires are grippier and offer superior traction due to a different rubber compound; the rim is also less likely to rotate inside RC tires if they are well-fitted.
* RC tires are softer, which means they grip obstacles better, but they have higher rolling resistance and become more significantly deformed under heavy loads (see Figure 5-14).
* RC tires come with foam inserts that you can remove to make them extra soft (see Figure 5-15).
* Most RC tires look more realistic due to more accurate proportions (taller and narrower) and due to treads modeled after real wheels (see Figures 5-16 and 5-17). However, different proportions can mean they're too narrow for a LEGO rim (see Figure 5-18).
* RC tires come in many shapes and sizes, but they usually cost more (note that most vendors sell RC tires by the pair).
* RC tires come in a greater range of sizes than do LEGO tires (see Figure 5-12).

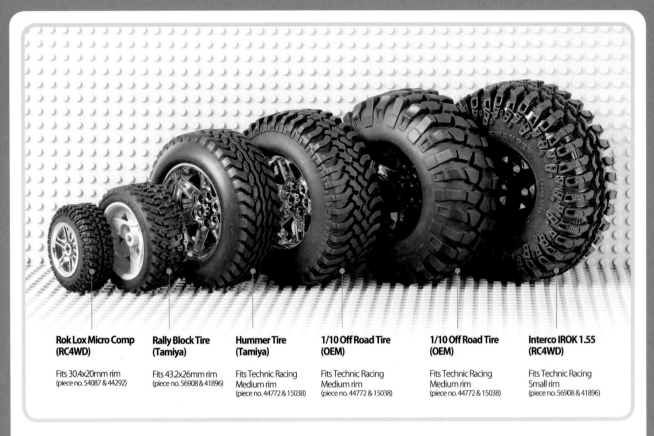

Rok Lox Micro Comp (RC4WD)	Rally Block Tire (Tamiya)	Hummer Tire (Tamiya)	1/10 Off Road Tire (OEM)	1/10 Off Road Tire (OEM)	Interco IROK 1.55 (RC4WD)
Fits 30.4x20mm rim (piece no. 54087 & 44292)	Fits 43.2x26mm rim (piece no. 56908 & 41896)	Fits Technic Racing Medium rim (piece no. 44772 & 15038)	Fits Technic Racing Medium rim (piece no. 44772 & 15038)	Fits Technic Racing Medium rim (piece no. 44772 & 15038)	Fits Technic Racing Small rim (piece no. 56908 & 41896)

Figure 5-12: Some popular RC tire/LEGO rim combinations

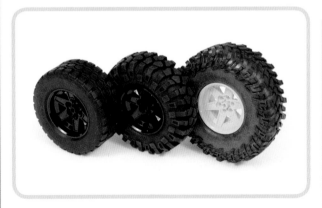

Figure 5-13: RC tires allow you to create bigger wheels at the cost of weight. Left to right are a LEGO Technic Racing Medium rim with a LEGO 94.3×38 R tire (diameter: 94.3 mm, total weight: 67 g), a ROCK CRUSHER X/T 1.9-inch tire by RC4WD (diameter: 108 mm, total weight: 107 g), and a Baja Claw TTC 1.9-inch tire by RC4WD (diameter: 122 mm, total weight: 126 g).

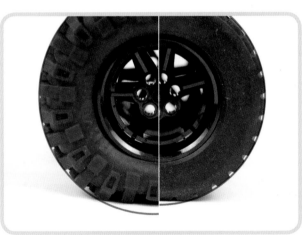

Figure 5-14: RC tires are softer and more prone to deforming than LEGO tires. Compare a ROCK CRUSHER X/T 1.9-inch tire by RC4WD (left) and a LEGO 94.3×38 R tire (right) with 2 kg of load applied.

* RC tires are usually noticeably heavier than LEGO tires of a similar size (see Figure 5-13), which can be a benefit because the weight lowers the vehicle's center of gravity.
* Their softer, stickier material makes RC tires wear down a little faster and get dirtier and harder to clean.
* RC tires rarely fit LEGO rims perfectly, meaning that two identical tire/rim combinations can look a bit different.
* RC tires are quite smelly when they're brand new.
* RC tires may be frowned upon by LEGO purists.

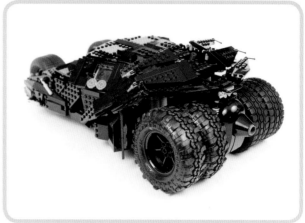

Figure 5-17: RC tires often look more realistic than LEGO tires, as evidenced by the 76023 Tumbler set, with a pair of LEGO 94.3×38 R tires on the right and a pair of Interco TSL SX Super Swamper XL 1.9-inch tires on the left. The Interco tires are actually miniature versions of the real Super Swamper tires used in the original Tumbler vehicle.

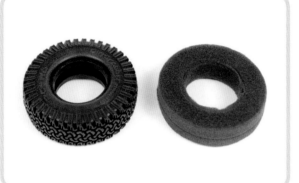

Figure 5-15: By default, RC tires come with foam inserts that you can remove to make them softer. Here's a Dirt Grabber 1.9-inch tire by RC4WD next to its foam insert. Note that the insert weighs just 3 g, so it's not worth it to remove it just to save some weight.

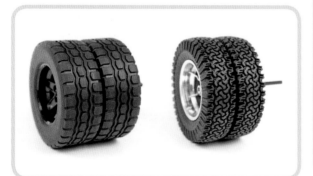

Figure 5-16: RC tires usually look more realistic than LEGO tires due to different proportions and treads. Compare the double LEGO 94.3×38 R tires (left) to the double Dirt Grabber 1.9-inch tires (right).

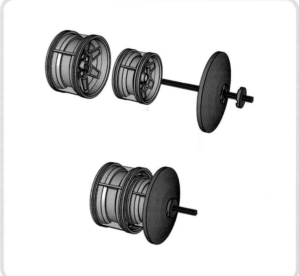

Figure 5-18: Because of its realistic proportions, a single Dirt Grabber 1.9-inch tire is too narrow—and two such tires are too wide—for a single LEGO Technic Racing Medium rim. Here's an exploded and assembled view of the combination of rims I've used for two Dirt Grabber 1.9-inch tires: The dark grey dish acts as an inner edge of the rim.

mechanics

6

gears and power transmission basics

Why do we need gears? An intuitive answer is that we need them to transfer drive from a motor to a receiving mechanism. While true, this is not the complete picture. The essential purpose of gears is to transform the *properties* of a power input to suit our purposes. Transferring drive is just a side effect of this process.

Gears can be driven by all kinds of inputs, from electric motors and manual cranks to wind turbines and mill wheels. Let's start by considering gears powered by electric motors, because unlike other power inputs, motors have constant, measurable properties.

Every motor has a certain mechanical power, consisting of two factors: rotational speed and torque. These are the two properties we can transform using gears. Both speed and torque are explained in detail in Chapter 1.

When do we need speed? When do we need torque? Each mechanism and model you build has unique needs. Some will need more speed and less torque than the motor provides, but for others, the reverse will be true. Using gears, we can transform torque into speed or speed into torque. There are two very important but very simple rules for this relationship:

* Driving a large gear with a small gear increases the torque but decreases the speed. This is called *gearing down* (see Figure 6-1).
* Driving a small gear with a large gear increases the speed but decreases the torque. This is called *gearing up* (see Figure 6-2).

Speed and torque are *inversely proportional*: If we decrease the speed by a factor of two, the torque is increased by a factor of two. We can't transform one property without affecting the other, unless we modify the power input by exerting more force on a manual crank or by providing an electric motor with a higher voltage.

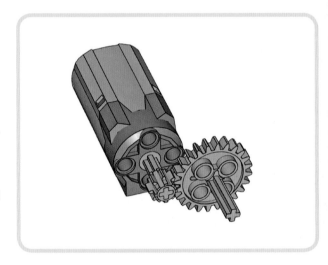

Figure 6-1: Gearing down

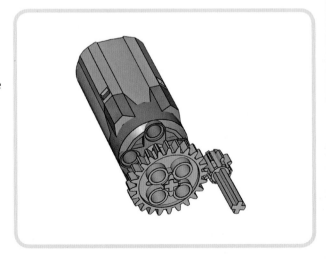

Figure 6-2: Gearing up

When propelling a vehicle that is light and needs little torque to move, we can transform the abundant torque into extra speed by gearing up. The amount of torque we can transform depends mainly on the vehicle's weight. Experienced builders can estimate the range of possible transformation knowing just the vehicle's weight and the type of motor used to drive it.

drivers, followers, and idlers

Let's consider a simple example of a geared power transmission, shown in Figure 6-3, in which the grey motor is connected to a wheel via two gears. The green gear that is closest to the power input (the motor) is called a *driver gear*. The red gear that receives the drive from the driver gear is called a *follower gear*. (Illustrations in this chapter will use the same color scheme: green for driver gears and red for follower gears.)

Whenever there is a pair of meshed gears on separate axles, one of the gears is a driver, and the other is a follower. The driver is the gear the drive is transferred *from*, and the follower is the gear the drive is transferred *to*.

As the gears rotate, so do the axles on which they are mounted. Therefore, a driver axle, called the *input*, and a follower axle, called the *output*, follow the rotation of the gears. Most mechanisms have a single input axle, but the output axles can be numerous. The common differential mechanism is a good example of one input with many outputs (see Figure 6-4).

In addition to driver and follower gears, we have *idler gears*. If there is a set of gears in a series, the first one is the driver gear and the last one is the follower gear. All the gears in between are called idler gears (see Figure 6-5), because they could just as well not exist. In other words, they don't affect how the torque and speed are transformed.

Idler gears are typically meshed with two or more gears at the same time, while the driver and follower gears are meshed only with one, as shown in Figure 6-6. Exceptions to this rule are shown in Figure 6-7.

Note that idler gears should be used only when absolutely necessary, as they add friction and need to be properly supported. An excess of idler gears is shown in Figure 6-8.

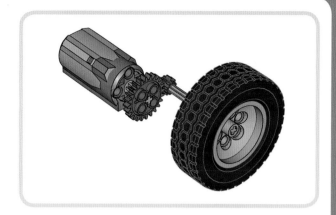

Figure 6-3: Driver (green) and follower (red) gears

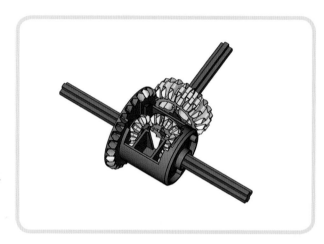

Figure 6-4: The differential has one green input axle but two red output axles.

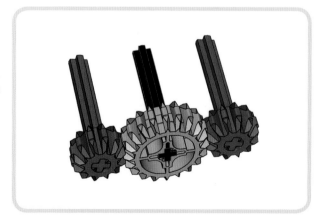

Figure 6-5: Three gears meshed one by one, with the idler gear in grey. The idler's axle serves only as its mounting point.

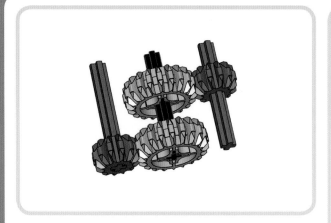

Figure 6-6: The middle gears in this picture are idler gears. Both are meshed with only one gear, but they are mounted on the same axle and are of exactly the same size, which means that they work just as a single gear would.

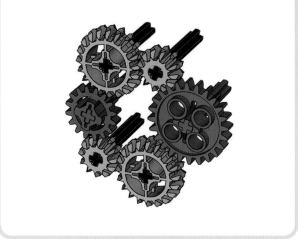

Figure 6-8: All the middle (grey) gears in this picture are idler gears. They do not affect how torque and speed are transformed between the driver gear and the follower gear.

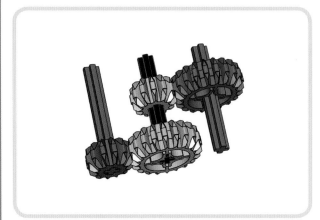

Figure 6-7: The middle gears in this picture are not idler gears. Both are mounted on the same axle, but they are of different sizes, which means that they affect how torque and speed are transformed. This is because the varying size of the gear affects the torque it transfers.

gear ratios

A *gear ratio* is the relationship between the number of teeth in two interacting gears. *Interacting gears* might refer to two gears that are meshed or otherwise connected, two gears connected by a roller chain, or even two pulleys connected by a drive belt. The gear ratio of two sprockets connected with a chain is exactly the same as the gear ratio of those sprockets directly meshed.

A gear ratio is defined as follows: *the number of follower gear's teeth* to *the number of driver gear's teeth*.

For instance, if we drive a 24-tooth gear with an 8-tooth gear, the gear ratio, also known as the *torque ratio*, is 24:8. However, we should reduce both numbers in a gear ratio until one of them is 1. To do this, we need to find a divisor, usually equal to the smaller number. As you can see here, if we divide both numbers in a 24:8 gear setup by 8, we get a 3:1 ratio, which is much more convenient and immediately shows us that three revolutions of a driver gear result in a single revolution of a follower gear.

So what good is this ratio? We can use it to easily calculate how speed and torque are transformed between the two gears. Looking at the 3:1 ratio, we can tell that the speed is reduced by a factor of three, and because torque is inversely proportional to speed, we can calculate that the torque is tripled.

Now consider an example where the driver has more teeth than the follower: We have a 20-tooth driver gear and a 12-tooth follower gear. The gear ratio is 12:20, which is equal to 0.6:1. This means that we need 0.6 revolutions of the driver gear to get a single revolution of the follower gear, so the speed is increased, but at the same time the torque of the follower is 0.6 of the driver's torque, so the torque is decreased.

Our gear ratio also reveals whether we're gearing down or gearing up. If the first number of the gear ratio is greater than the second (as in 3:1), we are gearing down—this is also called *gear reduction*. If the first number of the gear ratio is smaller than the second (as in 0.6:1), we are gearing up—this is also called *gear acceleration* or *overdrive*. If we have a 1:1 gear ratio, speed and torque remain the same.

What if we want to calculate the total gear ratio of a mechanism with many pairs of meshed gears? In this case, we ignore all the idler gears and calculate ratios for all pairs of driver and follower gears. Then, in order to get the final gear ratio of the entire mechanism, we simply multiply these gear ratios. Consider a mechanism with two pairs of 8-tooth drivers and 24-tooth followers. The gear ratio of the first pair is 3:1, and so is the ratio of the second pair. If we multiply these ratios, we get the final ratio of 9:1.

Now that we can calculate gear ratios, let's go back to the previous examples showing idler and non-idler gears.

Consider the first set of gears, shown in Figure 6-6. It consists of two pairs of gears: a 12-tooth driver with a 20-tooth follower and a 20-tooth driver with a 12-tooth follower. The ratio of the first pair is 20:12, and the ratio of second pair is 12:20. If we multiply these, we get the final ratio of 1:1. The idler gears did not change the ratio at all.

Now consider the second set of gears, shown in Figure 6-7. It consists of two identical pairs of gears, which have a 12-tooth driver with a 20-tooth follower. The ratio of each pair is 20:12, and if we multiply these, we get the final ratio of 2.779:1, which is not equal to 1.667:1 (the ratio of the first and the last gear only). Here, the middle gears are not idlers—they affect the final gear ratio of the whole set—and they can't be ignored.

Finally, how do we calculate the ratio if a worm gear is used? Well, that's even simpler: *the number of follower gear's teeth* to 1. That's because a single revolution of a worm gear rotates the follower gear by a single tooth. For example, it takes 24 revolutions of the worm gear to rotate a 24-tooth gear fully, and hence, we get the ratio 24:1.

gear ratio quick reference

Use Table 6-1 to find the resulting ratio when combining two gear wheels. First select the driver gear from the upper row, then select the follower gear from the left column, and then find the field where they cross. The value in that field is the gear ratio in *driver:follower* format.

Green ratios indicate gearing up (which results in more speed, less torque). For example, a gear ratio of 1:2 means that one rotation of the driver gear causes two rotations of the follower gear. You'll get double the speed but half the torque. Red ratios indicate gearing down (which results in less speed, but more torque). A gear ratio of 2:1 means that

two rotations of the driver gear cause one rotation of the follower gear. This is a *gear reduction*—you'll get half the speed but double the torque.

Visit *http://gears.sariel.pl* for an online, interactive gearing ratio calculator and other tools.

NOTE Only the most popular gears are included in the table, and only one gear is shown per tooth count. For example, there are three kinds of 16-tooth gear wheels but as they all produce the same ratio, only the standard type is shown in the table.

efficiency and gears

Every gear has weight and generates friction that has to be overcome if we want the gear to rotate. Every gear in our mechanism dissipates part of the drive motor's power, and the *efficiency* of the gear tells us how much power is transferred and how much is lost. Unfortunately, it's extremely difficult to calculate the individual efficiency of each gear, especially since gears wear over time. We do know, however, how power is lost in mechanical systems, so we can safely assume two basic rules for maximum efficiency:

* The fewer the gears we use, the better.
* The smaller the gears we use, the better.

In practice, low efficiency results in a loss of torque and speed. This loss happens because low efficiency generates resistance—resulting from friction, among other things—that a motor has to overcome. You can see this with motorized vehicles; in most cases their wheels rotate faster when you lift them off the ground. All of this means that the real, functioning mechanism is never as effective as the gear ratio alone indicates, and how much its efficiency is diminished is determined by the efficiency of the gears.

You can see the importance of efficiency in any mechanism that includes a worm gear. A worm gear's extremely high gear reduction comes at the cost of efficiency. Some sources estimate that a worm gear loses almost one-third of the motor's power due to high friction and the gear's tendency to slide along its axle. The friction is high enough to make worm gears hot if they handle high torque for a prolonged period of time, and the friction is also the reason why LEGO worm gears can't be follower gears. Worm gears are irreplaceable for some applications, but in general, they should be used in moderation.

table 6-1: gear ratio quick reference

driver gear / follower gear

	1:1	1:1.5	1:2	1:2.5	1:3	1:3.5	1:4.5	1:5	1:7	8:1
	1.5:1	**1:1**	1:1.33	1:1.67	1:2	1:2.33	1:3	1:3.33	1:4.76	12:1
	2:1	1.33:1	**1:1**	1:1.25	1:1.5	1:1.75	1:2.25	1:2.5	1:3.5	16:1
	2.5:1	1.67:1	1.25:1	**1:1**	1:1.2	1:1.4	1:1.8	1:2	1:2.8	20:1
	3:1	2:1	1.5:1	1.2:1	**1:1**	1:1.17	1:1.5	1:1.67	1:2.33	24:1
	3.5:1	2.33:1	1.75:1	1.4:1	1.17:1	**1:1**	1:1.29	1:1.43	1:2	28:1
	4.5:1	3:1	2.25:1	1.8:1	1.5:1	1.29:1	**1:1**	1:1.11	1:1.56	36:1
	5:1	3.33:1	2.5:1	2:1	1.67:1	1.43:1	1.11:1	**1:1**	1:1.4	40:1
	7:1	4.67:1	3.5:1	2.8:1	2.33:1	2:1	1.56:1	1.4:1	**1:1**	56:1

backlash and gears

For LEGO gears, we can simply assume that *backlash* is the free space between the meshed teeth of two adjacent gears. In an ideal situation, there would be no free space at all, but in practice, LEGO gears always generate some backlash.

The general rules are as follows:

* Old-type gears generate much greater backlash than the new bevel gears.
* The smaller the gear, the greater the backlash.
* The backlashes of any directly meshed gears sum up.

Why is backlash so bad? Consider, for example, any steering mechanism: Any significant backlash between it and the motor that controls it will not only degrade the accuracy of steering but also make the wheels have some margin of

freedom so that they may turn a bit when they meet an obstacle. This may cause your vehicle to waver out of a true straight line as it navigates bumps or create a noticeable delay as you steer a vehicle.

Backlash can become troublesome whenever accuracy is needed. Many sorts of cranes, drawbridges, and turntables suffer from backlash. The best way to avoid backlash is to use pneumatics instead of mechanics (see Chapter 10) or to use linear actuators, which currently have the least backlash of all the mechanical parts produced by LEGO (see Chapter 14).

How does backlash work with a worm gear? Again, this gear proves unique in generating nearly no backlash—except for the fact that it can slide along the axle a bit, being slightly narrower than 2 full studs. Now, that doesn't mean that mechanisms with the worm gear have *zero* backlash—unfortunately, there is still backlash from the follower gear. Therefore, a mechanism with a worm gear and a 16-tooth follower gear will always have greater backlash than one with a worm gear and a 24-tooth follower gear. And again, it is recommended that you use a worm gear with bevel gears due to their relatively insignificant backlash.

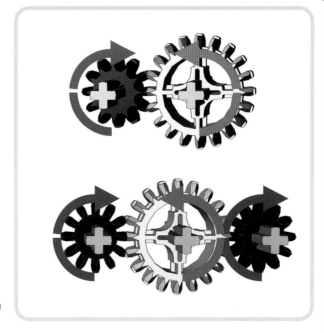

Figure 6-9: An even number of meshed gears (top) and an odd number of meshed gears (bottom)

controlling rotational direction

When gears are meshed directly, the driver gear affects the follower gear's direction of rotation. Whether the follower rotates in the same or in the opposite direction as the driver depends on the number of gears between them. When gears are in a parallel series, the rule is simple: With an even number of gears (2, 4, 6, and so on), the follower rotates in the opposite direction, and with an odd number of gears (3, 5, 7, and so on), the follower rotates in the same direction (see Figure 6-9). You may find yourself adding or removing idler gears to adjust the follower's direction.

Direct observation may be the quickest means of determining the output rotation of gears that mesh perpendicularly. For example, in a 4×4 vehicle's drivetrain with a longitudinal driveshaft, the front and real differentials must be oriented in opposite directions for the front and rear wheels to rotate in the same direction, as shown in Figure 6-10.

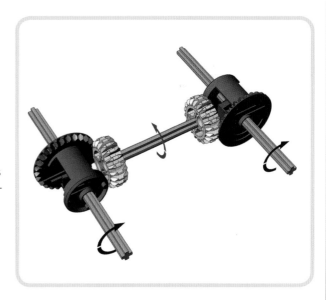

Figure 6-10: The proper orientation of differentials and bevel gears in a 4×4 drivetrain

an inventory of gears

The LEGO Group has released various types of gears throughout the history of the Technic line. The gears can be divided into a few different types, and I'll discuss them type by type, starting with the most common and familiar gears.

Figure 6-11 shows all types of gears. Some have additional variants not included in this figure. For example, the 8-tooth gear has three variants, but they all retain the same essential properties. Others, such as the three types of the 16-tooth gears shown in the figure, look similar but have somewhat different properties. The most essential difference between gears is the shape of their teeth. *Straight cut*, or *spur gears*, have distinctive rectangular teeth that can be meshed only in parallel with each other (see Figure 6-12). Spur gears are the only gears that can have LEGO chains or track links put on them.

There are also *bevel gears*; their teeth are rounded and chamfered. As Figure 6-13 shows, these gears come in two subtypes: single-bevel gears, with teeth chamfered on one side, and double-bevel gears, with teeth chamfered on both sides. Single-bevel gears can be meshed at right angles only, and only from their chamfered side, while double-bevel gears can be meshed at right angles from either side or in parallel. To keep it simple, just think of single-bevel gears as double-bevel gears that have been cut in half. And yes, you can mesh single- and double-bevel gears together.

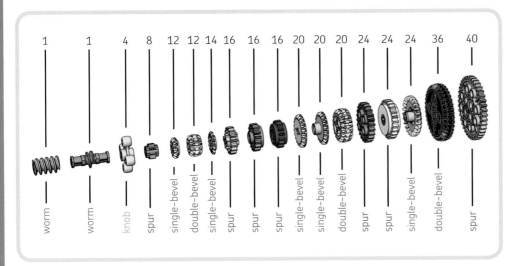

1	1	4	8	12	12	14	16	16	16	20	20	20	24	24	24	36	40
worm	worm	knob	spur	single-bevel	double-bevel	single-bevel	spur	spur	spur	single-bevel	single-bevel	double-bevel	spur	spur	single-bevel	double-bevel	spur

Figure 6-11: Types of LEGO gears and their respective numbers of teeth

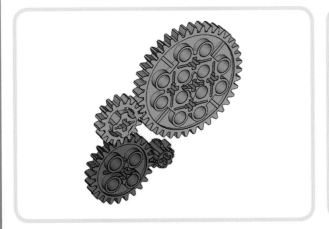

Figure 6-12: Spur gears are distinguished by their rectangular teeth that can be meshed only in parallel.

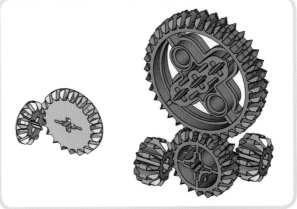

Figure 6-13: LEGO bevel gears and all the ways they can be meshed; single-bevel gears are marked tan, and double-bevel gears are marked light grey. Note that the first look and effectively act like halves of the latter.

Finally, there are worm gears and knob gears, which are purpose-built and mesh only with selected gears, as I'll discuss in detail in the following sections.

worm gear

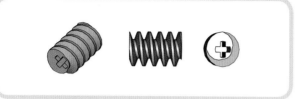

A worm gear is a purpose-built gear that has a number of unique properties. You can only use it as the driver gear, never as the follower. In other words, it can drive a gear but it can't be driven by a gear. This property comes in handy for mechanisms that need to lift something and keep it raised; in such cases, a worm gear acts like a lock that prevents the load from falling, because no matter how hard the load pulls on the mechanism's gears, these gears can't drive the worm gear. Such mechanisms include all sorts of winches, cranes, forklifts, railroad barriers, drawbridges, and so on.

The worm gear is also extremely useful for gearing down. Every revolution of the worm gear rotates the follower gear by just a single tooth, reducing the speed and increasing the torque drastically. Therefore, worm gears are used for gearing down whenever very high torque or low speed must be achieved within a small space. Additionally, as the worm gear rotates, it tends to push against the follower gear and slide along its own axle. Usually, this sliding movement must be stopped by placing a strong casing around it, but certain mechanisms use this sliding tendency (see Chapters 10 and 12 for examples). Despite its unusual appearance, the worm gear can drive any spur gear, and with proper spacing, it can drive bevel gears as well (see Figure 6-14).

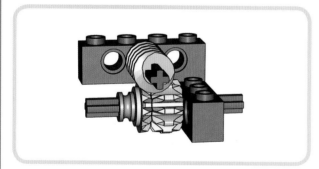

Figure 6-14: A worm gear driving single- and double-bevel follower gears

It's even possible to use a worm gear to drive racks, which results in a very compact boom-extending mechanism (see Figure 6-15). This can be useful in a crane or a telescoping forklift or in any other application where space is at a premium.

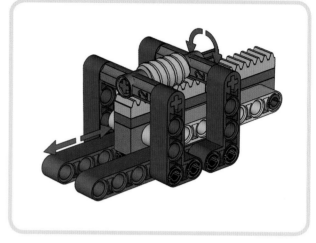

Figure 6-15: A worm gear driving a rack

3L worm gear

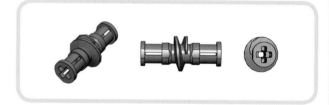

The 3L worm gear was introduced in early editions of three sets in 2014 (42023, 42026, and 42027). It's quite rare because it was later recalled by the LEGO Group, which claimed the gear suffered from structural problems. It's still available secondhand and offers unique properties. It consists of two 1-stud-long bushes with axle holes and a 1-stud-long worm section in the middle. Unlike a regular worm gear, you can't put a single axle through it because the worm section has no axle hole inside. It works with the same gears as the regular worm gear, but it can fit in tighter spaces due to a shorter worm section, and it doesn't slide on its axle.

8-tooth gear

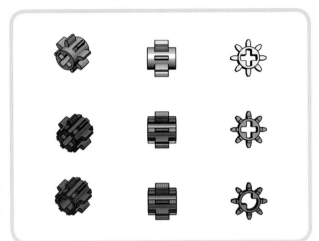

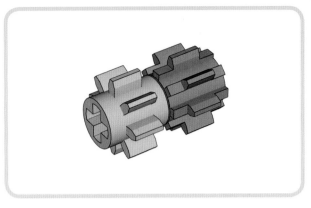

Figure 6-16: The reinforced 8-tooth gear (right) is much thicker than and looks different from the original variant (left). It still fits everywhere the original gear fits, making it a perfect replacement.

The 8-tooth gear is the smallest LEGO gear in existence, and it's a fragile one. It's not suited for high torque, but due to its size, it's very popular, especially for gearing down. Its primary disadvantage is that it generates severe backlash.

These are the three variants of the 8-tooth gear, from top to bottom:

original 8-tooth gear Its fragile teeth can be bent by excessive torque, and its thin center can get stuck in a pin hole.

reinforced 8-tooth gear Introduced in 2013/2014, it has a significantly reinforced central ring, making it more torque resistant and safe from pin holes.

sliding 8-tooth gear A very rare variant of the reinforced 8-tooth gear, it can slide freely along the axle. It was primarily designed to drive outriggers in the 42009 Mobile Crane Mk II set. The gear is held in place while the axle slides through it, allowing the outriggers to be lowered when they're extended, retracted, or somewhere in between.

The reinforced 8-tooth gear is in every way better than the original variant (see Figure 6-16), which it has effectively replaced. Still, it's interesting to note that there are at least three variants of the original 8-tooth gear that were produced from three slightly different molds (shown in Figure 6-17). Apparently, LEGO experimented with making this gear stronger before eventually replacing it with the reinforced variant.

Note that all 8-tooth gears are unfit for use with LEGO chains: The chain skips over the original gear and doesn't mesh at all with the reinforced one.

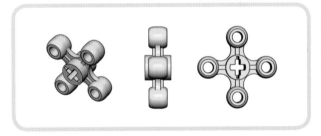

Figure 6-17: Three mold variants of the original 8-tooth gear

knob wheel

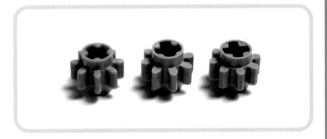

The knob wheel is an important and popular piece, even though it's technically not a gear. Knob wheels can mesh only with other knob wheels and can do so in both a perpendicular and a parallel manner. Their advantages are that they are much stronger than gears and they can handle significantly higher torque. They are most commonly used in a perpendicular setup, because the regular gears that can transfer the drive in such a setup are more likely to snap under torque than the knob wheels are. The disadvantage of knob wheels is that the unique shape of their teeth makes them

work unevenly. This is particularly apparent when a large torque is applied to a perpendicular setup of knob wheels; their speed of rotation starts to fluctuate. Also, because all the torque is applied to just a few contact points, knob wheels are prone to wear. Their contact points rub away over time, and worn knob wheels start producing a squeaking sound when working.

single-bevel 12-tooth gear

The single-bevel 12-tooth gear is the smallest of all the bevel gears. It's irreplaceable in differential mechanisms and very popular when you need to transfer the drive at right angles inside a tight space. However, it's easily broken under high torque, which has led many builders to exclude differentials completely from their off-road vehicles.

double-bevel 12-tooth gear

The double-bevel 12-tooth gear is much stronger than its single-bevel counterpart, and it's most often used with a double-bevel 20-tooth gear. It doesn't fit inside differentials or in tight spaces, which makes it less popular for perpendicular meshing.

14-tooth gear

The first gear used inside differentials, the 14-tooth gear proved so fragile that it was later replaced by the 12-tooth version. It is no longer used in the official LEGO models and is unpopular with builders.

16-tooth gear

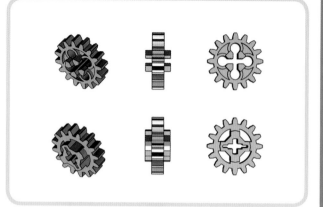

The 16-tooth gear is a reasonably strong and useful gear. It's the smallest gear that can be operated with a LEGO chain. Just like the 8-tooth gear, it comes in the original variant (top row), which was replaced in 2011 with a reinforced variant (bottom row). The new variant is much less fragile, but other than that, it's identical to the original one.

16-tooth gear with clutch

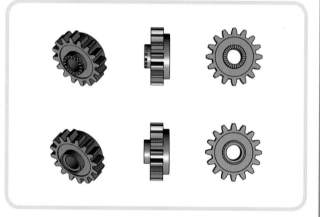

The 16-tooth gear with clutch was designed specifically for transmissions. It doesn't work well with a LEGO chain because its short teeth make the chain slip. Instead, it has the unique ability to be engaged or disengaged by the transmission driving ring (see Figure 6-18). We'll explore this property in more depth in Chapter 19. When disengaged, it remains loose on the axle. The original variant of this gear (top row) included tiny teeth around the central hole (see Figure 6-19) that could be meshed with an old-type half bush (the one with teeth) and thus lock the gear to the axle (see Figure 6-20). In 2011, it was replaced by a "smooth" variant without teeth (bottom row).

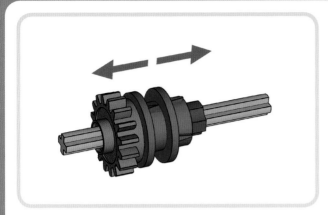

Figure 6-18: A 16-tooth gear with clutch can be engaged or disengaged by a transmission driving ring.

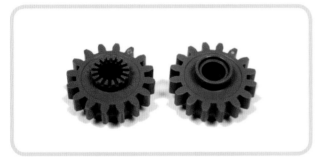

Figure 6-19: The original 16-tooth gear with clutch variant (left) has prominent teeth around the hole; the new one (right) is smooth.

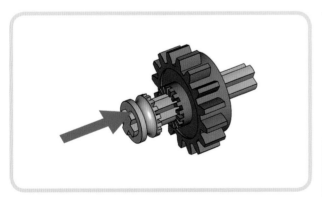

Figure 6-20: The original variant of the 16-tooth gear with clutch can be locked to the axle by meshing it with the old-type half bush with teeth. The smooth variant doesn't have this option.

double-sided 16-tooth gear with clutch

Introduced in 2015, the double-sided 16-tooth gear with clutch has a clutch on both sides and is apparently meant to replace the regular 16-tooth gear with clutch. It seems to have been created to help avoid building errors, because it has no "right" or "wrong" side: It will work no matter how you place it when you're building a transmission. It can only be engaged by the 3L transmission driving gear, not by the older 2L gear.

single-bevel 20-tooth gear

The single-bevel 20-tooth gear is a larger version of the single-bevel 12-tooth gear. It's relatively rare and not very popular because of its thin body, which makes it prone to snapping under high torque.

single-bevel 20-tooth gear with pin hole

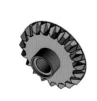

The single-bevel 20-tooth gear with pin hole is a modification of the single-bevel 20-tooth gear. Rather than replacing the original gear, it adds new possibilities. One feature is the

ability to rotate freely on an axle so you can use the gear to transfer drive "over" the axle without actually driving it and without adding the axle's friction to its own. The other is a half-stud-thick collar at its base, making it less prone to bending and snapping under torque. This gear is often used to drive linear actuators (see Chapter 14).

double-bevel 20-tooth gear

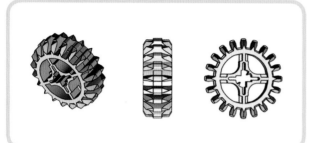

The double-bevel 20-tooth gear is very popular, strong, and reliable. It's most commonly used with a single-bevel 12-tooth gear, but it's useful in other setups, too.

24-tooth gear

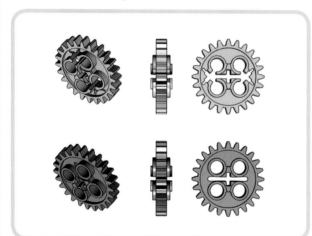

The popular, strong, and reliable 24-tooth gear comes in its original design (top row) and a reinforced variant (bottom row). It goes back to the '70s Technic sets and remains one of the most popular gears today.

24-tooth gear with clutch

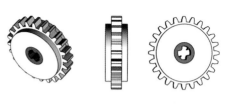

The 24-tooth gear with clutch is white with dark grey in the center; it has the unique ability to harmlessly slip around the axle if it can't make the axle rotate. It's most often used for end-to-end applications in which the motor only runs until it reaches a set point. This includes almost all steering mechanisms in which the wheels can be turned only within a limited angle, railroad barrier mechanisms by which the barrier can be raised or lowered only to a certain degree, and winches. In these types of mechanisms, the gear allows the motor to run even if the mechanism is stopped, preventing damage to the motor.

The moment when this gear starts to slip depends on how hard the axle resists the gear when it rotates. In most cases, you will want the gear to slip only when the axle is actually blocked and not when it's just stressed. You can achieve this by gearing down between this gear and the last axle it drives—in Figure 6-21, this is the red axle. Because there is 3:1 gearing between that axle and the gear, the red axle will have to resist three times more to make the gear slip than it would if it were connected to the gear directly.

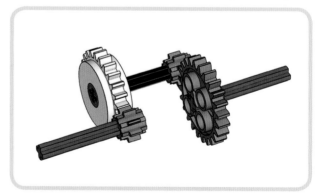

Figure 6-21: The 3:1 gearing between the 24-tooth gear with clutch and the mechanism it drives (the red axle) makes the gear more efficient. The red axle will need to resist it three times more to make the gear slip.

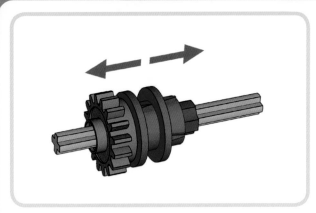

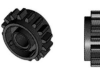

Figure 6-18: A 16-tooth gear with clutch can be engaged or disengaged by a transmission driving ring.

double-sided 16-tooth gear with clutch

Introduced in 2015, the double-sided 16-tooth gear with clutch has a clutch on both sides and is apparently meant to replace the regular 16-tooth gear with clutch. It seems to have been created to help avoid building errors, because it has no "right" or "wrong" side: It will work no matter how you place it when you're building a transmission. It can only be engaged by the 3L transmission driving gear, not by the older 2L gear.

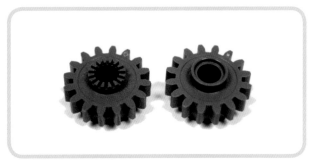

Figure 6-19: The original 16-tooth gear with clutch variant (left) has prominent teeth around the hole; the new one (right) is smooth.

single-bevel 20-tooth gear

The single-bevel 20-tooth gear is a larger version of the single-bevel 12-tooth gear. It's relatively rare and not very popular because of its thin body, which makes it prone to snapping under high torque.

single-bevel 20-tooth gear with pin hole

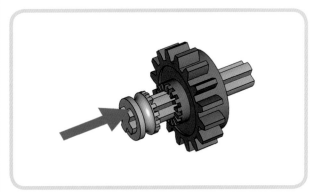

Figure 6-20: The original variant of the 16-tooth gear with clutch can be locked to the axle by meshing it with the old-type half bush with teeth. The smooth variant doesn't have this option.

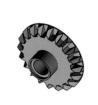

The single-bevel 20-tooth gear with pin hole is a modification of the single-bevel 20-tooth gear. Rather than replacing the original gear, it adds new possibilities. One feature is the

ability to rotate freely on an axle so you can use the gear to transfer drive "over" the axle without actually driving it and without adding the axle's friction to its own. The other is a half-stud-thick collar at its base, making it less prone to bending and snapping under torque. This gear is often used to drive linear actuators (see Chapter 14).

double-bevel 20-tooth gear

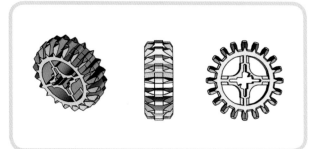

The double-bevel 20-tooth gear is very popular, strong, and reliable. It's most commonly used with a single-bevel 12-tooth gear, but it's useful in other setups, too.

24-tooth gear

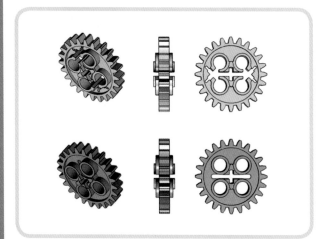

The popular, strong, and reliable 24-tooth gear comes in its original design (top row) and a reinforced variant (bottom row). It goes back to the '70s Technic sets and remains one of the most popular gears today.

24-tooth gear with clutch

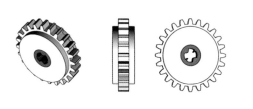

The 24-tooth gear with clutch is white with dark grey in the center; it has the unique ability to harmlessly slip around the axle if it can't make the axle rotate. It's most often used for end-to-end applications in which the motor only runs until it reaches a set point. This includes almost all steering mechanisms in which the wheels can be turned only within a limited angle, railroad barrier mechanisms by which the barrier can be raised or lowered only to a certain degree, and winches. In these types of mechanisms, the gear allows the motor to run even if the mechanism is stopped, preventing damage to the motor.

The moment when this gear starts to slip depends on how hard the axle resists the gear when it rotates. In most cases, you will want the gear to slip only when the axle is actually blocked and not when it's just stressed. You can achieve this by gearing down between this gear and the last axle it drives—in Figure 6-21, this is the red axle. Because there is 3:1 gearing between that axle and the gear, the red axle will have to resist three times more to make the gear slip than it would if it were connected to the gear directly.

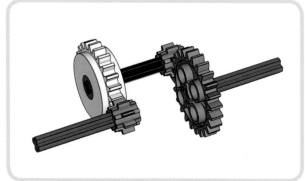

Figure 6-21: The 3:1 gearing between the 24-tooth gear with clutch and the mechanism it drives (the red axle) makes the gear more efficient. The red axle will need to resist it three times more to make the gear slip.

Not all of these gear wheels look identical or start slipping at the same moment. Most noticeably, this gear originally had *2.5*5.0 Ncm* written on one side, but newer versions are unmarked.

24-tooth gear with crown

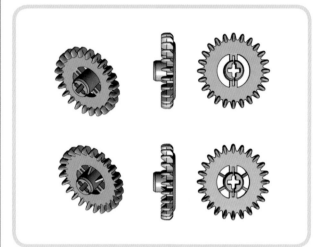

The 24-tooth gear with crown was an early attempt at bevel gears and is similar to the regular spur 24-tooth gear wheel. It too has an original (top row) and reinforced variant (bottom row). It can be meshed with spur gears in parallel or at an angle, as shown in Figure 6-22, but it's weak and inconvenient to use due to its shape and the protruding central hub. Modern bevel gears are more versatile.

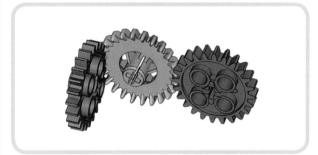

Figure 6-22: The 24-tooth gear with a crown (light grey) is a special gear whose teeth have a unique shape. It's designed to mesh in parallel and at an angle with regular spur gears.

36-tooth gear

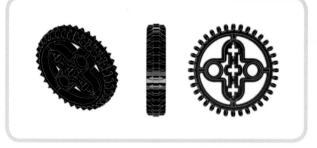

The 36-tooth gear is the largest bevel gear and the only one with no single-bevel counterpart. A convenient and surprisingly strong gear, though a rare one, it usually comes in black.

40-tooth gear

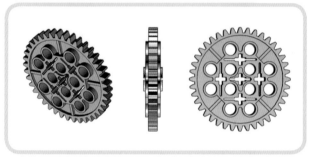

The 40-tooth gear is the largest regular gear. Although rare and seldom used because of its immense size, it's popular in tracked models as a sprocket wheel for the old type of tracks.

Hailfire Droid wheel gear

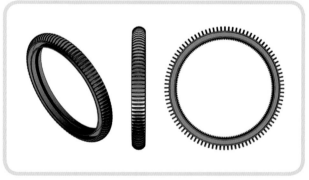

The extremely rare (4481 set only) and big (212 mm or 26.5 studs) Hailfire Droid wheel can be considered a gear, too, due to the 168 teeth on its inner ring. The whole wheel is 3 studs

thick, its inner teeth are 1 stud wide, and it has 1-stud-deep troughs on both sides. It's missing a central axle hole, so driving it requires a structure built inside or around it.

Hailfire Droid wheel gears are great for use as turntables in very large models. With two gears like this, it's possible to put them on top of each other, filling the troughs on their facing sides with up to 41 LEGO balls (see Figure 6-23). The resulting mechanism acts like a ball bearing, which makes it capable of rotating under significant loads; additionally, the sheer size of the gear makes it very stable.

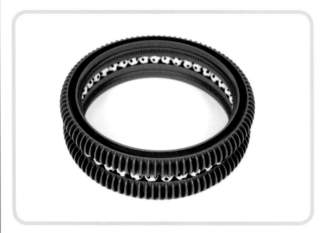

Figure 6-23: A turntable made by combining two Hailfire Droid wheel gears. It takes 41 standard LEGO balls to fill the Hailfire turntable entirely.

differential gears

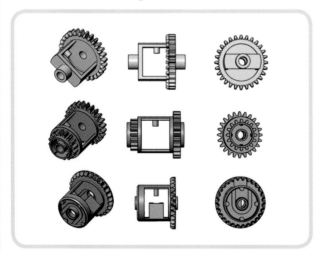

LEGO has produced three different differential gears. Let's review them starting from the top row.

old-type 28-tooth differential gear

The oldest differential gear, the old-type 28-tooth differential gear, is designed for use with 14-tooth gears inside but is also compliant with the single-bevel 12-tooth gears. It takes a lot of space and comes with 28 teeth that can be meshed in both a parallel and a perpendicular manner. It always comes in light grey.

16/24-tooth differential gear

The successor of the older differential gear, the 16/24-tooth differential gear is more universal and can be used in situations where other differential gears cannot be used. Its housing ends with a 16-tooth gear wheel on one side and a 24-tooth gear wheel on the other, both of which can be meshed in parallel only. The 24-tooth side can be driven with a LEGO chain. Additionally, both sides can be engaged by a transmission driving ring, locking the differential (see Figure 6-24). It comes almost exclusively in dark grey.

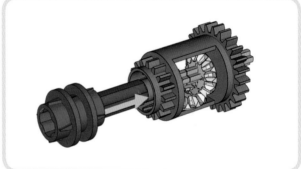

Figure 6-24: A 16/24-tooth differential gear locked by a transmission driving ring. Once locked on either side, it works like a solid axle, not like a differential. A lockable differential is useful in off-road vehicles.

new-type 28-tooth differential gear

The new-type 28-tooth differential gear is a variant introduced in response to the growing popularity of studless constructions in which a differential of even width is difficult to use. Its teeth can be meshed in a perpendicular manner only, and it's just 3 studs wide. Much less massive than the other differentials, it is surprisingly strong, especially when enclosed inside a 5×7 studless frame that was designed specifically for it (see Figure 6-25). Its inside is designed to work with the single-bevel 12-tooth gears only, and it includes a special structure that keeps them in place securely.

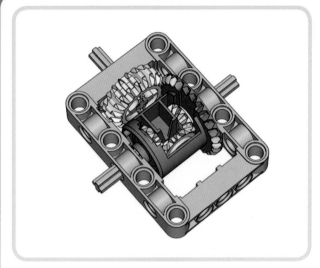

Figure 6-25: A new-type 28-tooth differential gear in a common and robust setup, enclosed inside a 5×7 studless frame and driven by a double-bevel 20-tooth gear

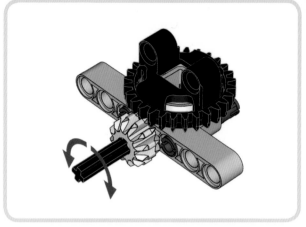

Figure 6-26: A small turntable can be meshed with a single- or double-bevel 12-tooth gear from the bottom, providing an easy way to make it rotate.

turntables

There are four variants of Technic turntables, one small and three big. Each is made of two halves (we'll call these *top* and *bottom*), which, once connected, are designed to stay together permanently with the top rotating around the bottom.

Note that the top and bottom of each turntable type always come in different colors, the most common of which are shown in the figures that follow.

small Technic turntable

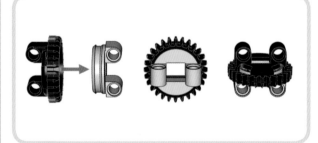

The small turntable is 3 studs tall, and its diameter is 28 mm or 3.5 studs. Its top has 28 teeth on its outer ring, all chamfered on the side that connects to its bottom (see Figure 6-26). The hole in its middle is a 1×1 stud square, which means you can put many things through it, including an axle, even with a bush or an axle joiner on it; a universal

joint; the rod of a pneumatic cylinder or of a linear actuator; up to four pneumatic hoses; or even a beam, although the beam's square profile will stop the turntable from rotating. However, you can't put wires through a small turntable because the wires' plugs are too big, nor can you put LEGO LEDs through a small turntable. It's very difficult to mesh this turntable with a worm gear.

big Technic turntable with 56 teeth and studs

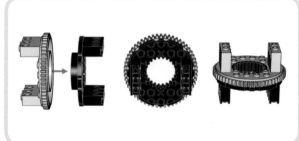

The oldest type of turntable is the big turntable. It is 5 studs tall (the pin holes on its top and bottom are 5 studs apart), and its diameter is exactly 7 studs. Its top has 56 spur teeth on the outer ring. The hole in its middle is exactly the size of a 24-tooth gear, with 24 inner teeth on the bottom piece. There are 4 studs of space between the "walls" on both the top and bottom. All in all, it's optimized for studfull constructions and thus is largely obsolete today.

big Technic turntable with 56 teeth and no studs

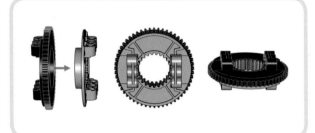

The newer version of the big turntable, introduced in 2004, is optimized for studless constructions. It's 3 studs tall, and its diameter is exactly 7 studs. Its top has 56 square spur teeth on the outer ring. The hole in its middle is almost the size of a 24-tooth gear, with two notches on opposite sides that make it slightly smaller. On the bottom piece, the hole has 24 inner teeth. There are 3 studs of space between the "walls" on both the top and bottom, which is less space than in the older turntable. Notches were needed in the inner ring to accommodate this change. In other words, you can put a 24-tooth gear inside the turntable with studs, but not inside this one.

big Technic turntable with 60 teeth and no studs

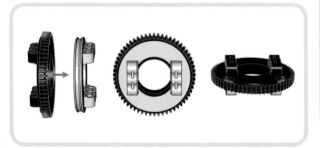

Introduced in 2015, the big Technic turntable with 60 teeth and no studs is closely based on the small turntable's design. It is 3 studs tall, and its diameter is 7.5 studs (60 mm). Its top has 60 teeth on the outer ring, all chamfered on the side that connects to the bottom, just like in the small turntable. The hole in its middle has a diameter of 3 studs and no inner teeth. There are 3 studs of space between the "walls" on both the top and bottom.

Similar to the small turntable, the advantages of this turntable are twofold: It can be easily driven with 12-tooth gears (see Figure 6-27), and the lack of inner teeth leaves more (and safer) room for pneumatic tubing or wires. It's also

optimized for high loads; its halves are harder to separate, and they generate much less friction when rotating than in both 56-teeth turntables. Just like the small turntable, it's very difficult to mesh with a worm gear.

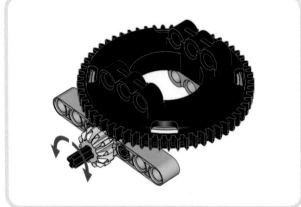

Figure 6-27: Similar to the small turntable, the big 60-tooth turntable can be meshed with a single- or double-bevel 12-tooth gear from the bottom.

obsolete gears

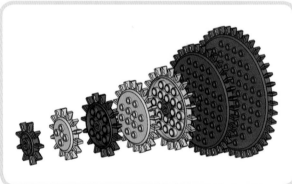

These gears are parts of two early systems of LEGO gears: the Samsonite system introduced in 1965 and the Expert Builder system introduced in 1970. They're predecessors of the Technic system, which replaced them in 1977. These gears have been absent from LEGO sets since then, but they're still relatively easy to find in secondhand sales.

They mesh in both parallel and perpendicular manners but only with other gears from this era. Just like knob wheels, they have teeth that make them work unevenly. Note that they're massive and are made from a very durable material. Some even have metal centers, which makes the smallest of them popular with builders seeking heavy-duty gears. The larger ones are rarely used because of their enormous size.

7

chains and pulleys

Transferring torque with LEGO pieces is possible not only with gears and axles but also with two additional systems: pulleys and chains. All of these systems work with similar principles.

LEGO pulleys are wheels that can be connected via strings or rubber bands, allowing for the transfer of drive and movement. You've seen similar pulleys in "belt" systems in real life. Pins without friction, bushes, and other circular elements can also be used as LEGO pulleys. A pulley system is particularly useful for lighter loads, transferring drive silently and over a long distance.

LEGO chains work similarly, though they're better suited for higher torque than a pulley. A chain replaces the rubber band of a pulley system, and gears replace the pulleys. The driver gear in a chain is known as a *sprocket*, just as in a tracked vehicle. Instead of being held by the frictional force of a string or rubber band, a chain is held by meshing its links with gears. Figure 7-1 shows the pulley and chain systems side by side.

Since the chain system is less versatile and therefore simpler, we are going to discuss it first. Then we will move to pulley systems and configuration. Keep in mind that the same configurations are possible for chain and pulley systems, though they're often more practical with pulleys.

chains

The LEGO chain system has been present in the Technic line since 1979, and despite its rarity, it's unlikely to go out of use. The chain consists of small, rigid links that can be connected so that every link can be tilted relative to the next one (see Figure 7-2). In this way, we can create a flexible but rigid chain of any length, which can be wrapped around gears. Figure 7-3 shows the size of the LEGO chain compared to a 1×2 brick. You may also recognize the chain link as similar to the LEGO track link (see Figure 7-4), which is used for tracked vehicles.

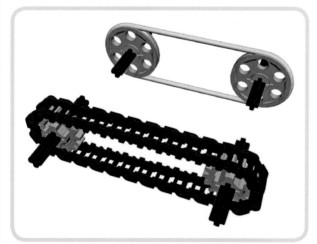

Figure 7-1: Two pulleys with a rubber band (yellow) and two gears with a chain (black). The two systems share the same working principles.

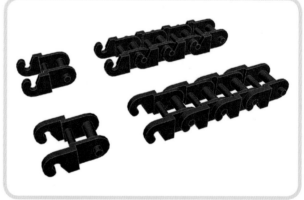

Figure 7-2: A single chain link and a section of four connected links, shown with slots facing upward and downward. In theory, the chain is less likely to come apart when its slots face the gear, but in practice, the difference is negligible.

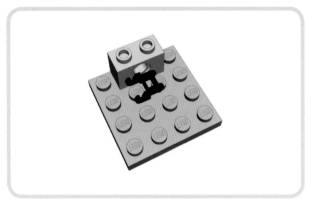

Figure 7-3: An individual chain link is very small and practically impossible to combine with any other type of LEGO piece.

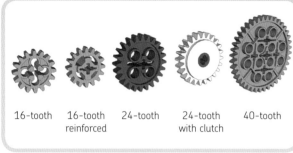

16-tooth   16-tooth reinforced   24-tooth   24-tooth with clutch   40-tooth

Figure 7-5: All the chain-compatible gears

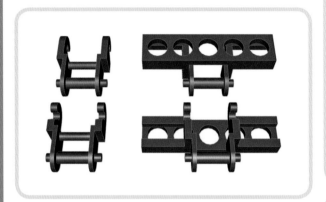

Figure 7-4: The chain link (left) is similar to the LEGO track link (right) and can be combined with it. To learn more about tracks, see Chapter 18.

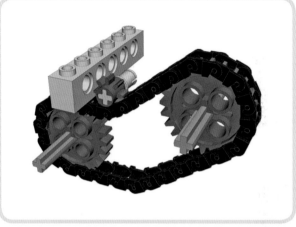

Figure 7-6: The 8-tooth gear also works with a chain but cannot drive it due to the gear's small size. It can still be used as an idler gear, adapting the shape of the chain to the surrounding structure.

Five different gears work with the chain, as shown in Figure 7-5. While the 8-tooth gear can work with the chain, too, it cannot drive the chain as it's simply too small (see Figure 7-6). Also note that by using the 24-tooth gear with clutch, you can make a chain slide when its output is stopped (for example, under load), meaning that the chain will behave just like a rubber band would over pulleys. Chains can also be wrapped around turntables to drive them, but they are rarely used this way as there are other, much less space-consuming methods of driving a turntable (for example, with a worm gear or an 8-tooth gear).

Even though the chain is rigid, it has a degree of elasticity because the links are made of thin material. This allows us to adjust the *tension* of the chain. In general, the chain should not be very tight, as a tight chain is more likely to come apart under torque. Some *play* in the chain is therefore desired. The section of the chain that makes contact with

the gear has no play; rather, the play of a chain accumulates between the gears, usually in the lowest section of the chain due to gravity (see Figure 7-7). This play allows the system to withstand more force and becomes a problem only when it's large enough to decrease the chain's area of contact with the gears, increasing the risk of links skipping their teeth, or when it's large enough to come in contact with the structure around the chain, where it can catch. When dealing with chains longer than 20 links, it's a good idea to add 1 extra link just to lower the tension. Soft shock absorbers can be used to add a bit of tension.

The chain can be used to change the gear ratio by simply connecting two gears of different sizes. Linking two gears via a chain works exactly like directly meshing them: The gear ratio is equal to the number of follower gear's teeth divided by the number of driver gear's teeth. For instance, by using a chain to drive a 24-tooth gear with a 16-tooth

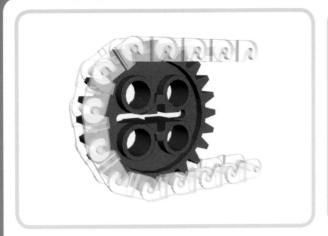

Figure 7-7: A close-up view of the chain wrapped around a gear shows that each link occupies two teeth. The section of the chain that has contact with the gear has no play in it, and its elasticity is minimized.

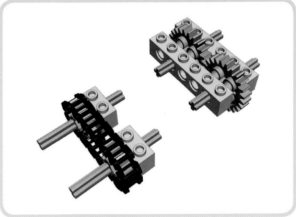

Figure 7-8: One major advantage of a chain (left) is that it does not require reinforced structure around it to handle high torque, unlike gears meshed directly (right).

gear, we obtain a 16:24 ratio, which can be reduced to 1:1.5, just as in a direct connection. And in the same way, the ratio of a chain system is not affected by idler gears. The only difference is that the chain keeps all the gears it's wrapped around rotating in the same direction, with the exception of idler gears that are located outside the chain rather than inside it (see the idler gear in Figure 7-6). Note that you can use one chain to drive several follower gears of various sizes, creating a different ratio for each of them.

The important characteristic of a chain is its behavior under torque. When a high torque is applied to gears meshed directly (shown at left in Figure 7-8), it pushes them apart, which may cause their teeth to skip. But when a high torque is applied to gears connected with a chain, it pulls them together. This means that a chain has an advantage in high-torque applications: Gears connected with a chain don't need a reinforced housing—the chain is something of a structural reinforcement itself.

pulleys

Pulleys are circular LEGO pieces designed to work with rubber bands or strings. They are distinguished by a groove around the rim, and there are only four types, as shown in Figure 7-9. Other LEGO pieces can be used as pulleys, too, but without a groove, they don't hold rubber bands or strings as securely. Note that many wheels without tires can also be used as pulleys.

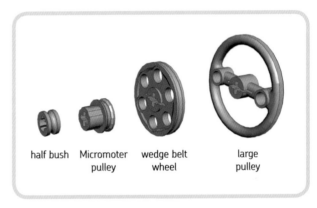

half bush   Micromoter pulley   wedge belt wheel   large pulley

Figure 7-9: All four LEGO pulleys

The two most common pulleys are the regular half bush and the wedge belt wheel (so named because of its resemblance to real-life wheels designed to work with wedge belts, which we replace with rubber bands). The large pulley is less common, and the Micromotor pulley is the rarest, as it was originally meant to be used only with the LEGO Micromotor. When we connect two pulleys with a rubber band or a string, we create a gear ratio between them, just as we do in a chain system. The ratio depends on the proportion of their driver and follower diameters, which are shown in Figure 7-10. By driving a wedge belt wheel with a half bush, for example, we get a 21:5.8 ratio, which is equal to 3.6:1. And by driving a Micromotor pulley with a large pulley, we get a 9:32 ratio, which is equal to 1:3.55.

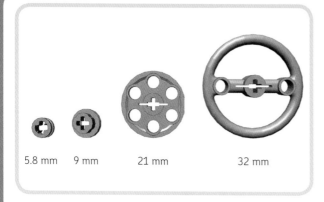

5.8 mm   9 mm   21 mm   32 mm

Figure 7-10: The diameters of the pulleys, which determine their ratios

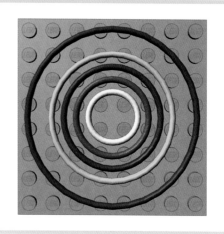

Figure 7-11: LEGO rubber bands come in five sizes, with diameters of 2, 3, 4, 5, and 7 studs. This figure also shows the most common color for each size.

However, ratios between pulleys are less reliable than ratios between gears because there is no solid connection between driver and follower, just an elastic rubber band or a string that can slip, extend, or retract under load, thus altering the ratio. We can actually use this lack of a solid connection to our advantage—for instance, such slippage could prevent a motor from stalling. The diameter-based calculation should, therefore, be considered just an approximate value. The *effective ratio* depends on a number of factors, including the torque transferred and the tension of the element connecting the pulleys, and it varies rather than staying at one fixed value.

Using pulleys with strings is the subject of the next section. For now, we will focus on rubber bands. It's perfectly possible to use any kind of thin rubber band, but the LEGO Group actually produces its own rubber bands, which work noticeably better. The rubber bands found in Technic sets are made of a high-quality silicone that rarely breaks and stays elastic for years, and their round cross section fits pulleys' grooves better than the square cross section of ordinary rubber bands.

The pulley-dedicated LEGO rubber bands come in five sizes, from a 2×2-stud band to a 7×7-stud band. Other than their size and color, the bands are identical, and each of them can be stretched to a larger size, with the bigger bands able to stretch more than the smaller ones. The various bands and their most popular colors are shown in Figure 7-11.

The general behavior of two pulleys connected with a rubber band is very similar to that of two gears connected with a chain: The rubber band acts as a belt, keeping all the pulleys inside it rotating in the same direction. Its shape can be changed with idler pulleys, and it pulls pulleys together when subjected to high torque. One band can also be used

to drive several follower pulleys of various sizes by a single driver pulley, effectively creating a different ratio for each of them.

The main difference between rubber band and chain drive systems is that the rubber band should be as tight as possible, because any play can stop it from transferring drive or even make it fall off the pulleys. Slippage in a pulley system isn't entirely negative—the fact that a band can slip when the follower pulley is stopped or blocked eliminates the need for a clutch of any kind. Note that when tight enough, the LEGO rubber bands can transfer surprisingly high torque without slipping, although they are generally considered less reliable than gears in high-torque applications. One problem is that bands are more likely to break, which can be disastrous when dealing with high torque.

Another advantage of pulley systems is their small size and thickness. The two most common pulleys—the half bush and the wedge belt wheel—are only a half stud thick, allowing two pairs of pulleys to fit where only one pair of gears would, as shown in Figure 7-12. That makes them a better choice than gears when space is limited and torque is low. Moreover, as long as the bands don't slip, they create practically no backlash, regardless of their number, which is a huge advantage over gears in mechanisms that need to react quickly and accurately. Finally, they are practically noiseless.

Also note that the band is more flexible than the chain and can be bent in any direction, allowing you to create mechanisms that are just not possible with a chain, such as pulleys that can be driven at an angle (see Figure 7-13).

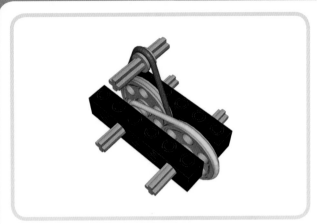

Figure 7-12: Two pairs of pulleys can fit into a 1-stud-wide space, which would be filled entirely by a single pair of gears.

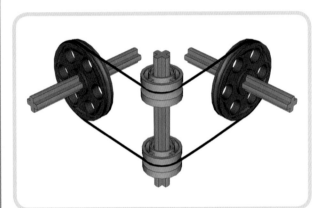

Figure 7-13: Two pulleys are connected by a rubber band at an angle, with two freely rotating rims on a vertical axle used as idlers to guide the band.

string and pulley systems

Using pulleys with strings is different from using pulleys with rubber bands. You can, of course, tie string into a loop and wrap it around two pulleys, but it won't work as well because it won't be as tight as a rubber band—string is simply less elastic and has much less grip. While rubber bands are used to transfer drive between two or more pulleys, string is best used to transfer the actual movement, that is, the displacement itself.

A perfect example of such a system is a winch in a crane, where string is wound on a reel and rotating the reel makes it pull loads up and down through a system of pulleys, as shown in Figure 7-14. In this case, the reel is the driver, and the movement is transferred to the hook at the end of the string. Without pulleys, the reel would have to be located on top of the crane, directly above the load. With pulleys, the string can be guided from the top of the crane to the back of it, where the reel is easily accessible and acts as the crane's counterweight.

There are numerous examples of mechanisms using string to transfer movement, including drawbridges, window blinds, and even cable railcars (where a car literally attaches to and detaches from a moving cable to travel). However, pulleys can do more than guide movement.

Pulleys and string can be combined into systems that realize mechanical advantage. *Mechanical advantage* is a measure that shows how much a given mechanism amplifies the force we apply to it. For example, a mechanical advantage of 2 means that the force is amplified twice. This is exactly the kind of speed/torque transformation we have discussed when dealing with gears, and mechanical advantage is simply another way of describing a ratio. So, a mechanical advantage of 2 is simply a ratio of 2:1.

The idea of mechanical advantage is well illustrated by the crane example from Figure 7-14. Let's assume that we have already installed in the crane a system of pulleys that

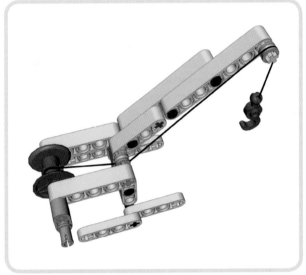

Figure 7-14: A simple crane uses a winch to pull a load on a hook up and down. The movement is transferred through a string, which is guided from the reel to the top of the crane by two half bushes acting as idler pulleys.

grants us a mechanical advantage of 2. This simply means that we have to apply half the force for twice as long—and that's because amplification of the force comes at the cost of the extra length of string to wind up. For example, to lift a 100 g load 1 m, we have to rotate the reel long enough to wind up 2 m of string using only enough force to lift 50 g. Trading torque for speed works to our advantage because how much we can lift is usually more important than how fast we can lift it. With enough mechanical advantage, we can lift or move any load, no matter how heavy—its weight affects only the amount of time it will take. (Obviously, it also requires a structure strong enough to support it.)

Pulley systems that realize mechanical advantage are usually installed just between the top of a crane and its hook. The invention of such pulley systems is attributed to ancient Greeks, and the systems were refined by ancient Romans. It is estimated today that the most advanced Roman cranes allowed a single person to lift up to 3 tons of load, which is quite impressive for simple machines made mostly of wood. This load capacity could be multiplied by using a number of cranes together to handle a single load. Many of the ancient buildings we admire today could not have been created without this invention that allowed human power to move extremely heavy objects.

A pulley system typically consists of at least one pulley that is fixed above the load and stays in place—for example, on the top of our crane—and at least one pulley that moves together with the load—for example, by being attached to the hook of our crane, as shown in Figure 7-15. So, there are two groups of pulleys, one fixed and another moving, and each can consist of many pulleys.

The way the two groups of pulleys are connected with string and how many times they are connected determines the mechanical advantage they provide. There are three categories of pulley systems, each with groups of pulleys connected in different ways, and we will discuss them starting with the simplest one.

simple pulley system

The simplest pulley system consists of two groups that are identical. The upper group is the fixed one. The string goes over the upper group's first pulley and then comes down to the lower group, which is moving, and wraps around the lower group's first pulley. Then it comes back to the upper group and is tied to it, or it can be wrapped around a second pulley and repeat the arrangement between the first two pulleys. This means that the string can't be tied directly to the hook after it comes from the first upper pulley, which is the main difference between the simplest pulley system and the lack of any such system, as Figures 7-16 and 7-17 show.

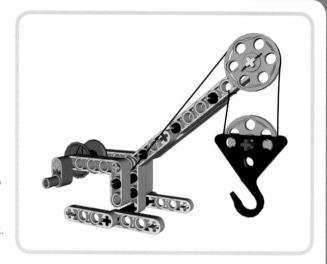

Figure 7-15: Our simple crane equipped with a pulley system. Two groups of pulleys are used, each consisting of a single pulley: The upper one stays on top of the crane, and the lower one moves up and down with the hook. This particular arrangement of string between the pulleys grants a mechanical advantage of 2.

As you can see in Figure 7-17, the simplest pulley system has two sections of string connecting the two groups. This means that in order to lift the load, we have to wind up twice as much string as without this system, but using only half the force. There's no free lunch: We are trading time for work, having to do less work but over a longer period of time.

But let's consider what happens if we add another section of string between the two groups. We will need one more pulley to prevent the sections from getting tangled up with one another, as shown in Figure 7-18.

As you see, the string is now tied to the lower group, but only after it goes through three pulleys: two upper ones and one lower one. Three sections of string connect the two groups, granting a mechanical advantage of 3. We need to wind up three times as much string but use only one third of the force. By now you have probably guessed that *the number of sections of string connecting the groups determines the mechanical advantage they realize.*

These simple pulley systems are commonly used in sailboats and have various names depending on how many sections of string connect the two blocks. The system with two sections is called a *gun tackle*, and the system with three sections is called a *luff tackle*. Other systems, shown in Figures 7-19 to 7-21, have up to six sections of string. As the number of sections increases, the whole system becomes less and less efficient, as each pulley creates additional friction and the significant length of string in the whole system is prone to stretching under load.

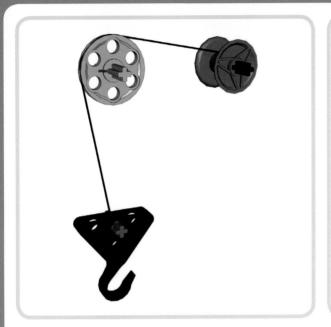

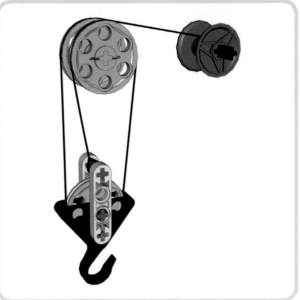

Figure 7-16: This arrangement has an upper group with a single pulley and no lower group. The string that comes off the pulley is tied directly to the hook. No pulley system is created, and no mechanical advantage is gained.

Figure 7-18: A pulley system with three sections of string between the groups, called a luff tackle. The upper group has string coming through it twice and hence two pulleys to prevent the string from getting tangled up. The string is then tied to the red axle in the lower group. This arrangement grants a mechanical advantage of 3.

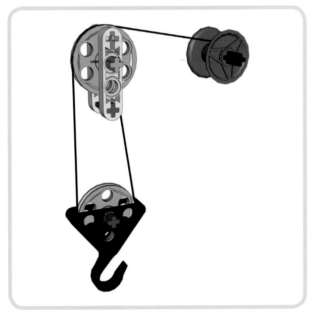

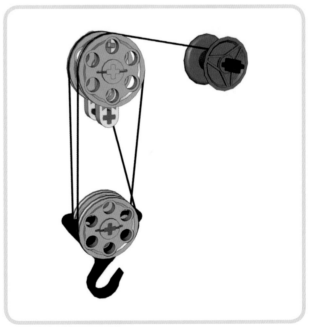

Figure 7-17: This arrangement, called a gun tackle, has two groups, each with a single pulley. The string comes off the upper pulley and around the lower pulley. It is then tied to the element that is part of the upper group and remains fixed to it. This is the simplest pulley system, with a mechanical advantage of 2.

Figure 7-19: This system, called double tackle, grants a mechanical advantage of 4.

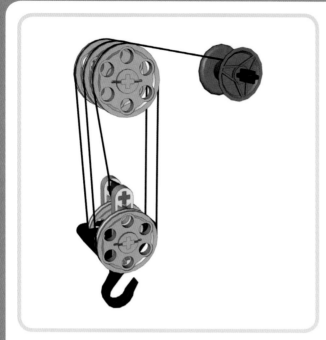

Figure 7-20: This system, called gyn tackle, grants a mechanical advantage of 5.

differential pulley system

Despite its name, the differential pulley system (also known as the *Chinese windlass*) does not use a differential gear. Instead, it uses an upper group with two different-sized pulleys rotating on the same axle, as shown in Figure 7-22. The string is arranged so the rotation unwinds it from one pulley while winding it on the other. The mechanical advantage is determined by the size difference of the pulleys and is greatest when the size difference is smallest. In fact, differential pulleys can achieve an extremely high mechanical advantage, far surpassing that of any other pulley systems. They are also safer to operate because the weight of the load can't unwind the string from the upper pulley. When a regular pulley is released while the load is midair (for example, when you disconnect it from a motor or simply let go of its crank), the load will unwind the string from the upper pulley and drop down. In a differential pulley system, the load pulls on both ends of the string, which are wound onto two coaxial pulleys from opposite sides. Thus, if a differential pulley is released, the load stays right where it is.

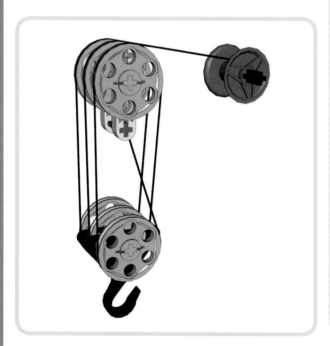

Figure 7-21: This system, called threefold purchase, grants a mechanical advantage of 6.

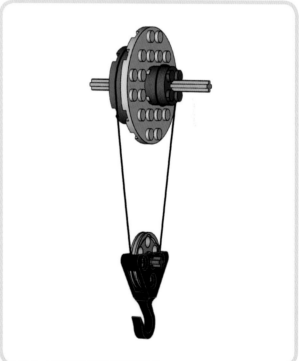

Figure 7-22: A differential pulley system producing a mechanical advantage equal to 4

If R is the radius of a large upper pulley and r is the radius of a small upper pulley, the mechanical advantage of the differential pulley is equal to $(2 \times R) / (R - r)$.

In Figure 7-22, R is 16 mm (2 studs) and r is 8 mm (1 stud), which gives a mechanical advantage equal to 32 / 8, which is 4. Using this formula, you can see that the mechanical advantage is bigger if the difference in the upper pulleys' sizes is very small. For example, if the smaller pulley had a radius of 1.5 studs (12 mm), the entire system would produce an advantage of 32 / 4, which is 8.

Note that the formula remains true regardless of the unit of measure used. You can simply use studs, which in the example in Figure 7-22 would be $(2 \times 2) / (2 - 1) = 4 / 1 = 4$.

Keep four details in mind when you're building a differential pulley:

* Because you're winding and unwinding a string, it's best to use reels or drums rather than pulleys. Smooth, round pieces of a fixed diameter, such as round bricks, are the best choice because you can combine several of them to obtain a reel of your desired width. Just don't forget to fasten the end of the string to them!
* Make sure you store some reserve of the string on the reels. Because the string is wound and unwound at varying rates, the amount of string in reserve limits the reach of the differential pulley: At some point, you'll simply run out of string.
* It's important to prevent the string from skipping from one reel onto the other. In Figure 7-22, the yellow round plate acts as a simple separator. The larger and smoother the separator, the lower the risk of the string winding up on it. In this example, the string could catch on one of the yellow plate's studs.
* Because the mechanical advantage depends on the relative radius of the reels, it can be affected by the amount of string on the reels. Make sure the extra layers of string don't make the reels equal in diameter, as this would effectively stop the pulley.

power pulley system

The power pulley system is the most complex and most effective of the three systems. It's distinguished by having one upper group and several lower groups that are connected in series, with the hook attached to the last one, as shown in Figure 7-23.

As you see, this system starts with one section of the string (black) coming off the reel, going through the upper pulley, going through the pulley of the first lower group, and then being tied to part of the upper group. Then the lower group has another section of string (green) attached to it.

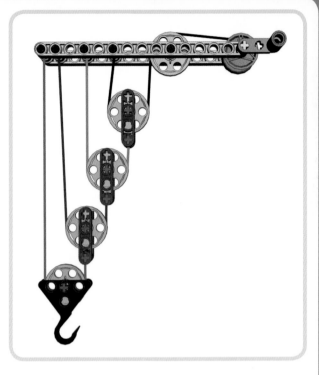

Figure 7-23: The power pulley system consists of one upper group and a number of moving lower groups connected in series. There are four lower groups here, granting a mechanical advantage of 16.

This string goes through the pulley of a second lower group and is then tied to part of the upper group, just like the first string's section. This series can continue until the final lower group, which has a hook attached to it and handles the actual load. In Figure 7-23, the hook is present on the 4th lower group, but it could just as well be present on the 20th one. Note that by moving the points where strings are tied to the upper group away from its pulley (to the left in Figure 7-23), it's possible to make the lower groups travel not only up and down but also forward and backward.

The mechanical advantage of the power pulley system is equal to 2^n, where n is the total number of lower groups. This means that the mechanical advantage increases rapidly with the number of lower groups, starting with 2 for one group, 4 for two groups, 8 for three groups, 16 for four groups, and so on. This may not sound impressive compared to the 22 we achieved with the differential pulley system, until you realize that the advantage in the power system exceeds 1,000 with 10 lower groups and 1 million with 20. And there is no technical limit on how many lower groups can be used, although just like the other systems, this one becomes inefficient with many pulleys adding friction and a lot of string stretching under load.

levers and linkages

Levers and linkages are some of the simplest machines and form the basis for countless more complex mechanisms. While levers are mostly used to provide a mechanical advantage that allows us to move heavy loads, linkages are mostly used to transform one type of a motion into another. Both are common in everyday life: If you have ever played on a seesaw or used pliers, you have relied on levers and linkages.

levers

A basic lever is simply a beam that has one point of support in the form of a hinge or a pivot, as shown in Figure 8-1. We will call this point a *fulcrum*. A lever also has input and output forces. We will call the applied, or input, force the *effort* and the reaction force the *load*. Finally, we will call the sections of the lever between its fulcrum and its ends *arms*.

When a lever provides a mechanical advantage, our input force is amplified. But that increase in force does come at a cost, just as it does with all other simple machines. A lever with a mechanical advantage of 2 allows us to move the load using half the force it would take without the lever but covering only half the distance (traveling at half the speed).

The mechanical advantage of the lever depends on the distances between the fulcrum, the load, and the effort. The so-called *law of the lever* states that the mechanical advantage of a lever is equal to d_e/d_l, where d_e is the distance between the effort and the fulcrum and d_l is the distance between the load and the fulcrum. For example, for the lever shown in Figure 8-2, d_e (indicated by the blue arrow) is 5 studs long, and d_l (indicated by the red arrow) is 3 studs long. Therefore, the mechanical advantage of this lever is 5/3, or 1.67. This means that in order to lift a 1 kg load 1 m with this lever, we have to apply the effort needed

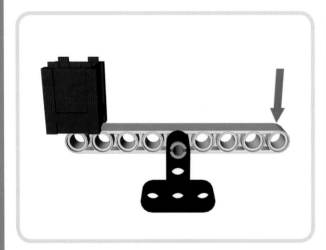

Figure 8-1: A simple lever, consisting of a beam (yellow) supported by the fulcrum (black). The brown crate is the load, and the green arrow represents the effort. When effort is applied downward, the load is lifted up.

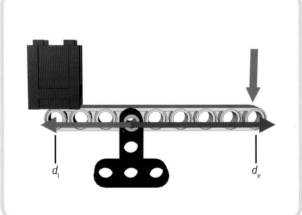

Figure 8-2: This lever has a mechanical advantage of 5/3, or 1.67, because the distance between the fulcrum and the effort is 5 studs and the distance between the fulcrum and the load is 3 studs.

to lift 0.6 kg and move the end of the lever 1.67 m. The mechanical advantage still benefits us because we're trading time, which we have plenty of, for force, which is limited.

The law of the lever also means that the force applied to the arm of a lever is *inversely proportional* to the arm's length. Therefore, it takes more force to move a lever with a short arm than it takes to move a lever with a longer arm. A lever with a 3-stud-long arm will take twice the force as a lever with a 6-stud-long arm to move the same load. The lever with the 6-stud-long arm, though, will move the load twice as far because of its longer length.

Figure 8-3 illustrates the distance/force proportion. We have a lever with a 3-stud-long arm and a 7-stud-long arm. If we apply force to the longer arm, the lever offers a mechanical advantage of 2.33 (7/3), and if we apply force to the shorter arm, the lever offers a mechanical advantage of 0.43 (3/7). If we put a 1 kg load on the longer arm and a 2.33 kg load on the shorter arm, the loads will balance each other.

Note that a lever can have equal d_e and d_l distances, resulting in a mechanical advantage of 1. This simply means that there is no mechanical advantage and the distance/force balance remains unaltered. Such a lever can still be useful, as it reverses the direction of movement (that is, by pushing down, you lift a load up).

Finally, note that a lever does not necessarily have to be a straight beam. It can be bent and work just the same. A simple crowbar is a good example of a bent lever (see Figure 8-4): It has a long arm, a short arm, and a central part that we put on the floor, thus creating a fulcrum. By shoving the short arm under the load, we are able to use the long arm to lift that load using less force than without the crowbar.

classes of levers

The positions of the fulcrum, the load, and the effort on a lever can vary. There are three possible combinations, which are called *classes*. Fortunately for us, the law of the lever is exactly the same for each class, meaning that the mechanical advantage is calculated in the same way for all of them.

The lever classes are as follows:

* Class 1 (see Figure 8-5): The fulcrum is located in the middle of the lever and the load and effort at its ends. This is the only class of lever where effort and load are applied in opposite directions (that is, to lift a load up, you have to apply effort downward). Examples: a seesaw or a crowbar.
* Class 2 (see Figures 8-6 and 8-7): The load is located in the middle of the lever and the fulcrum and effort at its ends. Example: a wheelbarrow, with the wheel being its fulcrum.
* Class 3 (see Figures 8-8 and 8-9): The effort is located in the middle of the lever and the load and the fulcrum at its ends. Because of this arrangement, class 3 levers have a mechanical advantage of less than 1 and are used to trade force for distance rather than the other way around. This makes them useful when there is plenty of force that can be used to move the load over greater distance. Example: a boom of a crane elevated by a pneumatic cylinder attached to its middle.

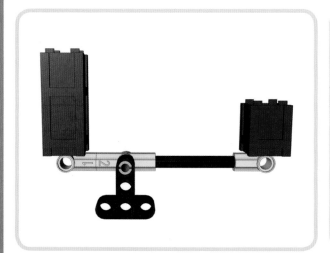

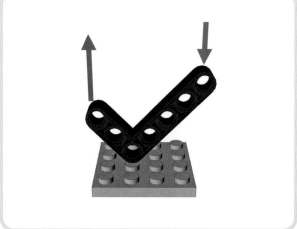

Figure 8-3: This lever has a mechanical advantage of 2.33, meaning that one of its arms is 2.33 times as long as the other one. Therefore, any load put on the longer arm can balance a 2.33 times heavier load on the shorter arm.

Figure 8-4: The bent 3×5 beam can work just like a crowbar.

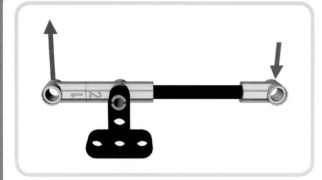

Figure 8-5: Class 1 lever with the fulcrum in the middle and the effort (green) and load (red) at its ends

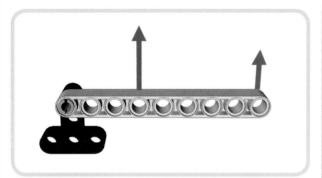

Figure 8-6: Class 2 lever with the load (red) in the middle and the fulcrum and effort (green) at its ends

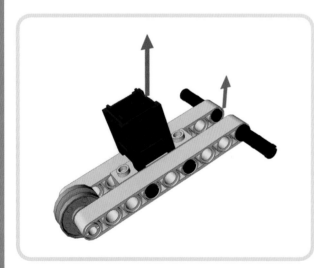

Figure 8-7: An ordinary wheelbarrow is an example of the class 2 lever, with its wheel being the fulcrum. The load is located in the middle of the wheelbarrow, and the effort is applied to the end of it. Wheelbarrows usually provide a mechanical advantage greater than 1, unless you apply the effort exactly where the load is located.

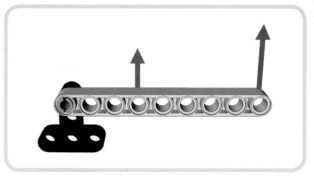

Figure 8-8: Class 3 lever with the effort (green) in the middle and the fulcrum and load (red) at its ends

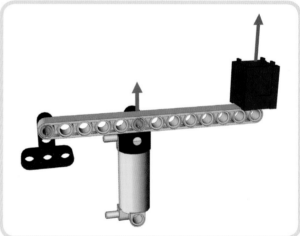

Figure 8-9: A boom of a crane is an example of the class 3 lever, with the load and the fulcrum at its ends and the effort applied to its center (in this case, by a pneumatic cylinder). Class 3 levers have a mechanical advantage less than 1, meaning that they require plenty of effort but can move loads over large distances. This is favorable when it comes to pneumatics, which can exert huge force but have limited reach.

from levers to linkages

An interesting thing happens when you connect ends of two identical levers located one above the other: The elements connecting their ends will maintain the same position as the levers move. This happens at every point in the levers' range of movement, regardless of their length. We can use this system of parallel levers, also known as a 4-bar linkage, to our advantage.

As Figure 8-10 shows, we can expand our crane's boom in Figure 8-9 by adding a parallel lever to it. This addition provides two advantages: First, we can move both levers by applying effort to only one of them because the elements connecting them will transfer the movement from one to the

other. Second, and more importantly, the element at the "load" end of the levers will move with the levers while maintaining constant orientation. This means that the load's angle won't change as it moves up and down with the levers, which is useful when moving loads that we don't want to tip over.

Many kinds of machines—front loaders and telescopic forklifts, for example—use parallel levers to handle loads. The 8265 set, shown in Figure 8-11, is an excellent example of a front loader: Its bucket is connected to arms that form parallel levers. Note that a linear actuator on each side acts as the lower lever, and by extending or retracting, it controls the bucket's height. When it extends or retracts to the point that its length differs from that of the upper levers, an additional

linkage between it and the bucket keeps the bucket level. The same additional linkage allows us to tip the bucket with another linear actuator. The bucket's orientation depends entirely on the lengths and locations of the levers.

For the orientation to be maintained, the two levers have to be of identical length, and their ends have to be connected with identical spacing, as shown in Figure 8-12.

Note that the levers connected in this way can't make a full rotation: They limit each other, colliding at a certain point. Therefore, their rotation is limited to a certain range, which can be adjusted by locating the levers not exactly one above the other but with a small displacement, as shown in Figure 8-13. Also note that the elements connecting the

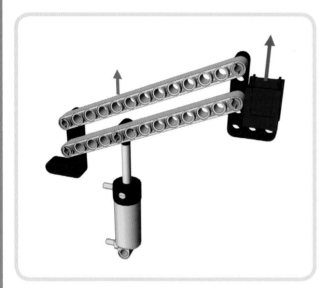

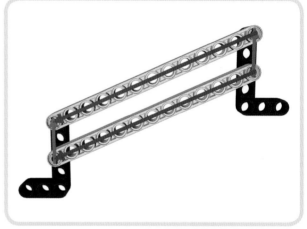

Figure 8-12: The parallel levers maintain the orientation of the elements at their ends only if the levers' length and spacing are identical.

Figure 8-10: A boom of a crane made of parallel levers. The parallel levers ensure that the element on the end of the levers maintains constant orientation as the levers move it up and down.

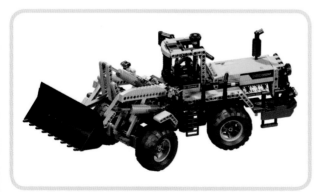

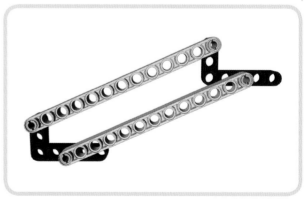

Figure 8-13: The parallel levers are displaced to adjust their range of movement. By moving the upper lever a little backward (left in the figure), we can increase the maximum reach upward at the cost of maximum reach downward.

Figure 8-11: The 8265 set features a complex front loader whose arms (elevating the bucket) form parallel levers.

two ends of the levers don't have to be identical, nor do they need to be set at the same angle—it's only the angle and distance between the points of attachment that matter (see Figure 8-14).

Other variations are possible with a parallel-levers arrangement. For example, the element connecting the levers at the fulcrum can be rotated, making the element at the other end rotate at the same angle, as shown in Figure 8-15. This is one way to tip the bucket of our front loader.

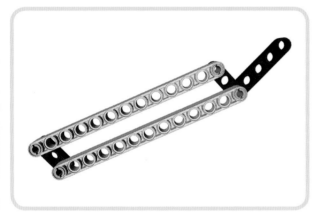

Figure 8-14: The functioning of the parallel levers relies on the positions of their points of attachment. These positions can be made identical on both ends using various elements set at various angles.

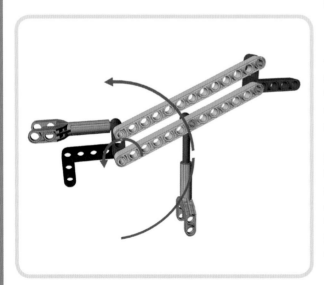

Figure 8-15: This boom variant uses one actuator to lower and raise the parallel levers (green arrow) and another to rotate the element that connects them at the fulcrum (red arrow), thus making the element at their other end rotate.

As Figure 8-16 shows, there is an interesting effect if the levers are not exactly parallel: Rotating the levers makes the element connecting their ends rotate slightly as well. This limits the levers' range of movement but can sometimes be desirable—in particular, when we want the element at the levers' ends to be oriented differently in the lowermost and uppermost positions. This is the case with the 8460 Pneumatic Crane Truck set, where such an arrangement is used to control the stabilizing outriggers. This arrangement makes the outriggers nearly horizontal when lowered and nearly vertical when raised, effectively increasing their reach.

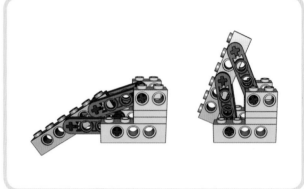

Figure 8-16: An outrigger mechanism from one of the LEGO mobile cranes uses levers that are not exactly parallel. The yellow part is the chassis, the levers are red, and the actual outrigger is grey.

Finally, you can use the fact that the parallel levers rotate relative to the elements that connect them to your advantage. By putting gears on the axles that rotate together with the levers, we can transfer that rotation through these elements (for example, to another pair of parallel levers connected to the first pair of levers).

Figure 8-17 shows two pairs of parallel levers connected in such fashion—gears that transfer the rotation of one pair (left) to another (right). All the levers are identical and the gears maintain a 1:1 ratio, the result being that the element at the end of the series moves along a horizontal line. There is technically no limit to how many pairs of levers can be used in a series; the only constraint is the friction and the sum of the gears' backlash.

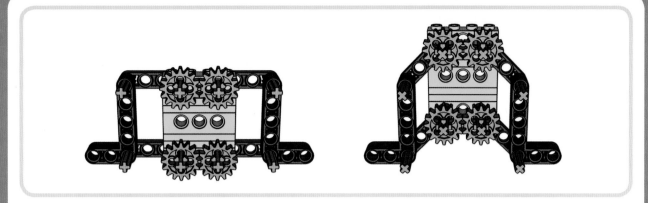

Figure 8-17: Two pairs of parallel levers connected by gears are installed on the element between them. The gears make the pairs rotate in opposite directions, moving the parts at both ends horizontally.

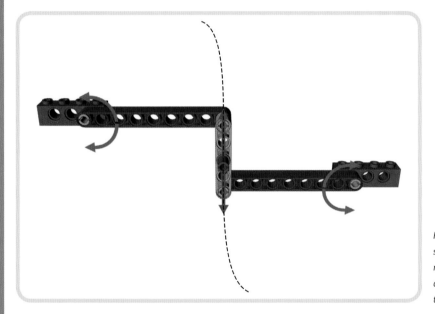

Figure 8-18: Watt's linkage consists of two long side links and one shorter central link. A rocking movement of any of the side links makes the central link move so that its center (marked by the red pin) follows a straight line.

linkages

Linkages are groups of rigid links connected by joints that allow them to perform certain restricted movements. They are mostly used to convert rotary or rocking motion into linear motion, allowing elements of various machines to move along straight lines. They can also be used to achieve mechanical advantage using the law of the lever. The lever is, in fact, the simplest linkage possible.

The key advantage of linkages is that their movement remains restricted without the need for external guiding elements, as shown in Figure 8-18. This makes them convenient for many uses. In the real world, linkages are used to control the movement of suspension components. Note also that usually only one particular point of a linkage follows the desired movement, and we can use pins located at this point to transfer this movement elsewhere—for example, to the base of the element we want to move using the linkage. A nearly infinite variation of motions can be achieved by varying the lengths and positions of just three or four beams!

NOTE In all the figures of linkages here, beams in the same color are of the same length. A dark grey color is used to mark the supporting structure, which remains stationary and to which the linkage is attached, and red pins mark the point of the linkage that performs the desired motion.

Chebyshev linkage

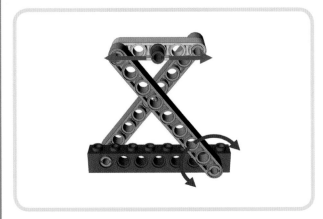

The Chebyshev linkage, also known as *Tchebycheff's linkage*, consists of three links and is driven by the rocking motion of the lower links (light grey). This motion makes the central link (yellow) move so that its center (marked by the red pin) follows a straight line. The motion continues to the point at which the central link becomes vertical. The central link needs to be the shortest of the three to prevent it from colliding with the supporting structure (dark grey).

Hoeken's linkage

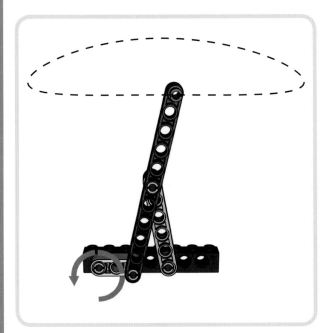

Hoeken's linkage consists of three links and is driven by the rotary motion of the shortest one (yellow). The proportions of the following three dimensions are crucial to make this linkage work: the length of the shortest link (yellow), the length of the medium link (light grey), and the distance between points of attachment to the supporting structure. The proportions should be 2 to 5 to 4. The longest link (blue) can be extended to any length beyond its upper joint. The tip of this link traces the shape of a flattened oval cut in half (the dotted line in the illustration), and the size of this oval is determined by the extended link's length. A little less than half of this link's movement is linear. Such an unusual motion pattern can be used, for example, to drive the legs of walking vehicles.

pantograph

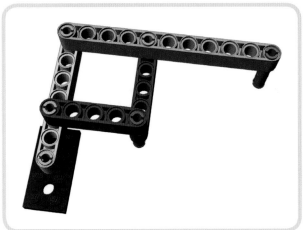

A pantograph is a particular type of linkage with four links and two points, and its movement is quite interesting. In a pantograph, the point marked by the green pin mimics every movement of the point marked by the red pin, but on a larger scale. The difference in scale depends on the length of the longest link (light blue) and on where other links are attached to it (note that the longest link actually works like a lever).

The most interesting and popular use of this property is creating enlarged or reduced copies of drawings by attaching pens to both these points and "drawing" with one of them manually. This also works with handwriting; Thomas Jefferson used this method to duplicate his correspondence. Today, scaled copies can easily be created using a computer. However, pantographs still remain in use where certain tools require accurate manual control, as in engraving and sewing.

Peaucellier–Lipkin cell

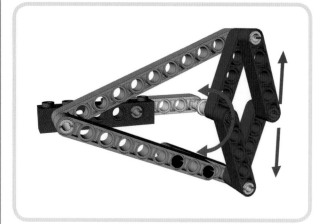

The Peaucellier–Lipkin cell, also known simply as Peaucellier's cell, consists of seven links and is driven by the rocking motion of the central link (yellow). Note that the spacing between the cell's two points of attachment to the supporting structure needs to be equal to the length of the central link.

The Peaucellier–Lipkin cell works on the principle of inversion of a circle (with the central link tracing part of it), and it was one of the first linkages capable of producing perfectly linear motion. Its invention was crucial for the development of 19th-century industry and, most notably, for its use in steam engines.

Sarrus linkage

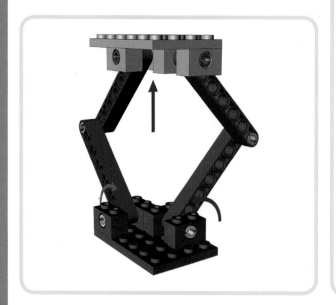

The Sarrus linkage consists of four links in two identical groups that are perpendicular to each other. All links are of equal length, and the linkage is driven by the rocking motion of both lower or both upper links. The advantage of the Sarrus linkage is that it can be used to lift the structure connecting the upper links, providing an impressive range of movement as seen in Figure 8-19). Note that the perpendicular links work in different directions and thus exert stress on each other, which is why they need to be very rigid and preferably several studs wide for the linkage to work properly.

The disadvantage of the Sarrus linkage is that it requires one link from one group to be moved simultaneously with a second link from a second group. In other

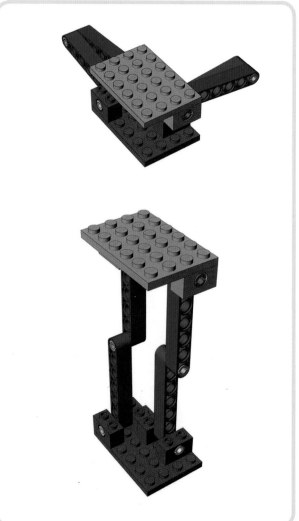

Figure 8-19: The Sarrus linkage's minimum and maximum range of lift

words, the motion of the links needs to be mechanically synchronized. Figure 8-20 shows one of the simplest synchronization methods. Note that the Sarrus linkage can consist of three or four groups as well, but two properly synchronized groups are enough to provide stable movement of the upper structure.

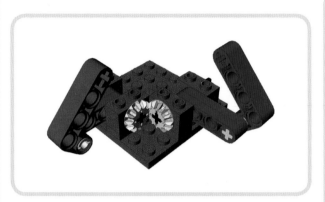

Figure 8-20: This Sarrus linkage uses mated bevel gears to synchronize links between the two groups.

Scott-Russell linkage

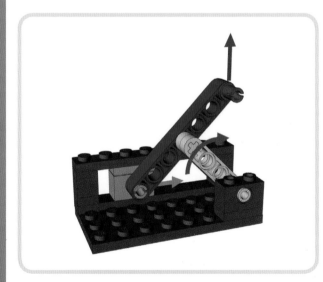

The Scott-Russell linkage consists of two links and is driven by the rocking motion of the shorter one (yellow). The longer link (blue) has one end attached to the supporting structure so that it can slide on it along a straight line. That makes the other end of that link move in a straight line as well. Both ends of that link move as if they were locked between guiding elements, but only one end actually is.

Note that the spacings between all joints of the linkage (marked by pins in the illustration) have to be equal. In this example, they are all equal to 3 studs.

scissor linkage

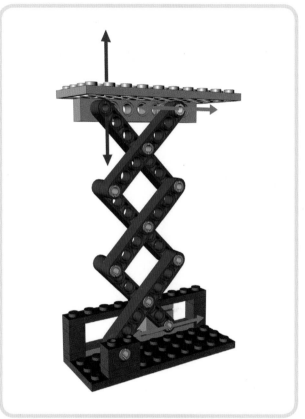

A scissor linkage, also known as a scissor mechanism, combines Scott-Russel and Sarrus linkages to create a compact mechanism capable of lifting with impressive range. It can consist of any even number of identical links—for example 2, 4, 6, and so on—and is driven by either the rocking motion of any link or by moving the end of the link that can slide within the supporting structure. Note that one of the top links also has an end that slides within the upper structure, but its movement can be restrained by simply making the upper structure's weight rest on it. In the illustration, the end has an axle pin with a bush attached to support the upper structure while sliding.

The two key advantages of the scissor linkage, its range (shown in Figure 8-21) and its stability, combined with its compactness, make it a very popular mechanical solution. For example, it appears in car doors to make windows move up and down; in so-called scissor lifts; and even in high-end

computer keyboards, where it's used to stabilize keys. There is no limit to how many links can be used in a scissor linkage, except that every joint adds extra friction. There are also no special length or distance requirements, except that all links have to be equal.

Watt's linkage

Watt's linkage (shown earlier in Figure 8-18) consists of three links: a short central link (light blue) and two longer side links (blue). The linkage is driven by the rocking motion of either side link. As the side links rotate, the central links move so that the mechanism's center follows the dotted line, which remains straight most of the time. Note that while the ends of that line deflect to the left and right, you can limit motion of the linkage to the straight part only.

Watt's linkage is sometimes used in suspension systems to keep suspension components moving up and down rather than sideways. In most configurations, its side links are two or even three times longer than the central link.

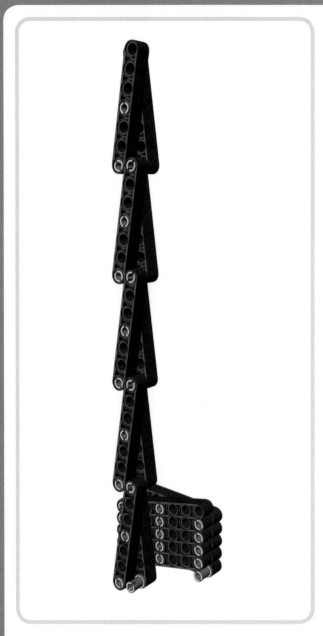

Figure 8-21: A comparison of the same 10-link-long scissor linkage in a fully retracted and a fully extended position

9

custom mechanical solutions

While the LEGO Group produces an incredible range of specialized Technic pieces, they won't always meet our needs.
Sometimes we'll need to combine pieces to create mechanical solutions we find in the real world. This is the subject of
this chapter: mechanisms that extend the functionality of
your constructions beyond the limits of ready-made LEGO
pieces. Here you'll find mechanisms that transform one
type of motion into another, that take basic LEGO lights and
transform them into sophisticated signaling systems, and
much more.

These mechanisms are fun to build just on their own as
explorations of mechanical engineering concepts, but you'll
also find them quite useful when building larger models.

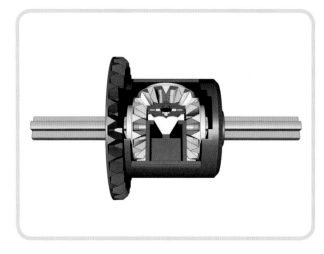

Figure 9-1: A ready-made LEGO differential, with the differential housing in
dark grey, three inner gears in tan, and two output axles in light grey

a stronger differential

Differentials are an essential part of every driven axle in
a vehicle with wheels. They're also important in large and
heavy LEGO vehicles. The prebuilt LEGO differential consists
of a housing with a ring gear and with places for two axles
and three bevel gears inside, as shown in Figure 9-1. This is
the mechanism that we'll re-create, stronger and better.

NOTE There are three variants of ready-made LEGO
differentials. They are all discussed in Chapter 6.

In automobiles, a differential is located between the
wheels. The differential's housing is driven, and the differential transfers the drive to the wheels through its two output
axles. Note that the differential transfers the drive from the
housing through the central bevel gear, which is meshed
with bevel gears on the two axles. The central bevel gear

can balance the drive between the output axles, meaning
that it can drive one axle faster than the other. This ability
to balance the drive enables the vehicle to turn smoothly.
Figure 9-2 shows that the wheels of a turning vehicle travel
along different arcs. As a result, the inner and outer wheels
have to travel different distances. A differential is able to
balance this difference by driving the outer wheel faster than
the inner one.

As ready-made LEGO differentials are torque sensitive
and rarely appear outside of big, expensive sets, we can
build our own differential using a large Technic turntable,
as shown in Figure 9-3.

This kind of custom differential is much larger and much
sturdier than a ready-made one. Using a turntable allows the
mechanism to transfer drive to the differential without using
bevel gears, instead using the much stronger knob wheel.

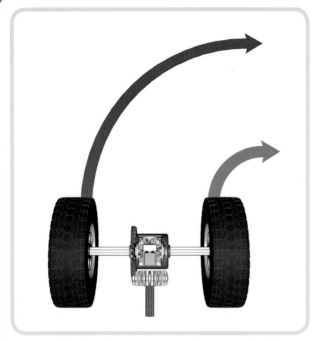

Figure 9-2: Differential in a turning vehicle. The red axle transfers drive to the differential housing, which then transfers it to the wheels.

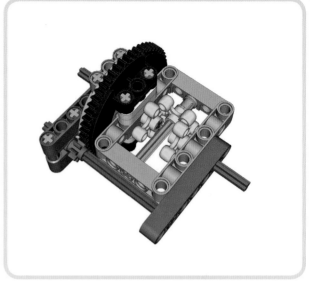

Figure 9-3: A custom differential made of a large Technic turntable connected to a studless frame. The input axle is shown in red, the output axles are shown in green, and the dark grey beams are parts of the chassis's structure around the differential.

At the same time, the turntable provides a robust mounting point, holding the differential firmly to the chassis.

It's possible to build a vehicle without using differentials, but there are some disadvantages. Without a differential, at least one wheel will slip while cornering a turn, increasing friction and tire wear and impairing the vehicle's maneuverability.

If there is no differential in a driven, nonsteered axle, that axle will also be prone to slipping while making a turn. This can actually be desirable if your intention is to build a vehicle whose rear end slides dramatically when turning. In the real world, small, lightweight vehicles, such as go-karts, are usually built without differentials because the advantages of a differential are not worth the increase in the drivetrain's complexity.

If there is no differential in a driven and steered axle (like the front axle of a front-wheel-drive car), turning becomes much more difficult. The difference in the inner and outer wheels' speeds while cornering is much greater in steered axles than in nonsteered ones, creating so much friction that it exerts significant stress on the drivetrain and can even stall the motor. At the same time, the minimum turning radius becomes larger because the wheels, forced to rotate at equal speeds, lose their grip.

differential locks

With all the advantages of using a differential, there is also one disadvantage that is particularly important for off-road vehicles. As a differential transfers drive between its two outputs, it tends to transfer more of it to the less loaded one. This works fine when turning, but it can stop a vehicle entirely if one of the wheels slips or loses contact with the ground. A so-called *slip situation* occurs, in which the differential transfers all the drive to the wheel that has lost contact, completely stopping the one that's still touching the ground. When this happens, we can use a *differential lock* to force the differential to drive both wheels, overcoming the slip situation.

A differential lock joins a differential's two outputs together, effectively disabling the differential so that it transfers drive but doesn't balance it. It's important to understand that a differential lock does not *prevent* a slip situation: The lock is used when a slip occurs and *fixes* the slip. This is because a differential lock and a differential can't work at the same time. As a result, the differential lock

a custom differential

1

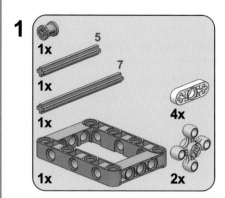

1x
5 1x
7 1x
4x
1x
2x

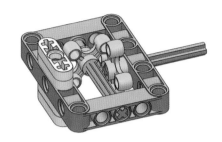

2

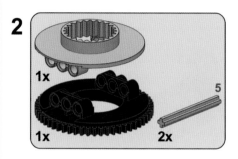

1x
5
1x
2x

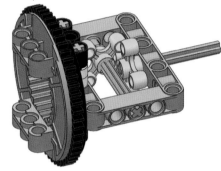

3

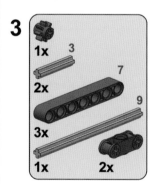

1x
3 2x
7 3x
9 1x
2x

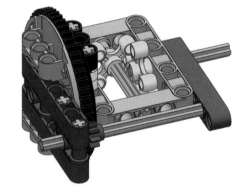

4

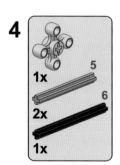

1x
5 2x
6 1x

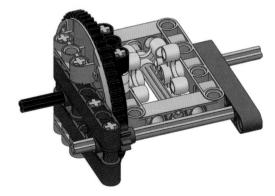

should remain disengaged to allow the differential to function normally and should engage only when a slip situation stops the vehicle. Real off-road vehicles come with manual or automatic locks that engage when a slip situation is detected and disengage when the vehicle drives out of it. LEGO differentials can be locked manually with relative ease; doing this automatically is also possible, but it's extremely complex and impractical. Figures 9-4 and 9-5 show simple manual differential locks for all three variants of ready-made LEGO differentials.

LEGO differential locks use transmission driving rings (#6539) that can be engaged and disengaged using a transmission changeover catch (#6641). The catch can be controlled remotely with a motor or with pneumatics. The latter solution is more convenient if there are many locks on your vehicle that move together with the suspension. Note that it's not necessary to put a lock on every differential on

a vehicle—just one is usually enough to make the vehicle drive out of a slip situation.

Figure 9-6 shows a compact, robust nonsteered axle design based on the 5×7 studless frame. It allows the differential to be driven with a 3:1 gear reduction from the front or rear so that the drive can be transmitted through this axle to the next one. It also allows for easy locking and unlocking of the differential, using a lever that can be motorized or—as in this example—controlled by a small pneumatic cylinder.

As you can see, differential locks add to a chassis's width significantly. This is why they are unpopular in complex LEGO suspension systems (see Chapter 17), which are quite wide themselves. Still, given the fact that locks are not required on every axle, it's a good idea to install them on nonsteered driven axles, where they fit more easily than on steered ones.

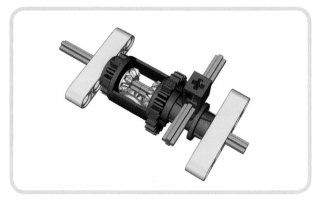

Figure 9-5: With the other LEGO differential variant, things are simpler: Each side of its housing can be engaged directly by a transmission driving ring, thus locking it to one of the outputs and efficiently disabling the differential.

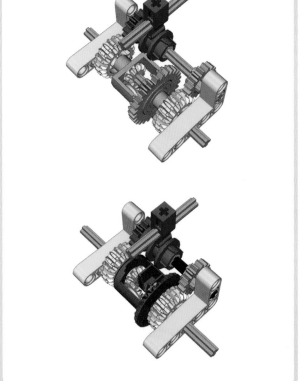

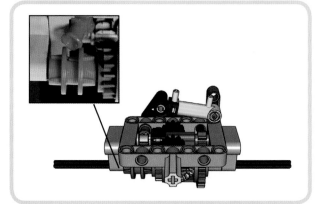

Figure 9-6: Compact nonsteered axle with a differential lock. Note that the transmission driving ring is moved by a common connector piece rather than by the changeover catch. The connector piece moves it without any backlash and is less likely to snap off under stress.

Figure 9-4: LEGO's oldest (top) and newest (bottom) differentials can have locks made of four extra gears and a transmission driving ring, which locks the two outputs together, disabling the differential. With the latest variant, the lock is 1 stud narrower than on the first.

a custom differential

1

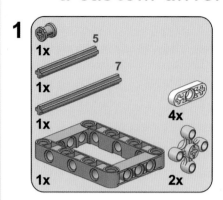

1x · 5
1x · 7
1x
4x
1x · 2x

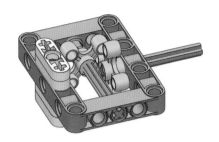

2

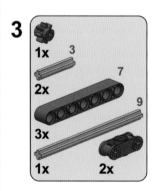

1x
1x · 2x · 5

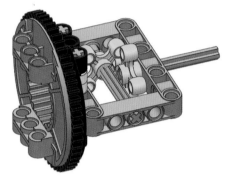

3

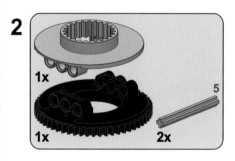

1x · 3
2x · 7
3x · 9
1x · 2x

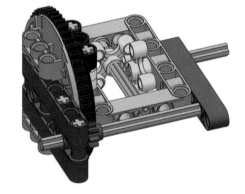

4

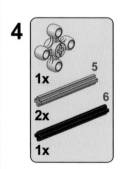

1x · 5
2x · 6
1x

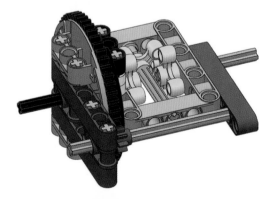

should remain disengaged to allow the differential to function normally and should engage only when a slip situation stops the vehicle. Real off-road vehicles come with manual or automatic locks that engage when a slip situation is detected and disengage when the vehicle drives out of it. LEGO differentials can be locked manually with relative ease; doing this automatically is also possible, but it's extremely complex and impractical. Figures 9-4 and 9-5 show simple manual differential locks for all three variants of ready-made LEGO differentials.

LEGO differential locks use transmission driving rings (#6539) that can be engaged and disengaged using a transmission changeover catch (#6641). The catch can be controlled remotely with a motor or with pneumatics. The latter solution is more convenient if there are many locks on your vehicle that move together with the suspension. Note that it's not necessary to put a lock on every differential on

a vehicle—just one is usually enough to make the vehicle drive out of a slip situation.

Figure 9-6 shows a compact, robust nonsteered axle design based on the 5×7 studless frame. It allows the differential to be driven with a 3:1 gear reduction from the front or rear so that the drive can be transmitted through this axle to the next one. It also allows for easy locking and unlocking of the differential, using a lever that can be motorized or—as in this example—controlled by a small pneumatic cylinder.

As you can see, differential locks add to a chassis's width significantly. This is why they are unpopular in complex LEGO suspension systems (see Chapter 17), which are quite wide themselves. Still, given the fact that locks are not required on every axle, it's a good idea to install them on nonsteered driven axles, where they fit more easily than on steered ones.

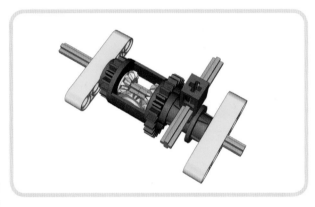

Figure 9-5: With the other LEGO differential variant, things are simpler: Each side of its housing can be engaged directly by a transmission driving ring, thus locking it to one of the outputs and efficiently disabling the differential.

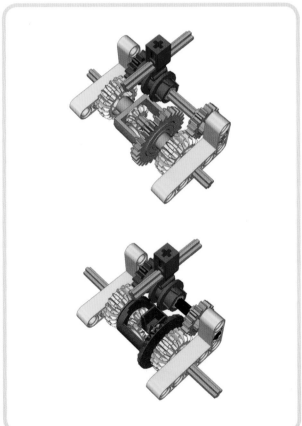

Figure 9-4: LEGO's oldest (top) and newest (bottom) differentials can have locks made of four extra gears and a transmission driving ring, which locks the two outputs together, disabling the differential. With the latest variant, the lock is 1 stud narrower than on the first.

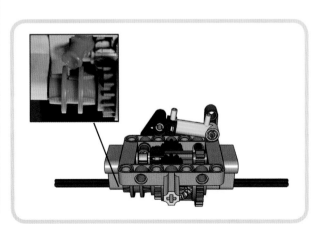

Figure 9-6: Compact nonsteered axle with a differential lock. Note that the transmission driving ring is moved by a common connector piece rather than by the changeover catch. The connector piece moves it without any backlash and is less likely to snap off under stress.

an axle with a differential lock

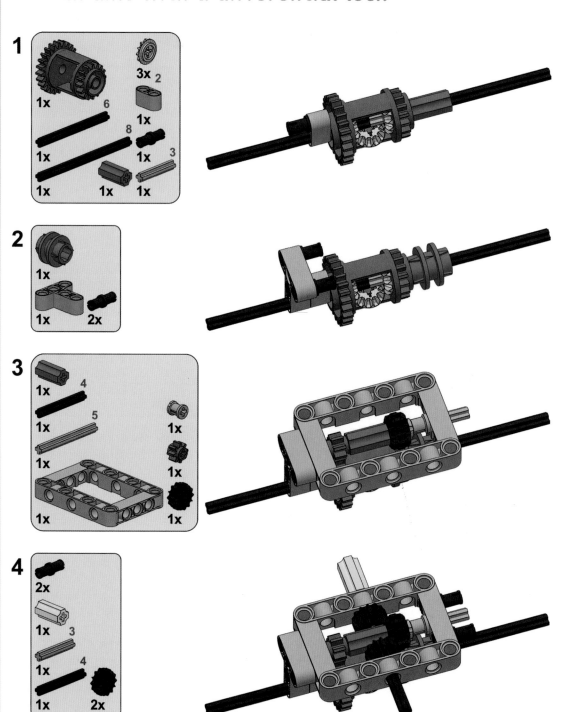

1

3x 2
1x
1x 6
1x 8
1x 3
1x 1x 1x

2

1x
1x 2x

3

1x 4
1x 5
1x 1x
1x
1x 1x

4

2x
1x 3
1x 4
1x 2x

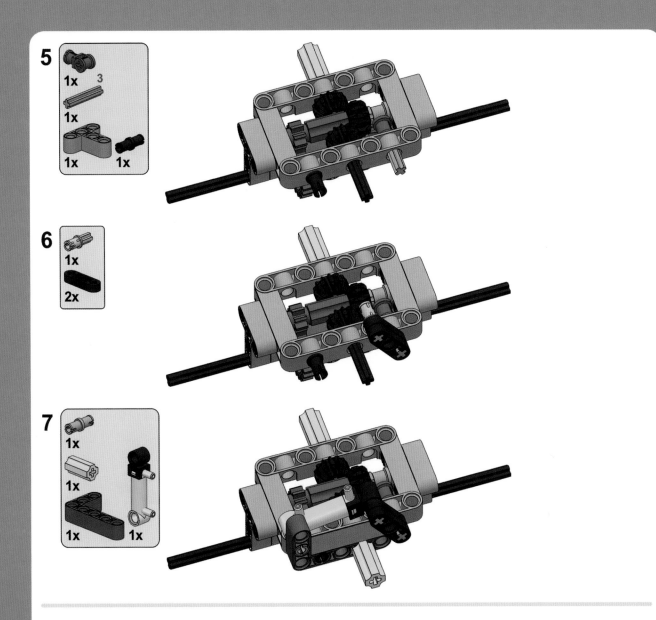

ratchets

We want certain mechanisms to remain locked once they have stopped—for example, a winch on a crane or a rail-crossing barrier. If such mechanisms are motorized, a stopped motor will keep them stopped, but only until the load on the mechanism overcomes the motor's resistance and starts to drive it backward. This scenario is likely in the case of a heavy load, such as what a crane might carry.

One way to lock a mechanism completely is by using a worm gear (discussed in Chapter 6), but a worm gear reduces your speed dramatically and lacks the ability to unlock a mechanism. One better alternative is a ratchet.

A LEGO ratchet has two elements: a freely spinning gear and a *pawl*, the small lever that stops the gear from spinning (see Figure 9-7). The pawl allows a gear to rotate in one direction but blocks it instantly when it starts to rotate in the opposite direction.

To work properly, a pawl needs to have a tip on its end that touches the gear's teeth at a specific angle. As Figure 9-8 shows, if we draw a line coming out of the mounting point of the pawl, this line should aim very slightly below the ratchet's rim. If the line aims too low, the ratchet will lock in both directions. If the line aims too high, the ratchet won't lock at all, bouncing off the teeth rather than stopping rotation.

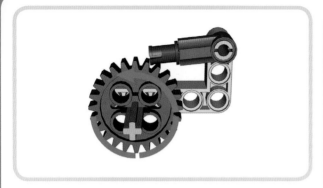

Figure 9-7: A simple pawl (red) securing a 24-tooth ratchet (grey). The ratchet is free to rotate counterclockwise, as indicated by the green arrow, but the moment it starts rotating clockwise, the pawl will lock itself against the nearest tooth (although it's still possible to unlock it by hand).

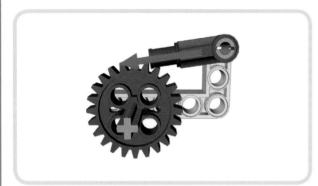

Figure 9-8: The angle of the pawl should be such that the line coming out of its mounting point aims slightly below the gear's rim.

The ratchet's shape also matters a good deal—luckily, a simple pin is perfectly suited for our needs. The pawl also needs to be *balanced* so that its tip tends to drop on the gear under its weight. Ratchets, therefore, are *gravity sensitive*.

NOTE It's possible to create a gravity-independent ratchet by attaching an elastic element, such as a rubber band, that keeps the ratchet pressed down on the wheel just as gravity normally would.

Figure 9-9 shows one possible use of a ratchet—as a means to store the potential energy of springs.

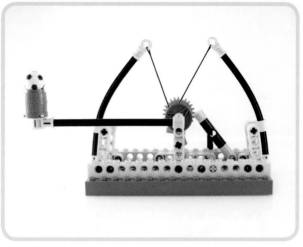

Figure 9-9: My working model of Leonardo da Vinci's leaf spring catapult used a ratchet as a trigger, keeping the catapult loaded and firing it when unlocked. The ratchet was strong enough to store the energy of two bent axles acting as a spring.

linear clutches

A linear clutch works just like the 24-tooth clutch gear described in Chapter 6—it slips under torque. By installing it between a motor and a mechanism, you can prevent the motor from stalling when the mechanism is blocked.

The difference between the linear clutch and the clutch gear is that the clutch gear needs to be meshed with a gear on another axle to work, whereas the linear clutch comes directly between two axles in single line. This saves a lot of space because the linear clutch can simply replace any axle that is at least 4 studs long. The linear clutch also fits between two universal joints that are at least 2 studs apart, and it doesn't need to be supported, so it can work at any angle.

The linear clutch makes use of axle pins with friction. As Figure 9-10 shows, two of these are inserted into a pin joiner, and then their axle ends can be inserted into axle joiners or universal joints, which can be connected to axles of any length. Note that using this clutch for a prolonged period of time will eventually wear down its parts.

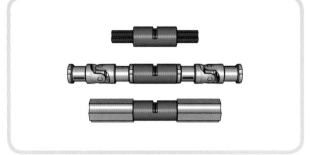

Figure 9-10: Two axle pins (blue) inserted into a pin joiner (red) are the core of the linear clutch (top). They can then be inserted between two axle joiners (middle) or two universal joints (bottom).

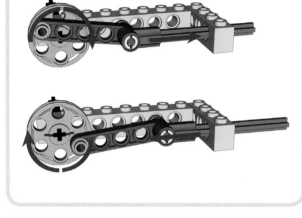

Figure 9-11: An eccentric mechanism with a disc (light grey), a beam (red), and a pushrod (green). The pushrod's travel distance is equal to 2 studs—that is, the disc's diameter minus 1 stud.

eccentric mechanisms

An eccentric mechanism, also called a *crank mechanism*, is used to transform rotary motion into reciprocating motion and vice versa. It's a vital part of almost every car's engine, transforming the linear movement of pistons into the rotation of the driveshaft.

A typical eccentric mechanism consists of a disc and a short beam that connects the disc to a pushrod. As the disc rotates, the beam makes the pushrod move forward and backward along a straight line, as shown in Figure 9-11. Note that if the green pushrod is guided, it has only linear motion. In this case, it is guided by the yellow Technic brick.

The distance the pushrod travels depends on the disc's diameter. The bigger the diameter, the longer the pushrod's travel distance. We can also provide rotational motion using a shorter beam instead of a disc, as shown in Figure 9-12. Here, the distance the pushrod travels depends on the length of the shorter beam.

An eccentric mechanism can also be used to transform rotary motion into rocking motion (that is, partial rotary motion). This type of mechanism, shown in Figure 9-13, has no pushrod; instead, it has a second disc that performs a partial rotation back and forth. The range of its movement depends on the relationship between the two discs' circumferences, and we can adjust the degree of movement by using different-sized discs. For this type of mechanism to work, however, the diameter of the second disc has to be larger than the diameter of the first disc, and the beam's length has to be larger than the first disc's diameter.

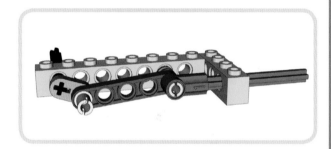

Figure 9-12: An eccentric mechanism with a shorter beam instead of a disc

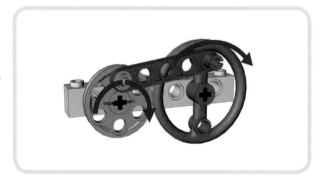

Figure 9-13: An eccentric mechanism with two discs connected by a beam. The smaller disc makes full rotations, and the larger disc makes only partial rotations back and forth.

As shown in Figure 9-14, we can also replace discs with beams in this type of eccentric mechanism. Because the second beam doesn't make a full rotation, the whole mechanism takes up less space. Note that this type of mechanism works only in one direction; you cannot drive the grey beam with the green beam.

Eccentric mechanisms can be put to a variety of uses, appearing in a car's windshield wipers, an oscillating fan, and so forth.

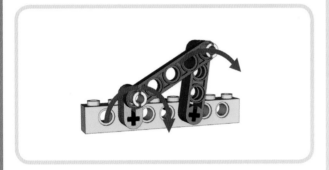

Figure 9-14: An eccentric mechanism with beams instead of discs. Because the second beam (green) makes only a partial rotation, the mechanism takes up less space.

Scotch yokes

A Scotch yoke is a simpler alternative to an eccentric mechanism. It does the same job—converting rotary motion into reciprocating motion and vice versa—while using a smaller number of moving parts. The parts, however, are less common than those in an eccentric mechanism. A Scotch yoke takes more space than an eccentric mechanism but is less likely to fail under high torque.

A Scotch yoke consists of a rectangular frame hung between two sections of an axle. The frame has a slot inside it into which a single pin located on a disc adjacent to the frame enters, as shown in Figure 9-15. As the disc rotates, the pin can go up and down freely inside the slot, but its sideways movement is translated directly to the frame and thus to the axles.

Each rotation of the disc makes the frame move forward and backward by a range equal to the disc's diameter.

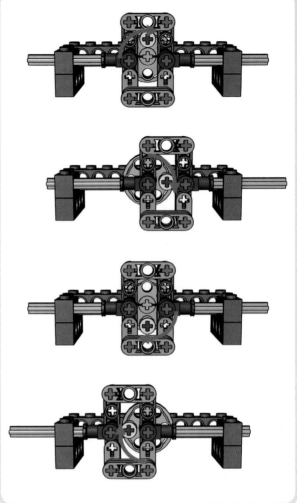

Figure 9-15: Working cycle of the Scotch yoke with a frame (green) and a disc with a single pin (yellow)

The Scotch yoke's range of movement is equal to the disc's diameter, which means that it transforms the movement more efficiently than an eccentric mechanism would. We can increase the range by using a bigger disc and increasing the size of the slot inside the frame accordingly. The height of the slot has to be at least equal to the disc's diameter, which also means that the yoke's movement range is the minimum height of its slot.

a Scotch yoke

1

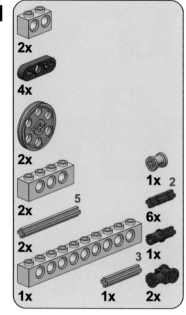

2x
4x
2x
2x
2x
1x

1x 2
6x
1x
3
1x 2x

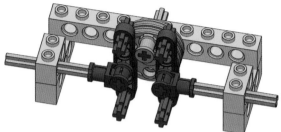

2

4x

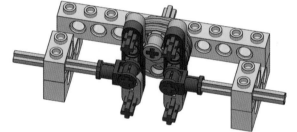

3

4x

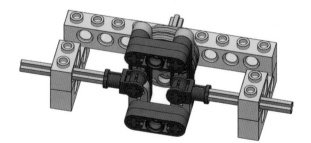

Oldham couplings

An Oldham coupling, also called an *Oldham joint*, is a coupling that transfers drive between an input and an output that are not aligned. While you can use universal joints or even gears to connect a misaligned output and input, these solutions may not always suit your needs. Using two universal joints tends to take a lot of horizontal space, and using gears may result in an unwanted change in torque and speed. An Oldham coupling maintains a 1:1 ratio and takes only a little space, though it is more complex, has a large diameter, and produces extra friction. To see an Oldham coupling in action, visit *http://www.youtube.com/ watch?v=2M9cp_IJ4_I.*

Oldham couplings consist of two identical attachments—one for the input and another for the output—and a single sliding element between them. In the real world, the major advantage of an Oldham coupling is how short it is; in the world of LEGO, we can make an Oldham coupling 3 studs long, which is still only half the space required by two universal joints.

The coupling shown in Figure 9-16 can transfer drive between an input and an output that are misaligned by 1 stud horizontally and 1 stud vertically (the location of the input and output axles is shown in Figure 9-17). It is possible to build such a coupling using longer axles and thus increase the maximum displacement of its input and output. While the coupling will remain 3 studs long, however, its diameter will get significantly larger.

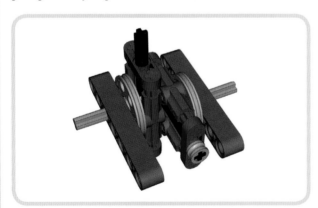

Figure 9-16: An Oldham coupling consists of two identical attachments (blue and red) and an element that slides between them. This Oldham coupling is only 3 studs long.

an Oldham coupling

1

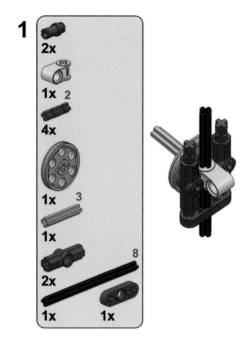

2

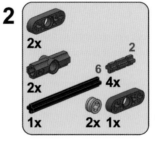
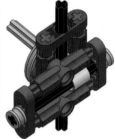

3

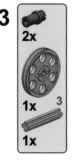
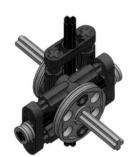

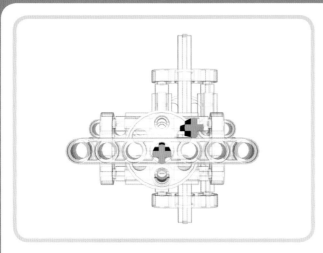

Figure 9-17: The maximum displacement between this Oldham coupling's input and output is 1 stud horizontally and 1 stud vertically. The coupling can be expanded to allow greater displacement at the cost of increasing its diameter.

Schmidt couplings

A Schmidt coupling, like an an Oldham coupling, transfers drive between an input and an output that are not aligned while maintaining a 1:1 ratio between them. It, too, is an alternative to using gears or universal joints to transfer drive.

A Schmidt coupling consists of three discs or triangles, each connected with three links to one another, making six links total. The first disc is attached to the input, the third disc is attached to the output, and the middle disc doesn't need any support—it can work while hanging in midair. Uniquely, this coupling's input and output can move relative to each other because the middle disc equalizes their movement. The coupling can therefore transfer drive between two elements while they are in lateral motion, which is not possible with traditional gearing or Oldham couplings.

We can build a Schmidt coupling with LEGO pieces by using piece #57585 as a base for the triangles, as shown in Figure 9-18 (note that only pins without friction should

be used). The coupling is 5 studs long, but it's extremely robust and can handle greater torque than any alternative solution, including universal joints. It's also mesmerizing to watch. The coupling shown in Figure 9-19 can be moved by up to 5 studs, and we can increase this value by making the triangles' arms longer. The links should be made longer accordingly—however, for the coupling to work, each link (shown in yellow) can be only a little longer than the radius of the triangle.

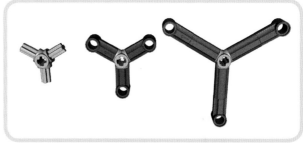

Figure 9-18: LEGO piece #57585 (light grey) can be used to create triangles of various sizes.

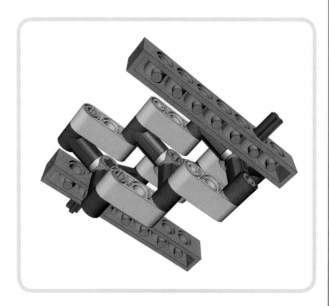

Figure 9-19: A Schmidt coupling with three triangles (in green, red, and blue) and six links (yellow). Note that the middle triangle (red) doesn't need any support—it can even move as the coupling works.

stepper motors

In the real world, stepper motors rotate by a constant angle every time they are turned on instead of rotating continuously. For example, we might have a stepper motor that performs one-quarter of a rotation every time its button is pressed. Such motors are very useful for complex automations of many sorts; real assembly lines are full of stepper motors.

While LEGO does not produce this kind of motor, we can build a custom one mechanically. By adding a simple mechanism to a motor, we can make it work like a stepper motor and use it for a variety of tasks; for example, we can control a sequential gearbox remotely.

To create a stepper motor, we need a knob wheel mounted on a motor's output axle and a beam fastened to that wheel with an elastic element, such as a shock absorber or a rubber band, as shown in Figure 9-20.

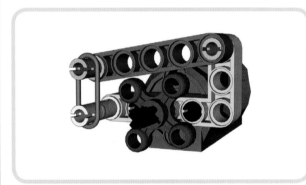

Figure 9-20: The knob on the motor's output axle (blue) has a beam (red) fastened to it at all times by a rubber band (green). This makes a regular motor behave similarly to a stepper motor.

By keeping the beam fastened to the knob at all times, we slow the motor down every quarter rotation (90 degrees). The motor takes a while to overcome the pressure and perform another quarter rotation; its constant rotary movement now becomes intermittent. By turning the motor on for just the right amount of time, we can control it precisely, making it turn by a desired number of rotations. To keep track of the number of rotations, we can watch the knob or simply listen to the sound of the motor, which is quite different from a motor running continuously. Note that this mechanism exerts some pressure on the motor, causing the motor's internal parts to wear down faster than usual.

Geneva mechanisms

A Geneva mechanism (see Figure 9-21), sometimes called a *Geneva drive* or *Maltese cross mechanism*, converts motion between its input and output so that every rotation of the input advances the output by a specific, constant angle. In plain English, that means it converts continuous rotary motion into intermittent rotary motion. A Geneva mechanism may appear odd, but it's quite common. For example, Geneva mechanisms appear in mechanical watches and movie projectors, where they stop every frame of the film for a fraction of a second.

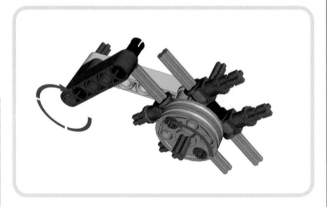

Figure 9-21: A simple Geneva mechanism with an input (red) and an output (green). Each rotation of the input advances the output by a quarter rotation—that is, 90 degrees.

Building a Geneva mechanism with LEGO pieces is a tough job since real Geneva mechanisms use complex circular elements to achieve the desired motion. The following BI shows a relatively simple and small model.

Note that the output of this mechanism can rotate freely when not engaged by the input, while in a real Geneva mechanism, the output remains locked when not engaged by the input. Building a model with LEGO mechanisms in which the output remains locked like this is extremely difficult, and any attempts to do so will result in very large and complex mechanisms. The Geneva mechanism can be simulated in a simple way, though, by putting lots of friction on the green axle. This friction makes the mechanism stop unless engaged by the input.

a Geneva mechanism

1

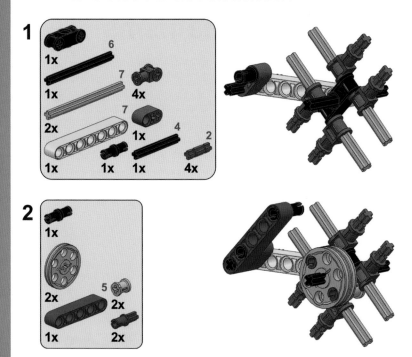

2

reverse lights

Let's assume we have a vehicle on which we want reverse lights that turn on and off automatically when the vehicle backs up. We can create such lighting with a single switch connected to a driveshaft; we just have to block that switch to limit it to the on and off positions only. The Power Functions switch has an *on-off-on* switching pattern, and by blocking one of its extreme positions, we can limit it to *on-off*, as shown in Figure 9-22.

With the switch blocked, all we have to do is connect the axle that goes through it to the driveshaft, using a gear with a clutch so that the switch won't stop the driveshaft once switched, as shown in Figure 9-23. Note that the gear ratio matters here: Any gear reduction from the driveshaft will slow down the switching, and we don't want that. For the switch to react to changes in the driveshaft's direction quickly, we need a 1:1 gear ratio or higher.

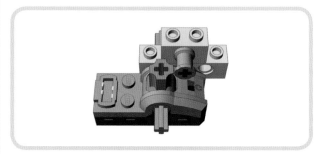

Figure 9-22: In this simple way to limit a Power Functions switch to the on and off positions, the pin prevents the orange switch from moving to the far right on position).

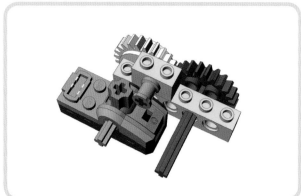

Figure 9-23: A blocked Power Functions switch is connected to a vehicle's driveshaft (red) through a 24-tooth gear with clutch (white).

Any lights connected to the switch in this setup will turn on when the vehicle drives in one direction and off when it drives in another. There's a chance we will get the directions wrong and our reverse lights will turn on when the vehicle goes forward; to fix this, simply change the direction the axle inside the switch rotates by moving the switch to the opposite side of the driveshaft or by adding one more gear between it and the driveshaft. Of course, this mechanism adds the friction of the clutch to the driving system of the gear while the vehicle is moving. This friction causes a loss of power in the drivetrain, a loss that gets bigger with higher driveshaft-to-switch gear ratios.

flashing lights

When we want LEGO lights to flash, we have two options: We can use old 9V bricks with lights (shown in Figure 9-24), which have the built-in ability to flash, or we can use LEGO LEDs from the Power Functions system, which require adding a custom mechanism.

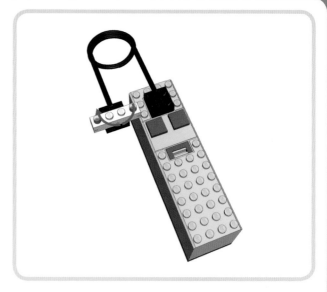

Figure 9-25: A 1×4-stud 9V brick with lights connected to a 9V battery box. By rotating the brick on the plug 180 degrees, we can switch between its lighting modes.

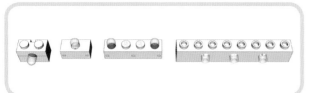

Figure 9-24 Four types of 9V bricks with lights

Depending on the polarity of the power supply, 9V bricks with lights are programmed to provide steady light or to flash. To switch between the two modes, change the orientation of one of the plugs of the wire connecting the brick to the power supply—or, more simply, rotate the brick on the plug 180 degrees, as shown in Figure 9-25.

Bricks with lights, however, have a number of disadvantages when compared to LEGO LEDs. Most importantly, they are long out of production, so it's difficult and expensive to find a brick in good working condition today. Secondly, they use tiny incandescent light bulbs, which means that they consume a lot power, are prone to failure, and produce a strong yellowish light in all directions, as shown in Figure 9-26. LEGO LEDs are free from all these disadvantages, and they fit in much smaller spaces. Their only drawback is the lack of a built-in ability to flash, which we can add mechanically.

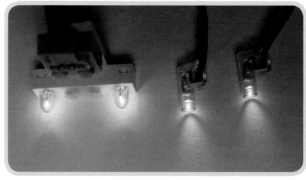

Figure 9-26: A 1×4-stud 9V brick with lights (left) and a pair of Power Functions LED lights (right). Note the difference in the color and direction of the light.

To make LEGO LEDs flash, we need a switch and a motor. Using an old 9V switch is the easy way, but we can use a Power Functions switch as well, which we can connect via an eccentric mechanism. Figures 9-27 and 9-28 show both versions.

With the old 9V switch, adding the ability to flash is simple: The switch can be connected directly to a motor whose rotary motion will keep turning it on and off, thus making the lights connected to the switch flash. The flashing frequency can be adjusted by adding a gear between the

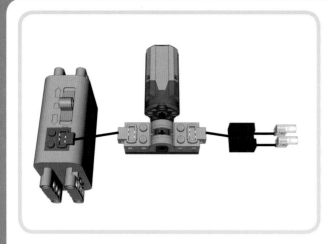

Figure 9-27: The old 9V switch

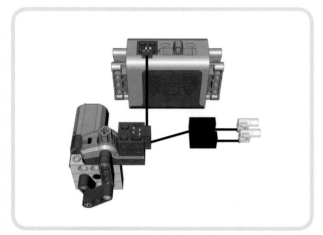

Figure 9-28: The Power Functions switch

motor and the switch or by changing the motor's speed. Note that Power Functions extension/adapter wires are needed to use the old 9V switch with Power Functions LEDs and power supplies. The old 9V power supply requires no adapter.

The Power Functions switch needs to be motorized through an eccentric mechanism to make the lights connected to it flash. The eccentric mechanism keeps the switch going back and forth through its three positions (*on-off-on*).

turn signals

Now that we've covered how to make LEGO lights flash, we can take this knowledge one step further and create turn signals for our vehicle.

To create turn signals, we need to extend our flashing-light mechanism by connecting two more switches to it. The resulting device will be controlled by a single motor and will have two groups of LEDs connected to it; one will flash or the other will, depending on the motor's direction.

Since we discussed how to make a flashing-light mechanism in the previous section, let's focus on the two extra switches. We need to hard-couple them so that turning one switch on turns the other off. The coupling can be done with two gears, preferably two 16-tooth gears (as shown on the left in Figure 9-29), because they are the smallest gears accurate enough, or two half bushes with teeth (as shown on the right in Figure 9-29). The important thing is to keep the two axles going through the two switches at slightly different angles so both switches can't be turned on or off at the same time.

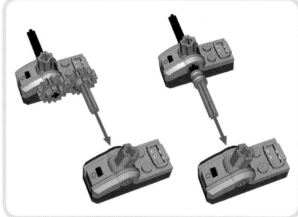

Figure 9-29: Hard-coupling two Power Functions switches with gears (left) and toothed half bushes (right). Note that the angle of axles coupled this way differs, preventing the two switches from being turned on or off simultaneously.

Next, with the two switches hard-coupled at different angles, we need to block one of them in the same way as with the reverse lights described earlier in this chapter (see Figure 9-30). We will limit the switching pattern from *on-off-on* to *on-off*. Since the switches are hard-coupled, both will be blocked.

Now we have to connect the axle of one of the switches to the input of the flashing-light mechanism. A gear with a clutch is needed to allow the input to keep running after the switches are switched, as shown in Figures 9-31 and 9-32.

The only thing left to do at this point is to connect all these elements electrically. A connection scheme for the variant with the 9V switch is shown in Figure 9-33. The

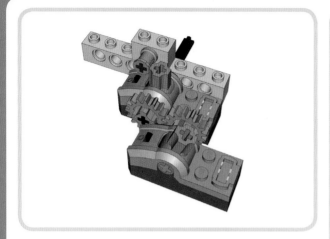

Figure 9-30: Two hard-coupled switches with one of them blocked. The hard-coupling makes the block work on both switches.

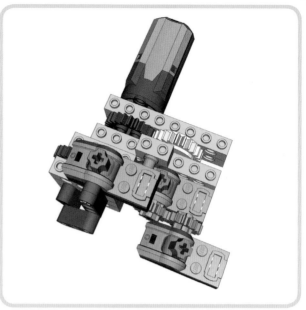

Figure 9-32: A more complex variant uses the Power Functions switch and an eccentric mechanism to make lights flash. The gear is identical to that of the previous figure.

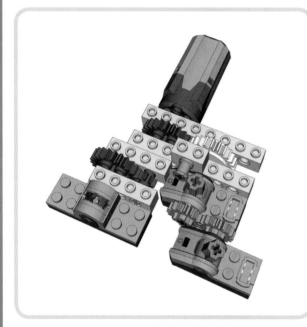

Figure 9-31: Two hard-coupled switches connected to a motorized flashing-light mechanism that uses an old 9V switch. Note the gear down between the motor and the 9V switch—it lowers the flashing rate of the lights to a realistic value.

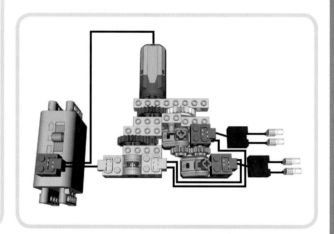

Figure 9-33: Electric connection scheme for the simpler mechanism variant. For a remote-controlled model, you should connect the master switch to the same IR receiver as the motor.

variant with the Power Functions switch follows the same pattern: The *master switch* (the one used in the flashing-light mechanism) is connected to the same power source/control module as the motor. The two *child switches* (the hard-coupled ones) are connected to the master switch and have lights connected to them. Thus, as the master switch creates a flashing effect, the child switches control which group of lights is flashing at the moment. You can switch between the two groups by changing the motor's direction.

Note that there is no limit to the number of flashing lights we can control with this method. And the same motor that controls this mechanism can be used to steer the vehicle that houses it, making the turn signals work automatically as you steer your model!

complex turn signals

1

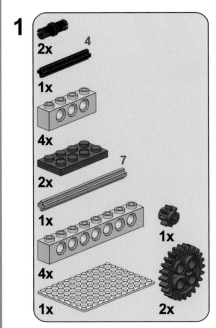

2x
4
1x
4x
2x 7
1x
1x
4x
1x 2x

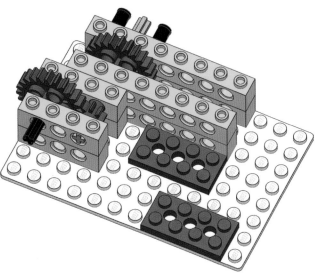

2

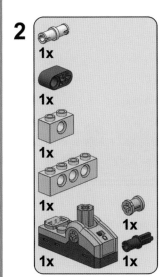

1x
1x
1x
1x
1x
1x 1x
1x

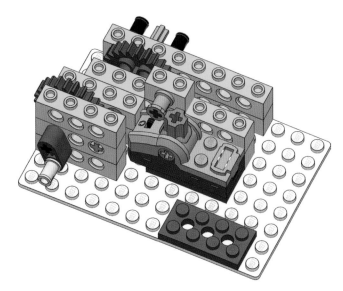

3

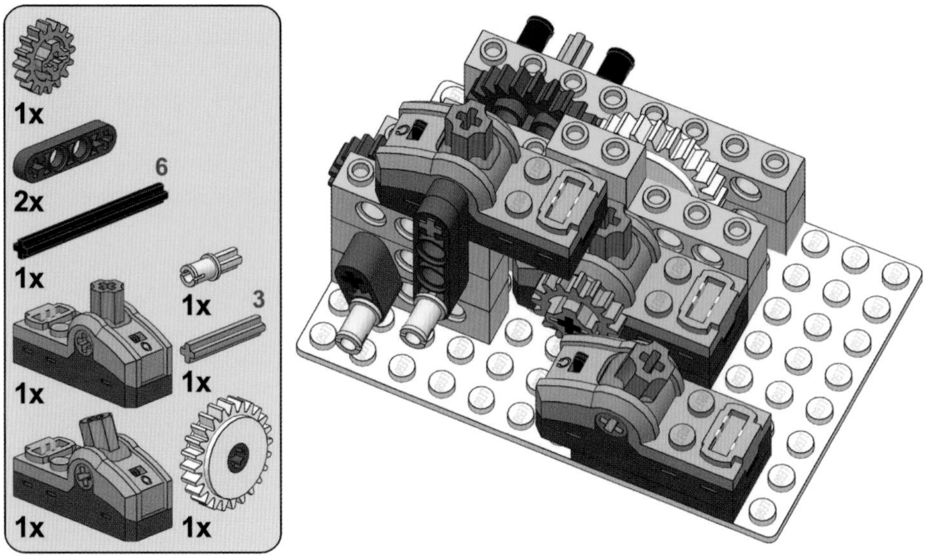

1x
2x   6
1x   1x   3
1x   1x

4

1x   3
1x   3
1x
1x

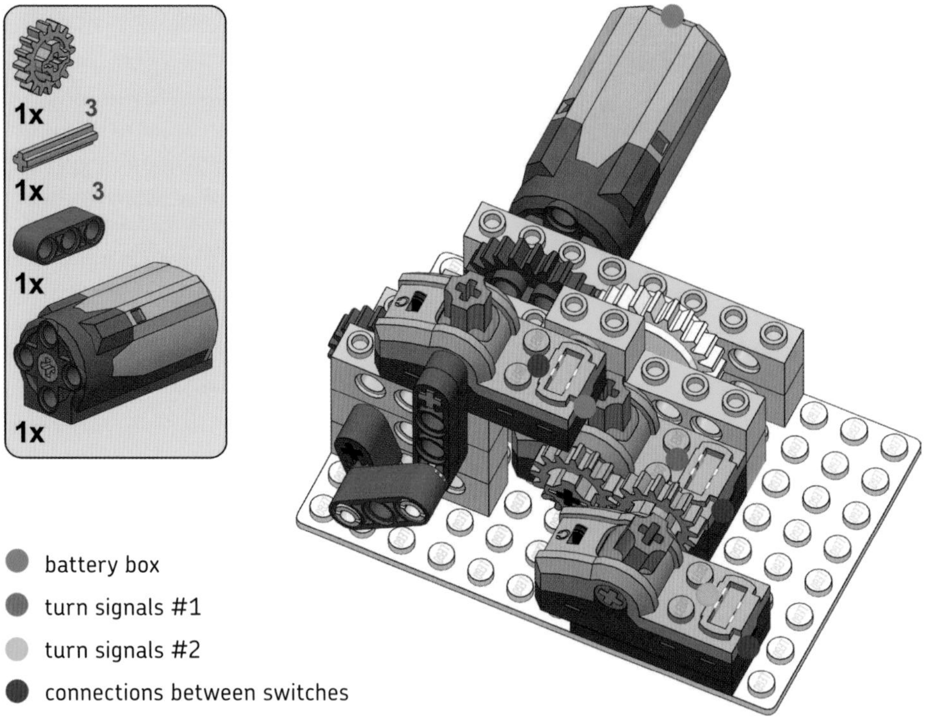

● battery box
● turn signals #1
● turn signals #2
● connections between switches

double-axle turntable transmission

Transmitting drive through a Technic turntable is quite easy with just one axle—we just have to put the axle through the turntable's center. However, one axle is not enough for some vehicles. Tracked excavators, for instance, need two separate axles to drive the right and left tracks, and their propulsion motors are often located in the superstructure, which is separated from the chassis by a turntable. In such a case, we can use a transmission driving ring (as shown in Figure 9-34) or an empty differential housing (as shown in Figure 9-35).

The disadvantage of such a transmission system, other than its complexity, is that when the superstructure rotates relative to the chassis, one of the axles is affected by its movement: the blue one in Figures 9-34 and 9-35. The axle is actually driven by the superstructure's movement, causing the whole chassis to turn. However, as the superstructure's rotation is usually slow, the effect is negligible, and it can be further minimized by gearing down both axles below the turntable. The advantage is that this transmission system allows you to build a tracked vehicle with all the electric elements in the superstructure. This means that no wires go through the turntable, which enables the superstructure to rotate any number of times without the risk of damaging any elements going through it.

Both variants can be built in a similar way. However, as the transmission driving ring variant is more practical, we will focus on it. The building instructions for this variant are shown next. Notice that the chassis and the superstructure can be easily built around this variant.

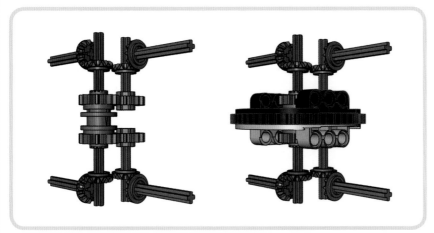

Figure 9-34: Scheme for transmitting drive through a turntable for two axles independently. Elements transmitting the drive are marked red and blue to show their independence. This variant uses a transmission driving ring to transmit drive over the blue axle that goes through the turntable's center. Note that there is no axle joiner inside the driving ring, so it rotates freely on the axle.

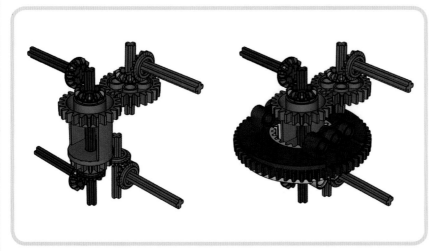

Figure 9-35: The same transmission system with an empty differential housing instead of a transmission driving ring. This variant is simpler but less practical because of the large 24-tooth gear on the housing.

a double-axle turntable transmission

1

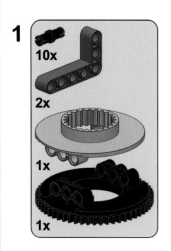

10x

2x

1x

1x

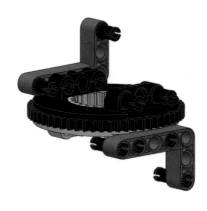

2

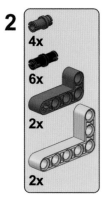

4x

6x

2x

2x

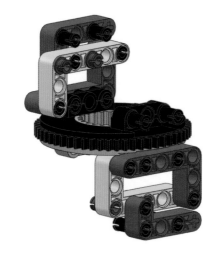

3

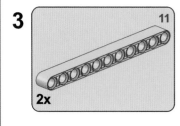

11

2x

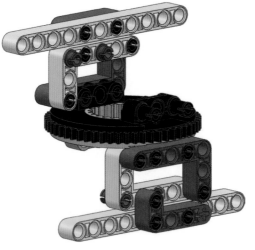

4

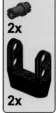

2x

2x

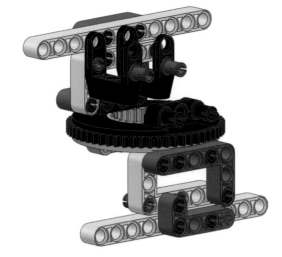

5

2x

1x

1x   3

1x

1x   7

1x   3x

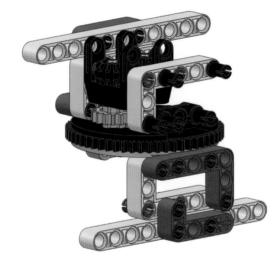

6

1x

1x   11

1x   2x

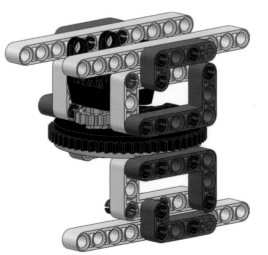

7

1x 7
1x 8 2x

8

2x
2x
1x

9

2x
1x 3
1x
2x 2x

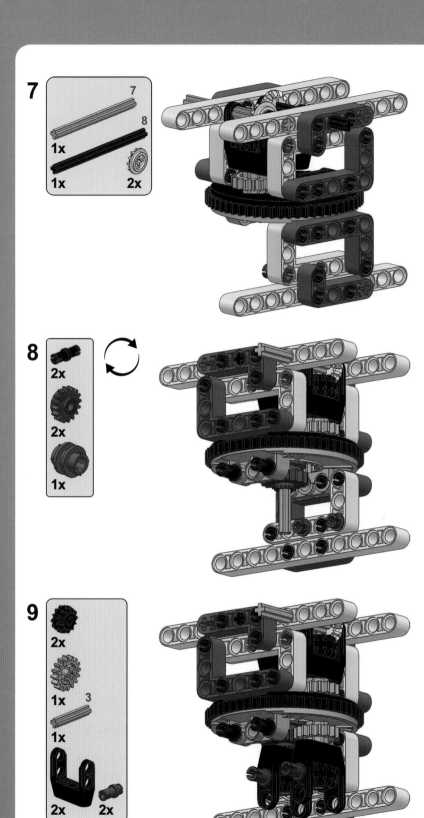

10

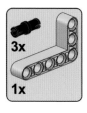

3x

1x

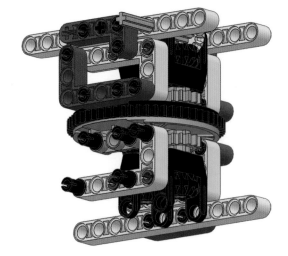

11

1x

1x

11

1x 2x

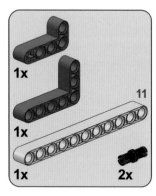

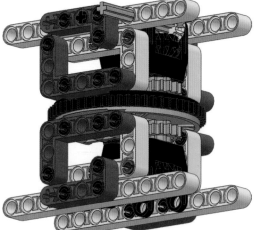

12

7

8

1x

1x 2x

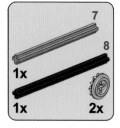

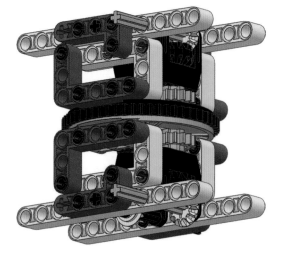

a sturdy
universal joint

While ready-made LEGO universal joints have a number of advantages, they are prone to failure when subjected to high torque. We can build a custom universal joint out of basic pieces that will act the same while being more robust, at the cost of bigger size (shown in Figure 9-36).

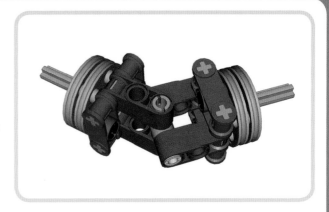

Figure 9-36: A custom universal joint is more robust but also larger than ready-made ones.

a universal joint

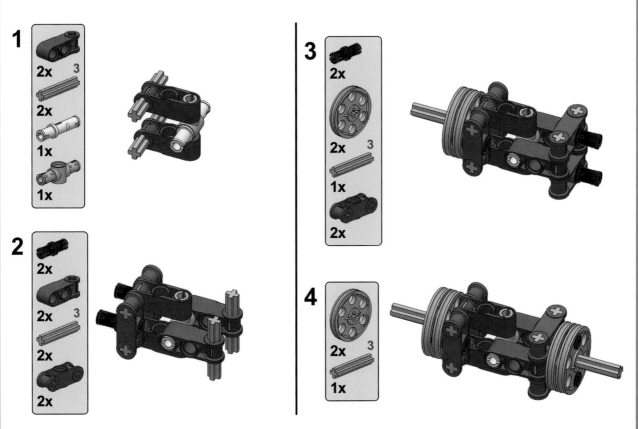

10

the LEGO pneumatic system

the Old system

The LEGO pneumatic system is a miniature model of real-life pneumatic and hydraulic systems. It consists of three basic modules: a *pressure generator*, such as a manual pump or a motorized compressor; a *control module*, which is one or more valves that direct the flow of air; and *cylinders*, which convert pressure to linear movement. The modules are connected by elastic pneumatic hoses that allow air to travel between them.

The basic working principle of a pneumatic system is based on the tendency of air to move from areas of high pressure to areas of low pressure. The pressure generator fills the pneumatic system with pressurized air, and then the air is directed to the cylinders using the control module, which makes the cylinders extend or retract. When the pressure of the system is equalized, all movement stops.

Every pneumatic system has limited capacity for air pressure. In LEGO models, that limit is normally three bars, which is roughly equivalent to three times atmospheric pressure. If a LEGO pressure generator exceeds this capacity, the pneumatic hoses may pop off the ports of pneumatic pieces.

Because the LEGO pneumatic system relies on hoses and ports, it is not perfectly airtight and is subject to leaks. Leaks usually occur at the ends of pneumatic hoses (or in the middle if they're damaged). These leaks result in reduced efficiency. And of course, as with any mechanical system, complexity is the enemy of efficiency in pneumatics.

NOTE Although LEGO connectors in the pneumatic system are technically called *inlets* and *outlets*, I'll call them *ports* for the sake of simplicity.

Three LEGO pneumatic systems exist: an Old, New, and V2 system. Each works a bit differently, as described in the following sections.

Introduced in 1984, the Old LEGO pneumatic system (shown in Figure 10-1) is relatively complex. Its control module includes two interconnected pieces and one pneumatic hose that connects the pressure generator to the cylinders. Although the last LEGO set that included the Old system was released in 1987, this durable system continues to be available secondhand.

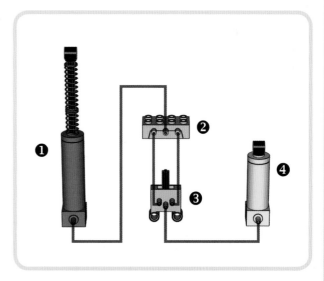

Figure 10-1: The Old-style pneumatic system uses two blocks to control airflow. The grey lines in this diagram represent hoses.

The *pump* shown in red at ❶ usually has a spring. When the pump is pushed, it pumps the surrounding air through its port; when the pump is released, the spring returns the pump to its initial rest position.

The light-grey element at ❷ is a *distribution block*, which includes a special *one-way valve*. Air is delivered from the pump into the distribution block's middle port, and the one-way valve forces the two side ports to pump air in only one direction: The port on the left takes air in, and the port on the right expels it.

The light-grey element at ❸ is a valve, which is connected to the distribution block by two hoses. A single distribution block can be connected to many valves using forked hoses. The total number of valves depends on how many pneumatic cylinders are meant to be controlled independently.

The valve has a lever that can be switched to one of three positions. One position extends all connected cylinders, another retracts the cylinders, and the third (middle) position cuts the connection that goes through the valve, effectively locking all cylinders. This third position is called *neutral*, and it's needed when you have many valves in a system because it prevents the valves from interfering with each other. The yellow element at ❹ is a cylinder; it extends when air is delivered to it and retracts when air is sucked from it.

NOTE When a cylinder is subjected to suction, the air pressure inside it drops until it becomes lower than the atmospheric pressure surrounding it (one bar), at which point the cylinder starts to retract. For this reason, the LEGO pneumatic system can exert up to three bars of pressure for extension but only up to one bar of pressure for retraction.

Compared to the other pneumatic systems, the Old system has the following advantages:

* It only takes one hose to connect a cylinder to a valve.
* Cylinders are available in both yellow and red.

The Old system also has the following disadvantages:

* The control module requires two hoses for every valve connected to the distribution block, making it somewhat complex.
* Cylinders are retracted with much less force than they are extended with, which can make some functions underpowered.

* Some unique pieces (like a distribution block) are needed that are only available secondhand because they haven't been produced since 1987.
* The system has limited compatibility with other systems.

the New system

The LEGO Group introduced the New pneumatic system (shown in Figure 10-2) in 1989. With its goal of simplicity and efficiency, the New system eliminated the distribution block and redesigned the pumps and cylinders, although it kept the Old valves. This New system is more similar to real pneumatic and hydraulic systems.

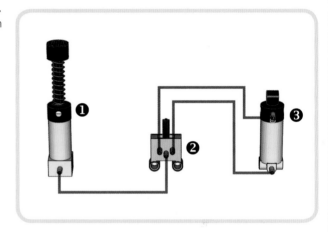

Figure 10-2: The New pneumatic system uses a simple design.

The yellow element at ❶ in Figure 10-2 is a spring-loaded pump. The light-grey valve at ❷ is the same as the valve in the Old system except it connects a bit differently: Air is delivered into it through the middle port, and its side ports are connected to the cylinder. Either valve's port can be connected to either cylinder's port; this connection determines which of the valve's two extreme positions makes the cylinder extend or retract.

The yellow element at ❸ is a cylinder. It extends or retracts depending on which port the air is delivered to.

Unlike the Old system, the New one expels air through the valves, resulting in distinctive hissing sounds when valves are switched under high pressure. Also, because the New system doesn't use suction, retraction is only slightly weaker than extension.

the LEGO pneumatic system

The LEGO pneumatic system is a miniature model of real-life pneumatic and hydraulic systems. It consists of three basic modules: a *pressure generator*, such as a manual pump or a motorized compressor; a *control module*, which is one or more valves that direct the flow of air; and *cylinders*, which convert pressure to linear movement. The modules are connected by elastic pneumatic hoses that allow air to travel between them.

The basic working principle of a pneumatic system is based on the tendency of air to move from areas of high pressure to areas of low pressure. The pressure generator fills the pneumatic system with pressurized air, and then the air is directed to the cylinders using the control module, which makes the cylinders extend or retract. When the pressure of the system is equalized, all movement stops.

Every pneumatic system has limited capacity for air pressure. In LEGO models, that limit is normally three bars, which is roughly equivalent to three times atmospheric pressure. If a LEGO pressure generator exceeds this capacity, the pneumatic hoses may pop off the ports of pneumatic pieces.

Because the LEGO pneumatic system relies on hoses and ports, it is not perfectly airtight and is subject to leaks. Leaks usually occur at the ends of pneumatic hoses (or in the middle if they're damaged). These leaks result in reduced efficiency. And of course, as with any mechanical system, complexity is the enemy of efficiency in pneumatics.

NOTE Although LEGO connectors in the pneumatic system are technically called *inlets* and *outlets*, I'll call them *ports* for the sake of simplicity.

Three LEGO pneumatic systems exist: an Old, New, and V2 system. Each works a bit differently, as described in the following sections.

the Old system

Introduced in 1984, the Old LEGO pneumatic system (shown in Figure 10-1) is relatively complex. Its control module includes two interconnected pieces and one pneumatic hose that connects the pressure generator to the cylinders. Although the last LEGO set that included the Old system was released in 1987, this durable system continues to be available secondhand.

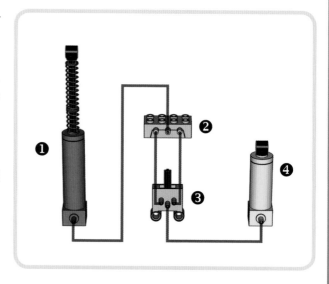

Figure 10-1: The Old-style pneumatic system uses two blocks to control airflow. The grey lines in this diagram represent hoses.

The *pump* shown in red at ❶ usually has a spring. When the pump is pushed, it pumps the surrounding air through its port; when the pump is released, the spring returns the pump to its initial rest position.

The light-grey element at ❷ is a *distribution block*, which includes a special *one-way valve*. Air is delivered from the pump into the distribution block's middle port, and the one-way valve forces the two side ports to pump air in only one direction: The port on the left takes air in, and the port on the right expels it.

The light-grey element at ❸ is a valve, which is connected to the distribution block by two hoses. A single distribution block can be connected to many valves using forked hoses. The total number of valves depends on how many pneumatic cylinders are meant to be controlled independently.

The valve has a lever that can be switched to one of three positions. One position extends all connected cylinders, another retracts the cylinders, and the third (middle) position cuts the connection that goes through the valve, effectively locking all cylinders. This third position is called *neutral*, and it's needed when you have many valves in a system because it prevents the valves from interfering with each other. The yellow element at ❹ is a cylinder; it extends when air is delivered to it and retracts when air is sucked from it.

NOTE When a cylinder is subjected to suction, the air pressure inside it drops until it becomes lower than the atmospheric pressure surrounding it (one bar), at which point the cylinder starts to retract. For this reason, the LEGO pneumatic system can exert up to three bars of pressure for extension but only up to one bar of pressure for retraction.

Compared to the other pneumatic systems, the Old system has the following advantages:

* It only takes one hose to connect a cylinder to a valve.
* Cylinders are available in both yellow and red.

The Old system also has the following disadvantages:

* The control module requires two hoses for every valve connected to the distribution block, making it somewhat complex.
* Cylinders are retracted with much less force than they are extended with, which can make some functions underpowered.

* Some unique pieces (like a distribution block) are needed that are only available secondhand because they haven't been produced since 1987.
* The system has limited compatibility with other systems.

the New system

The LEGO Group introduced the New pneumatic system (shown in Figure 10-2) in 1989. With its goal of simplicity and efficiency, the New system eliminated the distribution block and redesigned the pumps and cylinders, although it kept the Old valves. This New system is more similar to real pneumatic and hydraulic systems.

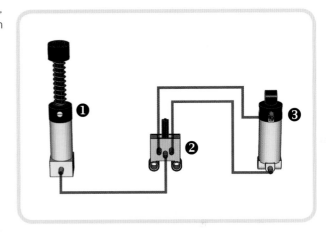

Figure 10-2: The New pneumatic system uses a simple design.

The yellow element at ❶ in Figure 10-2 is a spring-loaded pump. The light-grey valve at ❷ is the same as the valve in the Old system except it connects a bit differently: Air is delivered into it through the middle port, and its side ports are connected to the cylinder. Either valve's port can be connected to either cylinder's port; this connection determines which of the valve's two extreme positions makes the cylinder extend or retract.

The yellow element at ❸ is a cylinder. It extends or retracts depending on which port the air is delivered to.

Unlike the Old system, the New one expels air through the valves, resulting in distinctive hissing sounds when valves are switched under high pressure. Also, because the New system doesn't use suction, retraction is only slightly weaker than extension.

You can swap the cylinders between the Old and New systems, but the cylinders from the Old system will perform poorly due to their different internal construction.

Compared to the other pneumatic systems, the New system has the following advantages:

* A simple control module (no distribution block).
* Similar force is exerted by the cylinders when extending and retracting.
* Widely available and the most produced system to date.
* Two large cylinders can be joined together for doubled range.
* Fully compatible with the V2 system.

The New system has the following disadvantages:

* Uses two hoses to connect every cylinder.
* The cylinders are usually available only in yellow.

the V2 system

Introduced in 2015, the V2 system isn't a brand-new system: It's an update of the New system and is fully compatible with it. The ports in V2 pneumatic elements are stepped and have reinforced tops (see Figure 10-3), and there are new, longer cylinders. The pneumatic hoses are also made of more elastic material and connect more easily. But despite all of these improved features, the V2 system is 100 percent compatible with the New system and has the same working principles.

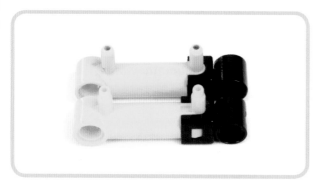

Figure 10-3: A small pneumatic cylinder from the New system (top) and one from the V2 system (bottom). They are identical in size, capacity, and performance, but the V2 version comes with a reinforced top and stepped ports that make connecting hoses easier.

Compared to the other pneumatic systems, the V2 system has the following advantages:

* Ports and hoses are easier to connect.
* Longer cylinders are available.
* Full compatibility with the New system.

The V2 system has the following disadvantages:

* Rare and expensive pieces; as of this writing, the V2 system is present in only two LEGO sets, the least expensive of which is $119.99.
* All cylinders are yellow.
* There's no way to join two long cylinders.

an inventory of pneumatic parts

Because most pneumatic parts are compatible with more than one system, the following inventory organizes them into four categories: pumps, control modules, cylinders, and miscellaneous pieces. The system from which a particular part comes is included in parentheses next to its name. The parts within a category are listed from oldest to newest.

NOTE Whenever possible, the pneumatic parts are shown fully extended for clarity. However, when length is given as part of the name (for example, the 6L pump), it refers to length of the part when retracted, not extended.

pumps

All pneumatic pumps can get hot from working fast for a prolonged period of time. Additionally, large pumps can generate higher pressure (over 30 pounds per square inch) than smaller pumps (up to 10-12 psi). For safety reasons, each pump type has a different threshold pressure that, when exceeded, makes air escape the pump.

large pneumatic pump (Old)

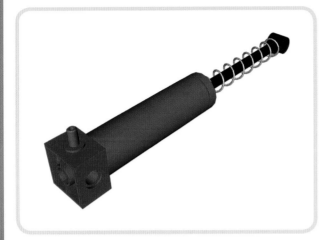

The large pneumatic pump (Old) is fitted with a single port and a spring-loaded rod. It comes in red and yellow, and it is 11 studs long (except for a rare variant with a 13-stud rod). It draws air in from the outside when the rod is pushed; when the rod is released, the spring returns it to its initial, neutral position.

The pump's bottom can be mounted on studs, and both sides have regular Technic holes. The size of the lower end (the one with the port) is 2×2 studs, and the upper end's is 1×1. The pump's upper end is ill-suited for manual pumping—it feels uncomfortable against a finger.

large pneumatic pump (New)

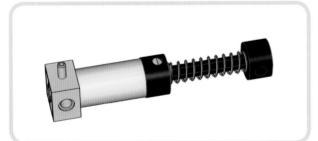

The large pneumatic pump (New) usually comes in yellow, but a rare, transparent light blue one is also available. Like the Old system's pump, it contains one port and a spring-loaded rod. It works just like the old pump does, and its dimensions are almost identical except for the addition of a contact pad on its upper end. This contact pad makes operating the pump with your finger more comfortable than operating the Old system's pump.

small 5.5L pneumatic pump (New)

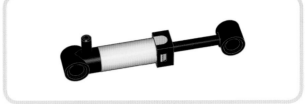

The small 5.5L pneumatic pump (New) with one port has a rod that extends by 2 studs and no spring. It works best when it's used with a motor rather than operated manually, which makes it perfect for motorized compressors. It has much lower capacity than larger pumps, which makes it less prone to overheating but also less efficient. This is why motorized compressors often include more than one such pump. It comes in yellow, blue, and transparent light blue.

small 6L pneumatic pump (New)

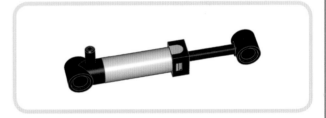

Introduced in 2011 to replace the 5.5L pump, the small 6L pneumatic pump (New) is identical except for its length. Its rod extends by 2 studs, too, but because it's 6 studs long, there is no half-stud displacement between its top and bottom, making it much easier to use. Despite its increased length, it has the same capacity and efficiency as the 5.5L version. It comes exclusively in light grey.

small 6L pneumatic pump (V2)

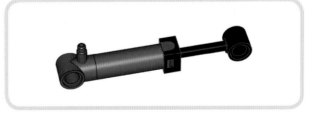

The small 6L pneumatic pump (V2) is identical to the New system's version except it has a stepped port. It comes only in blue, and unlike other small pumps, it has a blue bottom as well.

control modules

This section describes pieces created exclusively to control the movement of pneumatic cylinders—namely, the pneumatic valve, which has two variants. The Old pneumatic system also includes a special piece, the distribution block, but it has to do with management of the hoses and doesn't actually provide the means to control anything.

distribution block (Old)

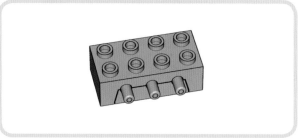

The distribution block is light grey and is the same size as a 2×4×1 LEGO brick. It's used exclusively in the Old pneumatic system for connecting a pump to valves and hasn't been produced since 1987. It has three ports on one side, and air is delivered to the middle port. An interior one-way valve affects how the ports work: The middle port allows air to flow both ways, the left port allows air to flow in only, and the right port allows air to flow out. If you use the ports incorrectly, the valve will close, stopping all air circulation inside the block. The valve will reopen when you connect the ports properly. Note that the block can work with any kind of pneumatic valve—Old, New, and V2 alike.

valve with studs (Old & New)

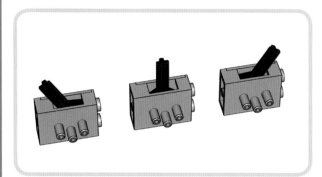

The valve with studs is the size of two 1×2 bricks and a 1×2 plate stacked, and it's always light grey. It has three ports on one side, and air is delivered to the middle port.

A lever (roughly 1.5 studs long) on one of the valve's narrow sides can be switched to one of three positions. The middle position, or *neutral*, cuts the connection inside the valve, effectively disconnecting the side ports from the rest of the pneumatic system. The left and right positions control the flow of air through the valve's side ports, as shown in Figure 10-4, making cylinders connected to these ports extend or retract. (The valve does not actively take in air; it only receives air through its ports and expels it through the hole that houses the lever.)

A valve can be attached on the top or bottom of any studded LEGO piece. It can also be braced between two 1×2 Technic bricks whose pin holes are then exactly 3 studs apart (see Figure 10-5).

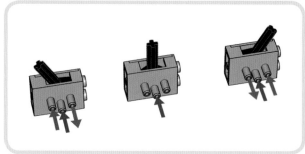

Figure 10-4: The direction of airflow through the valve's ports: Blue arrows show air coming from the pump, green arrows indicate air coming out of the valve to the cylinder, and red arrows indicate air returning from the cylinder to the valve.

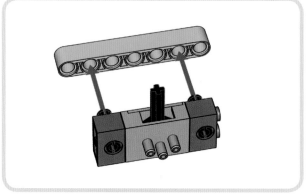

Figure 10-5: By placing a 1×2 Technic brick on each end of the valve, you can connect the valve to a brick or beam that is at least 5 pin holes long.

valve with no studs (New)

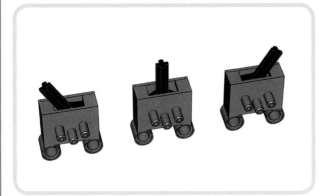

Introduced in 2003, the valve with no studs (New) works the same as the valve with studs. Aside from the color (dark grey only), the only difference is its lack of studs and the addition of two pin holes, 1 stud apart, on one side of the valve. These changes make it better suited for studless constructions. Also, because the valve's points of attachment are on one side and the valve's lever is on the other, the lever remains conveniently exposed when the valve is attached to something.

valve with no studs (V2)

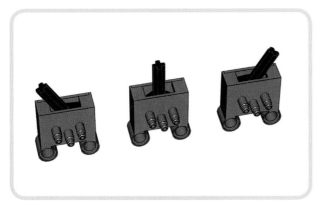

The valve with no studs (V2) is identical to the New system's valve except that it has stepped ports.

cylinders

The New and V2 system cylinders are fully compatible with each other and can be swapped between systems. However, the Old system cylinders have limited compatibility.

medium cylinder (Old)

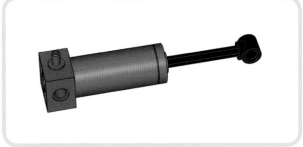

The medium cylinder (Old) includes a single port and a plastic rod that extends by nearly 4 studs. Its base can be mounted on studs or connected with pins. Available in yellow and red, its dimensions are the same as those of the Old large pump. However, unlike the Old pump, it has no spring. The cylinder's upper part expels air when extending and draws it in from the outside when retracting, and the cylinder exerts more force when extending than it does when retracting. It's only partially useful with the New pneumatic system because it can be extended but not retracted.

large 9L cylinder (Old)

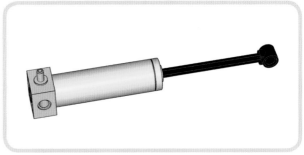

The large 9L cylinder (Old) is basically just a longer version of the Old system's medium cylinder. It has a single port and a plastic rod that extends by 6 studs. Its plastic rod and long reach make it more likely to break under stress than any other cylinder.

As with all Old-style cylinders, its upper part expels air when extending and draws it from the outside when retracting, and it exerts more force when extending than when retracting. And, just as with the regular large cylinder, its usefulness in the New system is limited because the New system doesn't allow it to retract.

small cylinder (New)

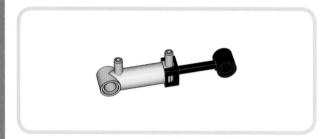

The New system's small cylinder has two ports and a plastic rod that extends by 2 studs. It comes in yellow and transparent light blue.

This rare and expensive pneumatic piece is easily confused with the small pneumatic pump. Despite its inability to exert large force due to its small capacity, this cylinder is valued for its small size.

medium cylinder with square base (New)

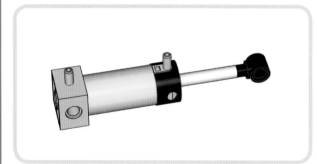

The New system's medium cylinder has two ports and a robust metal rod that extends by nearly 4 studs. It's similar in size to the large pneumatic pump. Its base can be mounted on studs or connected with pins.

medium cylinder with round base (New)

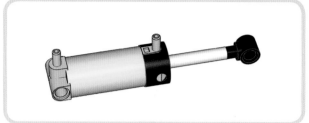

Introduced in 2002, the updated round-base version of the medium cylinder (New) has two ports and a metal rod that extends by nearly 4 studs. The only difference between this cylinder and the previous one is its round rather than square base; it can't be mounted on studs, but it can be connected with pins. The cylinder also needs less space around its base to pivot, making it more convenient than the square-based cylinder in most cases.

small cylinder (V2)

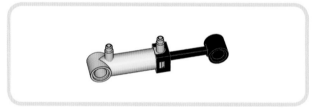

The small cylinder (V2) is identical to the New system's small cylinder except that it has stepped ports, its top part is reinforced, and—just like all V2 cylinders—it comes only in yellow.

large 1x1 cylinder (V2)

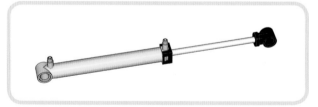

The large 1×1 cylinder (V2) is a new kind of part. It has two stepped ports and a metal rod. It's only 1 stud wide and deep, but it is 11 studs long and extends to a whopping 17 studs.

It's very robust and has impressive range, but its thin body exerts little force—in fact, roughly as little as the small cylinder. But it's still very useful when long reach is more important than force.

large 2x2 cylinder (V2)

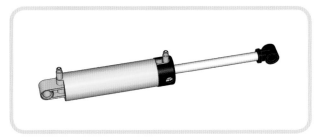

The large 2×2 cylinder (V2) combines features of the large 1×1 cylinder and the medium cylinders, but its base is slightly different. Just like the 1×1 cylinder, it has two stepped ports and a metal rod; it's 11 studs long when retracted and 17 studs long when extended. Due to its thick body, not only does it have great reach, but it also exerts plenty of force. Note that even though the body is 2×2 studs thick, both ends are just 1×1.

miscellaneous parts

This section covers an array of pieces that serve various purposes. Some of them, such as the hoses, are essential for any pneumatic system, and some are highly specialized and completely optional, such as the bracket for joining two medium cylinders.

pneumatic hoses and tubes

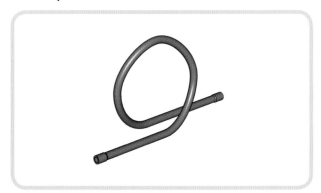

The 4 mm thick elastic rubber hose is a vital part of the Technic pneumatic system. It comes in various lengths and colors—black, grey, white, and blue—and is easy to insert through Technic holes and connect to the pneumatic system's ports.

When you're working with hoses, remember that LEGO pneumatic systems cannot maintain high air pressure for prolonged periods and each hose leaks somewhat, so the system becomes less and less efficient with each hose you add. Additionally, hoses tend to pop off ports when the pressure exceeds three bars, and if a hose is stretched or damaged, it can pop off even at a lower pressure. The oldest hoses, rarely found today, were made of a material that slowly broke down when it was exposed to UV light, causing the hoses to develop cracks and leaks. The newer hoses are made of silicone and are mostly immune to these problems. The hoses released with the V2 pneumatic system use a new kind of material that makes them more elastic and easier to connect to ports.

The 4 mm hoses make it easy to circulate air through any pneumatic system, no matter how complex, and they take up very little space in LEGO constructions. Their flexibility and resilience allows them to span components that need to have relative motion, but their inner ducts are narrow and can easily become blocked. To avoid blocking the tubes, be sure the surrounding structures do not press on a hose and that no hose is stretched or bent sharply.

Figure 10-6 shows a pneumatic hose connecting two pneumatic parts. Note that when a hose is attached to a port, it becomes thicker than 1 stud. As a result, the part of the hose with the port inside it can't fit through a Technic hole.

In addition to ports, pneumatic hoses can also be connected to 3 mm thick rigid tubes to join several pneumatic hoses to create longer ones.

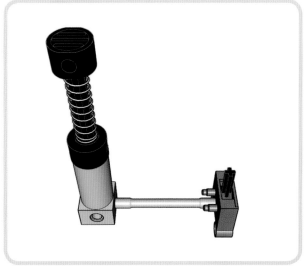

Figure 10-6: A hose connecting a large pump to a valve

In real hydraulic and pneumatic systems, *hose* always describes a flexible part and *tube* describes a rigid part. In keeping with this terminology, I'll refer to the flexible 4 mm parts as hoses and to the rigid 3 mm parts as tubes. Figure 10-7 shows how a 3 mm tube can connect two 4 mm pneumatic hoses. These tubes can also be connected to any studded structure, such as a brick, in a way that would not be possible with the regular pneumatic hose.

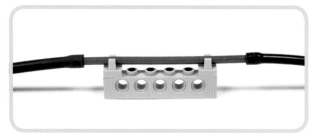

Figure 10-7: A tube connecting two hoses, connected to a Technic brick by two 1×1 tiles with clips

NOTE Real machines equipped with pneumatic or hydraulic systems often use rigid tubes to traverse structures that do not bend, such as a crane's boom. The 3 mm tube makes this type of construction easy to model with LEGO pieces.

T-pieces are used to split pneumatic hoses in two by connecting a hose to each port (see Figure 10-8). Two of the hoses act as a single section with the T-piece in the middle, and the third hose acts as its branch. Because every T-piece adds one new branch to a pneumatic hose, in order to split a hose into four, you need three T-pieces: one to split the hose in two and two more to split each of the two resulting hoses into two again. The rule is universal: Splitting a single hose into n hoses requires $(n-1)$ T-pieces.

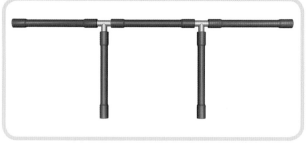

Figure 10-8: Two T-pieces allow a single hose (blue) to branch into three individual hoses (red).

NOTE Splitting hoses lessens the effectiveness of the entire pneumatic system because changing the direction of airflow by 90 degrees produces drag.

T-piece (Old)

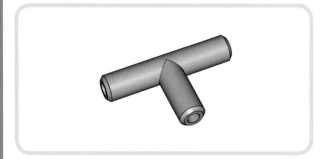

The Old version of the T-piece, which hasn't been produced since 1996, is simply a small, T-shaped piece with three ports. When air is forced into one port, it flows into the two other ports, making the T-piece work as a pneumatic parallel connector.

T-piece (New)

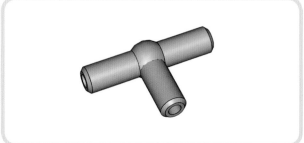

The updated version of the T-piece has a ball-shaped center, which makes it easier to disconnect from hoses. It works the same as the Old T-piece, but it's stronger and slightly more effective in reducing drag. Both types of T-pieces are always light grey.

hose connector with an axle hole (New)

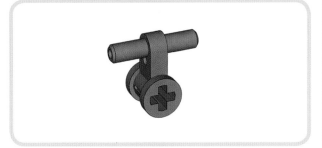

The hose connector with an axle hole (New) was introduced in 2011. Although it looks a bit like the T-piece, it's used to extend hoses, not to split them.

The purpose of this piece is to connect two sections of pneumatic hose so they're easy to remove. This allows you to easily connect or disconnect two pneumatic systems. This piece is especially well suited for creating a pneumatic *power take-off (PTO)*, a connection that powers removable external attachments, such as a pneumatic snowplow or a knuckleboom crane. Many agricultural machines also come with PTOs; for example, a tractor might switch between different attachments. With this piece, you can easily connect and disconnect various pneumatic attachments to the main pneumatic system.

cylinder bracket (New)

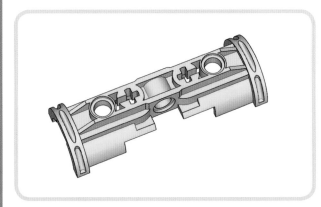

Medium cylinders, with their range of a bit less than 4 studs, are too short for many applications. One solution is to join two medium cylinders bottom to bottom using two brackets

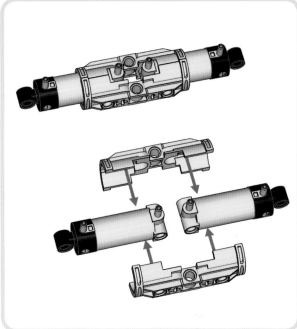

Figure 10-9: Assembled view (top) and exploded view (bottom) of two brackets securing two cylinders

(New), as shown in Figure 10-9. This allows them to work as one cylinder with rods extending from both ends, effectively doubling their length and reach. Note that these brackets work only with round-based medium cylinders, and they only come in yellow.

The brackets are symmetrical, so you can have one cylinder with ports facing up and the other with ports facing down. But having all ports on one side will make it easier to connect hoses. Their position matters because the cylinders won't work as one unless you couple their lower and upper ports with hoses split using T-pieces.

Figure 10-10 shows two brackets secured around two cylinders by two axles and two 3L beams with pins. The brackets are not physically attached to the cylinders or to each other. To attach them, either insert axles through their axle holes or add pins to their central holes and connect them with 3L beams. The pins-and-beams method is more reliable because it prevents the brackets from coming apart; however, it uses the brackets' central holes, which are often better used for routing hoses.

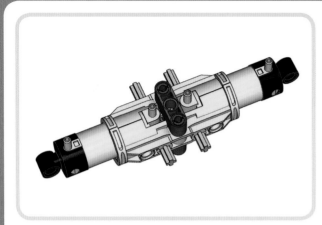

Figure 10-10: Two brackets secured around two cylinders

airtank (New)

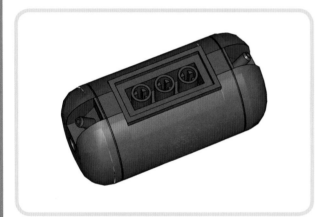

The airtank (New) stores compressed air. Available in blue and white, it comes in handy when you want to create a pneumatic system that doesn't require constant pumping. Even though with a little tinkering you can connect pneumatic hoses to plastic bottles or bags to store air, the airtank is the only original LEGO piece designed for this purpose.

NOTE Each pneumatic system has a capacity equal to the volume that can be filled with pressurized air. This volume is typically related to hoses, so adding several long hoses adds to the capacity significantly. However, the airtank's capacity is far greater than that of any number of hoses.

To make the air in the airtank available to the whole pneumatic system, place the airtank between the pressure supply and the control module. Keep in mind that there's nothing to limit how much air escapes the airtank. For that reason, you need to operate the valves carefully to unload the airtank gradually: A single mistake can send all the pressurized air into a single cylinder, resulting in a rapid movement.

According to LEGO, it takes 30 to 35 strokes of a large pneumatic pump to fill the airtank completely. At roughly 40 strokes, the pressure will reach the critical three bars, causing either the pump to stop working or the hose to pop off its ports. (If a breach occurs, the pressurized air will escape the airtank in a split second.)

Despite its apparent simplicity, the airtank's shape is actually complex. Its bottom has a 2×4 stud connecting area that can connect to studs from the top. This area is slightly recessed into the airtank's bottom, so to attach it to anything larger than 2×4 studs, you'll need a 2×4 plate as a buffer (see Figure 10-11). The airtank also has five 1-stud-deep axle holes that can connect to axles or axle pins. Three holes are in the bottom connecting area and one each in the center of both sides of the airtank.

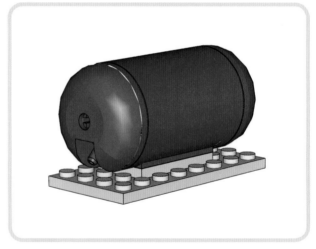

Figure 10-11: Because the connecting area is recessed into the airtank's bottom, a 2×4 plate is used as a buffer to connect the airtank to a 4×8 plate.

manometer (New)

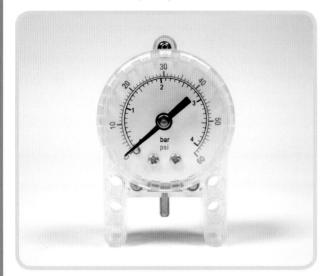

The manometer (New) is a rare part released in 2008. It's designed to measure the air pressure in a pneumatic system in psi and in bar units. Enclosed in a semitransparent 5×8×3 case, the manometer has a single metal port at the bottom. It connects using six pin holes that are each 2 studs deep.

To use the manometer to measure air pressure in the pneumatic system, place it between the pressure supply and the control module. You can connect it with a single section of pneumatic hose to practically anything, whether it's the airtank or any two sections of a hose using the T-piece. Figure 10-12 shows two examples of manometer placement.

The manometer works best with pneumatic systems that include an airtank or a motorized compressor, showing how much air is stored in the airtank or how much pressure the compressor generates. A system with a manual pump and no airtank simply won't generate enough pressure for long enough to make a manometer useful.

modding the pneumatic system

The pneumatic system is ripe for experimentation. The following sections describe some common ways to tinker with it.

non-LEGO hoses

It's easy to replace the original LEGO pneumatic hoses with custom hoses, as long as the custom hose is elastic and 4 mm thick (if you want to be able to insert it through Technic holes) and as long as it has reasonably large inner ducts. Some industrial hoses may come in handy for this purpose—for example, the fuel hoses used for radio-controlled models. Medical drip hoses—that is, IV lines—can be used too, but they tend to be sticky and to collect massive amounts of dust.

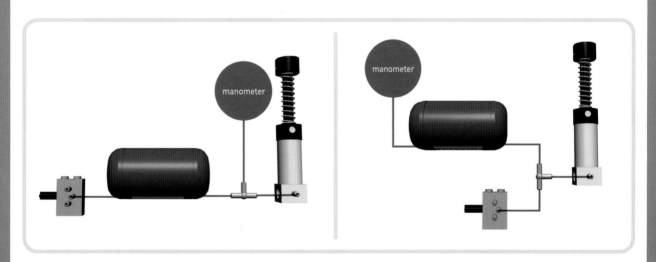

Figure 10-12: Two diagrams showing a pneumatic system with an airtank and a manometer. Notice that the airtank and the manometer work the same way in both cases.

non-LEGO airtanks

Although the LEGO airtank is quite useful, you can replace it with practically any airtight container. Plastic bottles or bags and even balloons can work well, as long as you connect them to the pneumatic system in a way that keeps them airtight.

removing springs to create motorized compressors

Because the large pneumatic pumps are much more powerful than the smaller pumps, you can use them to your advantage in motorized compressors. The one problem you'll encounter is that the spring in the large pump resists the force of the compressor's motor and slows down the entire mechanism. To solve this problem, remove the spring by pulling it off the Old large pump or, with the New pump, by cutting it (because the contact pad gets in the way).

pneumatic suspensions

In heavy models, you can use pneumatic cylinders instead of shock absorbers to create a kind of pneumatic suspension. Depending on the pressure of the air inside them, the cylinders will retract under the load and extend back to their neutral position once the load is reduced or eliminated.

The advantages of pneumatic suspensions are that they're tough and they allow you to adjust ground clearance simply by changing the air pressure. But they also have a few disadvantages: Their performance is worse than that of traditional shock absorbers, they're best used with heavy models, and their pneumatic system needs to be refilled from time to time due to microleaks.

turning your pneumatic system into a hydraulic one

In the real world, pneumatic systems are less popular than hydraulic systems. Liquid-filled hydraulic systems are widely used by machines that handle heavy loads, especially construction equipment such as excavators, cranes, front end loaders, backhoes, skid-steer loaders, forklifts, dump trucks, and so on.

If your constructions need to handle very heavy loads, you can turn the pneumatic system into a hydraulic one by replacing the air with liquid, although you must do this carefully.

The risks include damage to cylinders with metal rods: They can corrode depending on the fluid you use. Also, the rods are covered with grease for lubrication, which may react with the fluid you choose or be removed by it. And even if you use a "safe" fluid, there is still the matter of drying the cylinder after use—a difficult task given that the cylinder is almost fully closed.

The following is a list of tips for using fluids in LEGO pneumatic systems. However, I'm not recommending that you fill the system with fluid, and if you do so, you may damage your pieces in the process. Remember that if you decide to experiment with fluids, you do so at your own risk. Be advised that if something goes wrong, the result can get pretty messy!

* The best choice of liquid is a mineral oil—a noncorrosive, nonreactive, odorless fluid that is safe for human contact. Mineral oil is 20 percent thinner than water, inexpensive, and available at most drug stores.
* You should convert only the New or V2 LEGO pneumatic system to hydraulics because the valve is the only exhaust in the system; the fluid will exit only from there instead of exiting from cylinders, as in the Old system.
* You'll need a constant supply of fluid, and the LEGO pumps must be fully submerged in the fluid in order to pump it.
* The fluid's viscosity will improve the way the cylinders handle heavy loads, but this also means that you'll need to apply much greater force while pumping.
* The integrity of the seals in the pneumatic system is critical when you use fluid. Any leaks can introduce air into the system, which could block its function completely.
* Any leak in a fluid-filled pneumatic system can affect its surroundings. Make sure there are no electric or metal pieces near the pneumatic system in your construction. Also, try to build the system so that if a hose pops off, you can access the hose quickly and block it or lift its end to stop the fluid from leaking out.
* Never use the manometer with liquids; you're likely to damage it permanently.
* It's very difficult to dry the insides of pneumatic pieces unless you disassemble them. Pumping warm air through them continuously for a prolonged period of time will help; you can also try leaving them in a bag of uncooked rice for a while, because rice absorbs moisture.

pneumatic devices

This chapter presents devices that make creative use of pneumatic systems: motorized compressors, remote-controlled valves, and pneumatic engines. All these devices take advantage of the fact that the pneumatic system has been designed to be customizable, and there's almost no limit to potential modifications.

In this chapter, we'll start by discussing the most basic and versatile devices and then move on to more sophisticated and specialized ones.

motorized compressors

A *compressor* is a stand-alone mechanism that provides a continuous supply of pressurized air—for example, the massive air compressor you can find at the gas station (for reinflating tires) or the portable model you might use to inflate an air mattress. The most practical and popular method of building a Technic compressor is by driving small LEGO pumps with a motor. This method allows us to control a compressor remotely, and it ensures that the compressor works at a constant rate, making the cylinders in a pneumatic system move smoothly.

It's convenient to keep the motor attached directly to a compressor. This allows us to place the whole mechanism practically anywhere in our construction, as we are not bound by driveshafts, gears, or any other rigid elements. Our only limitation is finding a home for the electric wire and pneumatic hose.

There is one issue worth keeping in mind when building a motorized compressor: its *ripple*. LEGO pumps work in a cycle: They are retracted, pumping air into their outlets, and then extended, taking air from outside. In other words, they don't provide air constantly but only during exactly half of the

cycle. This cycle has two consequences that become more significant as the number of pumps working simultaneously increases: fluctuating air flow and vibrations, which result from the pumps' rods being repeatedly pushed back and forth.

Some builders are fond of building monstrous compressors with eight or more pumps driven by the RC motor (shown in Figure 11-1). This is not always the best solution, as RC motors are large, loud, and power consuming. Another solution is to divide pumps into groups that work alternately. For example, instead of four pumps working as one, we can use two pumps that are retracted while the other two are

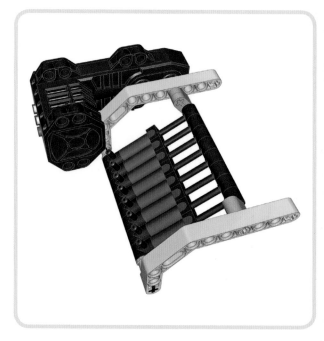

Figure 11-1: An eight-pump compressor driven by the RC motor. This design is a real monstrosity in the world of LEGO compressors.

extended. Ideally, we should have multiple pumps that are fully out of phase, because this limits both the load on the compressor's motor and the vibrations the compressor creates. Supporting the pumps' ends as rigidly as possible also reduces vibrations.

You might ask why we would want to use so many pumps in the first place. It's because a single pump has a very small capacity and is, therefore, not very powerful, taking quite a while to fill just a single large pneumatic cylinder. How fast your pneumatic system operates depends on the volume of pressurized air delivered to it, so using many pumps is a natural solution. The rule of thumb is that for a pneumatic system in which one or two large cylinders are working at the same time, it takes at least two pumps for a PF Medium motor to provide air pressure at reasonable rate.

NOTE All of the compressor designs in this chapter are intended for pumps that are 5.5 studs long when extended, not for the newer 6-stud-long version. This longer version is found only in a single set and is therefore quite rare.

Figures 11-2 through 11-6 show various compressor designs that drive more than one pump.

The rocking compressor, shown in Figure 11-6, can hold from 2 to 18 pumps, depending on the length of its axles. It moves the pumps in a reciprocating motion, rather than the rotary motion used in other compressors, which results in a more compact build. Moreover, it has a gearing with four possible gear combinations (see Figure 11-7).

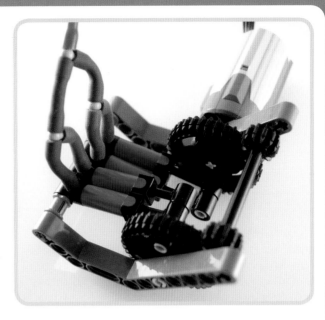

Figure 11-3: A compressor that can hold two or four pumps while making use of two 36-tooth gears. The orientation of the gears relative to each other is maintained by two 12-tooth gears on a separate axle, which also transfers drive between them. It's possible to connect two or more such compressors side by side to increase the number of pumps.

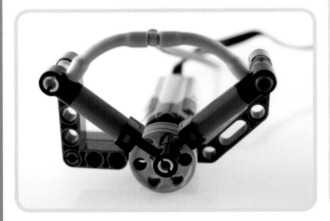

Figure 11-2: A compressor with two pumps that work alternately, both attached to two wedge belt wheels. The design is small, but it's difficult to add more pumps to it. In this compressor, the pumps are 90 degrees out of phase rather than 180 degrees, so the pressure is still "uneven." In other words, one pump is not fully extended while the other is fully compressed.

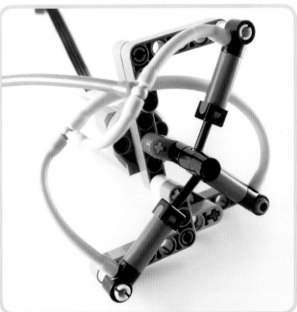

Figure 11-4: It's perfectly possible to split pumps in a compressor into three groups.

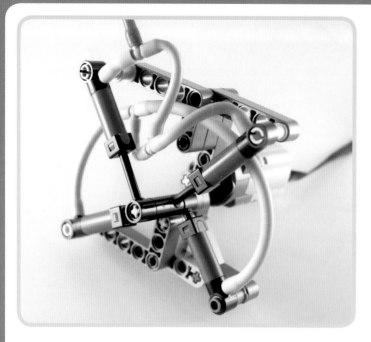

Figure 11-5: You can even split pumps in a compressor into four groups at various points of the working cycle. But such compressors are significantly more complex while working only a little more smoothly.

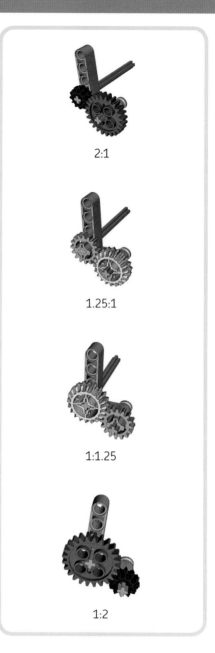

2:1

1.25:1

1:1.25

1:2

Figure 11-7: The four gear combinations suitable for the rocking compressor, with their ratios labeled

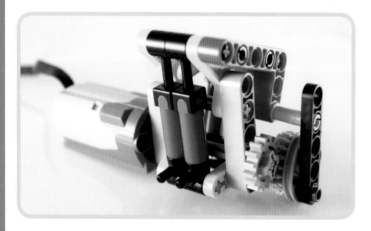

Figure 11-6: Finally, here's a design called a rocking compressor. While it doesn't extend pumps to their maximum, it can hold up to 18 pumps in two alternating groups.

a rocking compressor

Here's a look at the complete building instructions for a simple design. The blue axles limit the number of pumps, but making the axles 1 stud longer adds space for two more pumps. For clarity, the instructions show the compressor without pumps, but the pumps should be mounted on the blue axles.

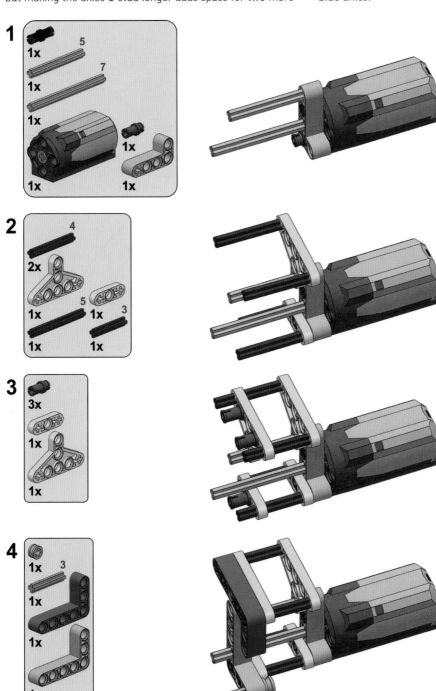

5

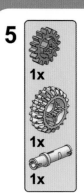

1x

1x

1x

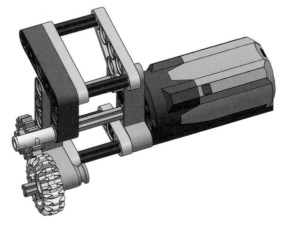

6

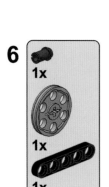

1x

1x

1x

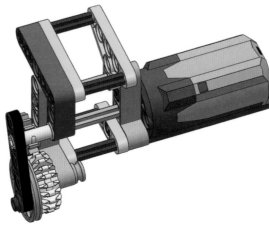

motorized valves

The purpose of motorizing a pneumatic valve is simple: remote control. A valve can be connected to a motor in a simple way, preferably with the use of a 24-tooth gear with a clutch, which prevents the motor from stalling (see Figure 11-8). Once the 24-tooth gear can no longer drive the valve, the grey circle inside the gear begins to rotate instead, which prevents damage to the motor or to the gearing.

Polish builder Maciej "dmac" Szymański discovered that if we use this exact combination of motor and gears with a regular 24-tooth gear (without a clutch), we'll get a return-to-center motorized valve—that is, a valve that returns to

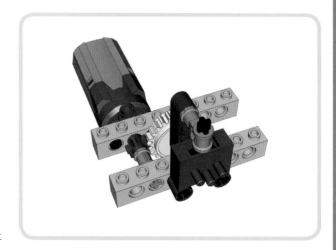

Figure 11-8: A simple way to motorize a pneumatic valve is to use a gear with a clutch for the motor's safety.

central position the moment the motor stops, thereby shutting down the valve (see Figure 11-9).

But precision is often crucial when switching pneumatic valves. The designs using a 24-tooth gear lack precision, while the design shown in Figure 11-10 offers plenty of fine-grained control. This is useful for retracting heavily loaded cylinders, when the valve has to be opened little by little to prevent cylinders from yielding to the load.

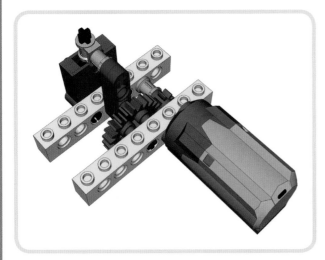

Figure 11-9: With a regular 24-tooth gear instead of the clutch gear, we get a return-to-center valve.

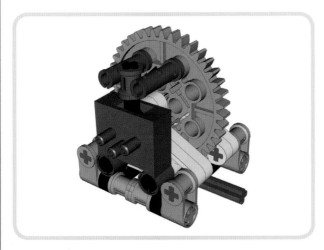

Figure 11-10: This high-precision valve-switching mechanism makes use of a worm gear and a 40-tooth gear to ensure accuracy. The red bush on the valve's lever improves it further by reducing backlash. Note that there is no safety clutch in this assembly; because the mechanism multiplies the motor's torque by a factor of 40, there is a chance that some pieces may be damaged if the motor doesn't stop at the right moment. To lessen this risk, a clutch can be added between the valve and the motor.

autovalve

An autovalve combines the functions of a motorized valve with those of a compressor. It makes use of the compressor's ability to function regardless of the input's direction of rotation—we'll use the motor's direction of rotation to control the valve itself. After switching, the motor can continue to drive the compressor as long as is needed.

The autovalve's working principle is based on a so-called *sliding worm gear*, as shown in Figure 11-11. The motor drives the compressor through an axle on which a worm gear is located. The worm gear drives one of two identical short axles with a 12-tooth gear and a short beam (shown in green). The beams act as pushing elements: Each of them can push the valve's lever in one direction and then continue rotating freely. But when driven in the opposite direction, the beam locks against the lever, stopping the respective axle and making the worm gear slide away from it. The worm gear slides until it meshes with the other axle's gear, at which point it starts to drive it and the other pusher located on it, effectively switching the valve.

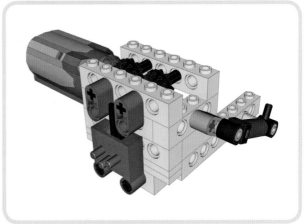

Figure 11-11: An autovalve uses a sliding worm gear to control a compressor and a pneumatic valve with just one motor.

The disadvantages of the autovalve include a long switching time, which can be remedied by driving the input faster, and the limit of one valve and one compressor per motor. Still, the compressor can be connected to any pneumatic system, with more valves controlled separately (see Figure 11-12).

To see an autovalve in action, visit *http://www.youtube.com/watch?v=OsDJ4iTs-P8*.

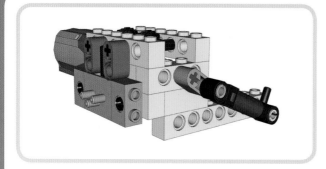

Figure 11-12: An autovalve can be created with both types of pneumatic valves (the older one is shown here) and with any compressor whatsoever—the single-pump compressor here is just an example.

a motorized valve

1
4x
2x 2
2x
1x
2x 5
3x

2
3
1x
2x

3
2x
1x

4
2
2x
2x
2x 2x

5
1x
1x

an autovalve

1

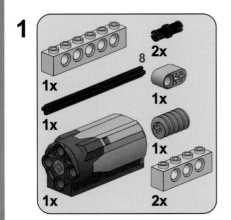

1x · 8 · 2x · 1x · 1x · 1x · 1x · 2x

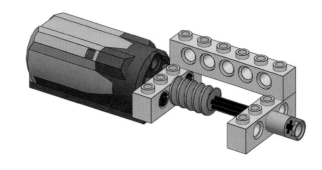

2

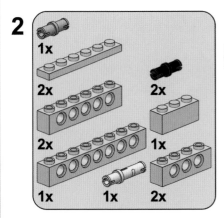

1x · 2x · 2x · 2x · 1x · 1x · 1x · 2x

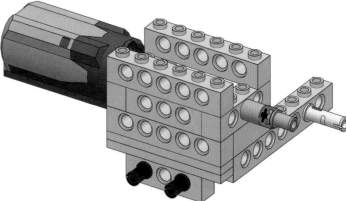

3

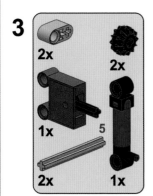

2x · 2x · 1x · 5 · 2x · 1x

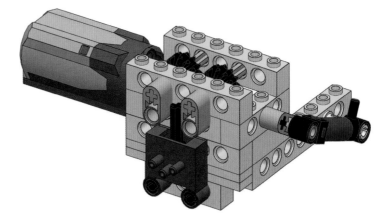

electro-pneumatic switch

The electro-pneumatic switch, which combines a PF switch with a pneumatic valve, can be a much simpler alternative to the autovalve when you have only one pneumatic circuit and compressor to control. If you have a motorized compressor, you need to connect the compressor's pumps to this device's pneumatic valve and the compressor's motor to this device's PF switch. As a result, a single manual lever (in this case, a 4L axle) will control the compressor and the valve at the same time. Moving the lever to one of the sides will start the compressor and make the cylinders connected to the valve extend or retract; moving the lever back to center will stop the compressor and shut the valve.

PF Servo-controlled valve

The PF Servo motors are well suited for controlling pneumatic valves because you can rotate them very precisely. The only problem is that the regular PF remote makes Servo motors rotate 90 degrees left and right, which is much further than a pneumatic valve can rotate. We can simply block the motor so it can only rotate to a certain point before being forced to stop, but a safer solution is to gear down the Servo, as shown in the following instructions. Note that because of the gear wheels, the valve will no longer be able to return perfectly to the middle; instead, it will stop a few degrees off-center. But it will still work correctly, because such a small difference is tolerable.

an electro-pneumatic switch

1
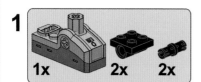
1x 2x 2x

2
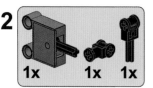
1x 1x 1x
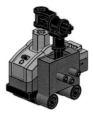

3

4
1x
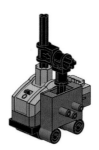

a PF Servo-controlled valve

1
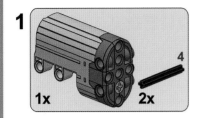
1x 4 2x

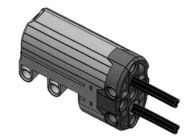

2
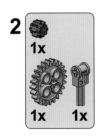
1x
1x 1x

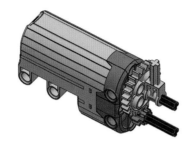

3
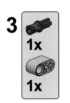
1x
1x

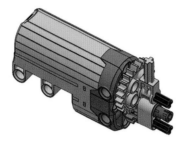

4
1x
2x
1x

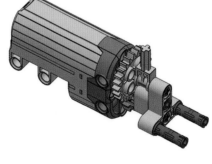

5
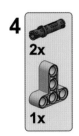
1x
1x

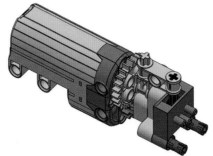

automated pressure switch

Having a motorized compressor in your pneumatic system doesn't necessarily solve your pressure problems. Complex pneumatic systems with many cylinders working in turns can require large amounts of pressurized air in the system at one moment and no air moments later. While the amount of air pressure that goes into a system can be managed by building a compressor fast and/or large enough, constantly turning it on and off can be an onerous task.

The solution to this problem is a pressure switch, also known as a pressure limiter. We can build one using a PF switch, a small pneumatic cylinder, and a rubber band.

How does a pressure switch work? Take a look at Figure 11-13, which shows how the switch connects the compressor motor to the power supply. The cylinder's lower port is connected to the pneumatic system, while the upper one is left open. A rubber band is put over the cylinder, keeping it retracted. If the pressure in the pneumatic system is high enough, the cylinder will overcome the rubber band and

extend. If the pressure drops, it will yield to the band and retract. This means that if we connect the cylinder to the PF switch, the switch can effectively control the compressor's motor, turning it on automatically when pressure is low and then turning it off when pressure's high enough. Such a mechanism is best used with an airtank, filling it automatically when necessary.

The pressure switch works best when close to the airtank, which, in turn, should be close to the compressor, as shown in Figure 11-14. Some builders create complete modules with the motorized compressor, airtank, and pressure switch all put together. I prefer to take advantage of the elastic elements—that is, the wires and hoses—to be able to adjust the location of these elements more freely. A singular module has fixed dimensions, while separate elements connected only by wires and hoses can be fitted into limited space in different ways, allowing for less massive and more creative housings.

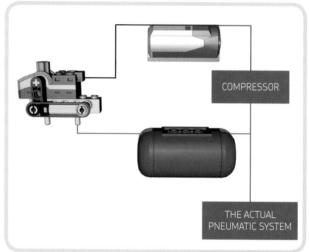

Figure 11-14: The general scheme of the pressure switch and its connections to other components of the pneumatic system. Black lines mark electric wires, blue lines mark mechanical connections, and green lines mark pneumatic hoses.

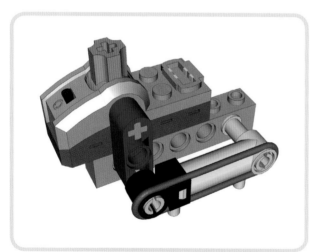

Figure 11-13: A close-up view of a pressure switch. The switch usually needs adjusting to activate at the desired pressure threshold. It can be fine-tuned by adjusting the rubber band's strength, the angle of the cylinder relative to the lever, and the length of the lever. It is also possible to use old 9V switches, which offer less resistance, or to use multiple cylinders. Large cylinders can be used as well, although their large capacity makes them less sensitive and therefore less useful in systems that must react to small changes in air pressure.

A properly built and adjusted pressure switch leaves you with only pneumatic valves to take care of; the compressor works automatically, and the pressure in the airtank is maintained at all times. Note that there is no particular place where the *switch-airtank-compressor* combination should be connected to the rest of the pneumatic system. Such a connection can be placed between the compressor and airtank, between the airtank and pressure switch, after the airtank

(as shown in Figure 11-13), or after the pressure switch—it will work the same regardless of placement. You can also connect a LEGO manometer to observe the relationship between air pressure and the functioning of the switch.

pneumatic engines

The functioning of pneumatic cylinders is somewhat similar to that of the pistons in an internal combustion engine, allowing us to build a compressed air engine with cylinders driving the crankshaft. Such an engine, sometimes called a *LEGO pneumatic engine (LPE)*, is powered by pressurized air delivered to the cylinders. Pneumatic engines are advantageous in terms of their performance, resemblance to combustion engines, and sound, which is quite loud and car-like compared to that of electric motors. What makes these engines appealing to many builders is their complexity, which creates almost endless possibilities for improvements. While the complexity of these engines may be appealing, they're also quite a challenge to build. Disadvantages of pneumatic engines include their size and their need to be constantly connected to a compressor. Moreover, pneumatic engines work only in one direction, and they get warm from the friction of many moving parts and from air being compressed inside the cylinders.

The working principle of a pneumatic engine is simple: A cylinder is connected to a shaft with a cam so that extending it rotates the shaft by a half rotation and retracting it rotates the shaft by another half rotation (see Figures 11-15 and 11-16). The same shaft uses another cam connected to a valve to switch the cylinder between extending and retracting continuously, thus creating a complete working cycle. The cycle, therefore, involves both cylinder and valve and goes as follows: Cylinder extends to maximum, valve is switched, cylinder retracts to maximum, valve is switched.

The problem with the cycle is that both cylinder and valve have *dead spots*, or points of the cycle at which they can stop, as shown in Figure 11-17. For a cylinder, it's the point when it's extended or retracted to maximum, and for a valve, it's the point when it goes through neutral position and no air comes through it. If we make an engine with just one cylinder and one valve, these dead spots will overlap and effectively stop the engine after it makes just half a rotation. This can be prevented by using a heavy flywheel and a modified valve.

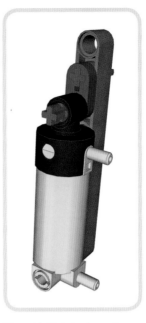

Figure 11-15: A simple way to connect the cylinder to a shaft is to use a cam made of a short beam. However, a cylinder can extend by 4 studs, but here it's allowed to extend by only 3.

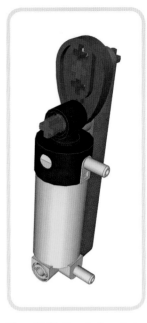

Figure 11-16: To make the cylinder extend fully, we need its tip to be mounted 1.5 studs away from the shaft. The Technic cam piece allows this.

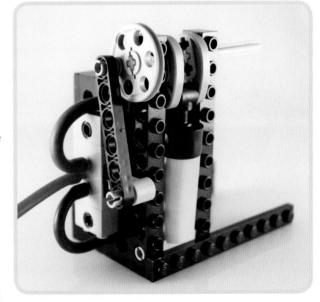

Figure 11-17: A simple cylinder and valve combination with two cranks: one made of Technic cams, converting the cylinder's motion into the crankshaft's rotation, and another made of a wedge-belt wheel, using the crankshaft's rotation to switch the valve back and forth. Note that both cylinder and valve are in dead spots here.

Modifying LEGO pieces is actually quite common among advanced LPE builders. The best pneumatic engines from these builders can far outperform any LEGO electric motor in terms of both speed and torque, but that performance comes at a cost. In such engines, cylinders' ports are often drilled to increase throughput; the valves' internal structure is cut to reduce their switching resistance; and many moving parts, such as cylinders and camshafts, are lubricated. Industrial tubing with clamps replaces LEGO hoses and is sometimes glued to the ports. Finally, these engines are powered with non-LEGO compressors, such as electric compressors for car tires. LEGO pneumatic pieces were simply not designed to move quickly, and there is a lot of friction involved in the many moving pieces of a pneumatic engine; these limitations justify modifications for some builders.

Getting back to our single-cylinder engine, a modified valve and a flywheel can make it work: The flywheel will provide the momentum necessary to get the engine through dead spots, while the valve will offer minimum resistance and thus minimum risk of getting stuck in a dead spot (see Figure 11-18). Such an engine needs to be started by spinning the flywheel manually, but it will keep running for as long as it receives sufficiently high air pressure.

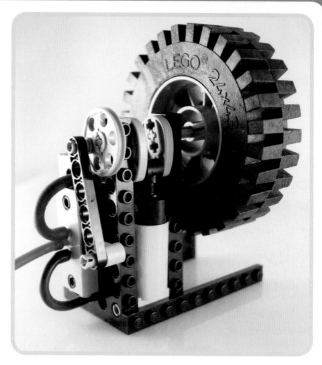

Figure 11-18: This is the engine from Figure 11-17 with a flywheel added to keep it running through overlapping dead spots. Starting such an engine is a little finicky, but it works fine once it gets going.

a single-cylinder engine

Here are the building instructions for the engine shown in Figure 11-18. Like every set of engine instructions in this chapter, these instructions have both the cylinder and hoses removed for clarity. In this BI, a photo shows the cylinder's position and a connection scheme for the hoses. Remember that engines like this work best with a large volume of continuous air pressure, and they are difficult to drive with a LEGO compressor.

1

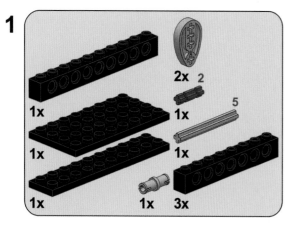

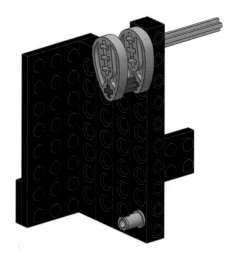

2

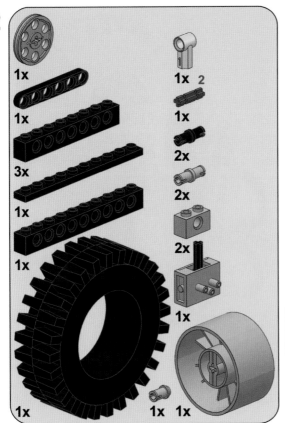

1x
1x
3x
1x
1x

1x   1x   1x

1x   2
1x
2x
2x

2x

1x

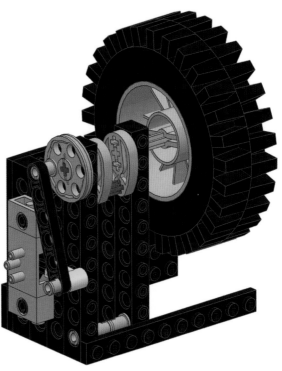

3

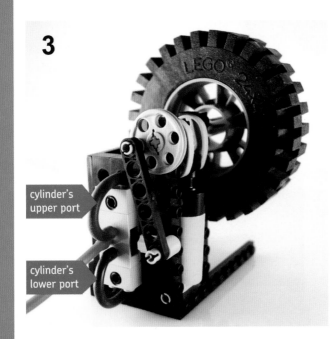

cylinder's
upper port

cylinder's
lower port

Engines with two, four, six, or more cylinders can be built as follows: The cylinders are split in two groups, with each group connected to one valve so that there are two valves in the engine for any number of cylinders. At any given time, one group of cylinders is retracting while the other is extending. These groups should be mixed so that no two cylinders of the same group are next to each other. All the cylinders are connected to a common camshaft, but with cams rotated 90 degrees relative to the adjacent ones (see Figure 11-19). This reduces the overlap of the cylinders' dead spots. Finally, each valve is connected to the end of the camshaft closest to the group of cylinders connected to the other valve, as shown in Figure 11-20. This arrangement ensures that we don't overlap dead spots between a valve and the cylinders connected to it.

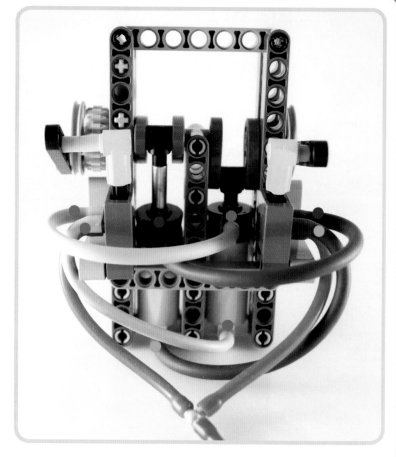

Figure 11-19: A two-cylinder engine built in accordance with the rules above. The colored dots show which ports are connected. Note the position of the cams. The engine can start all by itself and runs relatively smoothly. The tan gear can transfer drive from the engine. More cylinders can be added to the engine, and it reaches optimum smoothness with four cylinders, each with a cam rotated 90 degrees relative to the next one.

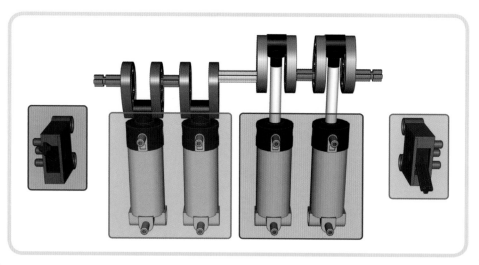

Figure 11-20: A simplified layout of a four-cylinder pneumatic engine. All cylinders, running the same camshaft, are split into two groups (marked green and blue), each connected to a single valve. The valves are connected to the sides of the camshaft nearest the opposite group.

a two-cylinder pneumatic engine

1

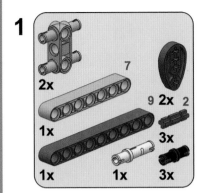

7
2x

9 2x 2

1x

3x

1x 1x 3x

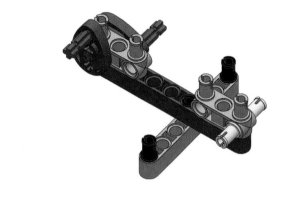

2

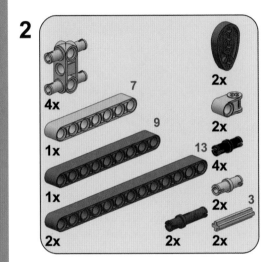

7
4x

2x

9
1x

2x

13
1x

4x

2x

2x 3

2x 2x 2x

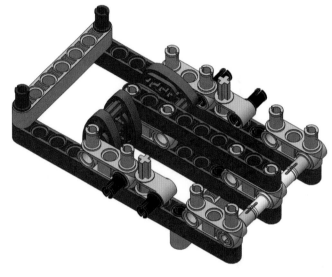

3

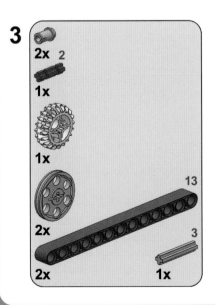

2x 2

1x

1x

13
2x

3
2x 1x

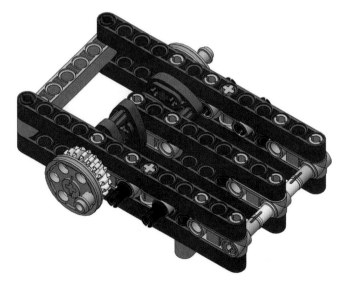

4

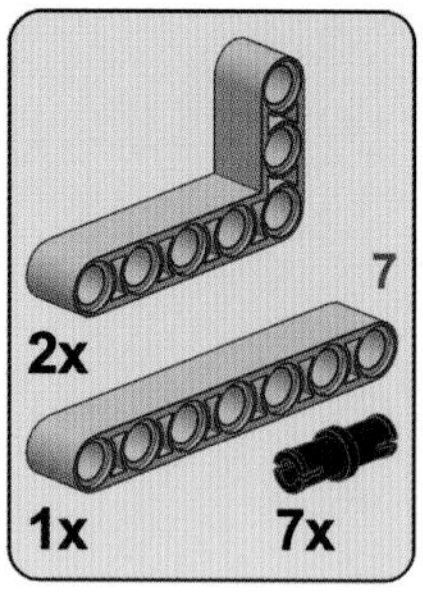

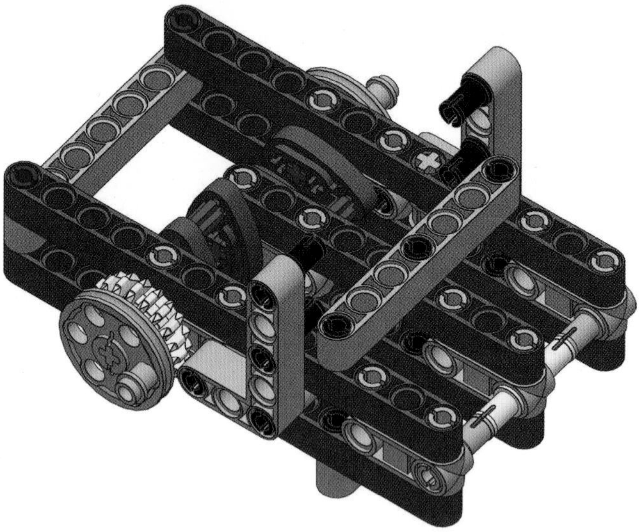

2x

7

1x   7x

5

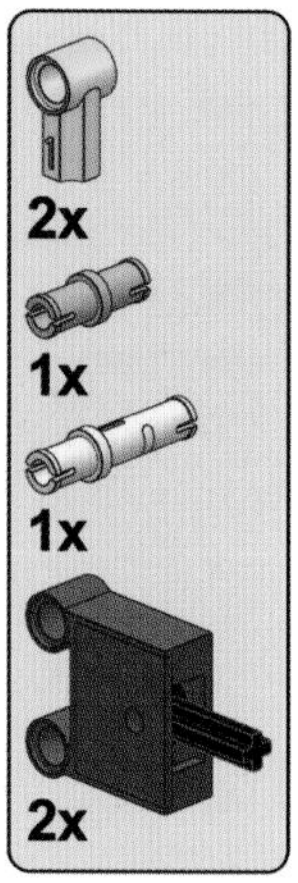

2x

1x

1x

2x

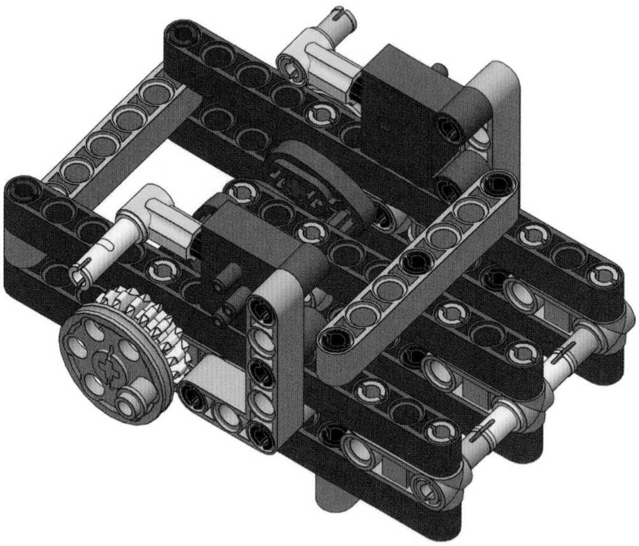

6

1x

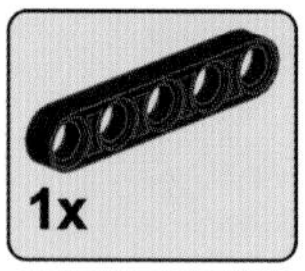

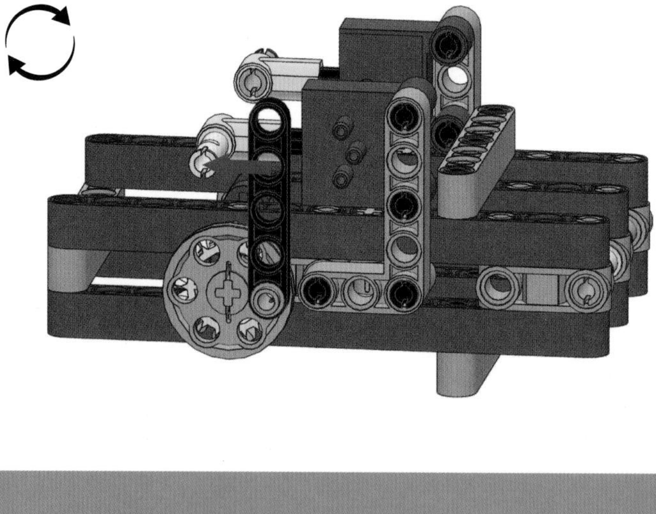

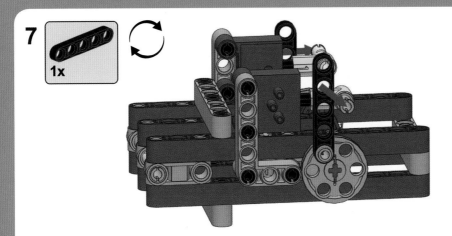

1x

In general, the more cylinders we add, the smoother the engine will run. The engine reaches optimum performance when we use at least four cylinders, each with its cam rotated 90 degrees relative to the adjacent ones (see Figure 11-21). On the other hand, adding more cylinders will result in a greater combined engine capacity, which will in turn increase fuel consumption. Note that the efficiency of LEGO compressors is poor compared to the capacity of such an engine. Note also that the engine's efficiency can't be improved by using airtanks because the engine needs a constant supply of equally pressurized air and airtanks provide only a single, short blast of very highly pressurized air. You can, of course, build an engine with a separate valve for each cylinder. Some builders do that for smoother operation, but it drastically increases the overall complexity of the engine.

One last issue is that cams are quite fragile when subjected directly to the cylinder's power. This problem can be remedied by using sliders—that is, elements that move together with the tip of the cylinder and thereby transfer movement to the cams (see Figure 11-22). Sliders keep a cylinder's tip moving in a straight line, and this creates a more favorable distribution of force, leaving the cams less stressed. The use of sliders is also more efficient because the cylinder's power is not wasted by tilting it sideways; instead, all of the power is transferred to the cam. Additionally, with cylinders maintaining the same position, it's possible to pack them more tightly. Sliders are very popular in complex engines—especially in those in the V system—as they allow a sturdier overall construction.

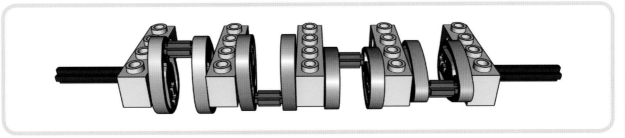

Figure 11-21: The "optimum crankshaft," with four cams, each rotated 90 degrees relative to the next one, provides the smoothest operation possible for a pneumatic engine.

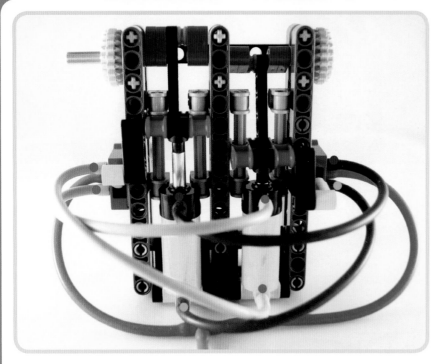

Figure 11-22: A two-cylinder engine with sliders. The colored dots show which ports are connected. The sliders are built around the red pieces, each moving along two light grey axles. They keep the cylinders' motion in a straight line and then transfer the motion to the cams (blue). Note that the extension of the cylinders is limited to 3 studs rather than 4, but thanks to this limitation, the sliders can also be used to control the valves.

a two-cylinder pneumatic engine with sliders

1

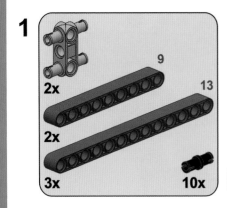

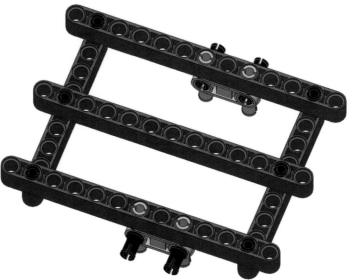

2

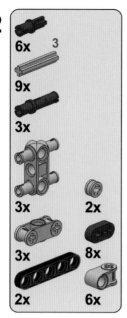

6x   3

9x

3x

3x   2x

3x   8x

2x   6x

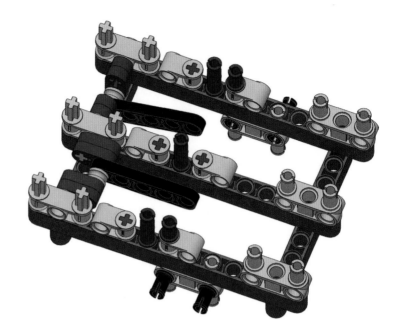

3

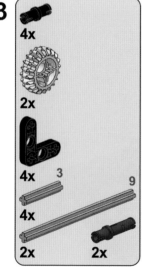

4x

2x

4x   3

4x   9

2x   2x

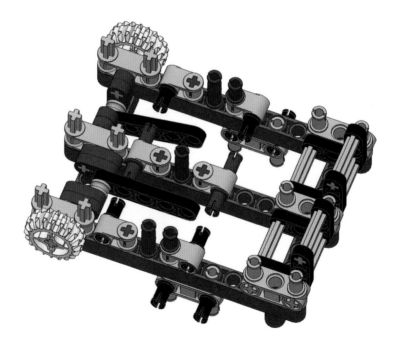

4

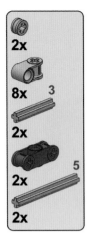

2x

8x 3

2x

2x 5

2x

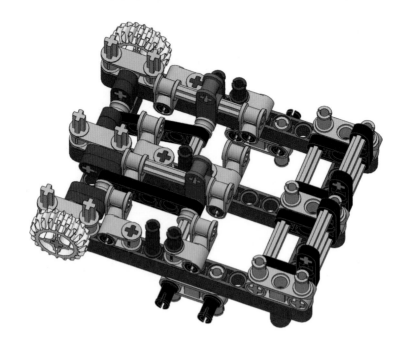

5

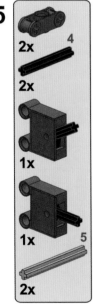

2x 4

2x

1x

1x 5

2x

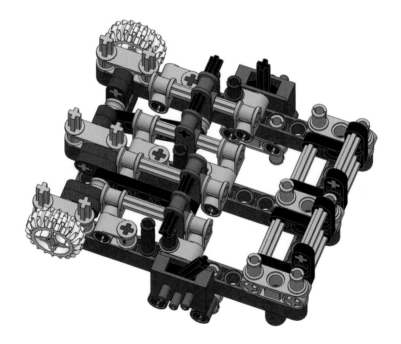

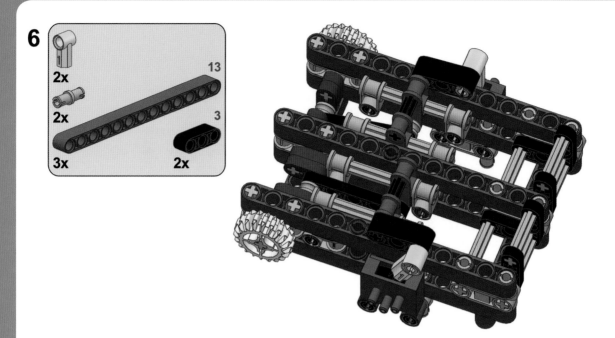

Engines in the V configuration are engines with cylinders aligned in two planes that form the shape of a letter *V* when viewed along the axis of their common camshaft. These engines can be built in two ways, both of which require building two identical modules with cylinders lined up and connecting them at a right angle. The first way is to build them with two separate crankshafts, each for one module, and to then use gears with a single central shaft to connect the modules. The second way is to use a single common crankshaft for both modules and to then connect two cylinders to each single crank pin. Since we want to keep the modules aligned (as they are in real engines), it's easier to use half-stud-thick beams to connect sliders to the cams rather than use 1-stud-thick cylinder tips (see Figure 11-23).

The possibilities with pneumatic engines are vast and include engines in W, boxer, and even radial systems. You can find many ingenious variants shown in detail by visiting Dr. Dude's YouTube channel: *http://www.youtube.com/user/ DrDudeNL/*. Dr. Dude, a Dutch builder, has been a fan of the LEGO Technic set—and of big Technic cars in particular—for over 30 years.

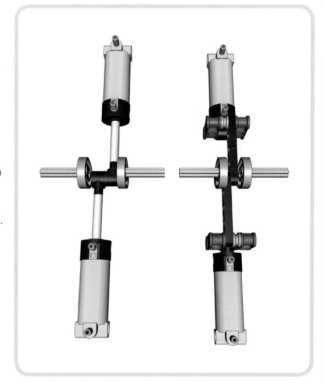

Figure 11-23: Two cylinders connected to a single cam directly (left) and through sliders (right). You can see that the sliders allow the cylinders to stay aligned, while direct connection forces one of them to be moved by 1 stud.

builder showcase

Many LEGO builders produce impressive pneumatic engines, but one of them is the unquestionable master in this field: Alex "Nicjasno" Zorko. Alex builds big and heavy models of sports cars and found LEGO motors too weak to drive them. He has developed incredibly advanced motors, including "simple" inline engines, a V6 that operates at speeds well above 2000 RPM, and a V8 strong enough to make even a very heavy model drift (shown in Figure 11-24). Alex shows his models at *http://nicjasno.com/* and sells his engines at *http://lpepower.com/*.

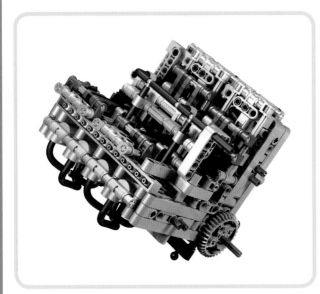

Figure 11-24: Alex "Nicjasno" Zorko's V8 motor

a working water pressure pump

While LEGO Technic creations don't mix well with fluids, it is possible to build a pneumatic pump that will work with water while ensuring that no sensitive pieces come into physical contact with liquid. This pump uses pressurized air to push water, making it fairly safe and simple to use in, for example, a LEGO fire engine model.

To create a water pressure pump, we need an airtight container that will initially be filled with water and will then have pressurized air delivered to it. Using LEGO pieces for such a container may not be the best idea; a small bottle with a metal or plastic cap is a better alternative.

The working idea of this pressure pump is that by delivering air into a closed, water-filled container, we can force the water out. The container therefore needs an entry for the air and an exit for the water. The entry can be anywhere in the container; the exit should be at the bottom to stay in contact with water as long as possible.

We can adapt our bottle by making two holes in the cap and putting two hoses through them, as shown in Figure 11-25. One hose (dark grey) will deliver air and can end just below the cap or go deeper into the bottle—it doesn't matter. The other hose (blue) will be the water's way out, and it should reach all the way to the bottom. It's a good idea to make the other hose stiff so that it doesn't float in the water; a rigid LEGO hose or a regular drinking straw can be used. The hardest part is making the cap airtight with hoses going through it. You can achieve this by using modeling clay, masking sol, or molten wax from a candle.

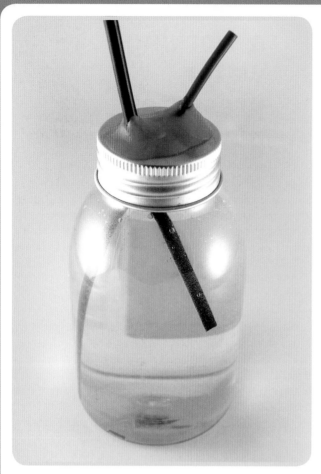

Now you can connect the first hose to any compressor, and the water will spurt from the other one. Note that water is much less compressive than air, so it will take very high air pressure to make water really spurt. You can make your pump more effective by delivering air to it faster and by making the exit hose narrow. You can also use an airtank full of pressurized air and connect it to the first hose through a pneumatic valve; opening the valve will empty it into the bottle in an instant.

Just make sure the water doesn't come out anywhere near the electric components of your construction!

Figure 11-25: A small plastic bottle with a metal cap makes for a very good container. The dark grey elastic hose delivers air, while the blue rigid one lets the water out (note that it can be extended by putting another elastic hose on its end). The cap was punctured in two places to let the hoses through and then sealed with modeling clay (pink).

12

building strong

There was a time when Technic bricks alone could support and hold together almost any motorized mechanism. But eventually LEGO introduced stronger motors with enough torque to push even Technic brick connections apart. Having more torque at our disposal is an advantage in all aspects except one—it requires *structural reinforcing*, adding extra pieces whose primary purpose is to hold other pieces together (see Figure 12-1). A properly reinforced mechanism stays together regardless of its motor's strength and how much load is applied to its output, even if the load stalls the motor.

This chapter explores how to find places in a structure where reinforcing is crucial; how to identify strong and weak LEGO pieces; and how to create casings, chassis, frames, and trusses to support your models.

why things fall apart

In order to find where and how to reinforce our structures, we first have to understand why pieces come apart. When we house a mechanism inside a structure, it has an input, an output, and points of attachment to that structure; most often this means we have axles with gears that are housed in a structure's pin holes, as shown in Figure 12-2. Whenever a mechanism works, it handles a load that exerts stress on its output and has to be overcome by the force applied to its input. For example, if our mechanism is a drivetrain, the motor driving its input has to overcome the stress exerted by its wheels—the rolling resistance and friction. This means that there are basically two forces in our mechanism, one applied to its input and one applied to its output, and that they work against each other. In other words, the output *resists* the input, creating stress that is carried through every component between them.

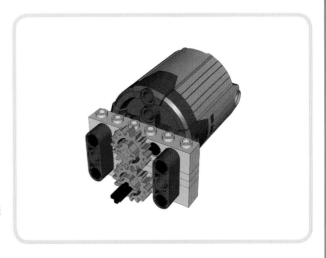

Figure 12-1: The two red beams hold the yellow Technic bricks together. Without these beams, the powerful PF XL motor would push the lower brick away the moment it started running.

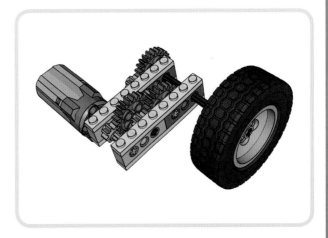

Figure 12-2: An example of a mechanism with a motor driving a wheel. The mechanism consists of six gears in three pairs on four axles, and it's housed inside Technic bricks held together by plates.

Let's think of this mechanism as a *chain*, with input and output being the first and last links. The initial force applied to the input (the first link) will be transferred through the chain and will stop on *the link of least resistance*. If the structure around our mechanism is solid, all links will have more resistance than the mechanism's output (the last link of the chain), and the mechanism will work as intended: Only the output will yield to the input. But if any link of our chain before the output has *less* resistance than the output, it will be dislocated and separated from the next link, thus breaking the chain and preventing the mechanism from working.

finding weak links

So let's find the weak link in our chain. In our example from Figure 12-2, we have a motor connected to the axle, an axle connected to the 8-tooth gear, an 8-tooth gear connected to the 24-tooth gear, and so on, all the way to the output and the wheel.

Most of the axle pairs (or other connections) in this chain are within a single LEGO brick. But the connection marked by red arrows in Figure 12-3 involves two 2×4 Technic bricks, meaning that when stress is applied, it can break apart (as shown in Figure 12-4). When deciding where to reinforce your model, look for the seams that could separate under stress.

Also note that a pair of gears that increases the gear ratio (the driver gear is bigger than the follower) is more likely to come apart than a pair that decreases the gear ratio (the driver gear is smaller than the follower). There is simply more force exerted on the follower gear when gearing up, and such a pair of gears is a good candidate for reinforcing.

Figure 12-5 shows one obvious way to reinforce our mechanism: We simply replace the two pairs of 1×4 bricks with two 1×8 bricks. On the upside, the weak seam is now gone, every link in our chain is solid, and we no longer need to use plates. Additionally, this solution adds no weight and takes up no extra space. The downside is that using long, solid bricks can be an invasive way of reinforcing, and building in this way is time-consuming and extremely inconvenient with complex gearing, as you'll have to place all elements at the same time.

Figures 12-6 and 12-7 show another way we can reinforce our mechanism: by adding support beams. This increases the weight of the mechanism and takes more space, but it involves only minimal changes to the original structure. Note that structures like the one shown in Figure 12-7 have the downside of added friction because the yellow bricks are partially supported by the axles—building compact mechanisms can come with a cost.

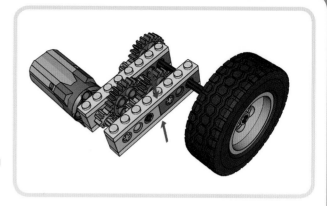

Figure 12-3: The critical connection in the mechanism from Figure 13-2 is marked by a red arrow here. This connection lies between two separate bricks and is held together merely by the clutching force of two 1×8 plates (yellow); therefore, it can be broken easily.

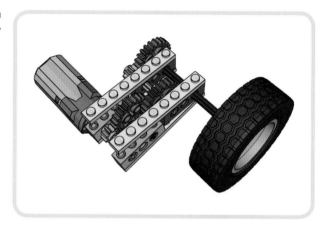

Figure 12-4: Without reinforcement, the weak link breaks apart the surrounding structure. The red gears are no longer meshed, and the mechanism fails.

understanding where to reinforce

The direction of a stressed gear's displacement depends on its location and its direction of rotation. When one gear drives another that resists it, the driver gear pushes against the follower gear just as the follower gear pushes back. This principle, which you might remember from high school physics, is a case of Newton's law of action and reaction, which states that forces are generated in equal and opposite pairs. Figure 12-8 shows a driver gear on top, rotating clockwise (as marked by the black arrow), and a follower gear on the bottom, being pushed down and to the side at the same time (as marked by the blue arrows).

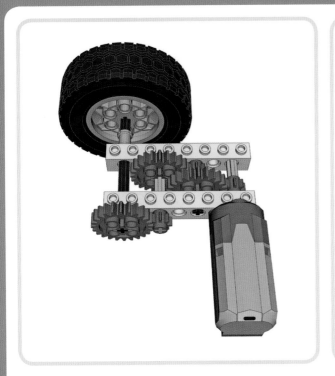

Figure 12-5: The two pairs of 1×4 bricks from our original structure have been replaced with two single, solid 1×8 bricks.

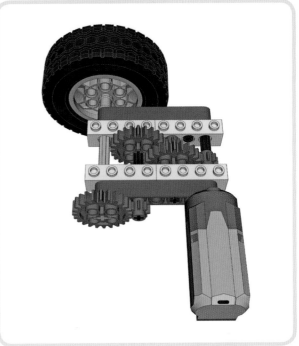

Figure 12-7: If vertical space is limited, horizontal beams (red) can sometimes be used. In this case, doing so requires using a few longer axles and moving the motor 1 stud away from the bricks. Note that in order to create a rigid connection, each of the bricks is attached to the beams at two points.

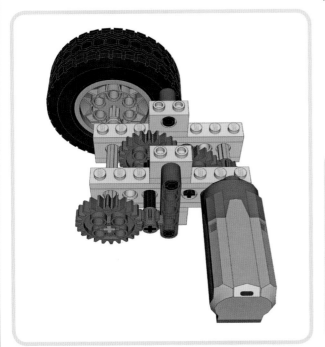

Figure 12-6: Vertical beams (red) are a popular means of reinforcement.

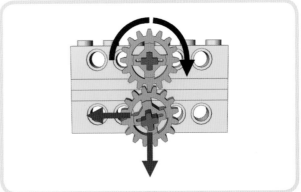

Figure 12-8: Directions of forces (blue) exerted by a driver gear (top) on the follower gear (bottom)

Now, if there were nothing holding the bricks in Figure 12-8 together, the follower gear would be pushed downward and to the left. The key to reinforcing properly is to limit displacement in *both* directions: Pieces that can't be separated can still be rotated, displacing and misaligning important elements of our drivetrain.

This same principle applies when two gears are mated at a different angle, as shown in Figure 12-9. Note that the gears in this figure can't come apart because their axles are both housed in a single L-shaped beam.

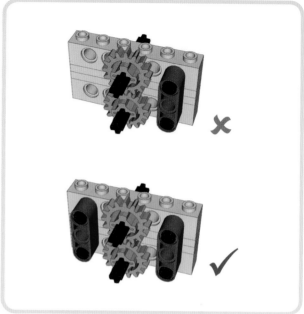

Figure 12-10: Holding one end of the bricks together doesn't create a rigid connection, but holding both does.

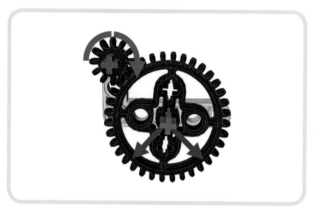

Figure 12-9: The directions of force exerted on the follower gear, which is located below and to the side of the driver gear

the right way to reinforce

Now that we know how to find weak links in our mechanisms, let's look at some examples of reinforcing. Figures 12-10 to 12-14 show reinforcing done poorly and done properly.

As you can see, reinforcing gears is about making sure the axles are securely supported. But since axles can be long and prone to bending, there are two rules to follow here:

* The axle should be supported at least at two points.
* The axle should be supported as close to the gears on it as possible, preferably from both sides of the gears.

Figure 12-15 illustrates the first rule, and Figure 12-16 illustrates the second rule. Axles are in fact much less rigid than beams or bricks, and they can bend, twist, or even slide through the gears when subjected to sufficient stress.

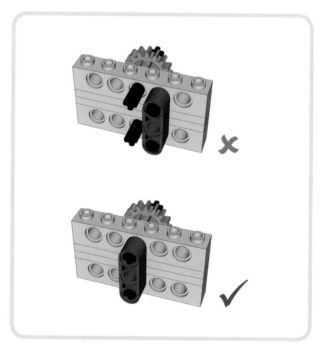

Figure 12-11: It's possible to reduce the number of reinforcing pieces by aligning them to the meshed gears rather than pairing them.

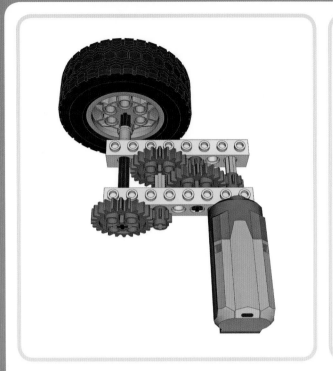

Figure 12-5: The two pairs of 1×4 bricks from our original structure have been replaced with two single, solid 1×8 bricks.

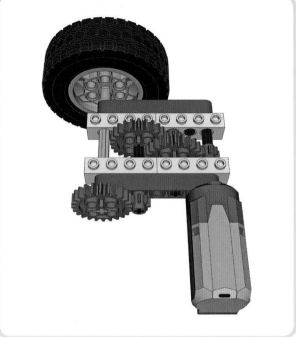

Figure 12-7: If vertical space is limited, horizontal beams (red) can sometimes be used. In this case, doing so requires using a few longer axles and moving the motor 1 stud away from the bricks. Note that in order to create a rigid connection, each of the bricks is attached to the beams at two points.

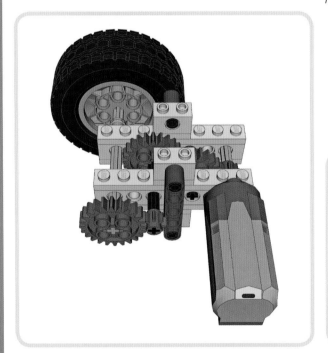

Figure 12-6: Vertical beams (red) are a popular means of reinforcement.

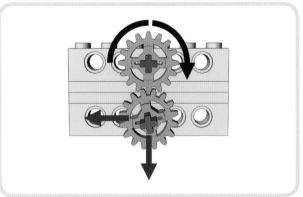

Figure 12-8: Directions of forces (blue) exerted by a driver gear (top) on the follower gear (bottom)

Now, if there were nothing holding the bricks in Figure 12-8 together, the follower gear would be pushed downward and to the left. The key to reinforcing properly is to limit displacement in *both* directions: Pieces that can't be separated can still be rotated, displacing and misaligning important elements of our drivetrain.

This same principle applies when two gears are mated at a different angle, as shown in Figure 12-9. Note that the gears in this figure can't come apart because their axles are both housed in a single L-shaped beam.

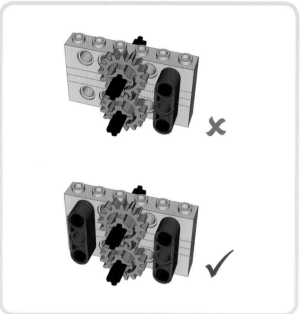

Figure 12-10: Holding one end of the bricks together doesn't create a rigid connection, but holding both does.

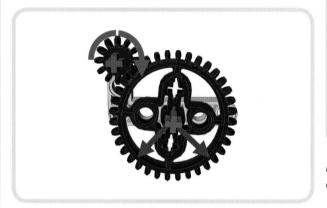

Figure 12-9: The directions of force exerted on the follower gear, which is located below and to the side of the driver gear

the right way to reinforce

Now that we know how to find weak links in our mechanisms, let's look at some examples of reinforcing. Figures 12-10 to 12-14 show reinforcing done poorly and done properly.

As you can see, reinforcing gears is about making sure the axles are securely supported. But since axles can be long and prone to bending, there are two rules to follow here:

* The axle should be supported at least at two points.
* The axle should be supported as close to the gears on it as possible, preferably from both sides of the gears.

Figure 12-15 illustrates the first rule, and Figure 12-16 illustrates the second rule. Axles are in fact much less rigid than beams or bricks, and they can bend, twist, or even slide through the gears when subjected to sufficient stress.

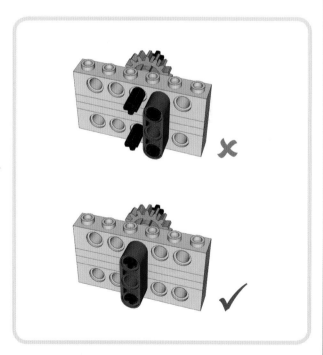

Figure 12-11: It's possible to reduce the number of reinforcing pieces by aligning them to the meshed gears rather than pairing them.

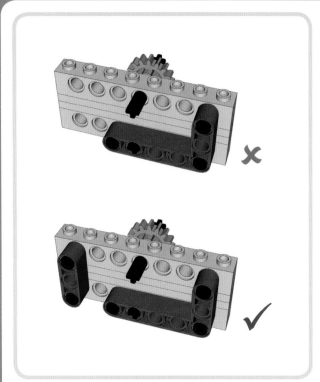

Figure 12-12: The L-shaped beam alone is not enough to create a rigid connection because it has only one point of attachment to the upper brick.

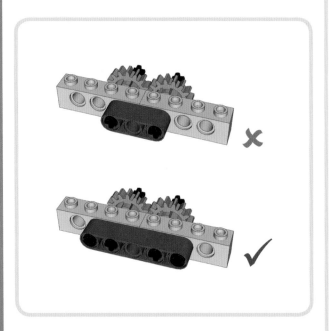

Figure 12-13: Beams that have only one point of attachment to adjacent bricks don't create a rigid connection. At least two points of connection to each brick are needed.

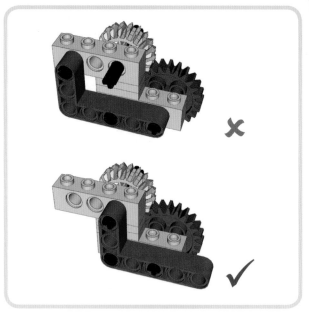

Figure 12-14: Plates help to create rigid connections. Use them as spacers between the points of connections of two bricks to prevent the bricks from oscillating.

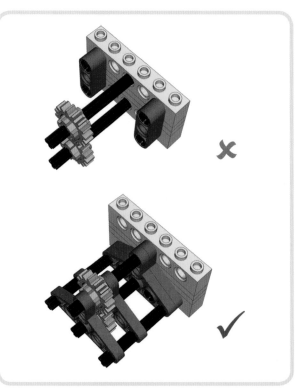

Figure 12-15: Both ends of the axles need to be reinforced to prevent the gears on them from coming apart.

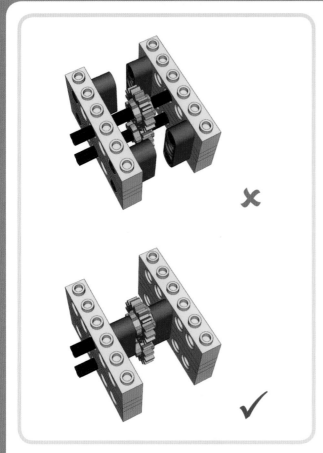

Figure 12-16: Empty space on the axles adjacent to the gears allows them to slide or enables the whole axle to bend. This empty space should be used for reinforcement.

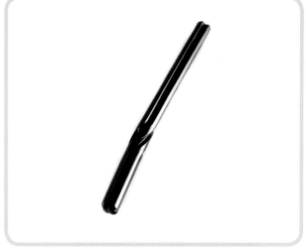

Figure 12-17: Axles are much more elastic than they might seem. This one has been twisted permanently by a PF XL motor.

Figure 12-17 shows a permanently twisted axle. Note that the longer the axle, the more easily it gets twisted—that's why it's always a good idea to swap a single long axle for a few shorter ones connected with axle joiners. Another good idea is to add substantial gear reduction near the output so that only a small portion of the drivetrain is subjected to high torque.

Reinforcing perpendicular bevel gears is a more difficult task, as even a minimal displacement in structure disengages the gears. This is because their teeth come into contact over a small area. We need to make sure the gears are firmly kept in place. A number of LEGO studfull and studless pieces are designed specifically to reinforce perpendicular gears, as shown in Figures 12-18 to 12-20.

When you have no dedicated LEGO pieces to reinforce perpendicular gears, you can still use basic pieces to do so. Figures 12-21 and 12-22 show examples of this approach using studfull and studless pieces.

things to remember when reinforcing

There are a few more rules of reinforcing worth keeping in mind:

* Minimal reinforcement is the best reinforcement. Extra pieces add weight and take up space.
* If a seam or joint can separate, it eventually will—and usually when you least expect it. (And Murphy's law says that it will be deep inside your MOC where you can't fix it!)
* Real reinforcement doesn't yield until pieces physically break.
* When building, think about disassembly, too. A reinforcement that has to be cut to be taken apart will cost you pieces.

The last rule is no less important than the ones preceding it. It's fairly easy to connect LEGO pieces in such a way that the resulting structure is impossible to disassemble without cutting some of the pieces. Figure 12-23 shows some examples. As you'll see, you should take precautions when inserting axles—always make sure it's possible to pull or push them out.

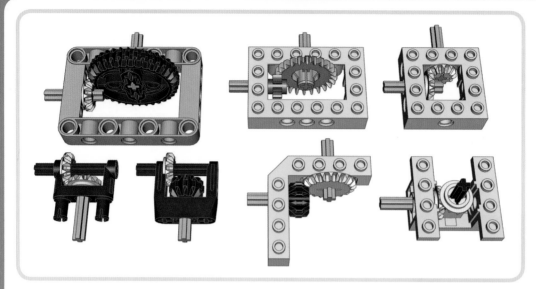

Figure 12-18: LEGO pieces for reinforcing perpendicular gears

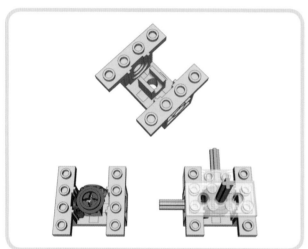

Figure 12-19: Piece #6585 is a particularly interesting brace that can reinforce both horizontal and vertical gears. Technic bricks and plates can be connected to it to support their axles.

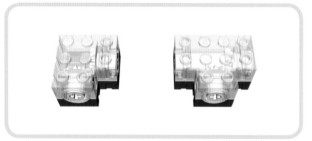

Figure 12-20: There are also so-called Technic gearboxes, which have special sturdy bevel gears enclosed. They are robust and can have axles inserted into them, but they are rare.

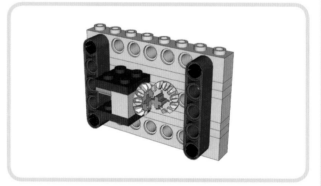

Figure 12-21: Perpendicular gears reinforced with bricks held together by beams. Note the use of 2×3 plates (blue) to hold the perpendicular brick.

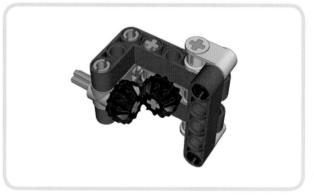

Figure 12-22: Perpendicular gears reinforced with L-shaped beams. Note that one end of the beams is held together by a vertical beam. This is because there are only axles on this end of the beams and the axles don't hold the beams together. The other end of the beams has a connector with pins that hold the beams together with a force very unlikely to be overcome by gears.

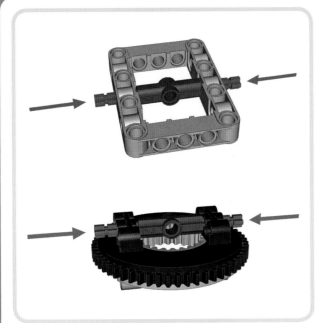

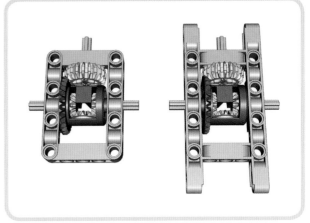

Figure 12-24: The studless frame comes in a regular (left) and an extended (right) variant. Both create a perfectly rigid reinforcement for the newest type of LEGO differential.

Figure 12-23: Dangerous structures: Once the axles marked by arrows are pushed in, these structures are impossible to take apart without cutting pieces.

reinforced differential casings

Differentials are often subjected to high torque because there is usually no gear reduction between them and the wheels. To make things worse, they are usually meshed using perpendicular gears. It was only in 2009 that LEGO released pieces designed specifically to remedy this problem: studless frames. But studless frames aren't very common and work only with the newest type of differential gear, as shown in Figures 12-24 and 12-25.

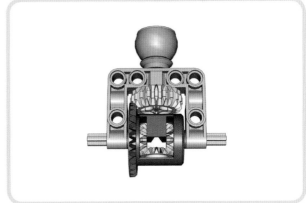

Figure 12-25: The larger part of the ball joint comes with an attached C-shaped frame, large enough to house the newest type of LEGO differential.

four reinforced differential casings

The following are examples of sturdy casings for all types of differentials, made of common pieces. They are inevitably inferior to studless frames because of their greater size and weight, but they are useful nonetheless.

1

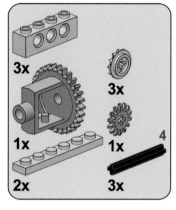

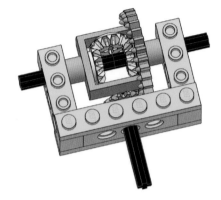

2

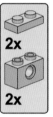

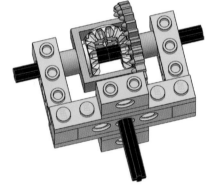

3

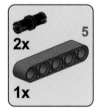

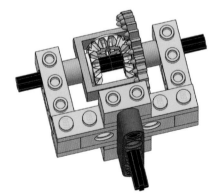

1

1x 6
1x
2x
2x

1x
5x
3x 4
1x

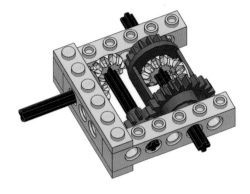

2

2x
2x

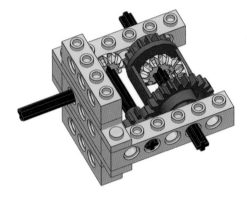

3

4x 5
2x

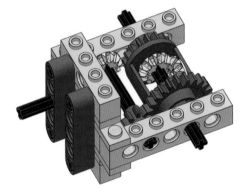

1

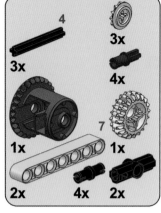

4
3x

3x

4x

7
1x 1x

2x 4x 2x

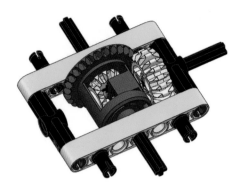

2

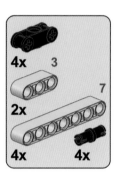

4x 3

2x

7

4x 4x

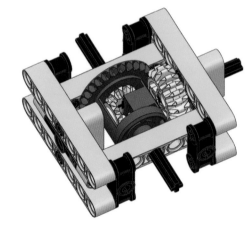

3

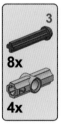

3
8x

4x

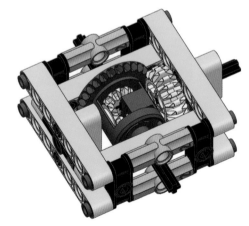

1

4

4x

3x

1x

1x   5   4x   3x

2x   2x   4x

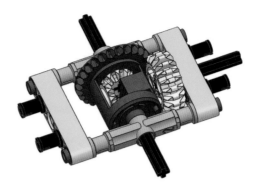

2

9

4x   4x

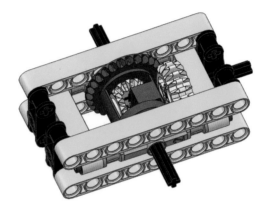

3

6

4x

4x

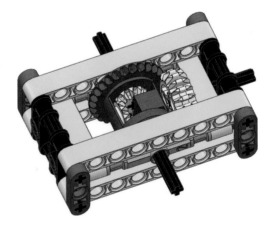

reinforced worm gear casings

Because of their unique design, worm gears need particularly solid reinforcement. As Figure 12-26 shows, apart from pushing the follower gear away, worm gears have a strong tendency to slide along the axle they're sitting on. This is a result of worm gears' enlarged axle holes. This lateral force can be strong enough to make a worm gear drill through adjacent pieces if sufficiently high torque is applied to it for a prolonged time!

LEGO released special casings for worm gears, but they are relatively large and work only with 24-tooth follower gears, as shown in Figures 12-27 and 12-28.

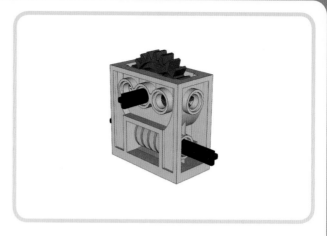

Figure 12-27: The LEGO casing for the worm gear is very sturdy and quite common, but it works only with a 24-tooth follower gear. It's also better suited for studfull structures than for studless ones.

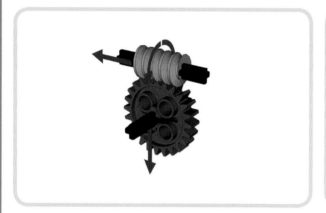

Figure 12-26: The directions of forces exerted by a worm gear. Unlike regular gears, a worm gear doesn't push the follower gear to the side; instead, it pushes itself against the follower gear along its axle.

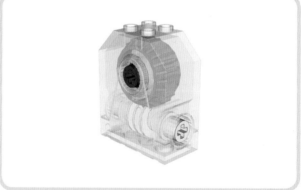

Figure 12-28: A gearbox with a worm gear and 24-tooth follower gear closed inside. It's even sturdier than the regular casing, but it's very rare.

three reinforced worm gear casings

Thankfully, if you have neither a casing piece nor a gearbox piece, you can easily build your own. Three designs for worm gear casings (using various follower gears) are shown here.

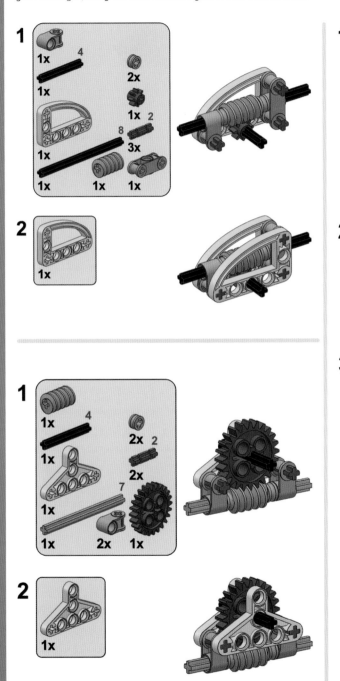

1

1x 4
1x
1x 2
1x 8
3x
1x 1x 1x

2

1x

1

1x 4
1x 2
2x 2
1x 2
7
1x
1x 2x 1x

2

1x

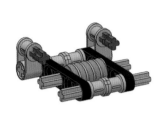

1

2
2x
1x
2x 5
3x 4x 2x

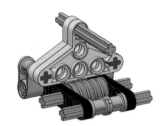

2

2x 5
1x

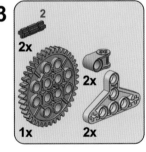
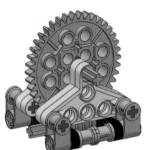

3

2
2x
2x
1x 2x

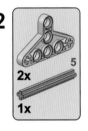
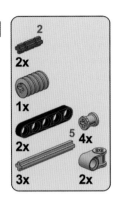

load-bearing structures

Load-bearing structures are the "skeletons" within our models. You might think of these structures as the framing of a house, the pylons of a suspension bridge, the chassis of a car, or even the bones of the human body. They support a construction's weight and maintain its rigidity, and they may have no other purpose beyond structural reinforcement.

rails, chassis, and body frames

A chassis is the type of a load-bearing structure most commonly used in vehicular models. A properly built chassis is sturdy enough to support the weight of the vehicle and rigid enough to maintain its shape as the vehicle negotiates obstacles and carries loads.

We're going to focus on the most convenient and commonly used way to build a chassis: *rails*, also called *stringers*. Almost all LEGO Technic sets use this method.

Rails are longitudinal members that span most or the entire length of the vehicle. Since one rail is not rigid enough to support a vehicle's weight, most body frames have two parallel rails, which are joined together with crossbeams so they act as one element. You can add other elements of the construction both in the gap between the rails and in the space around them.

Figure 12-29 shows a small, lightweight studless LEGO truck with two rails visible from the bottom. Note that elements are placed both on the sides of the rails (wheels, bumpers, side curtains) and between them (differential, piston engine).

Figures 12-30 and 12-31 show examples of simple studless and studfull rail/crossbeam configurations.

Configurations like these, which form a "skeleton" that supports other parts of the model, are called *body frames*. If you expect particularly large stress to be exerted on your model's chassis, you can add another pair of rails above the first one and connect the two pairs. Figures 12-32 and 12-33 show examples of a studless and studfull body frame, and Figure 12-34 shows a studfull body frame at work in my Tow Truck 2 model.

The most common gap size between rails is between 3 and 6 studs. A gap this size is big enough for most of the heavy elements you may want to place in the center of your model, such as big motors and power supplies, but not so wide as to affect the frame's rigidity.

Finally, we can build rails with more complex shapes to accommodate elements like pendular suspension components. Figure 12-35 shows examples of body frames with irregularly shaped rails.

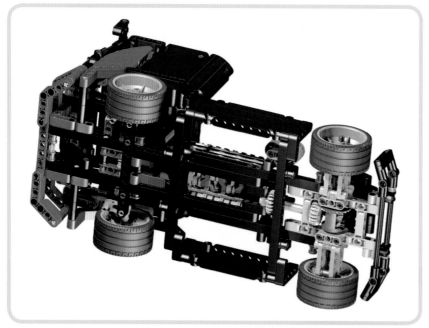

Figure 12-29: The 8041 set, a small racing truck, is a good example of a model built around two parallel rails.

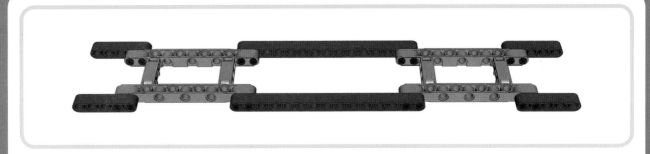

Figure 12-30: A simple combination of rails made of studless beams, with extended body frames working as crossbars. The frames provide space for differentials for front and rear axles, and there is plenty of space between the rails for a propulsion system or a power supply.

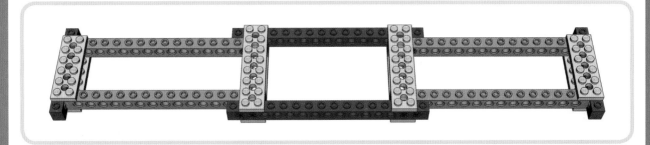

Figure 12-31: A simple studfull chassis combining bricks, pins, and plates

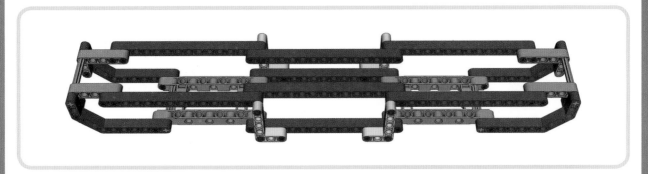

Figure 12-32: A studless body frame with two pairs of rails, one above the other. The upper pair is supported at the ends and in the middle. Studless frames work well with smaller, compact models where the ability to add many elements to the chassis is more important than its rigidity.

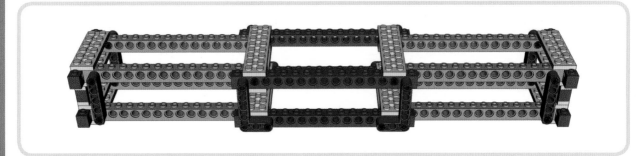

Figure 12-33: A typical studfull body frame, reinforced with vertical beams. This kind of frame works well for big, heavy models where rigidity is of primary importance.

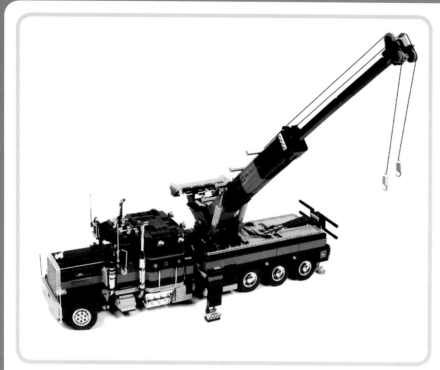

Figure 12-34: My Tow Truck 2 model was very heavy and almost 0.8 m long. It was held together by a massive studfull body frame with two pairs of rails, rigid enough to allow the model to be lifted by hand without any problems. The boom of the truck had its own frame of four studless rails, with the extendable section placed in the middle. It was covered with a studfull shell, which not only made it look better but also improved its rigidity.

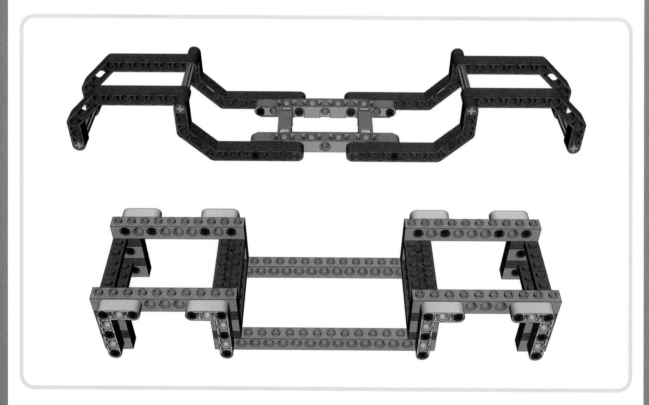

Figure 12-35: Examples of studless and studfull body frames with rails of complex shapes

trusses

A truss is a particular type of load-bearing structure that consists of beams that form repeated triangles, as shown in Figure 12-36. The triangles are often identical in size, but they don't have to be. The joints connecting these elements in a truss are often called *nodes*. Trusses are ubiquitous in the construction of buildings and machines—for example, tower cranes are built almost entirely with trusses. The advantage of trusses is that they can form large, lightweight, and very sturdy structures while using only a handful of basic pieces to build. Figure 12-37 shows a LEGO set that makes use of simple trusses.

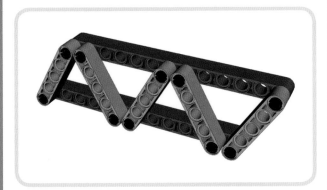

Figure 12-36: A simple truss

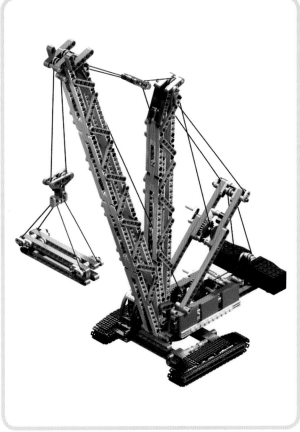

Figure 12-37: The 8288 Crawler Crane set comes with two booms (greyish in this image) made entirely of simple trusses.

Trusses can be divided into two categories: *planar trusses*, with all nodes within a single plane (like the truss in Figure 12-36), and *space trusses*, in which nodes extend in all three dimensions (like the truss in Figure 12-38). Space trusses are generally sturdier than planar trusses, and their simple construction allows for modular building. As Figure 12-38 shows, a simple space truss can actually be a combination of two or more planar trusses.

Just like any other load-bearing structures, trusses can be subjected to as many as four types of stress: *compression*, *tension*, *bending*, and *torsion*, as shown in Figure 12-39. It's possible to build a truss that can resist all four types of stress, but such a truss is heavy, complex, and takes lots of pieces to build. A more "economical" approach is to choose the type of truss that can handle only the kinds of stress we expect it to experience.

There are more than 20 types of trusses in the world. However, their complex geometry makes many of them difficult to reproduce with LEGO pieces, so we'll limit our discussion to three practical designs.

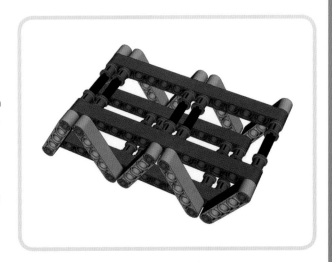

Figure 12-38: Two planar trusses, connected using axles and pins with bushes, create a basic space truss.

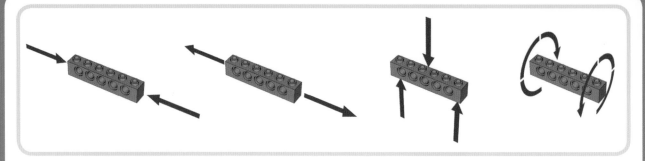

Figure 12-39: From left to right: compression, tension, bending, and torsion

Brown truss

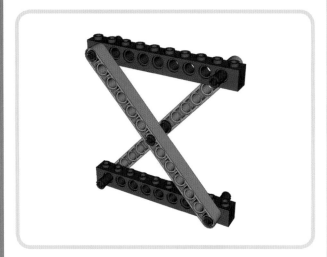

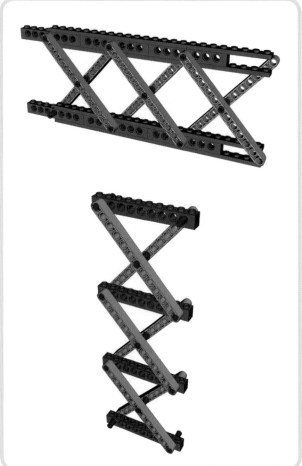

The Brown truss uses an X-shaped reinforcement between two horizontal members. If there is only one reinforcement between these members, its slant beams must be connected in the middle. If there are multiple Xs, this connection is not needed, as shown in Figure 12-40.

The length and angle of beams in the Brown truss module can be adjusted as needed, but the module is strongest with crossbeams exactly perpendicular to each other. Our example above, with 12-stud-long horizontal beams and 13-stud-long crossbeams, is of a convenient size: The gap between the pin holes of the upper and lower horizontal beams is exactly 10 studs tall.

The basic building block of the Brown truss, the planar X, can be combined into planar trusses similar in construction to a scissor mechanism, as shown in Figure 12-40. A more interesting solution is to combine the planar X into a space truss, as shown in Figure 12-41. The space combination can also be used to build modules that can easily be stacked on top of one another, as shown in Figure 12-42.

Figure 12-40: Planar combinations of the Brown truss module

The Brown truss is resistant to compression and torsion. Its resistance to tension and bending depends on the strength of connections between its modules.

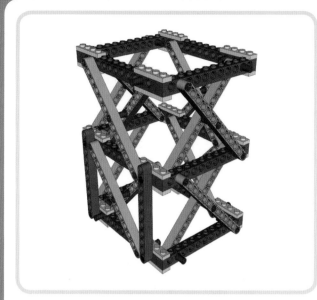

Figure 12-41: Space combination of the Brown truss module. Note that vertical beams (red) can be added for further reinforcement.

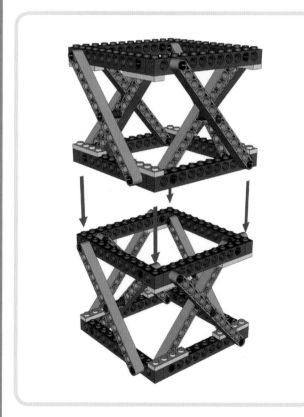

Figure 12-42: The Brown module is shown here combined into space modules that can be stacked on top of one another. This arrangement allows you to easily adjust the height of the resulting structure.

Warren truss

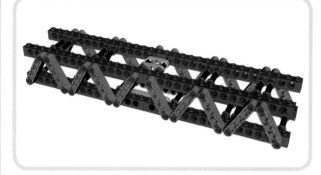

The Warren truss combines two simple planar trusses. The length and angle of the slanted beams (light grey) can be adjusted as needed. The slanted beams also don't have to be adjacent—small gaps between them are acceptable. The horizontal beams (dark grey) can be studless, as in Figure 12-38, or studfull, as shown above (in which case they can be further reinforced with plates).

The Warren truss is resistant to compression, tension, and bending. Torsion affects connections between its planar trusses and can lead to disintegration.

triangular Warren truss

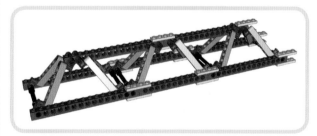

The triangular Warren truss, shown in Figures 12-43 and 12-44, combines two simple planar trusses to form the shape of a triangular prism. The truss has two lower beams but only one upper beam, which makes it weigh less than the regular Warren truss, though its construction requires additional connectors (red in the illustration and in Figures 12-43 and 12-44). This variant is nearly as robust as the regular Warren truss, except that its lower beams are subjected to more stress than the upper beam. Also, pressure on the upper beam can push the two lower beams apart unless they are connected (by perpendicular plates, for example).

The triangular Warren truss is resistant to compression, tension, and bending. With lower beams firmly connected by crossbeams, it is also considerably resistant to torsion.

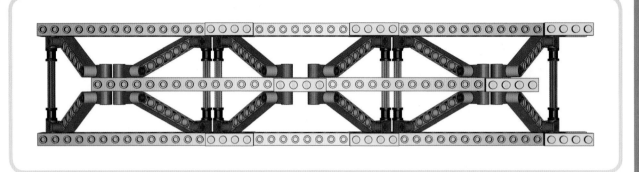

Figure 12-43: Top view of the triangular Warren truss

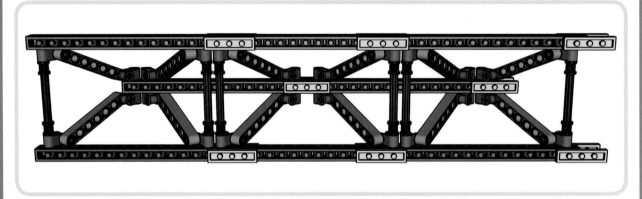

Figure 12-44: The bottom view of the triangular Warren truss shows that the lower beams (horizontal, top and bottom) are held together only from the inside of the truss. This means that they can be pushed apart by a sufficiently high load on the top beam (horizontal, middle).

simple triangular truss

A very effective way of employing a triangular truss was demonstrated in the 42042 Crawler Crane set. It consists of identical, 15-stud-long modules connected together with beams and pins with a stop (see Figure 12-45). The modules, which are exceptionally simple, light, and strong, are similar to simplified Brown truss modules with alternating members instead of crossed members. The entire design is ingenious in its simplicity: There's simply nothing redundant here! The resulting truss is resistant to everything except torsion.

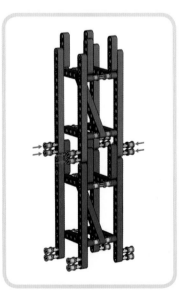

Figure 12-45: Two identical modules of simple triangular truss (red and blue) are joined by pushing in pins with bushes, as marked by red arrows.

a simple triangular truss

1

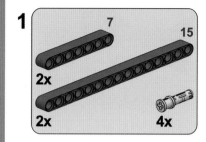

7
2x

15
2x

4x

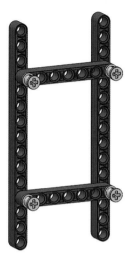

2

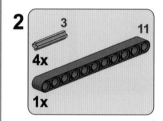

3
4x

11
1x

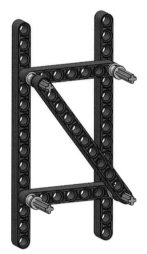

3

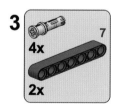

4x

7
2x

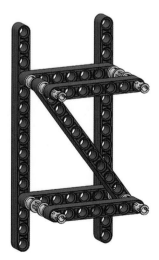

4

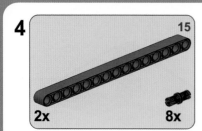

15

2x   8x

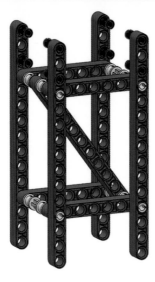

5

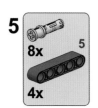

8x   5

4x

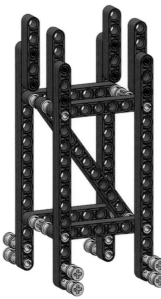

choosing the right truss

A truss made of firmly connected Brown modules can withstand all types of stress. It is, however, complex and heavy, so you'll want to use it only if it's absolutely necessary. This section explores how to determine which truss will work best for various vehicles.

Let's first consider a bus, which has a large gap between its front and rear axle. Its axles support it from the bottom, while its weight presses from the top on the middle of its chassis, as shown in Figure 12-46. This means that the chassis is subjected to bending. A regular Warren truss will easily

handle that stress while also resisting the minor compression and tension that occur when the bus starts and stops.

An off-road truck, on the other hand, is less subject to bending due to its shorter length. But such a truck is designed to negotiate difficult obstacles, which will make its suspension work hard, making the wheels go up and down. It's very likely that the front and rear axles of our truck will oscillate in opposite directions while traversing an obstacle, which will exert torsion on the chassis, as shown in Figure 12-47.

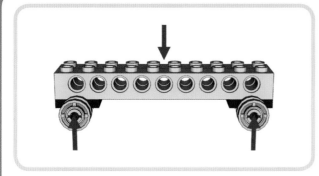

Figure 12-46: Forces exerted on the chassis of a bus. The chassis is primarily subjected to bending.

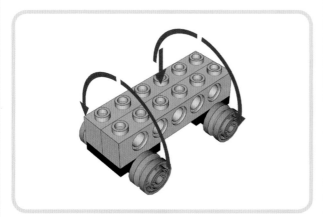

Figure 12-47: Forces exerted on the chassis of an off-road truck. The chassis is subjected primarily to torsion but also to bending.

We can use Brown modules in our truck's chassis if we want it to be extremely sturdy, but we can also use the triangular Warren truss to save some weight and space. With its lower beams held together, the triangular Warren truss will handle both torsion and bending.

Our last example is a tower crane, which has several elements that could use reinforcing. We'll see how different sections of the crane will benefit from using different kinds of trusses.

As Figure 12-48 shows, we can break our crane into four parts. First is the part that supports the entire crane, called the *tower mast* (yellow). As the weight of the crane rests on it, the tower mast is subjected to compression. Lifting loads also makes the crane tip a bit, so the structure is subject to some bending. Finally, the upper portion of the crane can rotate while the yellow truss remains fixed to the ground—this exerts torsion when rotation starts and stops.

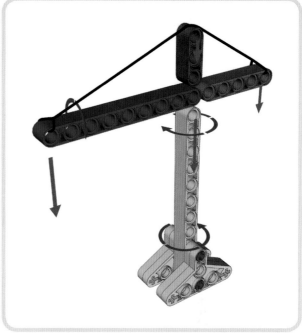

Figure 12-48: Forces exerted on various parts of a tower crane

So we know our yellow tower mast truss must withstand all types of stress except tension. A truss made of space Brown modules will be a good choice.

Our second truss (blue) is called the *jib*. It's the part directly responsible for moving loads. As one end is fixed to the center of the crane, the other has loads suspended on it and is supported by a cable called the *jib tie*, which exerts some compression on it. As the crane rotates, the loads swing a little below the jib, exerting some torsion on it as well. Note that the jib is the second-largest part of the crane, and it can add a lot of weight. We want the jib to weigh as little as possible, so the triangular Warren truss will be a good choice here, resisting both compression and torsion while adding less weight than other options.

The third part (green) is called the *counterjib*. The counterjib is fixed to the center of the crane at one end and supports the crane's counterweight at its other end. It is therefore subjected to bending, just like the jib, but to a smaller degree because of its shorter length. Its counterweight doesn't swing during rotation, so it isn't subjected to torsion. We can use the triangular Warren truss here as well, or we can instead choose the simpler regular Warren truss—the counterjib is so short that the difference in weight will be minimal.

Finally, the grey part, called the *top mast*, simply supports the cable that connects opposite tips of the jib and counterjib. The jib tie exerts compression on the top mast and slight bending on the counterjib, which we've already accounted for. The top mast is small and little stress is involved, so we can use a small section of the Warren truss; alternatively, we can give up on trusses and use any structure capable of supporting some weight put directly on top of it. Figure 12-49 shows an example of a real tower crane built the same way as our model.

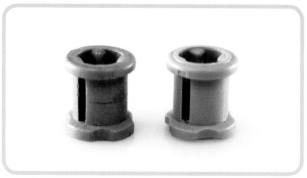

Figure 12-50: A bush: roughly 20 years old (left) and 1 year old (right). Note the crack in the old bush's side; under torque, this crack will soon lead to the bush's disintegration.

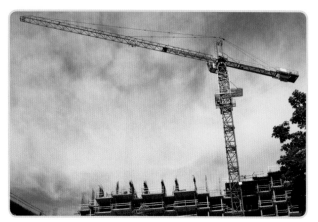

Figure 12-49: A real tower crane at work. As you can see, its tower mast is built with a Brown truss, and its jib is built with a triangular Warren truss, just like in our model.

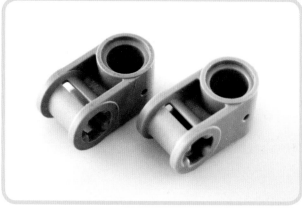

Figure 12-51: A connector: old (left) and new (right). Even though the old piece is free from damage or visible wear, the difference is obvious.

choosing the strongest pieces

Although LEGO pieces are known for their lasting quality, they are prone to aging and wear. This means there are two things you should avoid when picking pieces for a tough job: aged pieces and physically worn pieces.

It's safe to assume that LEGO pieces fully maintain their quality for at least 5 to 10 years, unless damaged. As your collection ages, or is supplemented with older pieces and garage sale treasures, you should carefully select the pieces that will handle high stress. The easiest way to determine a piece's age is to keep a few new pieces for comparison. LEGO pieces, particularly white and grey pieces, yellow over time. Figures 12-50 to 12-52 show the difference.

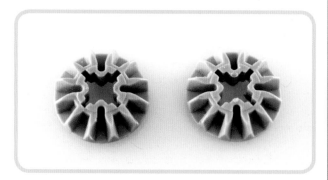

Figure 12-52: Two gears of the same type made roughly 10 years apart

Pieces that are physically worn aren't too difficult to spot. The wear can vary from very subtle—negligible for our purposes—to obvious damage. You should look for wear on the surfaces that contact other pieces, such as the teeth of gears or the area around the pin hole in a brick. Wear occurs more often on pieces that are subjected to high stress, such as knobs, small gears that are crucial for high gear reduction, or various pieces that work with worm gears. Figures 12-53 to 12-55 show typical examples of wear.

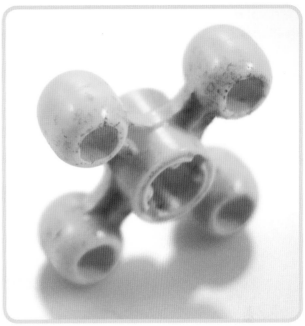

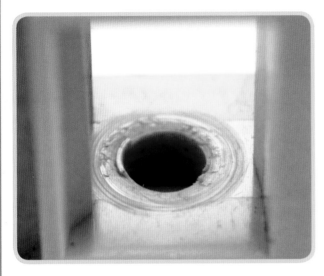

Figure 12-53: A close-up view showing the inside of a LEGO casing for a worm gear. Here, a worm gear has partially drilled into one of the casing sides.

Figure 12-55: This visibly worn knob has polished edges where the material has been rubbed away. Knobs transfer high torque over very small areas of contact, resulting in intense wear. Worn knobs produce a distinctive squeaking when working under stress.

Finally, note that differently colored pieces actually have different properties. The exact variations are difficult to measure, but I have observed that red pieces are particularly weak while yellow pieces are particularly strong. The difference isn't big, but it can manifest when pieces are subjected to prolonged stress.

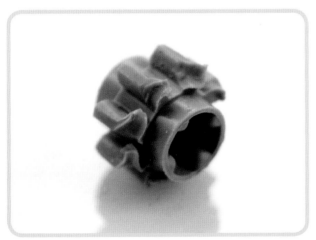

Figure 12-54: This gear's teeth were ground away when it was misaligned to a larger, stronger gear. While the piece itself is new and most of it remains intact, this kind of wear makes the gear unusable.

motors

13

an inventory of LEGO motors

Electric motors are the muscle of most Technic creations. While it's perfectly fine to build mechanisms driven by hand, and some builders actually specialize in human-powered models, the most impressive constructions are motorized. Motors can be used for almost anything, from driving and steering to rotating, elevating, extending, and even controlling other electric components. In this chapter, we'll explore which LEGO motors are best suited for which purposes.

LEGO has been making electric motors since 1965, and they can be classified into three general categories. The first motors were 4.5V motors, but they're rare, old, and inferior when compared to the newer motors, so let's move straight to the next category.

In 1990, LEGO introduced a second line of motors, running at 9V on six AA batteries (shown in Figure 13-1). These motors are considerably more powerful and convenient to use than their predecessors. The 9V line also has greater variation, including motors for boats with propellers and watertight housings. The 9V motors are widely available and highly popular. We'll discuss this line of motors in this chapter, with the exception of some specialized ones, such as the Trains and Monorail motors, which are very difficult (or downright impossible) to use outside their intended applications.

The third category of motors is the *Power Functions (PF)* line, introduced in 2007 (shown in Figure 13-2). These motors are designed to use a 9V power supply as well, but unlike the previous category, they are part of a carefully planned and currently developed system of motors and specialized parts. The Power Functions line includes just a few motors, which are designed to complement each other. Each motor is suited for different tasks, and the characteristics of the motors vary considerably. PF motors are well suited to studless building because they have odd widths and pin holes, and their torque is optimized for high-load applications. Additionally, the Power Functions system comes

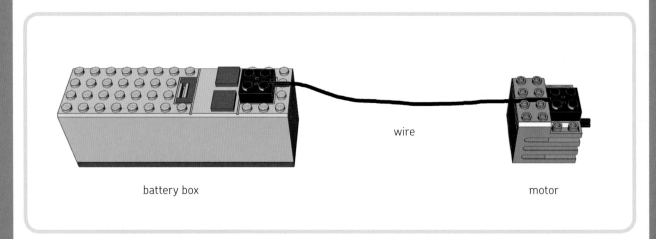

battery box   wire   motor

Figure 13-1: The 9V line is powered by a battery box, which also functions as a basic switch.

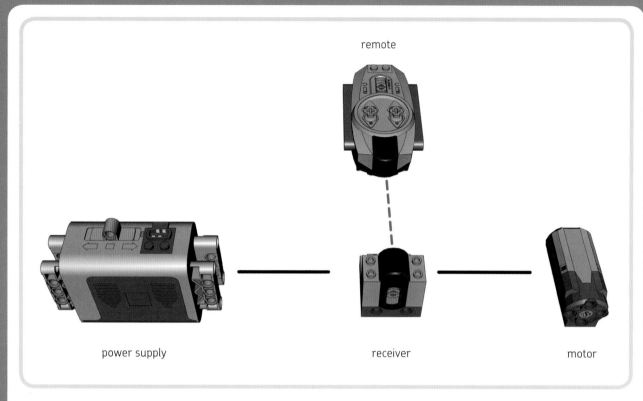

remote

power supply   receiver   motor

Figure 13-2: The Power Functions motor system can be controlled remotely.

with control elements that enable wireless remote control and adjust the speed of all motors connected to them. We'll explore the Power Functions system and its controls in Chapter 14.

The following list includes speeds of motors at both 9V and 7V whenever such data is available. (Rechargeable AA batteries and the rechargeable Power Functions battery provide a 7V power supply.) Also, note that motors are prone to wearing down over time; thus, the exact characteristics of any two motors of the same type can vary.

While there is no official technical specification for the LEGO motors, LEGO enthusiast Philippe "Philo" Hurbain has spent a lot of time performing many complex measures on them. This chapter's measurements are derived from his work and used with his kind permission. (Read more about Philippe's work at his site, *http://www.philohome.com/motors/motorcomp.htm*.)

2838, the first 9V motor

Torque: 0.45 N•cm
No-load speed at 7V: 1000 RPM
No-load speed at 9V: 2000 RPM
Dimensions: 6×4×3 studs
Produced: 1990 to 2002

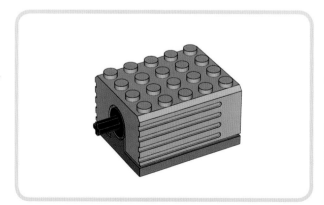

The first motor in the 9V line, the 2838, is relatively large and has no internal gearing, which results in very high speed and low torque. It's ineffective in high-load applications, where it requires substantial gear reduction, often including one or more worm gears. This motor is also prone to overheating. The motor has a 1L axle protruding out of it and connects to the power supply through a 2×5 contact area in the middle of its bottom surface.

71427, a popular and powerful 9V motor

Torque: 2.25 N•cm
No-load speed at 7V: 160 RPM
No-load speed at 9V: 250 RPM
Dimensions: 5×4×4 studs
Produced: 1997 to 2004

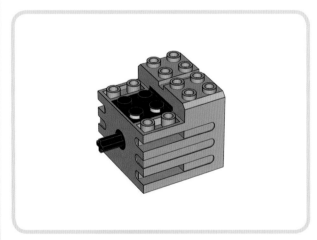

The 71427 is a popular 9V motor due to its reasonable size and favorable characteristics. It's a very quiet motor with substantial internal gearing, whose inertia means that the motor doesn't stop immediately when turned off. The motor has a 1L axle and connects to the power supply through a 2×2 contact area on top. Its upper surface is conveniently shaped: It has one recess for the power plug and another for routing the wire backward. Its lower surface has a 1-plate-tall 2×2 bulge in the back.

43362, a lighter 9V motor

Torque: 2.25 N•cm
No-load speed at 7V: 140 RPM
No-load speed at 9V: 219 RPM
Dimensions: 5×4×4 studs
Produced: 1993 to 2004

Externally identical to the 9V 71427 motor (shown previously), the 43362 motor is almost one-third lighter at the expense of slightly reduced speed. The difference in weight makes it more sought after than the original 71427 motor, so it sells for significantly higher prices. The motor has a 1L axle and connects to the power supply through a 2×2 contact area on top. Its upper surface is conveniently shaped and has one recess for the power plug and another for routing the wire backward. Its lower surface has a 1-plate-tall 2×2 bulge in the back. Just like the 71427 motor, this motor can be mounted on rails using the slots on its sides (shown in Figure 13-3).

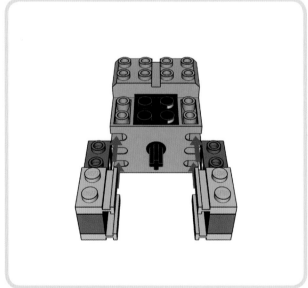

Figure 13-3: The slots on the sides of the 71427 and 43362 motors fit plates with rails. Each motor can be firmly secured using two or more of these plates. The red arrows show that the plates slide into slots in the motor's housing.

47154, a 9V motor in a semi-transparent housing

Torque: 2.25 N•cm
No-load speed at 7V: 210 RPM
No-load speed at 9V: 315 RPM
Dimensions: 4×4×4 studs
Produced: 2003 to 2006

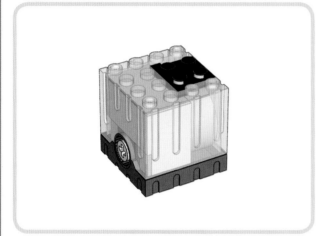

The 47154 motor is similar to the 71427 motor except that it has a higher speed and is louder. Its top and bottom are completely flat. The motor has a 1-stud-deep axle hole and connects to the power supply through a 2×2 contact area on top.

Micromotor

Torque: 1.28 N•cm
No-load speed at 9V: 16 RPM
Dimensions (with braces and pulley): 3.5×3×2 studs
Produced: 1993 to 2001

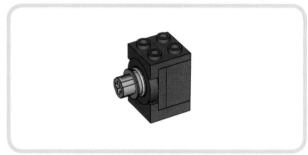

The 9V Micromotor is exceptional for its small size. It's rare, highly sought after, and expensive. Its speed is so slow that it doesn't usually need external gear reduction, but its torque is quite high for a motor of this size (higher than the 2838 motor's torque, for example). A complete Micromotor consists of four individual pieces: an upper and lower brace, a "Micromotor pulley," and the actual motor. The motor is rarely used without these pieces, although it can be operated without the braces if it is connected to something by its power plug (which connects to studs). The motor connects to the power supply through a 2×2 contact area at its back. Figure 13-4 shows an exploded view of the Micromotor and its parts.

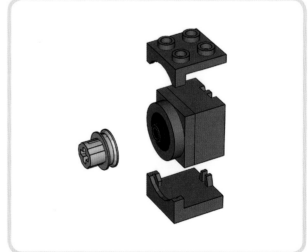

Figure 13-4: An exploded view of the Micromotor showing its upper and lower brackets, pulley, and motor

The Micromotor's specially designed pulley has a 1-stud-deep axle hole and a belt groove for a rubber band. The pulley allows the motor to be connected to an axle. The pulley also works like a slip clutch, preventing the motor from stalling. It's a crucial piece: Using the motor without the pulley is a sure way to destroy it!

MINDSTORMS NXT motor

Torque: 16.7 N•cm
No-load speed at 7V: 82 RPM
No-load speed at 9V: 117 RPM
Dimensions: 14×6×5 studs
Produced: 2006 to 2011

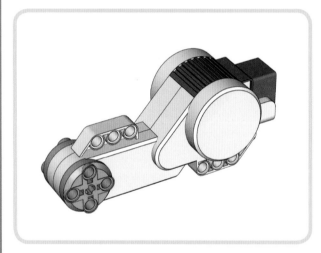

The MINDSTORMS NXT motor was designed specifically for the MINDSTORMS NXT set. It's distinguished by very high torque and power consumption. It includes a rotation sensor with a one-degree resolution, which is useful when you're designing robots that require precise control.

However, its shape and size are disadvantages when you're not using it with MINDSTORMS constructions, and it connects to the power supply through a MINDSTORMS-type plug, which means it requires a special converter cable to connect it to regular 9V or Power Functions power supplies. Unlike other motors, its output is a 3-stud-wide ring (orange in the preceding figure) with four 1-stud-deep pin holes around the center. It also has an empty 3-stud-deep axle hole in the center through which you can insert any axle. It's compatible with NXT and EV3 units.

MINDSTORMS EV3 Medium motor

Torque: 6.64 N•cm
No-load speed at 7V: 120 RPM
No-load speed at 9V: 165 RPM
Dimensions: 9×4×3 studs
Produced: 2013 to present

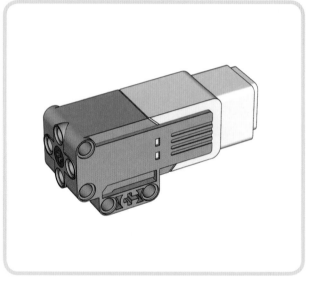

A MINDSTORMS equivalent of the popular PF M motor, the MINDSTORMS EV3 Medium motor is much slower but nearly twice as strong. It's very popular due to its modest size and convenient frontal 1-stud-deep axle hole, which allows it to connect in the same manner as PF motors. It includes a rotation sensor, it connects through a standard MINDSTORMS plug, and it's compatible both with EV3 and NXT units.

MINDSTORMS EV3 Large motor

Torque: 17.3 N•cm
No-load speed at 7V: 78 RPM
No-load speed at 9V: 105 RPM
Dimensions: 14×7×5 studs
Produced: 2013 to present

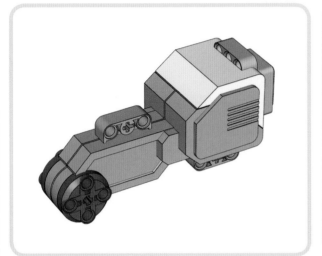

The MINDSTORMS EV3 Large motor is an updated version of the MINDSTORMS NXT motor and is a bit slower and stronger than its predecessor. It also has more pin holes and is generally easier to mount and use. It includes a rotation sensor, and it connects through a standard MINDSTORMS plug, which makes it compatible with EV3 and NXT units.

Power Functions E motor

Torque: 1.32 N•cm
No-load speed at 7V: 300 RPM
No-load speed at 9V: 420 RPM
Dimensions: 6×4×4 studs
Produced: 2010 only

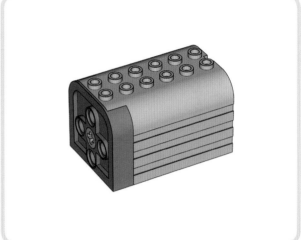

The unusual Power Functions E motor was designed for LEGO Education sets. It has low internal gearing, which allows it to be easily driven and to act as a power generator. However, its large size, poor speed, and low torque make it practically useless when compared to other Power Functions motors. The motor has a 1-stud-deep axle hole and an integral wire.

Power Functions M (Medium) motor

Torque: 3.63 N•cm
No-load speed at 7V: 185 RPM
No-load speed at 9V: 275 RPM
Dimensions: 6×3×3 studs
Produced: 2007 to present

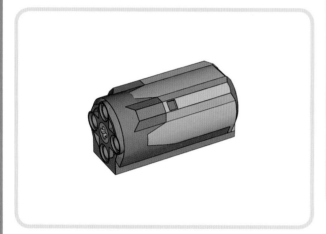

With a diameter of only 3 studs, the popular Power Functions M motor takes up little space and fits studless constructions exceptionally well while offering very good torque. The only downside to this motor is its length; other than that, it's easy to use, powerful, and versatile. This motor has a 1-stud-deep axle hole and an integral wire. It connects either from the front using four pin holes or from the bottom using studs.

Power Functions L (Large) motor

Torque: approx. 6.48 N•cm
No-load speed at 7V: 203 RPM
No-load speed at 9V: 272 RPM
Dimensions: 7×4×3 studs
Produced: 2012 to present

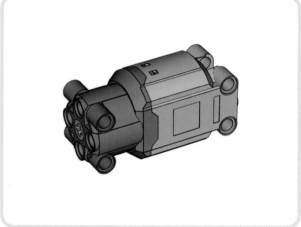

The L motor excels where the Medium motor is too weak and the XL motor is too big. Only slightly larger than the Medium motor, but faster and almost twice as strong, it has significantly higher power consumption and requires a V2 PF IR receiver to run at full power (see Chapter 14 for more information). This motor has a 1-stud-deep axle hole and an integral wire. It connects using pin holes: four in front and on either side and two at the back.

Power Functions XL motor

Torque: 14.5 N•cm
No-load speed at 7V: 100 RPM
No-load speed at 9V: 146 RPM
Dimensions: 6×5×5 studs
Produced: 2007 to present

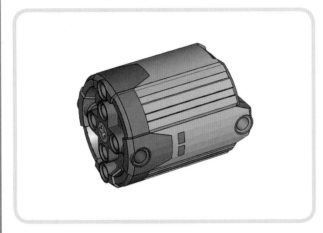

The XL is the most powerful Power Functions motor. It shares some essential internal parts with the NXT motor but has lower torque and higher speed. The XL motor is popular for its high torque, and it's more common and easier to use than the NXT motor. Still, its large size makes two coupled PF L motors a better choice in many cases. The XL motor has a 1-stud-deep axle hole and an integral wire; it also has six pin holes on its front and two on either side, which allow it to be firmly braced in a construction to handle its considerable output torque.

Power Functions Servo motor

Dimensions: 7×5×3 studs
Produced: 2012 to present

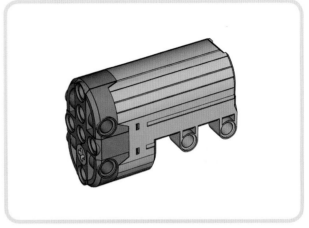

The Servo motor is designed specifically for steering systems. It can't rotate continuously; instead, it rotates 90 degrees clockwise or counterclockwise from its central position. Its low speed allows it to be used with most steering systems directly with no gearing in between, and it has enough torque to steer even heavy vehicles.

When used with a basic PF remote, the Servo motor rotates 90 degrees in one direction or the other when you push the remote's lever, and it returns to the central position when you release the lever. When used with the speed control PF remote or directly with the rechargeable PF battery, the motor follows the rotation of the speed dial, meaning that it provides proportional steering with seven steps in either direction and one neutral position (which it returns to after you press the remote's stop button). In other words, it uses the PF speed control feature to break its 180 degrees of total rotation range into 15 steps of 12 degrees each while its speed remains constant at all times.

This motor has a bulge on the bottom with a 1-stud-deep axle hole on the front and another on the back. Thus, you can insert the motor between two axles; it will keep them 1 stud apart and rotate them as one in the same direction. It also has an integral wire and six pin holes in front and four on either side.

RC motor

Torque (inner output/outer output): 4.22 N•cm/5.7 N•cm
No-load speed at 7V (inner output/outer output):
    783 RPM/580 RPM
No-load speed at 9V (inner output/outer output):
    1053 RPM/780 RPM
Dimensions: 11×6×5 studs
Produced: 2002 to 2006

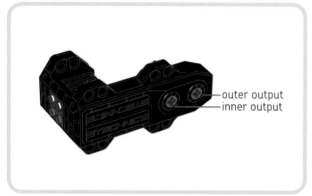

outer output
inner output

The 9V RC motor, also known as an "RC buggy motor," was originally designed for a discontinued series of fast radio-controlled cars (see Chapter 15 for more). As such, it has an unusual shape, good torque, and very high speed. Unfortunately, it is also very noisy and has extremely high power consumption; in fact, most power supplies can't run it at full power. In theory, its speed and torque make it the most powerful electric LEGO motor, and with efficient external gearing, it can outperform XL or NXT motors. However, it does tend to overheat under prolonged stress, which causes its internal electronic protection to shut off the power until the motor cools down. It works best when it's powered from a special LEGO RC unit (see Chapter 15) or from any PF power supply using a PF V2 IR receiver.

The RC motor is unique because it has two outputs. Both are empty 2-stud-deep axle holes that run in the same direction, but the motor's internal gear ratio is different for each of them: the inner output is geared up relative to the outer one by a ratio of 17:23. For this reason, the inner output has 1.35 times the speed and 0.74 times the torque of the outer one.

watertight motor (old)

Dimensions: 16.5×4×4 studs
Produced: 2003 to 2005

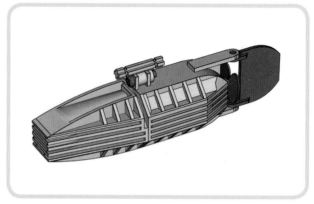

The rare watertight motor was specially created for propelling LEGO boats; in fact, it's hard to use it for anything else. It's a completely stand-alone element that needs no external power supply or a remote. Instead, it's powered by a single AA battery that fits inside and is turned on and off by rotating the front part of its housing. It ends with a three-blade propeller and a simple rudder. The rudder can be moved left or right, and it will maintain its position. The propeller is attached permanently and is impossible to remove without damaging it. Thus, the motor can't drive anything other than the propeller, and its exact parameters are unknown. A single metal screw secures the housing, which is then connected to the boat using an axle-like protrusion on top.

watertight motor (new)

Dimensions: 19.5×4×4 studs
Produced: 2006 to 2008

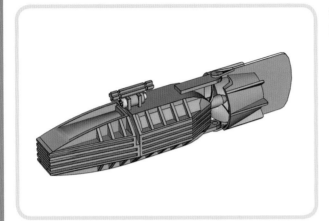

The revised watertight motor retains the same working principle as the old one, with room for a single AA battery inside and a housing with a screw and axle-like protrusion to connect to a boat. The difference is a new, two-blade propeller and a much larger rudder. The rudder makes the whole unit 3 studs longer and includes a tunnel-like structure that partially shields the propeller.

The exact parameters of the motor are unknown. It seems to have the same internals as the old version, but the propeller and rudder were redesigned for higher efficiency.

LEGO Power Functions system

The LEGO Power Functions system (or *PF* for short), introduced in 2007, is a combination of LEGO elements that allows you to motorize your constructions, equip them with lights, move them with linear actuators, and, above all, control them remotely. In this chapter, we will learn how this system works and how its elements can be combined.

The core parts of the Power Functions system can be divided into three groups: power supplies, control elements, and motors. There are several types of motors in the Power Functions system, and all of them are described in Chapter 13. The Power Functions system allows us to control motors with more flexibility, offering fine-grained control of speed and the ability to control multiple elements at once.

NOTE One of the novelties of the Power Functions system is that the majority of its elements have been released as stand-alone, separate LEGO sets. A list of these sets can be found at the end of this chapter.

manually controlling motors

To control a motor by hand with the Power Functions system, you need only two elements: a power supply and a motor, as shown in Figure 14-1. All Power Functions power supplies come with controls on them, some basic and some advanced, and these controls affect any and all motors directly connected to the power supply.

Note that the plugs of the Power Functions wires are *stackable*, and we can connect many wires to a single outlet, as shown in Figure 14-2.

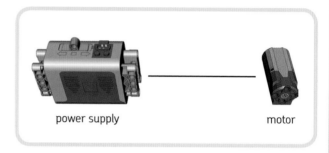

power supply   motor

Figure 14-1: The simplest Power Functions motor configuration

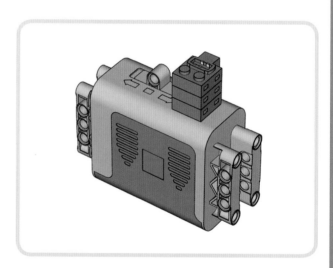

Figure 14-2: A regular Power Functions battery box with three plugs stacked on its outlet. Three elements can now be powered and controlled from this box at the same time.

The simple *power supply and motor* configuration has one serious disadvantage: If many motors are connected to one power supply, they will all work as one. This is inevitable when using the power supply as a control mechanism,

which is why the Power Functions system includes a separate group of control elements. The simplest element from this group is a switch, shown in Figure 14-3.

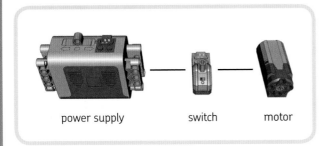

power supply   switch   motor

Figure 14-3: A slightly more complicated configuration for the Power Functions system

Just like all control elements, the switch is connected between the power supply and the element we want to control. It has three positions—forward, stop, and reverse—and they affect all elements connected to the switch.

Note that in this configuration, the controls of a switch and the regular battery box can work at the same time, so either can be used to control the motor. (But if the power supply is set to off, obviously, the setting of the switch won't affect the motor.)

remotely controlling motors

While direct manual control is a nice option, the key advantage of the Power Functions system is the ability to control motors remotely. This is done by a pair of elements: a remote and a receiver (see Figure 13-2 on page 184).

You can think of the remote and receiver as a switch split into two parts. One part, the receiver, is between the power supply and the elements we want to control, just like a switch. It also has a wire just as a switch does. The other part, the remote, has no wires and isn't physically connected to anything. It sends commands to the receiver using an invisible infrared link, just as most TV remotes do. It also houses batteries, just as TV remotes do, so it needs no external power supply. Your construction, with the receiver integrated into it, can be controlled from a distance using the remote.

It's important to remember that the infrared link between remote and receiver has its limitations. The black, semitransparent parts of both remote and receiver house infrared sensors that need to be exposed and within a line of sight of each other to maintain a link. The remote is actually sending out invisible light signals, and they won't reach the receiver if something blocks their way or if they are sent in the wrong direction. They can, however, bounce off walls and ceilings; so as long as you remain indoors, pointing the remote in the receiver's general direction is sufficient. You can also cover up the receiver almost entirely in constructions intended for indoor use, as Figure 14-4 shows. A 2×2 opening around or slightly above the receiver's top will do the job. Outdoors, maintaining the link between remote and receiver is more difficult: The remote has to be aimed with good precision, and its range can drop to as little as 1 m if the receiver's sensor is exposed to strong sunlight.

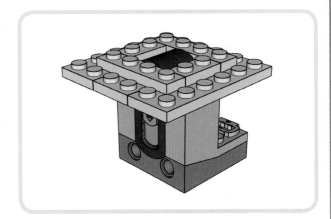

Figure 14-4: An IR receiver doesn't have to make your construction ugly. You can cover it up almost completely, leaving only the 2×2 opening around the sensor. The cover can end up level with the sensor or even slightly above it and still work, as long as you hold the remote higher than the receiver.

As Figure 14-5 shows, a receiver has two levers, one blue and one red, along with two outlets colored the same way. The levers and outlets correspond—the blue lever controls everything connected to the blue outlet, while the red lever controls everything connected to the red outlet. The remote comes with two pole reversers, one for each outlet/lever. The reversers' function is simple: They determine whether pushing a lever forward makes a motor connected to the corresponding outlet rotate forward or in reverse. The blue/red elements are independent and can work at the same time. In other words, the blue lever doesn't interfere with the red lever, and the blue pole reverser doesn't interfere with the red pole reverser.

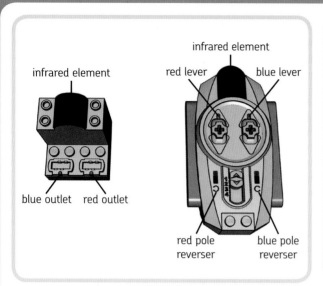

Figure 14-5: The receiver and basic remote

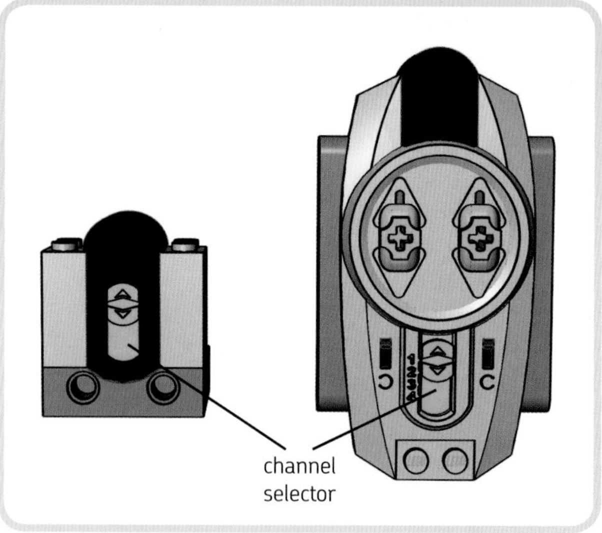

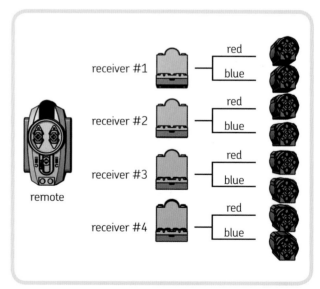

Figure 14-6: The channel selectors on a receiver and basic remote

There is a reason why we said that a lever controls *everything* connected to its corresponding outlet. Since the Power Functions plugs are stackable, you can connect as many motors or other elements to an outlet as you want—all of them will be controlled simultaneously by the corresponding lever. This means that you can control more than two motors using a single receiver, and the motors connected to the same outlet will work as one. For example, you can drive your vehicle with two motors together when one is too weak, or you can have the headlights in your vehicle turn on as it drives.

NOTE The actual number of elements that can run off a single power supply simultaneously is limited by their total power consumption. If it becomes too high, the power supply shuts down. This is most likely to happen with motors and least likely to happen with LEDs.

This limits us to controlling two functions independently per one individual receiver. We can, however, control more functions using many receivers and just a single remote. As Figure 14-6 shows, both receiver and remote come with a simple orange switch called a *channel selector*. It has four positions numbered from 1 to 4. With a channel selector, we can use a single remote with up to four receivers.

Imagine that we have four receivers, each set to a different channel: the first receiver set to channel 1, the second to channel 2, and so on. If you set the channel selector on the remote to 1, only the first receiver will react to the remote and the other three will not. Similarly, if you set the remote's selector to 2, only the second receiver will react to it; if you

set it to 3, only the third one will react; and if you set it to 4, only the fourth one will react. This way you can control up to eight functions independently with a single remote, but since the remote can only be set to one channel at a time, you can control only two functions at the same time. Controlling another two functions requires switching the remote's channel selector to a different position. Figure 14-7 shows the 1 remote / 4 receivers / 8 motors arrangement.

Figure 14-7: Each receiver is set to a different channel and has one motor connected to each of its outlets. In this way, eight motors can be controlled independently.

Controlling just two functions simultaneously is clearly a limitation—but one that can be overcome with additional remotes. You can use many remotes at the same time, even four, each tuned to a different channel. Many builders prefer to use several remotes at once rather than a single remote that needs switching between channels. It's even possible to use many remotes set on the same channel with a single receiver, for example, to let several people control the same construction.

Note that when many remotes are sending commands at various channels at the same time, receivers react more slowly. This is because each receiver reads commands from all four channels all the time, and its channel selector tells it only which to ignore and which to accept. When there are many commands to read simultaneously, the receiver is slowed down.

Now that we know how the Power Functions system works, let's take a look at its individual elements.

power supplies

The power supplies of the Power Functions system come in several variants, allowing us to choose between two types of batteries or even freeing us from the need for regular batteries at all. Every power supply can have many elements connected to it, but if too many elements are running off a single supply simultaneously, the electronic countermeasures in it will shut it down. This is most likely to happen with power-costly elements, such as motors. When it does, simply turn the supply off and on again.

AA battery box

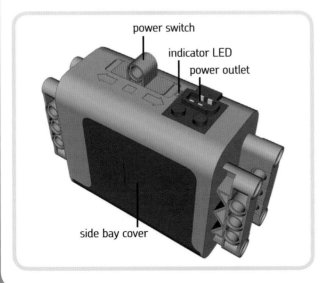

This simple box contains six AA batteries, with two side bays for three batteries each. The box is 11×4×7 studs, with an orange power switch protruding by 1 stud on top of it. The switch has three positions—forward, stop, and backward—and the indicator LED adjacent to the switch shines green on the first and last position. The box is completely studless and connects by pin holes on its sides.

AAA battery box

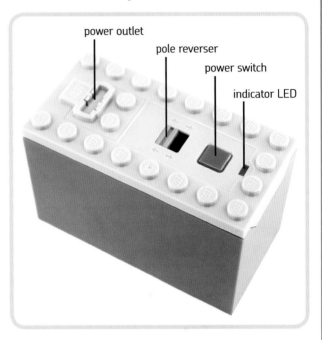

The box contains six AAA batteries, which are inserted by unscrewing the box's bottom. The box is 8×4×5 studs, with a studfull bottom and top. Its power switch has the form of a simple green button. Pushing the button toggles the box between *on* and *off*. The box also has an indicator LED that shines green when the box is on and a simple orange pole reverser that determines whether turning the box on makes motors connected to it run forward or backward. The AAA batteries are smaller and lighter than AA ones; they can't power as many elements simultaneously, and they last roughly a third as long.

NOTE This box comes with a timer: Once turned on, it will turn itself off after 2 hours. You can stop the timer by holding the power switch down for 3 seconds. Turning the box off and on again resets the timer. This feature, intended to prevent the batteries from running dry if you forget to turn the box off, can be mistaken for a malfunction or battery failure.

rechargeable battery

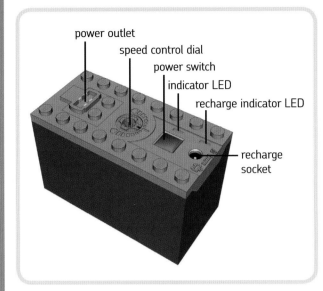

power outlet
speed control dial
power switch
indicator LED
recharge indicator LED
recharge socket

This self-contained battery with rechargeable power cells can be recharged using a transformer, without the need for replaceable batteries of any type. It's 8×4×5 studs, with a studfull bottom and top. Unlike regular battery boxes, it does not open. Its power switch has the form of a simple green button, and pushing it toggles the battery between *on* and *off*. Next to the power switch, there is an indicator LED that shines green when the battery is on and an orange speed dial with 15 positions: 7 forward, 7 backward, and 1 stop position. Turning the dial controls the speed of all motors and the brightness of all lights connected to the battery. It does not affect receivers connected to it. On the other side of the power switch, there is a recharge socket for the transformer, and an adjacent indicator LED blinks red during recharging and shines red when recharging is complete.

The battery houses two lithium ion polymer cells with a total capacity of 1100 mAh, providing a constant voltage of 7.4 V. The LEGO Group recommends recharging it with a dedicated transformer, sold separately, and defines the full recharge time as 4 hours.

While costly, the battery can be attractive to builders who use plenty of standard batteries. It allows them to build lighter and simpler because it weighs under 80 g (the AA battery box can weigh over 200 g, depending on the batteries' make). This battery can also be integrated into your construction permanently, with only a 2×2-stud opening to access its power switch and recharge socket. It provides lower voltage than standard batteries do (9 V) but higher voltage than rechargeable AA batteries do (7.2 V). Its capacity is smaller than that of most AA batteries, meaning that it runs dry more quickly, but it makes up for this by never needing a battery replacement. When empty, it can be recharged inside your construction by simply connecting the transformer to it, while the battery boxes usually need to be taken out of your construction to replace batteries.

NOTE This battery also comes with a timer: Once turned on, it will turn itself off after 2 hours. Unlike the timer in the AAA battery box, this timer can't be stopped. Turning the battery off and on again resets the timer.

receiver

The Power Functions receiver, shown in Figure 14-8, is 4×4×5 studs and requires at least a half stud of space at the back for plugs connected to it. It has a studfull bottom and top and two pin holes in front. It also has a four-position channel selector in front and an indicator LED adjacent to it, which shines green when the receiver is under power and blinks when the receiver accepts commands from its selected channel.

In 2012, a version with upgraded electronic components was released. This version is distinguished by the *V2* printed on the front (see Figure 14-9) and is otherwise identical externally. It delivers more power to the motors, meaning that it can fully power two PF L motors through a single outlet. You can connect two L motors to a single outlet of the older version, too—they just won't run at full power. Note that using a V2 receiver with PF M motors is not recommended.

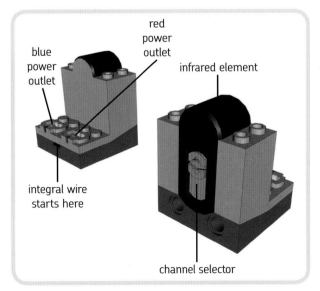

blue power outlet
red power outlet
infrared element
integral wire starts here
channel selector

Figure 14-8: A front and back view of the Power Functions receiver

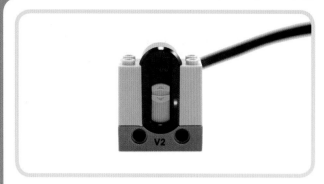

Figure 14-9: The V2 Power Functions receiver. Note the shining indicator LED.

remotes

As shown in Figure 14-10, there are two types of Power Functions remotes: a basic remote and a less common speed control remote. They work in a slightly different ways:

basic remote   The *go* command makes motors run until the *go* command is no longer received.
speed control remote   The *go* command makes motors run until the *stop* command is received.

The key difference is that when the basic remote stops sending the *go* command, the motors stop. This means that we must maintain an infrared link between remote and receiver as long as we want the motors to go. Note that while moving the remote's lever to the stop position stops motors immediately, breaking the infrared link means losing control over the motors. With the link broken, they carry on the last received command for 2 seconds and then stop—unless we manage to reestablish the link during these 2 seconds.

With a speed control remote, we just have to send the *go* command to start motors and the *stop* command to stop them. There is no need to maintain a constant infrared link between sending these two commands.

Another difference is how the remotes send commands. The basic remote keeps sending a command continuously for as long as you keep its lever in forward or reverse position. The speed control remote sends a command just once for every turn of a dial and once for pressing the stop button.

NOTE   It's not recommended to use both types of remotes with the same receiver simultaneously. They will interfere with each other, causing all motors connected to the receiver to stop or to behave erratically.

This limitation becomes complicated when we want to drive and steer a model with a speed control remote, which is well suited for controlling drive but ill suited for controlling steering (unless you're using the Power Functions Servo motor, as explained in "The Speed Control Feature" on page 199). The best solution, then, is to control steering with the basic remote on another channel by connecting

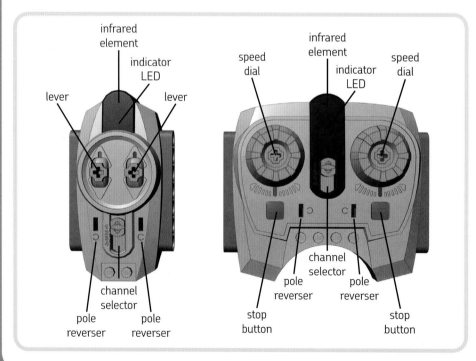

Figure 14-10: The Power Functions remotes: basic (left) and speed control (right). Each is powered by three AAA batteries.

the steering and driving motors to two separate receivers set to two different channels. The steering can be controlled by one receiver set to channel 1, and the drive can be controlled by a second receiver set to channel 2. There will be no interference as long as the remotes are set on proper channels.

basic remote

The basic remote comes with two levers: red and blue, each with forward, stop, and reverse positions. The levers return to the stop position when released. The basic remote also has two pole reversers, one for each lever. The remote is 10×6×4 studs and has a channel selector and an indicator LED that shines green for as long as a command is being sent. The remote is powered by three AAA batteries inserted by unscrewing a cover on its bottom. Both its sides have seven pin holes each, allowing you to connect several remotes side to side with pins.

speed control remote

The speed control remote comes with two dials: red and blue. The dials have no definite positions and stay in place when released. This remote, too, has two pole reversers (one for each dial), two red stop buttons (one for each dial), a channel selector, and an indicator LED that blinks green when a command is sent. The remote is 10×12×4 studs and powered by three AAA batteries inserted by unscrewing a cover on its bottom. Both its sides have seven pin holes each, allowing you to connect several remotes side to side with pins.

Note that this remote works in a special way with the Power Functions Servo motor: Instead of controlling the motor's speed, the speed control remote controls the angle of its output. So rotating the dial 30 degrees right makes the Servo motor's output rotate 30 degrees right, too—or left, depending on how you set the remote's pole reverser.

the speed control feature

There are 15 possible speeds in the Power Functions system: 7 forward, 7 reverse, and 1 "zero" speed, which stops the motors. Speed control is carried out by changing the voltage, meaning that speed control can affect not only a motor's speed but also the brightness of the lights.

The basic Power Functions remote uses only three speeds: top speed forward, zero speed, and top speed reverse. The speed control Power Functions remote, on the other hand, comes with dials that can be rotated in one direction or another. Rotating a dial in one direction sends a *speed +1* command; rotating it in another sends a *speed –1* command, but the rotation has to stop for a moment for the remote to finish sending the command. This means that the dials' rotation is intermittent, not continuous.

POWER FUNCTIONS ELEMENTS AS LEGO SETS

The following Power Functions elements have been released as separate LEGO sets:

* 8869: switch
* 8870: LED lights
* 8871: extension wire, long
* 8878: rechargeable battery
* 8879: speed control remote
* 8881: AA battery box
* 8882: XL motor
* 8883: Medium motor
* 8884: receiver
* 8885: basic remote
* 8886: extension wire, short
* 8887: rechargeable battery transformer
* 88000: AAA battery box

You can rotate a dial through all speeds, from +7 to –7, but note that dials don't stop even when maximum speed is reached. Since dials have no definite positions and can rotate infinitely, sending one command after another, it's impossible to change speed very quickly or to tell the current speed from the dials' position. This is why the speed control remote comes with separate stop buttons, one for each dial. While it's possible to rotate a dial to stop a vehicle, it takes some time and precision; you have to watch the vehicle itself to know when you're changing the speed to zero, for example, and not to –1. The stop buttons are the quick and sure way to go—you'll see why when your model is heading fast toward the edge of a cliff!

Note that the rechargeable Power Functions battery has a dial that does have definite speed positions. This control affects all motors and lights connected to the battery directly or through a switch but not through a receiver, as the receiver ignores the battery's dial.

modifying the remotes

Many possible modifications can make the remotes better suited for our needs. Let's look at three of them.

a basic remote with steering wheel

This simple, robust modification is suitable for driving and steering.

1

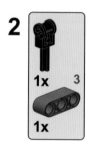

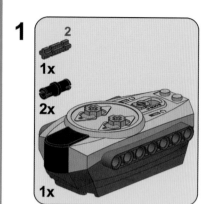

2

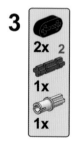

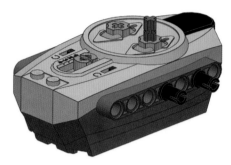

3

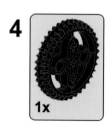

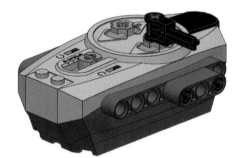

4

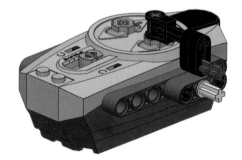

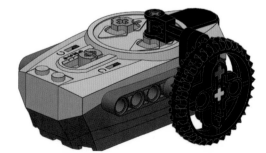

a basic remote with sideways lever

This more complex and less robust modification uses links.

1

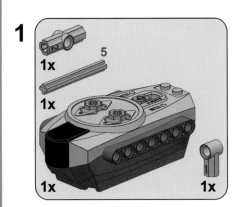

1x
5
1x
1x
1x

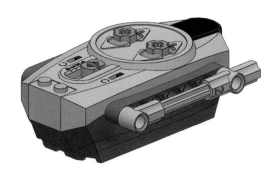

2

2x

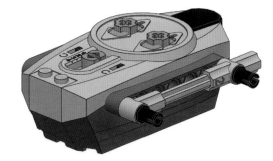

3

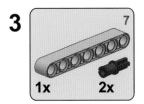

7
1x
2x

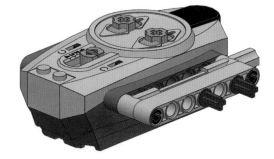

4

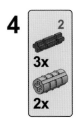

2
3x
2x

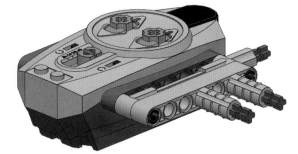

5

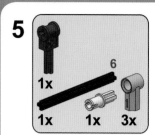

1x

6

1x   1x   3x

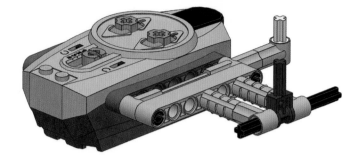

6

1x

2x   2x

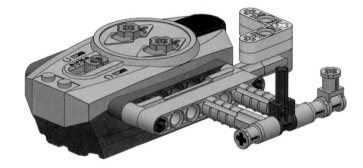

7

4x

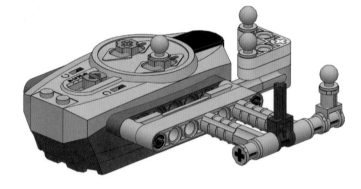

8

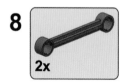

2x

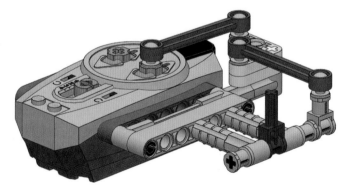

a basic remote with sideways lever

This more complex and less robust modification uses links.

1

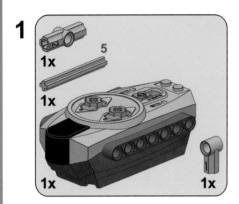

1x
5
1x
1x
1x

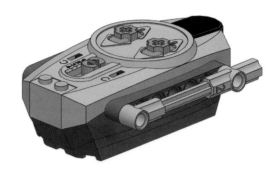

2

2x

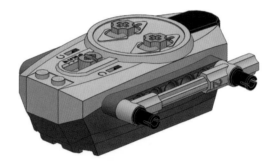

3

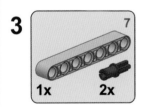

7
1x   2x

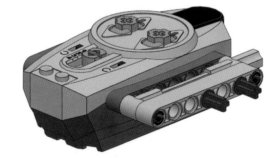

4

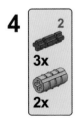

2
3x
2x

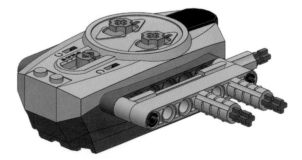

5

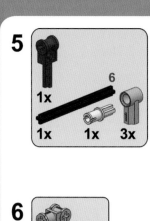

1x
1x 1x 3x

6

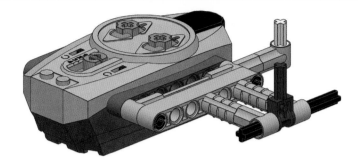

6

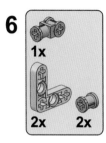

1x
2x 2x

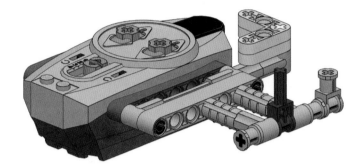

7

4x

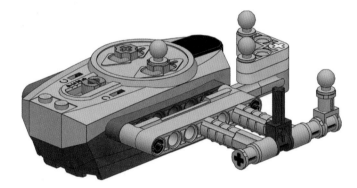

8

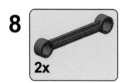

2x

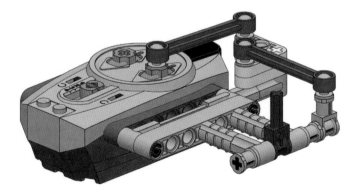

a speed control remote with central steering wheel

This modification is designed to control tracked vehicles, with each speed dial controlling a single track. Two speed dials are connected by a central steering wheel, which can be rotated as well as tilted forward and backward. With properly switched pole reversers, the steering wheel tilt controls drive, and the steering wheel rotation controls steering. To make the vehicle drive forward and then turn right, for instance, you would tilt the steering wheel forward and then rotate it right.

Note that this modification is subject to the disadvantages of the speed control remote—that is, it is limited to sending no more than two commands per second. It works best when operated carefully and not too fast.

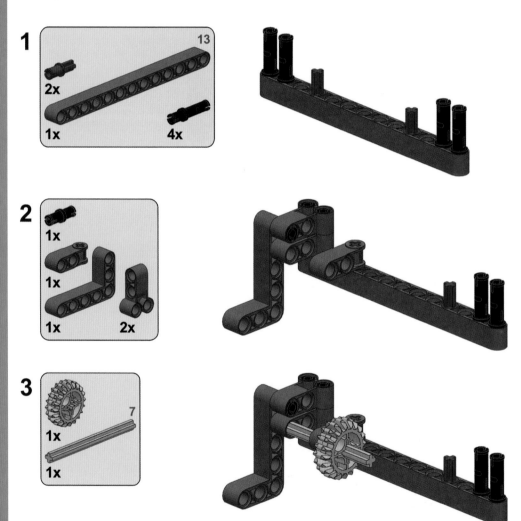

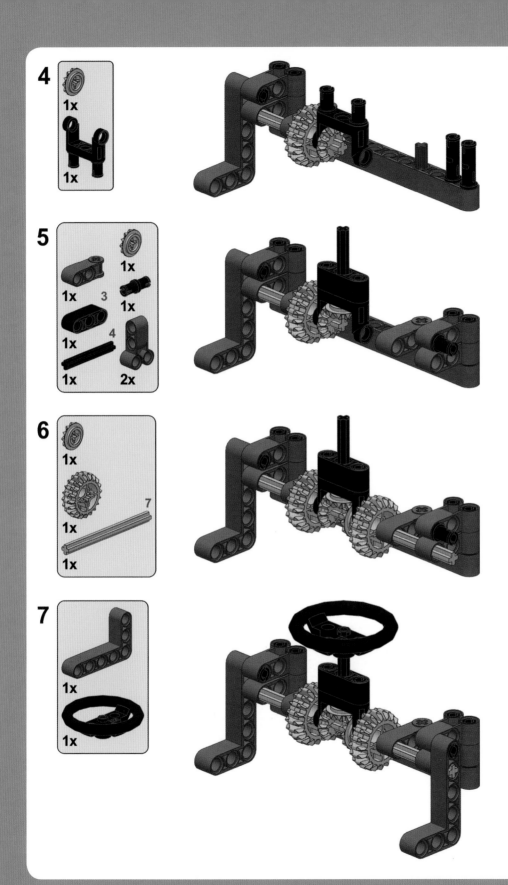

4

1x
1x

5

1x
1x

3
1x

4
1x
2x

6

1x
1x
1x

7

7

1x
1x

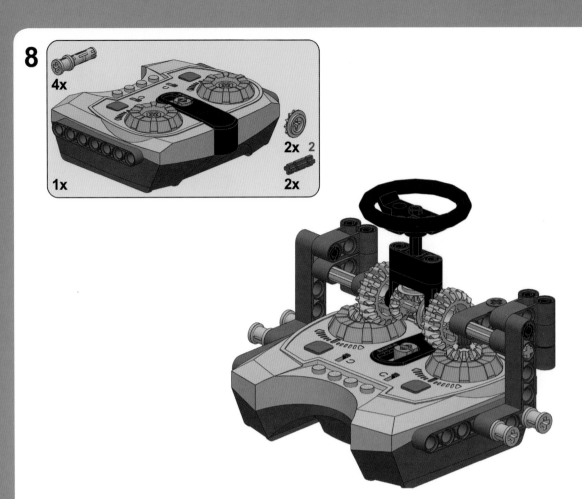

8

4x

2x 2

1x

2x

linear
actuators

Linear actuators, designed as supplementary parts of the
Power Functions system, are an interesting alternative to
the LEGO pneumatics. They come in two variants, large and
small, and both work thanks to inner screws. Each actuator
has an input whose rotation makes the actuator extend or
retract, depending on direction. When an actuator is extended
or retracted to maximum, its inner clutch engages, allowing
the input to continue rotating without damaging the actuator.

The actuators can thus be motorized without external
clutches, and their inner gear ratio makes them work well
with Power Functions motors without the need for external
gearing. Their performance differs from that of LEGO pneumatics, so they can replace LEGO pneumatics in some applications and complement them in others. Let's have a look at
linear actuators and then compare them to pneumatics.

large linear actuator

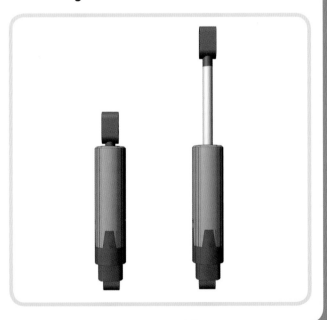

A large linear actuator is 11 studs long when fully retracted and 16 studs long when fully extended. It has a diameter of 2 studs, and it comes with two types of brackets (shown in Figure 14-11) that increase the diameter to 3 studs. One bracket provides an articulated mounting for the actuator, and the other provides a fixed one. It takes one or two 2L axles to firmly attach a bracket to the actuator. Examples of driving an actuator are shown in Figures 14-12 and 14-13.

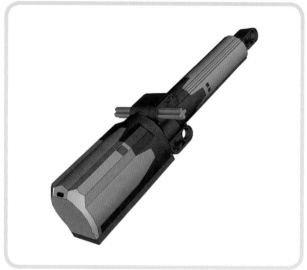

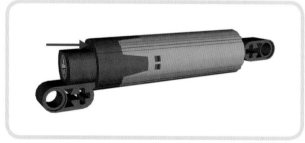

Figure 14-13: The bracket with fixed mounting can connect a motor and actuator as a single unit that can pivot around one of the mounting axles (light grey).

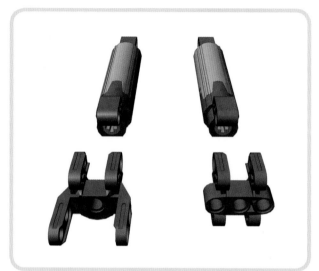

Figure 14-11: A large linear actuator plus bracket with articulated (left) and fixed (right) mounting

In 2010, LEGO announced that the actuators released earlier had a design flaw that could result in high friction occurring inside them when under load and lead to slow and coarse operation. A new design was introduced in September 2010. Actuators produced after this date are externally identical to the older ones, so the easiest way to distinguish them is by checking the production code on each actuator, shown in Figures 14-14 and 14-15.

Figure 14-14: The location of the production code on the actuator is shown by the red arrow. Look for three digits and the letter X minted on the flat dark grey surface.

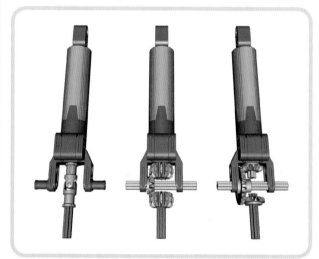

Figure 14-12: Three examples of transferring drive to the small linear actuator. Note that all three have a 1:1 gear ratio.

The production code consists of three digits and the letter X—for example, 36X0. The first two digits mark the week of the actuator's year of production, and the last digit is the ending digit of the year of production. So the

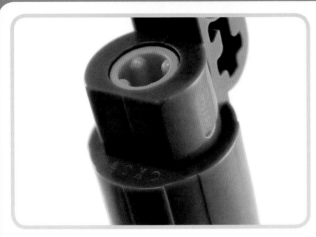

Figure 14-15: A close-up view of a linear actuator. The production code is 40X0, which means the 40th week of 2010, or 4 weeks after the improved design was introduced.

36X0 production code means the 36th week of 2010; this is exactly when the new design was introduced. Actuators produced before this date—for example, 29X0—are of earlier design; actuators produced after this date—for example, 40X0—are of improved design. Keep in mind that even if you have "flawed" actuators, it doesn't necessarily mean that failure will occur.

The large linear actuators can handle impressive loads. Their disadvantage, however, is their inner clutch, which creates significant noise and vibration when engaged.

small linear actuator

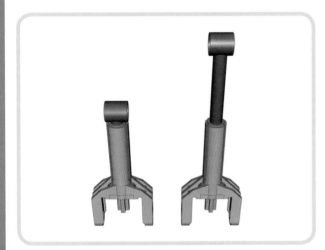

A small linear actuator is 7 studs long when fully retracted and 10 studs long when fully extended. It has a diameter

of a single stud and a fixed bracket that is 3 studs wide. Instead of an axle hole, it has input in the form of a 1L axle. Figure 14-16 shows simple ways of driving a small linear actuator.

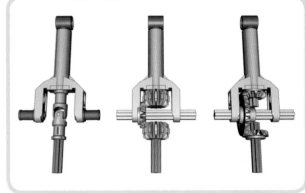

Figure 14-16: Three examples of transferring drive to the small linear actuator. Note that all three have a 1:1 gear ratio.

The load capacity of the small linear actuator is much smaller than that of its larger variant but still impressively useful given its size. Unlike the large actuator, the small one comes with a plastic internal shaft, which is less robust than the large actuator's metal one. The clutch in the small linear actuator works very smoothly and engages almost seamlessly. The small actuator can be very space efficient when combined with the Medium motor.

linear actuators vs. pneumatics

Linear actuators can do most of the tasks that pneumatic cylinders can, but they were not designed to replace them. The two systems differ in many areas, and the best results can be achieved by combining them so that they complement each other's advantages. Linear actuators have the following advantages when compared to pneumatics:

* Have a higher load capacity
* Can be motorized directly, without the need for compressors or valves
* Maintain better accuracy in all positions, as they don't depend on air pressure
* Maintain their position under any load; their inner screws lock them once stopped so they can't be moved by the weight of the load
* Don't have pneumatic hoses, just driveshafts

But they also have the following disadvantages:

* Can be difficult to transfer drive to, as driveshafts are less versatile than pneumatic hoses; this disadvantage grows with more complex systems and with the number of actuators
* Move with constant speed, lacking the smoothness of movement that can be achieved with pressure-dependent pneumatics
* Are generally larger in size
* Large actuators can cause problems when their inner clutches engage, as they produce lots of vibrations
* Are much more difficult to pair
* Resemble real-life hydraulic systems significantly less than pneumatics do

extension wires

We already know that the vast majority of the Power Functions electric components come with integral wires that are permanently attached to them on one end and have a plug on the other. These wires are obviously limited in length, which is why two kinds of extension wires were introduced: a 20 cm wire and a 50 cm wire (see Figure 14-17).

Beyond the obvious goal of adding extra length to any PF electrical connection, the extension wires have one very important feature: Each comes with one *adapter plug*. An adapter plug is a special variant of the Power Functions plug that can have regular PF plugs attached on top of it and old 9V system plugs attached to the bottom of it (see Figures 14-18 and 14-19). This way, each extension wire allows you to connect elements of the Power Functions and old 9V systems together.

A variety of 9V elements can be controlled with the Power Functions system, including all motors (the speed control feature works with them as well) and all types of lights. It is also possible to integrate PF elements into the 9V system to a limited degree. For example, the PF motors can be controlled with 9V battery boxes and switches, but PF receivers work only with PF power supplies.

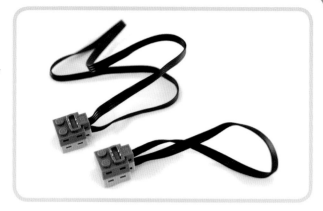

Figure 14-17: Power Functions extension wires: 50 cm long (top) and 20 cm long (bottom)

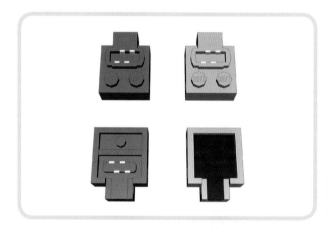

Figure 14-18: Top and bottom view of a regular Power Functions plug (left) and the adapter plug (right). Each extension wire comes with one plug of each type.

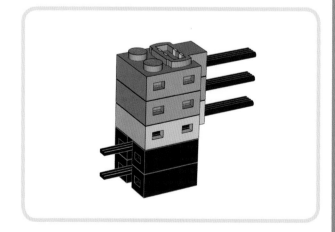

Figure 14-19: The Power Functions adapter plug (light grey) can have an unlimited number of Power Functions plugs (dark grey) attached on top of it and an unlimited number of 9V plugs (black) attached to its bottom.

miscellaneous elements

There are just a few more elements of the Power Functions system, and most of them are highly specialized—for example, train sets—so we will omit them here. That leaves just two elements so universal that they deserve to be described.

switch

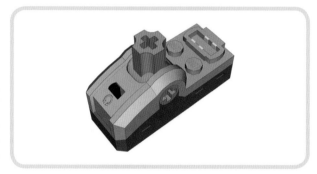

As mentioned earlier, the switch is the simplest control element. It is 5×2 studs and has a 1-brick-tall base, and it comes with an integral wire, one power outlet, one pole reverser, and an orange lever. The lever is identical to the one on the basic remote, with three positions—forward, stop, and backward—except that it doesn't return to the central position. It also has an axle hole through which any axle can be put—this comes in handy, for example, when we want to motorize the switch.

LED lights

The PF system's lights, shown in Figures 14-20 to 14-22, are a pair of LEDs with a piece of wire and a regular Power Functions plug. At half of its length, the wire enters a black 2×2×1 brick that separates in two, so the two LEDs can be placed relatively far from each other. Note that the black brick is not a plug of any kind: It's fully closed, just like a standard LEGO brick. The LEDs are enclosed in transparent housings that are less than 2 studs tall and less than 1 stud wide and that have protruding tubes with LEDs inside that fit perfectly into a pin hole.

The LEDs provide bright white light, directed only forward. Their power consumption is minimal, and their brightness can be controlled with the Power Functions speed control feature. Note that the type of LEDs used by LEGO has changed over time: The glow of older batches is slightly yellowish, while the glow of newer batches is bluish.

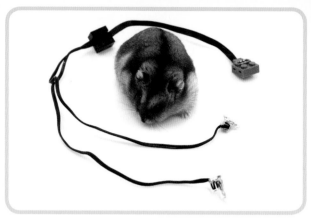

Figure 14-20: The Power Functions LEDs with a hamster provided for scale

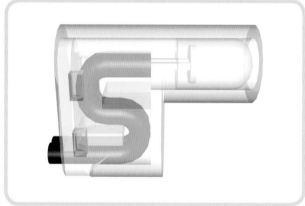

Figure 14-21: Side view of the LEGO LED. You can see part of the wire tucked in to prevent it from being ripped off. The actual LED is located in a protruding tube that fits into a pin hole and is slightly less than a single stud long.

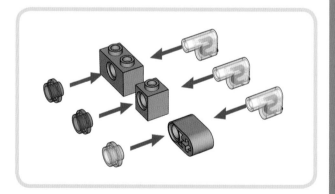

Figure 14-22: The most common examples of installing LEDs in other LEGO pieces. The LEDs fit perfectly into a pin hole. Since their protruding part is less than a stud long, there is still enough room to put in, for example, semitransparent round plates from the other side, creating lights in various colors.

the RC system

Despite being discontinued in 2003, the LEGO Radio Control (RC) system remains exceptional in many respects, most importantly in its motors' high performance. Its strength makes it popular with builders who are not satisfied with the limitations of the Power Functions system. Constructions that rely on the RC system are still published on a regular basis, and the system's components are still available on the second-hand market. Because no replacement for the RC system seems to be imminent, it's worth learning about this valuable alternative to today's PF system. This chapter helps you understand how the RC system works and what makes it unique.

overview of the LEGO RC systems

The LEGO Group has been experimenting with RC systems since 1998, ultimately abandoning them for the infrared or IR-based PF system. Out of several RC systems, one system has retained its popularity ever since: We'll call it the *RC proper*.

The RC proper system has two features that make it a builder favorite: You can combine it with regular LEGO pieces, and it can control any LEGO motor. This makes it unique in the RC family, which can be divided into four groups:

* Early RC system (1998–2001): One-piece chassis complete with four wheels, motor, steering, receiver with antenna, and battery box. Included a small remote with antenna. Incompatible with other systems. *Sets: 5599, 5600 (re-release)*

* RC proper (2002–2003): Central control unit complete with steering, receiver with antenna, and battery box. Compatible with regular LEGO pieces, motors, and wheels. Included large remote with antenna. The 8366 and 8376 sets also included an extra pair of solid plastic wheels for drifting. As mentioned, this is the system this chapter focuses on. *Sets: 8475, 8366, 8376*

* Mid-late RC system (2004–2006): Used a number of modules (one for steered axle, one for driven axle, and one for battery box/receiver with antenna) and the same remote as RC proper. Most elements, including body and wheels, were not compatible with standard LEGO pieces and were made exclusively for these sets. Equipped with a 7.2V battery pack and charger and a 9V battery for the remote. *Sets: 8369 (originally with yellow body, re-released in 2006 with blue body), 8675*

* Late RC system (2004–2006): Used the same non-standard body pieces and wheels as the mid-late system plus a new, smaller remote and one-piece chassis complete with motor, steering, receiver with antenna, and battery box. *Sets: 8378, 8676*

With the exception of the RC proper, the RC systems simply weren't versatile enough to attract builders: They either relied on a one-piece ready-made chassis or on pieces that didn't connect to regular LEGO pieces. It's interesting to note that the LEGO Group tried the one-piece chassis solution again in the PF era with the 8183 and 8184 sets, both released in 2009. Both sets featured various bodies built on top of a chassis that combined the motor, steering, battery box, and IR receiver and could be controlled with a standard PF IR remote.

RC proper system and its components

The RC proper system was designed as a combination of three elements: a control module, a steering attachment, and RC motors that were designed specifically for this system and were covered in Chapter 13. A typical set using this system would include two RC motors that were hard-coupled for propulsion, and the design and shape of all these elements made it easy to build a regular rear-wheel-drive (RWD) car around them, as shown in Figures 15-1 and 15-2.

Before we examine all these elements separately, it's important to understand that the heart of the system is the control unit—all other elements are optional. The control unit can work with any LEGO motor, and its steering output can be used with a custom steering system. The remote is also a crucial part of the system, because it works in conjunction with the control unit.

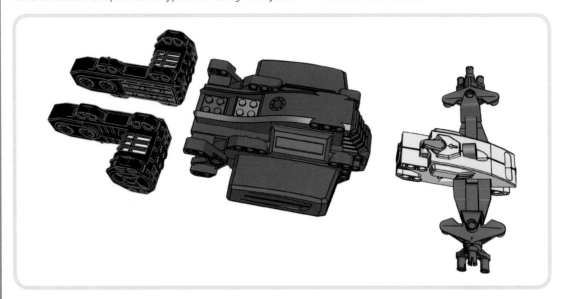

Figure 15-1: The key elements of the LEGO RC proper system: RC motors (black), control module (blue, antenna not included), and steering attachment (yellow) with suspension arms (red). Note that in reality all these elements are black.

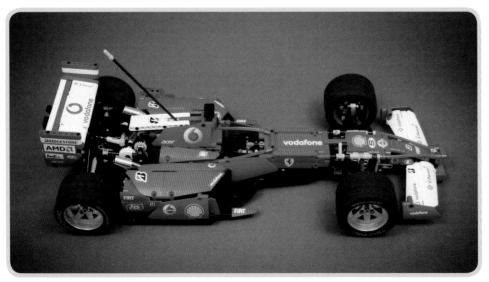

Figure 15-2: My F1 car model fits the RC elements within the slim body of the modern F1 racer. The control unit is located directly behind the driver's seat, and two RC motors are hidden behind the side air intakes. A PF M motor, also connected to the RC control module, is used to remotely shift the car's two-speed transmission built around the rear axle.

the control unit

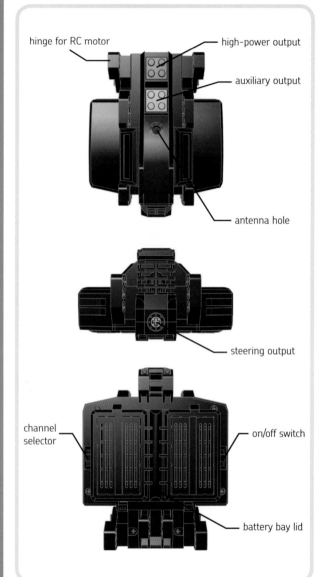

hinge for RC motor
high-power output
auxiliary output
antenna hole
steering output
channel selector
on/off switch
battery bay lid

by a push-in lid) are on the bottom. The outputs on top are simply contact areas for LEGO 9V plugs, whereas the steering output is just an axle hole that can rotate 90 degrees right or left and return to the center. Additionally, a hinge on each side of the module's back is designed as an easy mounting point for one RC motor. With shock absorbers added, this can serve as a simple rear suspension.

NOTE A rare version of the control module with no auxiliary output exists. It was included in the 8376 set, and except for the missing output, it's identical to the regular version.

the remote

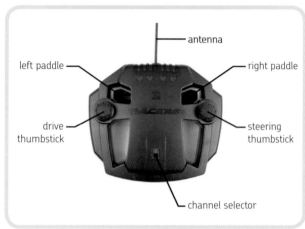

antenna
left paddle
right paddle
drive thumbstick
steering thumbstick
channel selector

The remote comes with a screwed-in antenna on the top, which is identical to the one on the control module; two thumbsticks; a three-position channel selector on the front; two paddles; and a 9V battery bay on the back. The left thumbstick controls motors that generate the unit's high-power output; the right thumbstick controls the motor's steering output. Both thumbsticks allow limited proportional control: There are three motor speeds and three steering output positions, determined by how far you tilt the given thumbstick. Both thumbsticks return to a neutral position when you release them. The channel selector is identical to the one on the control unit, and a remote will only work with the control unit set on the same channel. The paddles control any elements connected to the control unit's auxiliary output; for instance, if the element is a motor, one paddle makes it rotate right and the other makes it rotate left. Both paddles return to the off position when you release them. A single screw secures the battery bay lid.

The RC control unit is commonly referred to as the *RC unit*. It combines a battery box (six AA batteries), an RC receiver, and a steering servo with return-to-center function. A metal antenna is screwed into a hole on its top. The unit can work without an antenna, but that reduces its receiving range to nearly zero versus roughly 10 m with an antenna. Also on the top are a high-power output (red) and auxiliary output (grey). A steering output is on the front; an on/off switch, a three-position channel selector, and a battery bay (closed

the steering attachment

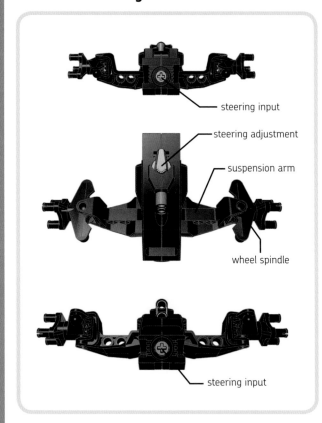

- steering input
- steering adjustment
- suspension arm
- wheel spindle
- steering input

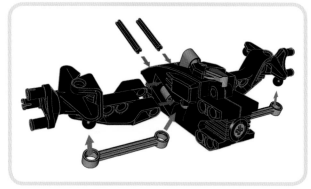

Figure 15-3: Exploded view of the RC steering attachment showing how two steering links and two axles connect steering arms and wheel spindles to the actual attachment.

The steering attachment connects to the control unit's steering output and combines several unique pieces in addition to regular LEGO pieces. The unique pieces are two suspension arms and two wheel spindles; two regular axles and two regular steering links are needed to connect them together, as shown in Figure 15-3. The attachment has a steering input in front and back, which are 1 stud deep and connected together. Also on top is an adjustment dial that can be used if the attachment bears to the left or right.

Note that the steering attachment has its own return-to-center function, which works just like the one in the control unit and allows the two units to work in unison. But whereas the control unit relies on an internal servo, the attachment's function is spring-loaded. It works very feebly in most used attachments due to prolonged wear.

Also note that regular pin holes connect suspension arms to the attachment, making it possible to build custom suspension arms and use them instead. Any suspension arms, custom or not, are kept at an angle to the attachment, producing a caster angle for the wheels; whether the angle is positive or negative depends on whether the attachment is facing front or back.

motors

Although you can connect the RC proper system to any motor, it was designed specifically to work with the RC motors and to let them run at full power (see "RC Motor" on page 191).

putting it all together

The 8475 set's building instructions (available online) are the best reference material for the RC proper system's elements. They demonstrate how to use hinges on the control module and how to add a working suspension to the steering attachment. Although you can enjoy the advantages of this system using nothing more than the control module and remote, it's useful to have all the pieces. You can experiment to make the elements of this system better suit your constructions, as shown in Figure 15-4. For example, you can bend the control unit's antenna or hide it entirely inside a model's body (neither seems to have any significant impact on the RC system's range).

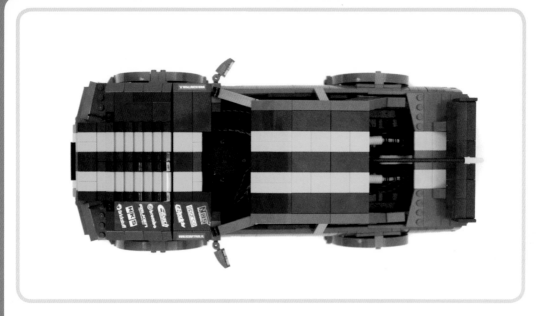

Figure 15-4: At 45 studs long and 18 studs wide, my Nissan Skyline GT-R model was probably one of the smallest cars ever built using the RC proper system. The body had a number of thin panels covering the control unit, and the steering system was entirely custom-built to make it small enough to fit. Additionally, the antenna was bent at a right angle to make it come out the rear windshield.

RC system vs. PF system

The RC system and PF system are strikingly different despite being released just a few years apart, and not just because of the different control medium (RC versus IR). The RC system is more specialized and was designed for high performance and ease of use with simple cars that could be built quickly and played with outdoors. The PF system, on the other hand, sacrifices performance for versatility and introduces a whole array of parts that are much less specialized and thus much more flexible: LEGO explicitly states that this system is not intended for outdoor use.

Perhaps the most important feature for the RC system's popularity is the famously powerful RC motor designed to work with it. The RC unit is the only original LEGO power supply designed to cope with the enormous power consumption of two of these motors at a time. Although it's entirely possible to operate RC motors using a PF battery, some of their power will go unused. The PF system comes with safety measures that limit the current

drawn from a power supply to prevent electrical elements from overheating. The PF motors were built to work under these restrictions; the RC motors were not and are limited as a result.

Let's look at the pros and cons of the RC system compared to the PF system. The RC system has some considerable advantages, including the following:

* Superior range up to roughly 10 m, both indoors and outdoors.
* No interference from sunlight, and no need to maintain a clear line of sight between the remote and the receiver.
* Limited proportional control—the RC system has only three motor speeds (the PF system has seven). Although this seems like a drawback, it comes with the benefit of working immediately without the lag inherent in the PF system.
* More power, meaning better performance.
* A larger, more comfortable remote that is also more intuitive to use.
* A control unit that comes with integrated steering output that acts very much like the PF servo motor. The unit also comes with a robust attachment that makes adding a positive-caster steered axle easy.

* Batteries that can be replaced without removing the entire control unit.
* A whole system that is well suited for fast, simple cars, and whose components easily come together in a durable, off-road capable chassis.

But the RC system also has a few downsides:

* Overall, the RC system is much less versatile, and it's difficult (but possible: see Figure 15-5) to use for anything other than a RWD car.
* The control unit is bulky, heavy, and difficult to integrate into many constructions, and its antenna is especially tricky to work around.
* The higher power consumption means shorter battery life.
* Powerful motors create high stress on drivetrain pieces along with the risk of permanent damage.
* The remote has no room for modifications and doesn't have an indicator to show whether it's working.
* The remote only lets you control two motors independently per one power supply because the power supply is also the receiver (a problem that doesn't exist for the PF system thanks to separate power supplies and receivers).
* The control unit's on/off switch is difficult to use.
* Replacing batteries requires access to almost the entire bottom of the control unit.
* The steering attachment has a fixed track of wheels (but this limitation can be circumvented by adding custom-built suspension arms to the attachment).
* The system has been out of production for more than a decade, and all its elements are rare, expensive, and often in deteriorating technical condition. The control units in particular are known for breaking down, so buyer beware.

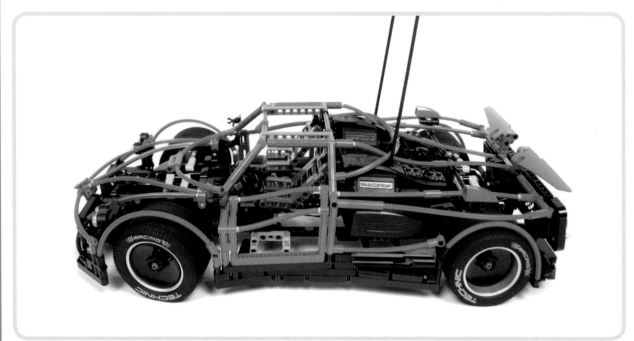

Figure 15-5: My Pagani Zonda model combined a lightweight skeletal body with two RC control units that powered four RC motors. Both units were set on the same channel so I could control them with a single remote, and one unit's auxiliary output was used to allow steering with a PF M motor. The car needed 12 AA batteries but reached speeds over 15 km/h, despite weighing 2 kg.

advanced mechanics

wheeled steering systems

The steering of wheeled vehicles is a complex subject in automobile design. While some real-life issues are of lesser importance in LEGO models because of their limited size and weight, it still pays to understand the principles at play.

In this chapter, we're going to learn how to build typical LEGO steering systems as well as how to implement optional features, such as return-to-center steering. We'll also explore issues of steering geometry and multi-axle steering.

Note that this chapter omits vehicles with fewer than four wheels. Steering bikes or trikes is elementary, so we are moving straight to where the real challenges begin.

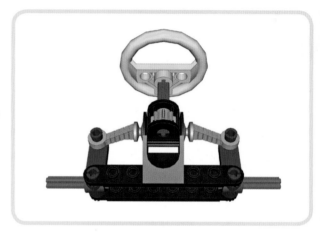

Figure 16-1: A typical LEGO steering mechanism

basic LEGO steering systems

The steering systems in LEGO constructions can be built with a number of specialized pieces, but it's also perfectly possible to rely only on common pieces. Let's start our exploration of steering by examining a typical steering mechanism, shown in Figure 16-1.

Note that we will be using colors consistently throughout this chapter: The black pieces are parts of the chassis, and the yellow one is obviously a steering wheel. That leaves four other important parts:

a steering shaft (red)   This is an axle that connects a steering wheel or a motor to the pinion of the rack-and-pinion gearset.

a rack-and-pinion gearset (grey)   This gearset consists of a pinion (here, an 8-tooth gear) and a rack, which is a toothed plate, below it (see Figure 16-4); when the pinion rotates left or right, it makes the rack slide.

steering arms (blue)   These arms rotate around the connection to the chassis, and their rotation is controlled by the rack.

spindles (green)   These are the axles in the steering arms on which the wheels are mounted.

Figure 16-2 shows our mechanism in action. Rotating the steering arms makes the entire vehicle turn. And obviously, to turn, the vehicle needs at least one more axle, as Figure 16-3 shows.

In Figure 16-2, the rack gear is a specialized piece (#2791) that is slightly elastic, allowing it to bend to stay mated with the round pinion gear as the steering wheel turns. The pinion gear can be used with other gears, but we'd have to compensate for the rotation of the steering arms. Figure 16-4 illustrates the problem.

When the steering arms are turned, the pins that connect them to the rack actually trace part of a circle. This causes the rack to move in two dimensions: not only left and right but also forward and backward. Only the

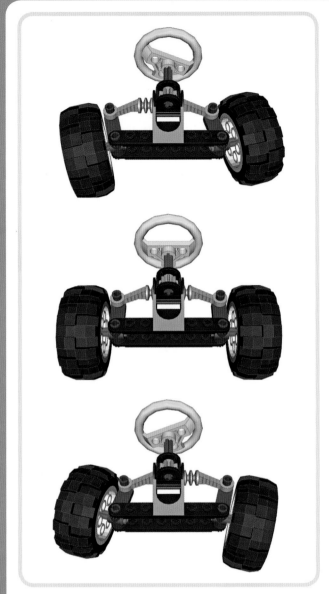

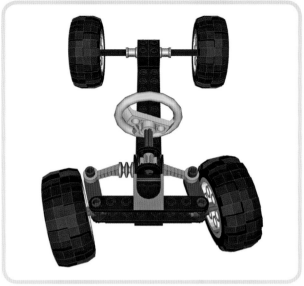

Figure 16-3: A LEGO vehicle with two axles: one fixed and one steered

Figure 16-2: Our simple steering mechanism in extreme left, straight, and extreme right positions

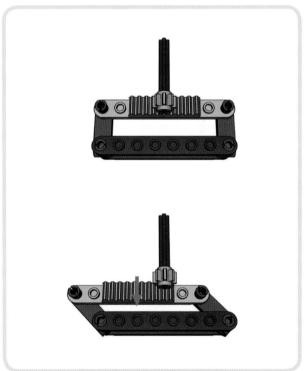

Figure 16-4: The rotation of the steering arms (blue) makes the rack (light grey) move not only side to side but also forward and backward.

lateral movement is desired, as the forward-and-backward displacement can disengage the rack from the pinion. Figure 16-5 shows the simplest solution to the problem: adding an extra pinion.

Another solution is to place the pinion in the middle of the rack's path of forward-and-backward motion, as shown in Figures 16-6 and 16-7.

These figures also introduce a new, simple element of the steering system. When we use nonspecialized pieces to build a steering system, we'll use two pieces: a *rack gear* (shown in light grey under the pinion), which is a 1×4-stud plate with teeth on top of it, and a *tie rod* (shown in light blue). A tie rod connects the ends of the steering arms to the rack gear.

As you can see, the tie rod travels forward and backward, requiring a margin of free space—the 2-stud-wide gap around it. But we may not want to waste space for such a gap; another solution is to make the rod more complex, as shown in Figure 16-8.

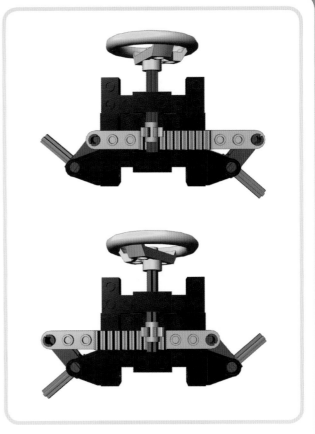

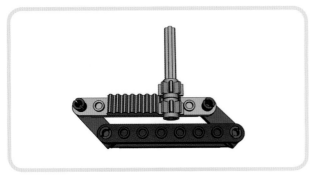

Figure 16-5: The simplest solution to an "escaping" rack is using two pinions so that when the rack moves away from one, it will be meshed with the other.

Figure 16-7: A steering mechanism in extreme right and extreme left positions. Note that the tie rod moves forward inside the 2-stud-wide gap around the pinion.

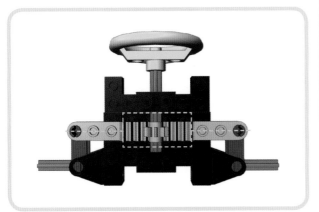

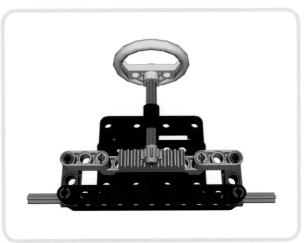

Figure 16-6: A steering mechanism in straight position. Note that the light blue tie rod is located in the center of the 2-stud-wide gap around the pinion.

Figure 16-8: A steering mechanism with a three-piece tie rod. The short, articulated sections on the sides pivot to accommodate the rotation of the steering arms.

Here the tie rod consists of three sections: a long central one (with the rack) and two short ones on its sides, connected by pins. These short sections pivot to accommodate the rotation of the steering arms and reduce the central section's forward-and-backward travel to zero, as Figure 16-9 shows.

The three-piece tie rod is a reliable and popular solution, but its side sections must be shorter than the central one. The whole assembly is rather wide and thus not suited for narrow vehicles. We can solve this by building a very simple steering system in which the rack gear is replaced by a lever, as Figure 16-10 shows.

You now know three solutions to the problem of a tie rod's travel, and you have seen examples of simple steering systems built with a handful of common pieces. Now that your steering system is working, you may want to add features to it.

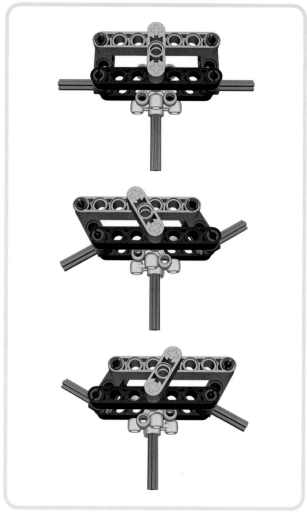

Figure 16-10: A steering mechanism without a rack. Instead, it uses two knob wheels and a short lever (grey) to transfer movement from the steering shaft to the tie rod.

return-to-center steering

Return-to-center steering is just what the name implies: a mechanism that returns the steering system to the center (straight) position when the system is released. Such a mechanism is best placed between the steering system and a motor controlling it, and such a "self-centering" design complements the use of remote controls. It allows you to build a steering system that steers to extreme left or extreme right when you push levers on your remote and that returns to center when you release it.

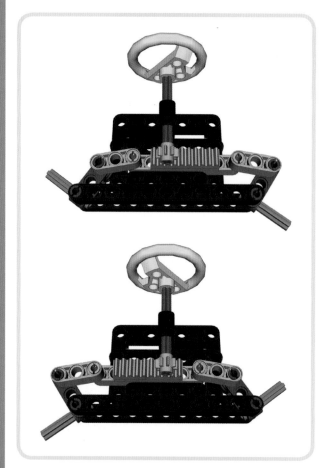

Figure 16-9: A steering mechanism with a three-piece tie rod in extreme left and right positions. Note that the longitudinal travel of the central section is zero.

NOTE These mechanisms use the basic Power Functions remote and a regular motor. You can use the speed control PF remote and PF Servo motor instead, which together provide not only a return-to-center system but also proportional steering. See Chapter 13 for details.

The easiest way to build a self-centering steering system with LEGO pieces is to use a rare specialized piece, #x928cx1, often called a *hockey spring*. It comes with a spring inside and can be attached to a PF Medium motor (as shown in Figure 16-11). In such a configuration, it will backdrive the motor to the central position every time the motor stops.

If you cannot find this specialized piece, you can use a rubber band as a simple centering mechanism. Shown in Figure 16-12, the mechanism consists of the band (white), which squeezes two beams (yellow) together to the sides of a connector sitting on the steering shaft (red). As the motor starts to rotate the shaft, the connector pushes the beams apart. If the rubber band is strained enough, it will stop the connector quickly, and when the motor stops, it will squeeze the beams back together, returning the connector and the shaft to the central position. Note that you have to find a rubber band providing just the right tension for this mechanism to operate smoothly.

As with any mechanism, return-to-center steering has its pros and cons. It works fast and simplifies the control of a

model, but it doesn't allow accurate maneuvering because it only has three possible positions. This makes it better suited for fast models where a steering system has to react quickly, rather than for slower ones that benefit from a steering system that allows for greater accuracy. It's also risky to use return-to-center steering with a large steering lock because rapid wide turns can make a vehicle unstable. (Steering lock is the maximum angle that wheels on a steered axle can be turned, as described in Chapter 1.) In my experience, any model that isn't built specifically for speeding will be better off with a regular steering system that allows you to adjust the driving direction accurately. In most cases, the PF Medium motor geared down to a 9:1 gear ratio provides optimum speed/accuracy balance for a regular steering system.

Ackermann steering geometry

When a wheeled vehicle makes a turn, its inner and outer wheels follow circles of different radii because the width of the vehicle separates them. If the inner wheels follow a circle of radius r_1, then the outer wheels follow a circle of radius r_2 (equal to r_1 plus the width of the vehicle), as Figure 16-13 shows.

A regular steered axle turns both left and right wheels at exactly the same angle, which means that none of the wheels follows exactly its proper radius. This creates additional friction and tire wear. Ackermann steering geometry corrects that by turning wheels at different angles. More

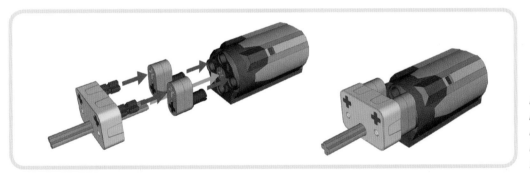

Figure 16-11: The hockey spring (yellow) and a schematic for attaching it to a PF Medium motor

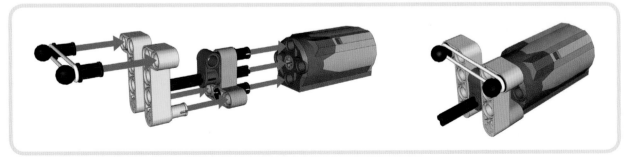

Figure 16-12: The rubber band–based return-to-center steering attachment for a PF Medium motor

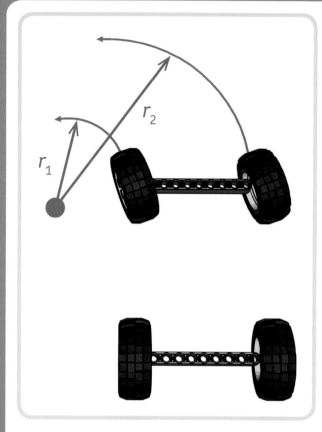

Figure 16-13: The inner and outer wheels of a steered vehicle follow circles of different radii: r_2 is equal to r_1 plus the width of the vehicle.

specifically, it turns them so that they are perpendicular to the center of the vehicle's turning radius, as shown in Figure 16-14.

This geometry, which makes the wheels follow correct radii, is achieved by modifying the steering arms so that they point at the middle of the rear axle, as Figure 16-15 shows.

When it comes to LEGO vehicles, this additional friction and the tire wear are negligible, except for very heavy and large models. The improved handling that comes with Ackermann geometry is advantageous but only noticeable with large vehicles with significant steering lock. Ackermann geometry is important enough to be used in many high-end RC cars, and two official LEGO Technic supercars use it: the 8865 and 8880 sets (shown in Figure 16-16). Both use independent steered suspension, which is also driven in the 8880 set.

Both the 8865 and 8880 sets use special steering arms with shifted pivot points, shown in Figure 16-17. Both are rare pieces by now, but we can build our own custom steering arm using other pieces, as shown in the building instructions on page 226.

There is one more way to achieve Ackermann geometry: We can use a three-piece tie rod with a longer central section and with the two side sections set at an angle, as shown in Figure 16-18. Such a tie rod has little travel, and it should be placed in front of the front axle. Note that with this solution, the steering arms don't point at the middle of the rear axle, so it's difficult to see whether the proper geometry is achieved. This solution puts very high forces in the tie rods.

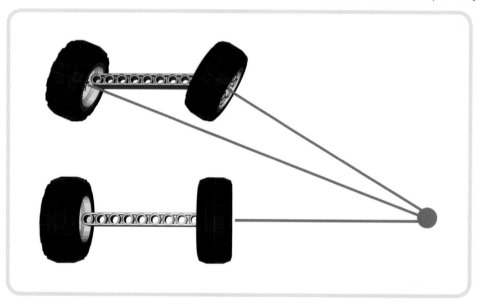

Figure 16-14: Ackermann steering geometry keeps the wheels on the steered axle perpendicular to the center of the turning radius when making a turn.

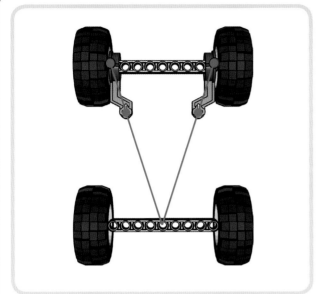

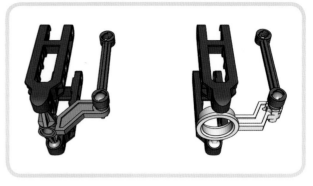

Figure 16-17: Steering arms from the 8865 (left) and 8880 (right) sets, mounted in suspension arms (blue). Both have shifted pivot points to allow Ackermann geometry; the 8880 arm also allows the wheels to be driven.

Figure 16-15: A proper Ackermann geometry: The front axle's steering arms point at the center of the rear axle.

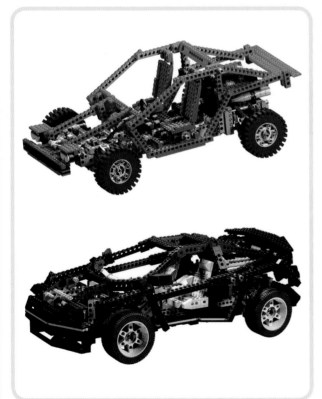

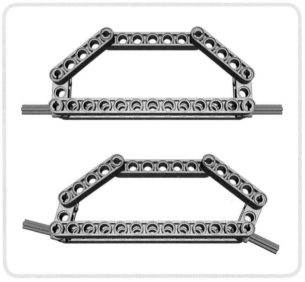

Figure 16-18: Ackermann steering geometry achieved by using a three-piece tie rod with a longer central section

Note that the central gear rack needs to be guided to keep it perpendicular to the chassis.

Ackermann steering geometry was included in the official LEGO sets as an additional technical highlight rather than for its actual advantages. Given the weights and sizes of most LEGO models, the benefits of such a sophisticated solution are negligible. Still, many builders consider including it in a model a great display of skill.

Figure 16-16: The 8865 and 8880 sets are designed with Ackermann geometry in mind.

a simple steering arm with Ackermann geometry

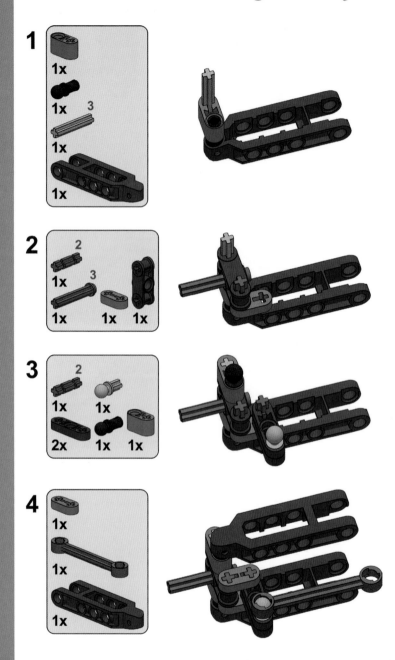

1
1x
1x 3
1x
1x

2
2
1x
3
1x 1x 1x

3
2
1x 1x
2x 1x 1x

4
1x
1x
1x

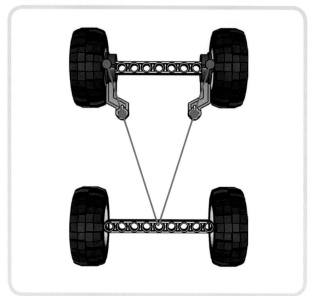

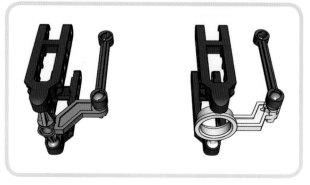

Figure 16-17: Steering arms from the 8865 (left) and 8880 (right) sets, mounted in suspension arms (blue). Both have shifted pivot points to allow Ackermann geometry; the 8880 arm also allows the wheels to be driven.

Figure 16-15: A proper Ackermann geometry: The front axle's steering arms point at the center of the rear axle.

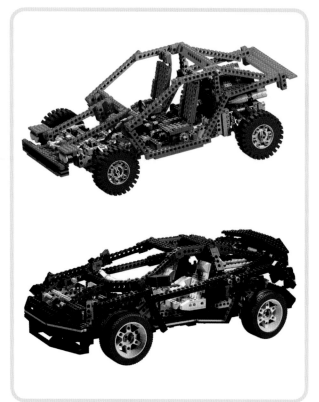

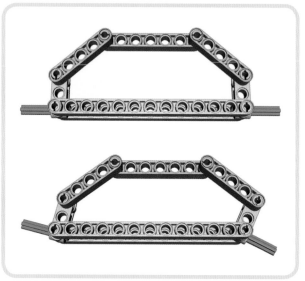

Figure 16-18: Ackermann steering geometry achieved by using a three-piece tie rod with a longer central section

Note that the central gear rack needs to be guided to keep it perpendicular to the chassis.

Ackermann steering geometry was included in the official LEGO sets as an additional technical highlight rather than for its actual advantages. Given the weights and sizes of most LEGO models, the benefits of such a sophisticated solution are negligible. Still, many builders consider including it in a model a great display of skill.

Figure 16-16: The 8865 and 8880 sets are designed with Ackermann geometry in mind.

a simple steering arm
with Ackermann geometry

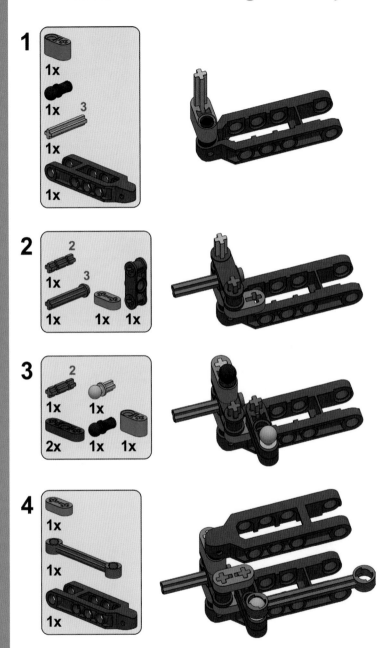

1
1x
1x 3
1x
1x

2
2
1x 3
1x 1x 1x

3
2
1x 1x
2x 1x 1x

4
1x
1x
1x

convergence of axles

While discussing Ackermann steering geometry, we learned that every vehicle has its *center of turning radius*. When the wheels are turned, the center is where lines perpendicular to each wheel meet (ignore the outer steered wheels if you use a regular steering geometry), as shown in Figures 16-19 and 16-20. The center can be closer or farther from the vehicle, depending on how much the wheels are turned.

Now, consider a line that points at the center and at the same time is perpendicular to the chassis of the vehicle. In Figure 16-21, that line goes exactly through the rear, fixed axle. No matter how much the steered wheels are turned, this line will always cross the chassis in the same place. We call it *the convergence line*.

When the axles of a vehicle are convergent, the vehicle turns easily and with little friction. The exact placement of the convergence line depends on the nonsteered axles. For example, when there is one such axle, the convergence line agrees with it; when there are two such axles, the convergence line is exactly between them (as shown in Figure 16-22). When there are three such axles at equal intervals, the convergence line agrees with the middle one, and so on.

When we have more than one steered axle, the convergence line helps to determine the proper spacing between the axles and the difference in their steering locks. For example, if we have steered axles in the front and rear of the vehicle, they should be symmetrical to the convergence line, which

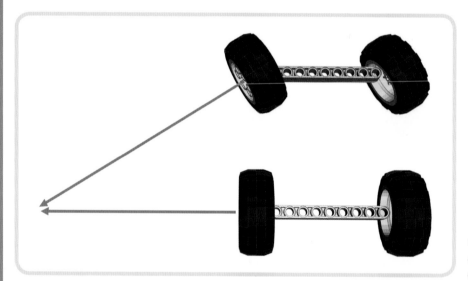

Figure 16-19: The center of turning for a vehicle with regular steering geometry: The outer steered wheel is ignored.

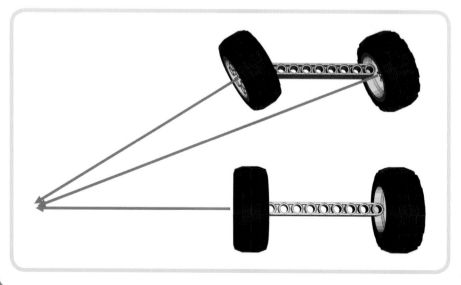

Figure 16-20: The center of turning for a vehicle with Ackermann steering geometry: All wheels "point" at it.

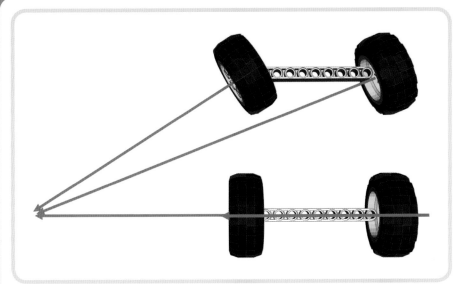

Figure 16-21: Blue marks the convergence line—the line that is perpendicular to the chassis while pointing at the center of turning.

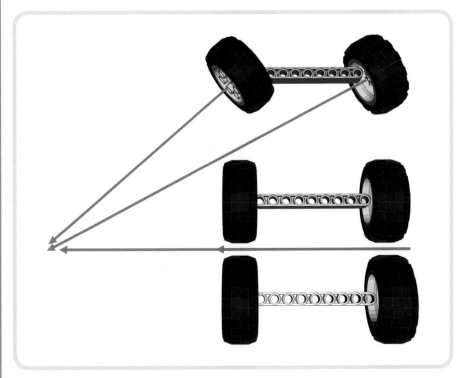

Figure 16-22: For a chassis with a single steered axle and two rear nonsteered ones, the convergence line lies exactly between the rear axles. In this example, since the rear wheels do not point at the rotation center, they will scrub in a turn. This is a big problem for vehicles and trailers with many nonsteered axles. It's also a big problem for airplanes, which turn very tightly.

means that the front axle should steer in the opposite direction of the rear axle, as shown in Figure 16-23.

The most complex case is when we have two or more steered axles next to one another; to maintain convergence, they need different steering locks. It is possible to calculate this difference, but it involves using trigonometry to calculate an inverse tangent.

Figure 16-24 shows a chassis with two steered axles and one nonsteered axle. We know that in this case, the convergence line agrees with the only nonsteered axle. We need to calculate the relationship between the angles of both steered axles, and to do this, we need to know these angles. This can be done by comparing distances between the steered axles and the convergence line for a given angle

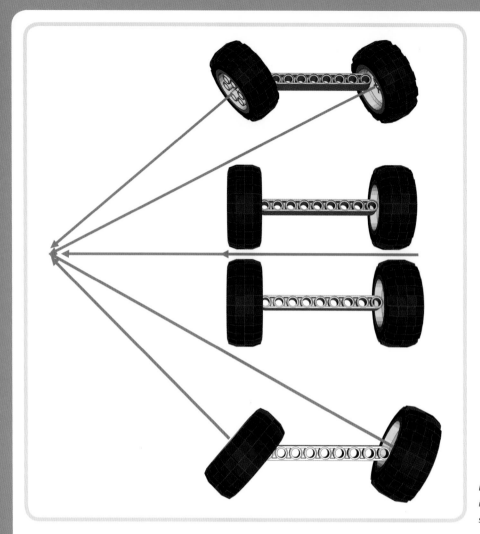

Figure 16-23: If there are steered axles in the front and rear, they should be symmetrical to the convergence line.

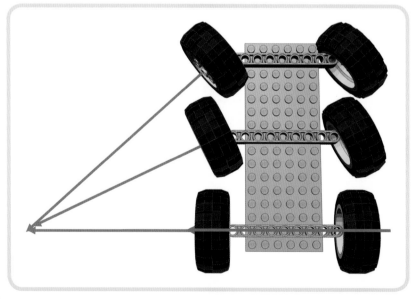

Figure 16-24: The steering locks of the two front axles of this chassis should differ to maintain convergence.

of the front wheels. In this example, let's assume the angle is 45 degrees. As we can see, the front axle is 13 studs away and the middle one is 7 studs away from the convergence line. We need to calculate the relationship between the shorter and longer distances:

$$\frac{7 \text{ studs}}{13 \text{ studs}} = 0.54$$

Next, we need to find the inverse tangent (arctangent) for this relationship.

$$\tan^{-1}(0.54) \approx 28 \text{ degrees}$$

We have just calculated the angle at which the middle axle should be steered, and we know that the angle of the front axle is 45 degrees. Now we need to compare these angles to know the difference between angles and translate it into gearing in the steering system.

$$\frac{28 \text{ degrees}}{45 \text{ degrees}} = 0.622$$

We can round the result to 0.6. This means that the middle axle should steer at 0.6, or about 60 percent of the front axle's angle. Therefore, the steering on the middle axle should be geared down to 0.6 as compared to the front axle. We can do this in two ways:

* Use a single steering shaft for both axles but with pinions of different sizes on each rack (see Figure 16-25).
* Use the same pinions on both axles but with two steering shafts with gearing between them (see Figure 16-26).

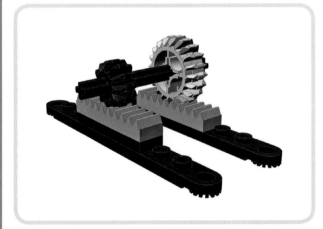

Figure 16-25: First method for two axles with different steering locks: a single steering shaft with two pinions of different size

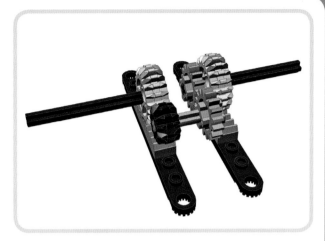

Figure 16-26: Second method for two axles with different steering locks: two identical pinions but two separate steering shafts with gearing between them

Whichever way we choose, it all comes down to the gear sizes. If we use a 20-tooth gear on the front axle, here's how we calculate the middle one:

$$20 \text{ teeth} \times 0.6 = 12 \text{ teeth}$$

As you see from the calculation, we need a 12-tooth gear. When assembling the model, we also need to make sure that the two steered axles are aligned.

Finally, a simple (and math-free!) alternative is to make a simple mock-up of the chassis showing just the distances between axles. You place the mock-up on a sheet of paper, turn the wheels so that they point at the center of the turning radius, and physically draw the lines and measure the angles. If you find any of these methods troublesome, you can always ignore convergence completely. It won't stop your models from driving or turning—they just won't handle as well as they would with convergent axles.

steering with virtual pivots

When a wheel is steered, it turns around an axis called the wheel's *steering axis*, or simply a *pivot* (see Chapter 25 for a more detailed explanation). Steering systems perform best when the pivot goes through the center of the wheel, but most LEGO wheels have pivots closer to the wheel's inner side, which impairs the steering performance of the entire vehicle. This placement also means that LEGO wheels don't

fit under realistic, tight fenders because they need a large margin of free space surrounding them to be steered.

One solution to this problem is to employ a steering system with virtual pivots that use a linkage to turn the wheel as though the pivot were located close to its center, as shown in Figure 16-27. This system works with most wheels. The main disadvantage is that the linkage makes it extremely difficult to add suspension between the chassis and the wheels; however, you can add suspension between the steering system and the rest of the chassis.

Virtual pivots are particularly useful in small-scale models where there is little room between the front wheels and the vehicle's body. Consider the model in Figure 16-28: It's very small, and the front fenders almost touch the front wheels. Yet it's fully remote controlled, and the front wheels can be steered without touching the fenders due to a small version of the virtual pivot steering system.

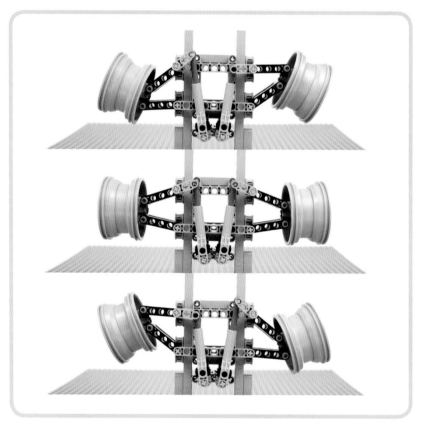

Figure 16-27: A top-down view of a steering system with virtual pivots. The tires have been removed from the rims for clarity.

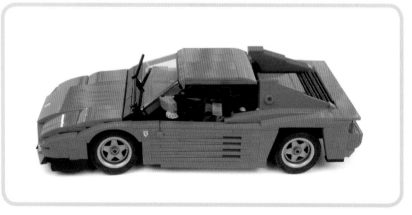

Figure 16-28: My Ferrari Testarossa model is small, at only 37 studs long, yet it has steered front wheels that fit under the front fenders because of the virtual pivot steering system.

a small virtual pivot steering system

In a small virtual pivot steering system, the wheels are turned by pulling and pushing the green beam (step 8). The system can be used with a motorized linear actuator or directly with a PF Servo motor.

1

2x 2x 2x 3 2x

2

4
1x 2x 1x 2x

3
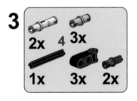
2x 4 3x
1x 3x 2x

4
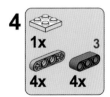
1x 3
4x 4x

5
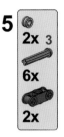
2x 3
6x
2x
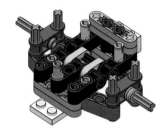

6
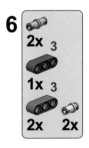
2x 3
1x 3
2x 2x
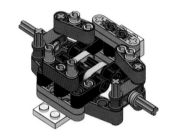

7
2x
2x
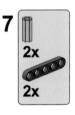

8
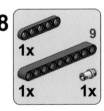
1x 9
1x 1x
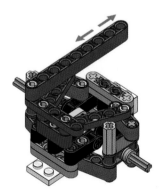

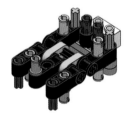
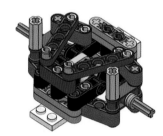
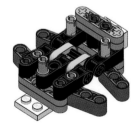

9

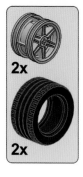

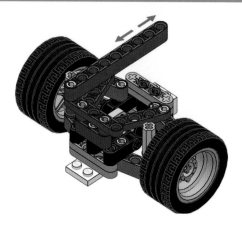

a large virtual pivot steering system

In a large virtual pivot steering system, the wheels are turned by two small linear actuators that are coupled and driven by a single motor. This system is best used with the PF M motor for light models and the PF L motor for heavy models.

1

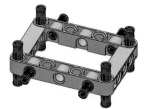

2

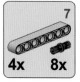

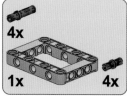

3

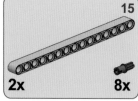

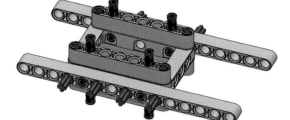

4

2x
4x
2x 9
3x 2x

5

5
1x
9
1x

6

8x
5
2x

7

3
2x
2x
2x

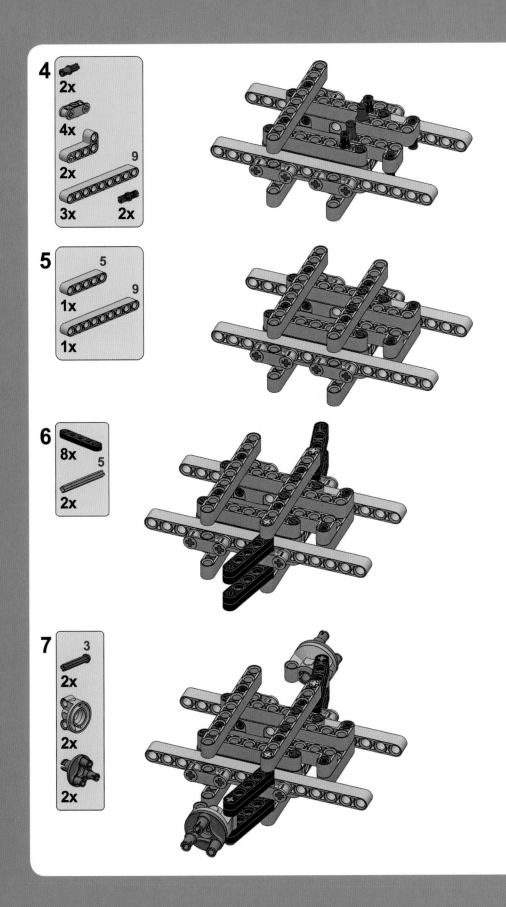

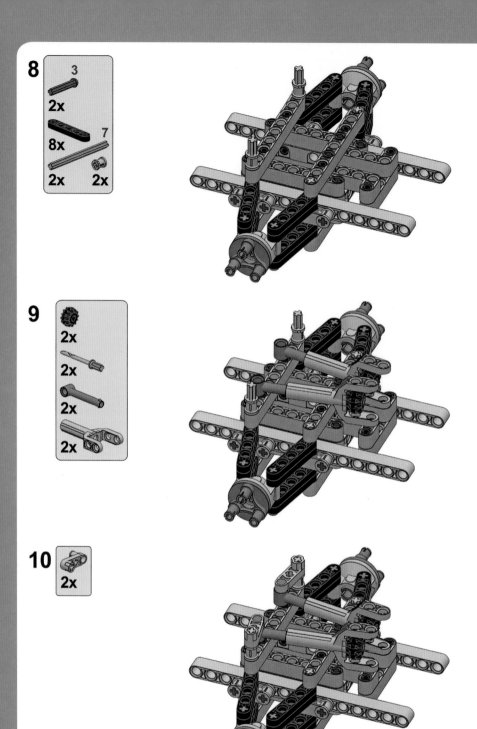

11

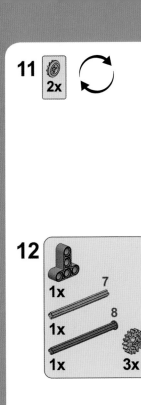

2x ↻

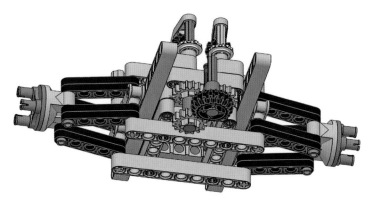

12

1x
1x
1x 7
  8
3x

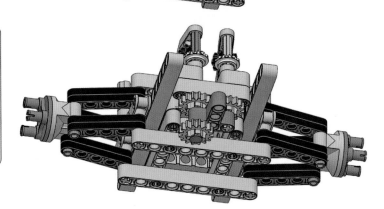

13

1x
1x 4
1x

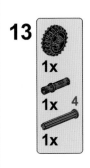

14

1x

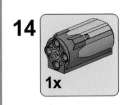

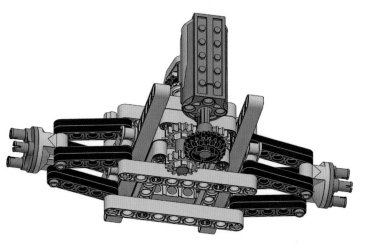

17

wheeled suspension systems

The previous chapter introduced us to the principles of steering in wheeled vehicles. Now, we'll take a look at two topics that are inextricably linked to steering axles: suspending axles and driving them. These interrelated mechanisms are frequently "separate," yet because they affect the same final element, the wheels, they can be built only in a limited number of combinations. For example, a suspension of a given type will work only with certain steering and drive systems.

Any axle of a wheeled vehicle can be suspended, driven, and steered at the same time. An axle can, of course, do none of these things and merely hold wheels together, but since such an axle is very simple to build, this chapter will focus on axles that are at least driven. We're going to discuss axles in four groups of increasing complexity:

* Driven axles (those that receive power)
* Driven and suspended axles
* Steered and suspended axles
* Driven, steered, and suspended axles

After going through the first group, we'll focus on the concept of suspending wheels; we'll learn how suspension systems work, how they are categorized, and how to choose the suspension that best suits our needs.

driven axles

A driven axle is a mechanism that connects two wheels while transferring drive to them from the chassis. The power is usually received from a driveshaft that is longitudinal to the chassis and perpendicular to the axle. Connecting these two elements is necessary, and a pair of bevel gears is the simplest solution. But in practice, bevel gears are prone to skipping under high torque, and a driven axle is where we can expect high torque. This leaves us with two other options: a differential or a pair of knobs. A differential is less likely to

skip, especially if braced inside a proper structure (shown in Figure 17-1), and knobs are extremely unlikely to skip at all thanks to their design (shown in Figure 17-2).

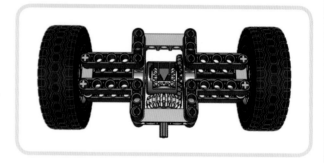

Figure 17-1: This is what a simple driven axle, also known as a live axle, can look like. The driveshaft (red) drives the 20-tooth double-bevel gear meshed with a differential case. The 5×7 studless frame braces the differential and prevents it from skipping. Note that there are two separate 7-stud-long axles connecting the differential to the wheels—axles used in this way are called halfshafts.

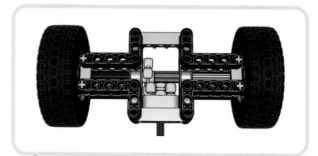

Figure 17-2: The same simple driven axle with a pair of knob wheels instead of a differential. The knob wheels are very unlikely to skip even if braced in a weak structure. Note that the two wheels' axles are now connected with an axle joiner (green), so they work like a single axle. For more information about using differentials, including their pros and cons, see Chapter 6; for ways of creating a custom differential, see Chapter 9.

suspension systems: concept and categories

A suspension is a system of linkages that connects the chassis of the vehicle to the wheels. Its primary purpose is to keep all wheels in constant contact with the ground, thus ensuring stability and proper traction of the vehicle. The suspension can also isolate the chassis from bumps and vibrations generated by the ground—but this is actually its secondary function, and it's not even present in all types of suspensions.

In order to maintain stability, a vehicle needs to be supported at no fewer than three points. For example, a bicycle is supported at just two points—where its wheels touch the ground—and it will fall over unless you support it at another point or drive it fast, in which case the stability comes from the gyroscopic effect of a wheel's rotation. So a vehicle needs at least three points of support, and we'll call these points *fulcrums* in our suspensions. Sometimes they are simply called *points*—hence the term *3-point suspension* for a suspension that provides three fulcrums for a vehicle and *4-point suspension* for one that provides four.

It's important to understand that with a suspension system, the number of wheels and the number of fulcrums differ. An unsuspended axle provides two fulcrums (one at each wheel), while a suspended axle provides just one, at the point of its attachment to the vehicle. For instance, a vehicle with four wheels can have one suspended and one unsuspended axle to get three fulcrums (Figure 17-3). A six-wheeled vehicle will also have three fulcrums if all three axles are suspended (Figure 17-5).

Consider a few simple examples in Figures 17-3 to 17-7 of chassis with various numbers of wheels and three (or more) fulcrums (fulcrums are marked with red arrows, chassis are black, and oscillating suspension parts are blue).

The way the wheels move in relation to each other is the first way to categorize a suspension:

* A suspension is *independent* when one wheel on a given axle can move without affecting the other one.
* A suspension is *dependent* when it's impossible to move one wheel on a given axle without affecting the other one.

In dependent suspensions, when one wheel of the axle goes up, the other one goes down, and vice versa. All the simple examples here are *dependent* (Figures 17-3 to 17-7).

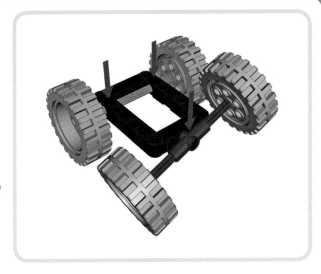

Figure 17-3: A simple chassis with four wheels, including two on a suspended axle

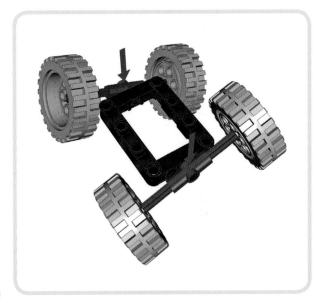

Figure 17-4: It's possible to build chassis with just two fulcrums, like this one with two suspended axles, but the chassis will need elastic elements supporting it against the axles to prevent it from falling to the side.

Also note that suspension types can vary between different axles. One vehicle can have, for example, an independent front suspension (on the front axle) and a dependent rear suspension (on the rear axle). Such a combination is actually quite popular because it allows you to build vehicles that are only as complex as necessary. In many cases, there is simply no need to use advanced suspension systems on all axles.

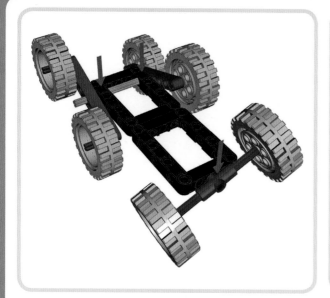

Figure 17-5: A chassis with six wheels, all suspended

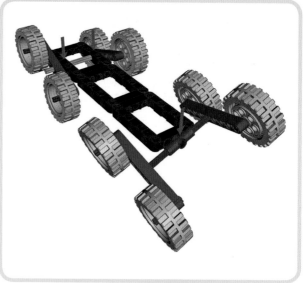

Figure 17-7: Even with many wheels, the number of fulcrums can be reduced by using more complex suspension systems that oscillate around more than one axle. This allows the wheels to adapt to the shape of obstacles in more planes.

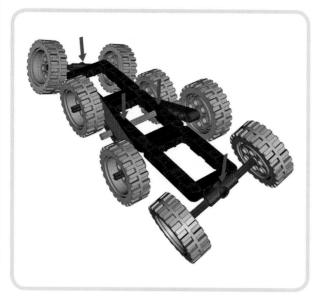

Figure 17-6: A chassis with eight wheels and four fulcrums, meaning it has a 4-point suspension. Long, multiwheeled vehicles often have more than three fulcrums.

* A suspension is *unsprung* when the chassis is supported by the given axle directly so the shocks from the axle are fully transferred to the chassis.

The easiest way to tell a sprung suspension from an unsprung one is by trying to press the vehicle's body down on its wheels. A sprung suspension will make the body yield, while an unsprung suspension will not. This is because a vehicle with unsprung suspension maintains *constant ground clearance*, which means that the middle of the chassis always stays the same distance from the ground. That makes unsprung suspension commonly used in heavy machinery, as it does not yield under heavy loads.

types of suspensions

Secondly, we can categorize suspensions by how they transfer shock from the road surface:

* A suspension is *sprung* when the chassis is supported by elastic elements attached to the given axle so the shocks from the axle are partially absorbed.

Of the many real-world suspension systems, we will learn to build four with LEGO pieces:

* Basic independent suspension
* Tatra-type suspension (a special kind of independent suspension developed and patented by the Tatra company)

* Pendular suspension (a very simple, dependent suspension based on a single axle's rotation)
* Floating axle (an axle with no rigid connections to the chassis whatsoever)

We will now discuss these suspension types using simple models of each. After that, we'll look at actual suspension designs.

double-wishbone independent suspension

Type: Independent, sprung

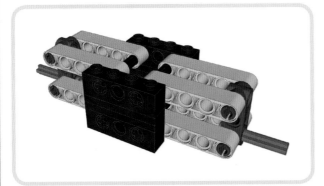

The chassis is black, the suspension arms are yellow, the steering arms (not steered in this case) are blue, and the spindles are green. As you see, each steering arm is suspended on four parallel levers that allow it to move up or down relative to the chassis while keeping the wheel in a vertical position. Consider the examples in Figures 17-8 and 17-9.

One element is missing from these images—the suspension arms need to be actually suspended. In other words, the chassis needs some elastic elements to support it against the suspension arms, or else the entire suspension will collapse. Shock absorbers are well suited and popular in this role (see Figure 17-10). Figure 17-11 provides an example of a model that uses independent suspension.

* **Advantages:** Best suspension type in terms of stability and traction; the orientation of the wheels is maintained at all times
* **Disadvantages:** Large width; relatively fragile construction

Note that it's possible to use the same elastic elements for the suspension arms for both wheels, but this will make the suspension dependent—causing one wheel to go up while the other one goes down (see Figure 17-12).

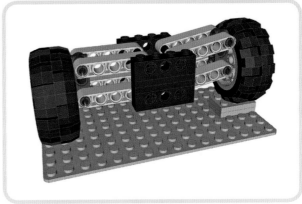

Figure 17-8: Independent suspension with one wheel on an obstacle. Note that the position of the other wheel is unaffected, as it should be with an independent suspension.

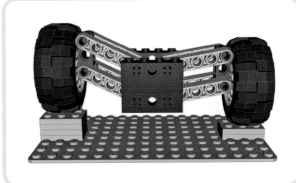

Figure 17-9: Independent suspension with both wheels on obstacles. Both wheels negotiate obstacles independently; hence the name of the suspension type.

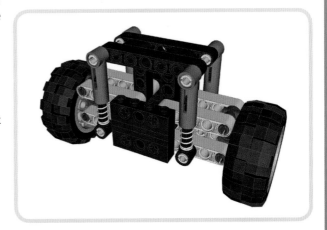

Figure 17-10: Independent suspension with four shock absorbers supporting the chassis against the suspension arms

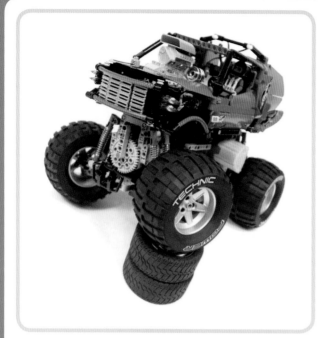

Figure 17-11: My Monster Truck model was a good example of independent suspension. Note that the vertical orientation of both front wheels was identical despite the extreme difference in their heights.

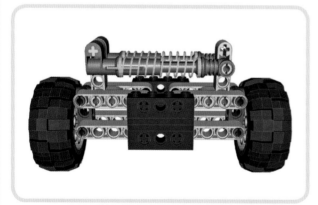

Figure 17-12: A suspension with shock absorbers supporting the suspension arms against each other (left and right). This solution will keep the chassis stable, but the suspension will become dependent.

Tatra-type suspension

Type: Independent, sprung

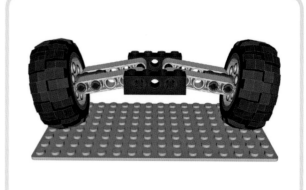

The Tatra-type suspension, also known as a swing-arm suspension, was developed and patented by the Tatra company, which uses it almost exclusively. The Tatra-type suspension is a simpler variant of the independent suspension that uses only two levers per wheel as suspension and keeps the spindles perpendicular to the suspension arms at all times. This means that the orientation of the wheels changes as they negotiate obstacles. By default, the wheels are tilted, as shown in Figure 17-13, a feature unique to this suspension type.

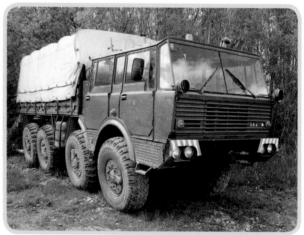

Figure 17-13: The default position of the Tatra-type suspension offers extra ground clearance. This "bowed" look can be mistaken for damage or warping.

Other than the tilting of the wheels, the Tatra suspension, shown in action in Figure 17-14, shares all the qualities and properties of a regular independent suspension. It is valued for the robustness coming from its simplicity, and it performs very well on rough terrain (Tatra off-road trucks are nothing short of legendary); its only downsides are inferior sideways stability and poor tire wear. Such a suspension is viable only for heavy off-road vehicles.

* **Advantages:** Simpler, more robust than a typical independent suspension
* **Disadvantages:** Slightly inferior traction because of the wheels' changing orientation; inferior sideways stability

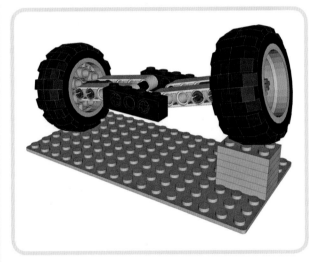

Figure 17-14: The Tatra-type suspension negotiating an obstacle with one wheel. Note that the orientation of the wheels changes in the process, which is why this suspension requires tires with a round profile (balloon tires) to maintain good traction.

pendular suspension

Type: Dependent, unsprung

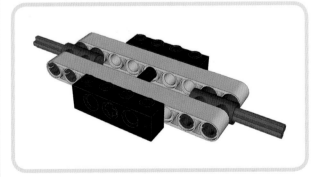

A pendular suspension is the simplest and the most robust kind of suspension: It allows the axle to swing back and forth on a single point just like a pendulum. As it's only one solid element, it can be very narrow and built with just a few pieces. Figure 17-15 shows a pendular suspension in action.

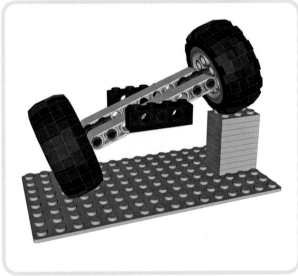

Figure 17-15: A pendular suspension negotiating an obstacle with one wheel. Note that the chassis, which is connected to the axle by the axle going through its center, is raised by 50 percent. This is generally bad for stability and for the driver's comfort.

On the downside, pendular suspension systems take a lot of space in the chassis, requiring the model to have a large gap in order for the suspension to fit. The pendular suspension system can't be sprung, but it often requires shock absorbers (see Figure 17-16) or other elastic elements to keep it stable—unless you arrange the suspended axles of your vehicle so as to provide three or more fulcrums. The longitudinal axle that goes through it is also the only way to transfer the drive to the suspension from the chassis. So the longitudinal axle is used as the driveshaft, which means that this suspension is mounted on the driveshaft and presses on it, creating extra friction.

* **Advantages:** Simplest and most robust suspension type; can be very narrow
* **Disadvantages:** Unsprung; takes a lot of space in the chassis; adds extra friction on the drivetrain (see "Pendular Suspension with Turntables" on page 252 for a means of mitigating this effect)

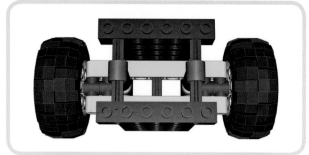

Figure 17-16: A pendular suspension stabilized with a pair of shock absorbers. Note that the shock absorbers work against each other and need to be half compressed when the suspension is level. When one wheel goes up, the absorber close to it is compressed more, and the other one is compressed less.

trailing arm suspension (floating axle suspension)

Type: Dependent, sprung

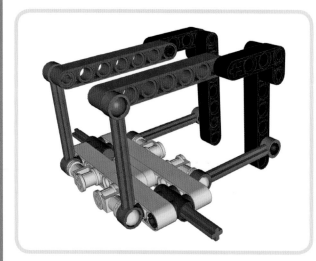

A floating axle suspension (or live axle) is a sprung variant of the pendular suspension. It's a single solid element that has no rigid connections to the chassis whatsoever; instead, it is connected to it by a number of links that form a linkage allowing it to move up and down and tilt to the sides. It can be just as narrow and robust as a regular pendular suspension, and it doesn't press on the driveshaft. However, it takes an extreme amount of space in the chassis because of the linkage that comes between it and the chassis.

Floating axles can be extremely complex. The variant we will focus on is a simple one (see Figure 17-17): It uses four links and two independent suspension arms above the actual axle that need to be supported by some elastic elements. It also uses a driveshaft with a single universal joint on it to keep the axle aligned with the chassis.

* **Advantages:** Combines all the advantages of pendular suspension with being sprung and usually more stable
* **Disadvantages:** Takes a lot of space in the chassis

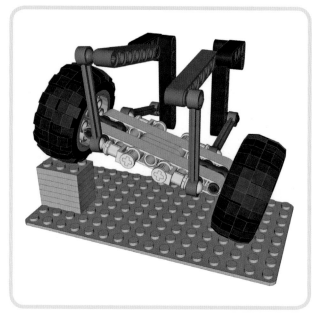

Figure 17-17: A floating axle negotiating an obstacle with one wheel. Note that the orientation of all four links is changed, while the chassis' orientation remains the same.

Choosing the best type of suspension for the job is always a little tricky, but your decision can be made easier by considering what is used in real vehicles. For example, luxury cars usually have full independent suspension to improve passengers' comfort, while construction vehicles—such as front-end loaders, for instance—usually have pendular suspension because the heavy loads they are handling would affect a sprung suspension too much.

wheel hubs and how to use them

The most natural way to connect a LEGO wheel to the suspension and then to the chassis is by using an axle—but that's not necessarily the best way. There are a number of elements called *wheel hubs* that allow you to make a sturdier, more secure connection. They are designed to act similarly to bearings—reducing the friction and stress between the wheel and the chassis while keeping the wheel stable, aligned, and firmly attached. In this section, I'll discuss one old wheel hub and the three modern hubs, all of which are shown in Figure 17-18. Note that each of these hubs can be driven or nondriven, and with the exception of the regular hub, they can all be steered.

Each of the modern wheel hub variants consists of two pieces: a dark grey connector that attaches to the wheel and rotates with it and a light grey holder that attaches to the chassis and remains stationary while the connector rotates inside it. The large contact area between the connector and the holder ensures a rigid connection with low friction. The old hub acts in a similar way; it has a rotating connector and

stationary holder, but it has a much smaller contact area between them, making the hub less rigid and less effective.

Note that the steered hub also exists in a newer black variant shown in Figure 17-19. The new variant was introduced in late 2016 to allow for more connections: The standard steering hub has two towballs, which connect only to steering links, while the black variant has axle holes instead of towballs. It's a small difference but one that creates countless new possibilities; with the black variant, you can connect much more than just steering links. The 42056 Porsche 911 GT3 RS set, for example, makes use of the variant's axle holes to install fake brake calipers on the front wheels. It appears that the newer variant is meant to replace the older one in LEGO sets.

The common feature of the modern wheel hubs is that they allow the same axle to go through them and through the wheel, but they also connect to the wheel with three pins around that axle. The old hub lacks the axle hole—it connects to the wheel using only the three pins. The most common Technic wheels feature three or six pin holes around the axle hole. The reason for six-hole variants, which were added recently, is that they're easier to connect to the hubs. With six pin holes, the wheel's pin holes and its axle hole are always aligned with the pins and axle hole of the hub. With three pin holes, you need to rotate the wheel relative to the hub until all the holes are aligned (see Figure 17-20).

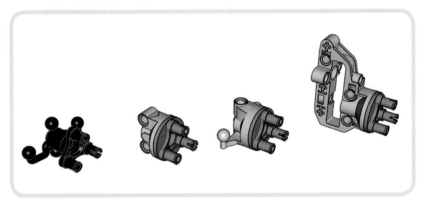

Figure 17-18: Four wheel hub variants (left to right): an old hub, a regular hub, a steered hub, and a portal hub.

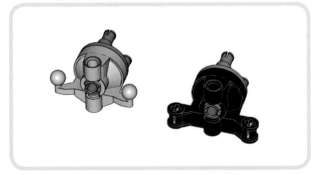

Figure 17-19: The standard steering hub (left) and its newer black variant (right), shown from behind. The only difference is that the newer variant uses axle holes instead of towballs.

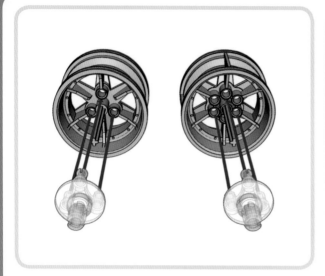

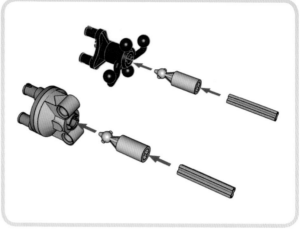

Figure 17-20: When you're using an axle, the way the wheel hubs (shown semitransparent here for clarity) connect to the rims can be tricky. With rims of the three-pin-hole variant (left), it's necessary to align the axle holes and the pins/pin holes between the rim and the hub. With rims of the six-hole variant (right), only the axle holes need to be aligned.

Figure 17-21: Other than the portal hub, all wheel hubs are driven by connecting a CV joint, which creates an articulated connection and can have a regular axle inserted into it. Rotating the axle then drives the wheel.

To drive a wheel hub, a special piece called a *CV (constant velocity)* joint is inserted into it and then a regular axle goes into that piece (see Figure 17-21). The CV joint connects a regular axle to the wheel hub in a way that allows the hub to be steered, to be driven, and to move up and down with the suspension. As the CV joint rotates, so does the connector part of the hub and the wheel attached to it. The only exception is the portal hub, which is driven using universal joints instead (see the building instructions).

The following building instructions show you how to use various types of wheel hubs to connect wheels to the chassis, forming an independent suspension with a driven wheel.

a pre-2011 wheel hub

1

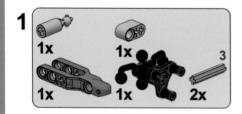

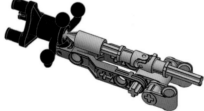

2

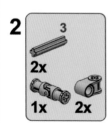

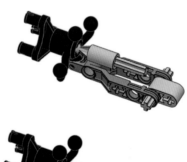

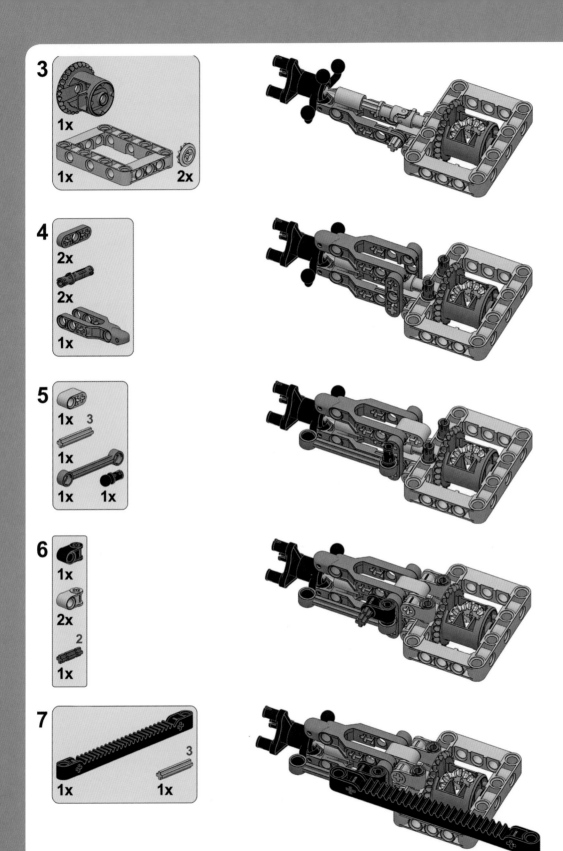

3

1x

1x   2x

4

2x

2x

1x

5

1x   3

1x

1x   1x

6

1x

2x

2

1x

7

3

1x   1x

a regular wheel hub

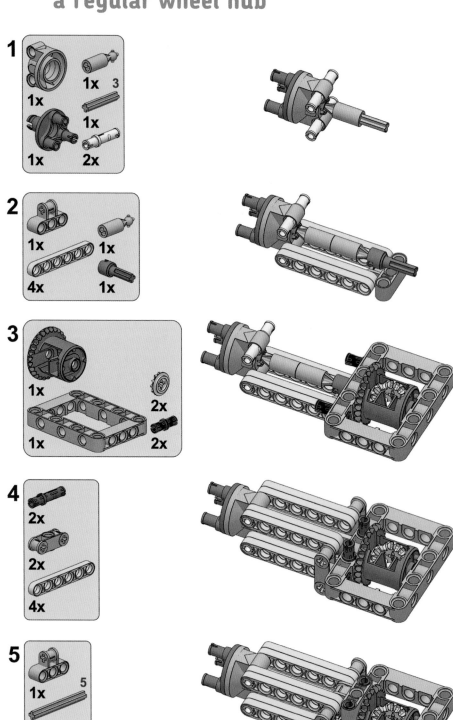

1
1x   1x   3
1x   1x   2x

2
1x   1x
4x   1x

3
1x   2x
1x   2x

4
2x
2x
4x

5
1x   5
2x

a steered wheel hub

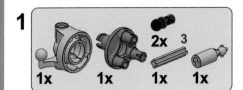

1

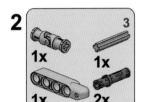

2x 3

1x   1x   1x   1x

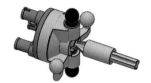

2

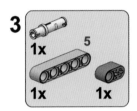

3

1x   1x

1x   2x

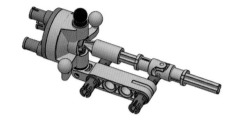

3

5

1x

1x   1x

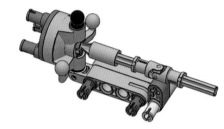

4

5

2x

1x

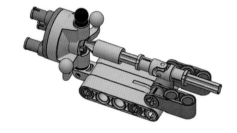

5

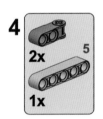

1x

2x

1x   1x

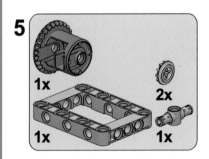

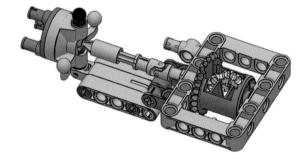

6

4x

1x

1x

7

4

2x 5 1x

1x 2x

1x 1x

8

1x

2

1x 5

1x 1x

9

1x

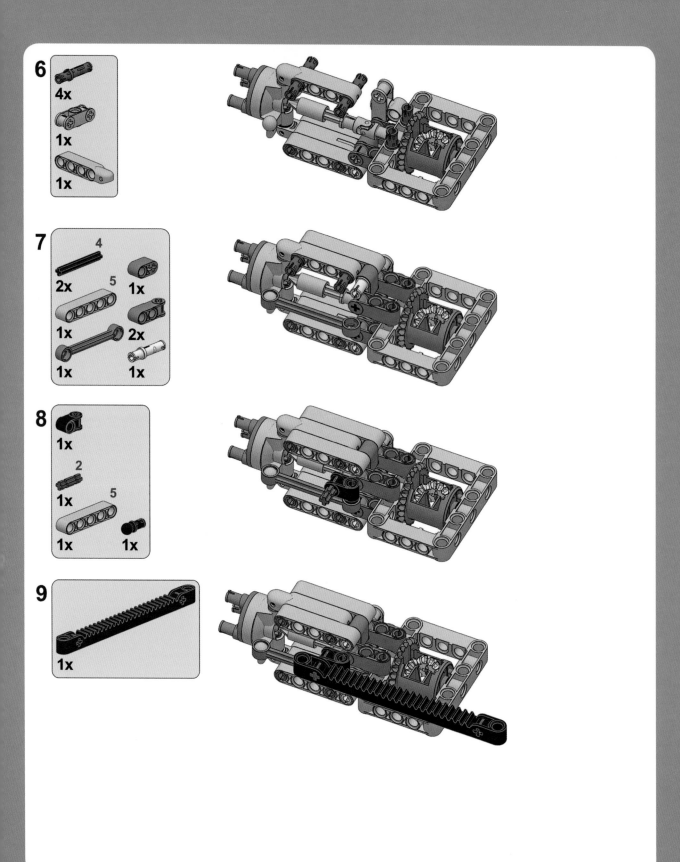

a portal wheel hub

1

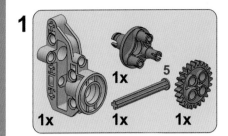

1x 1x 5 1x
1x 1x 1x

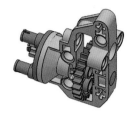

2

1x 2
1x 3
1x 2x 2x

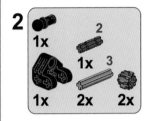

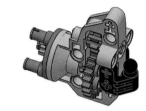

3

1x
1x 1x 2 1x

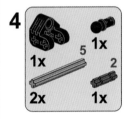

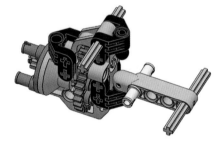

4

1x 5 1x
2x 2 1x

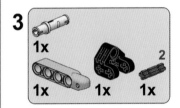

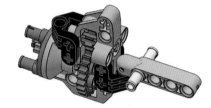

5

2x
1x

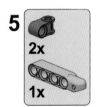

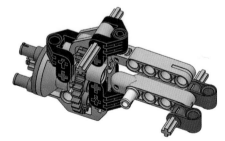

6

2x

1x

2x 1x 2

7

1x

1x

1x

8

1x

1x 2x

9

1x

2x 3 1x

2x 1x

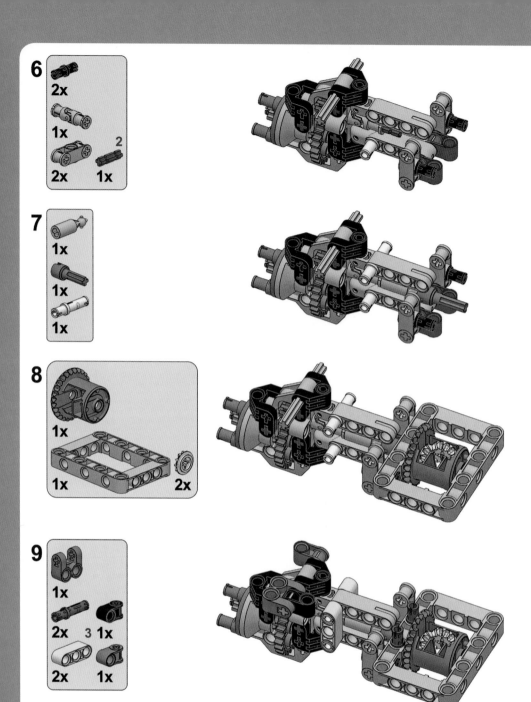

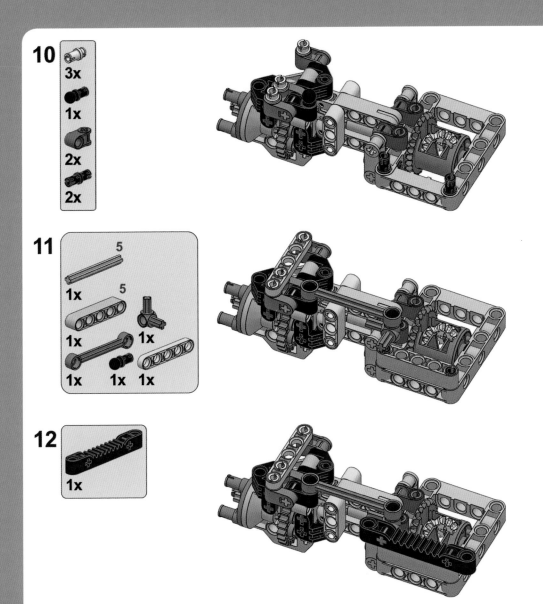

driven and suspended axles

Axles that are driven and suspended at the same time are relatively easy to build, and they're important because the vast majority of vehicles have at least one.

pendular suspension with turntables

As explained earlier, the pendular suspension has the disadvantage of being attached to the chassis by the driveshaft, which is subject to stress generated by the vehicle's weight. This single point of stress creates additional friction; however, this problem can be prevented almost completely by using a Technic turntable to attach the suspension to the chassis (see Figure 17-22), as an alternative to using ball

joints. The turntable then supports the weight of the vehicle, while the driveshaft can go through the middle of the turntable nearly unburdened.

Note that the large diameter of the turntable is bad for ground clearance, so it's a good idea to use this design in concert with portal axles. Also note that the hole in the turntable is large enough to install a differential case in it, which can be used to transfer both drive and steering through a single turntable (see Figure 17-23).

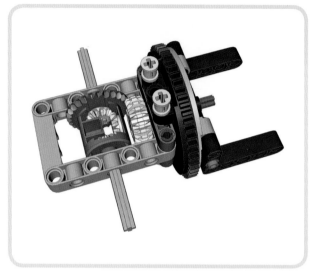

Figure 17-22: The newer type of Technic turntable is used to attach the suspension (the light grey frame) to the chassis (the black L-shaped beams). A turntable is a very rigid structure capable of supporting huge loads while adding minimum friction to the driveshaft (red) that goes through it.

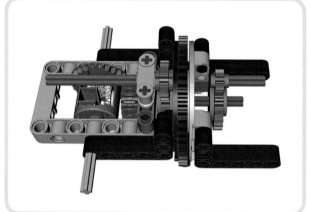

Figure 17-23: As an empty differential case rotates freely on an axle, it can be used to transfer steering over the driveshaft. Here, red pieces are acting as a driveshaft and green pieces are acting as a steering shaft without interfering with each other. Note that the steering shaft is slightly affected when the suspension tilts and the turntable rotates. Still, it's a useful solution when the driveshaft and steering shaft need to be connected to the suspension from the same side.

a stabilized pendular suspension

This is a simple, robust, and compact suspension kept stable by four shock absorbers. Keep in mind that absorbers of various length and hardness can be used.

1

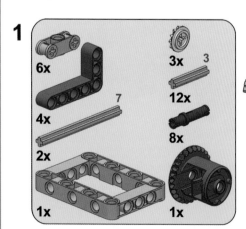

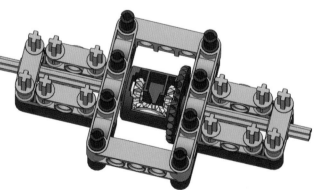

2

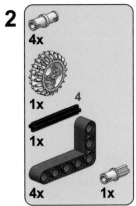

4x

1x 4

1x

4x   1x

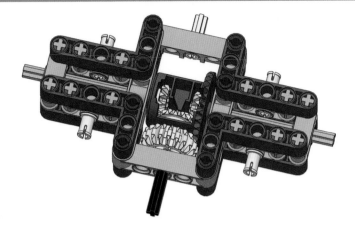

3

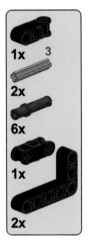

1x 3

2x

6x

1x

2x

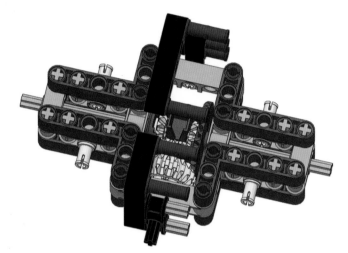

4

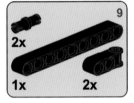

2x 9

1x   2x

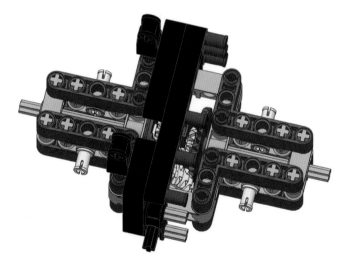

5

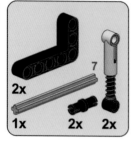

2x
1x 2x 2x

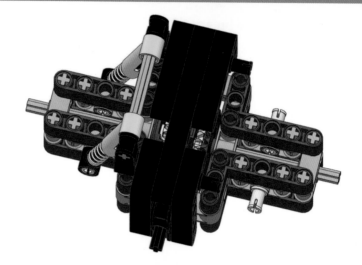

6

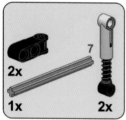

2x
1x 2x

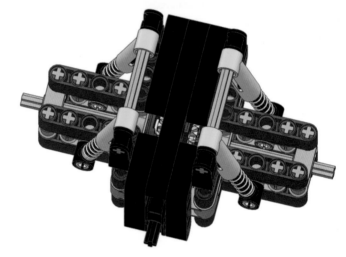

7

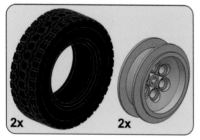

2x 2x

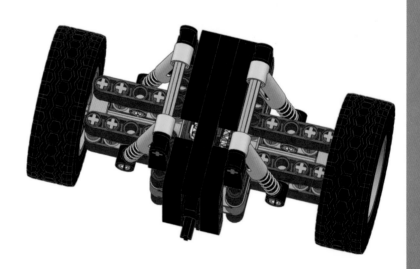

portal axles (geared hubs)

Portal axles use gear hubs on the wheels that increase both ground clearance and the gear reduction of the drivetrain, as Figure 17-24 shows. Practically any axle, including a steered one, can have gear hubs and become a portal axle at the cost of increased width. The most popular are hubs with a 24-tooth and 8-tooth gear combination, providing a 3:1 gear reduction. The 3:1 gear reduction means not only that torque on the wheels is increased three times but also that other parts of the drivetrain handle only a third of the overall load. This is very useful for steered axles because it allows us to use universal joints, which could otherwise be damaged by the load.

There are a number of ways to build narrow, strong gear hubs. The easiest one, however, involves a ready-made LEGO gear hub housing: a #92908 piece, into which a #92909 is inserted to support the wheel (see Figure 17-25). We will refer to this very convenient combination as a *LEGO hub*. Figure 17-26 shows a model that makes use of LEGO hubs.

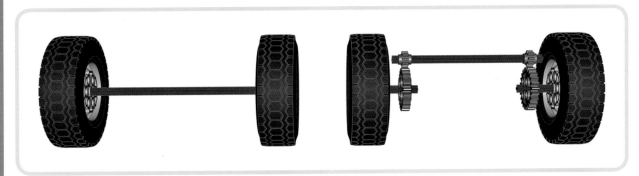

Figure 17-24: A regular axle (left) and portal axle (right)

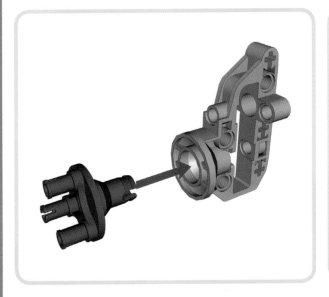

Figure 17-25: Pieces #92909 (left) and #92908 (right) together form a so-called LEGO hub.

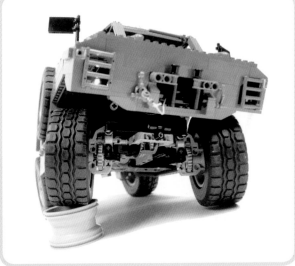

Figure 17-26: My model of the RG-35 4×4 MRAP vehicle made use of LEGO hubs to achieve an impressive ground clearance exceeding 6 studs.

a stabilized pendular suspension with a portal axle

This is a variant of the previous design with hubs added to make it a portal axle.

1

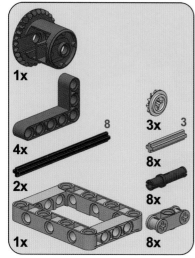

1x
4x
2x
1x

8
3x 3
8x
8x
8x

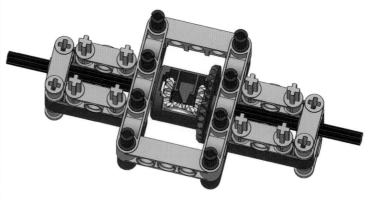

2

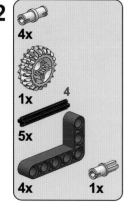

4x
1x 4
5x
4x 1x

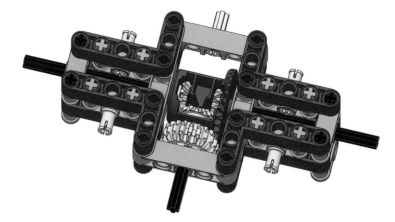

3

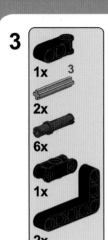

1x 3
2x
6x
1x
2x

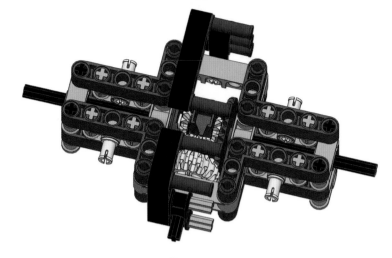

4

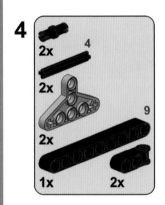

2x 4
2x
2x 9
1x 2x

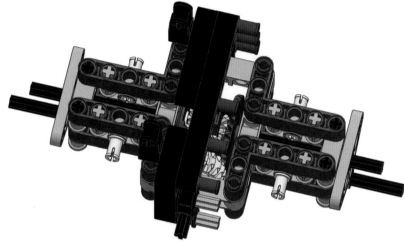

5

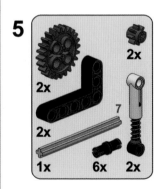

2x
2x 7
2x
1x 6x 2x

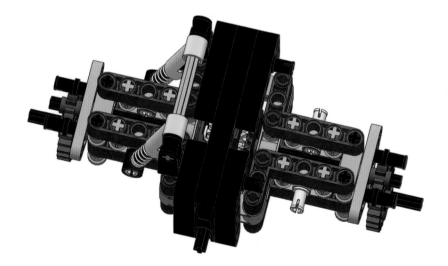

6

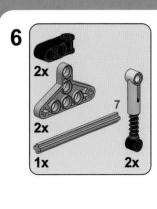

2x
2x
1x
2x

7

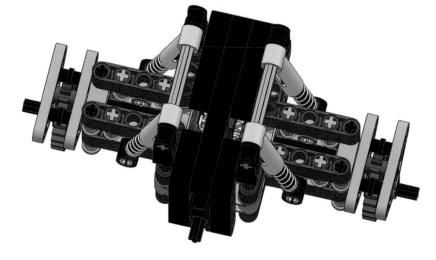

7

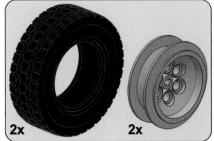

2x
2x

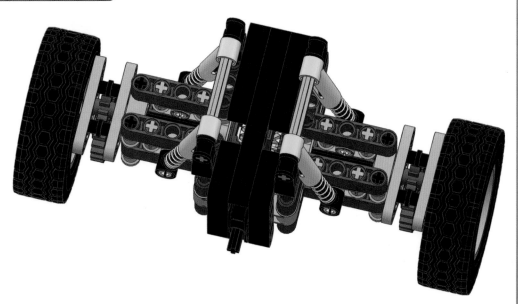

a Tatra-type suspension stabilized with four shock absorbers

This is a simple, robust suspension without a differential, well suited for rough terrain. Remember to set up the shock absorbers so that the wheels are tilted slightly downward when the suspension is unloaded.

NOTE It's possible to convert this design to use a portal axle, but it's not recommended with this suspension as doing so would decrease its sideways stability.

1

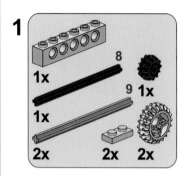

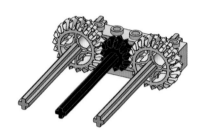

2

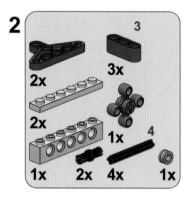

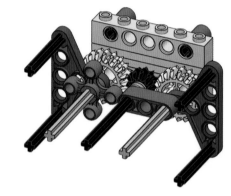

3

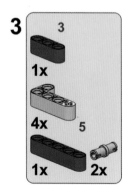

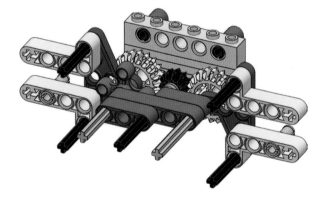

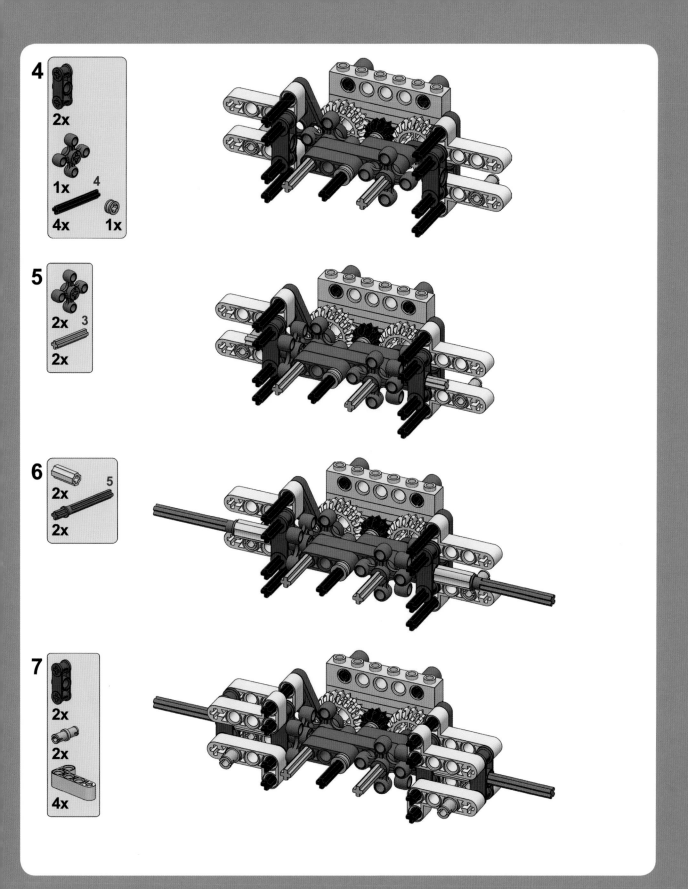

4

2x

1x   4

4x   1x

5

2x   3

2x

6

2x   5

2x

7

2x

2x

4x

8

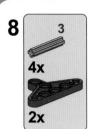

3

4x

2x

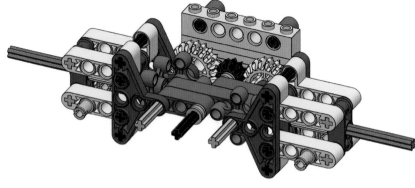

9

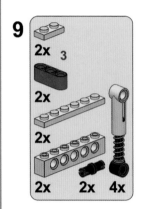

2x

3

2x

2x

2x   2x   4x

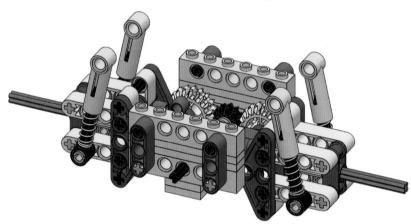

10

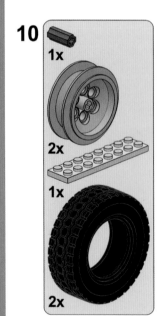

1x

2x

1x

2x

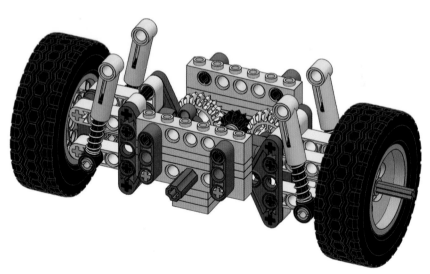

an independent suspension

This is a typical independent suspension. It's wide but
provides good overall performance.

1

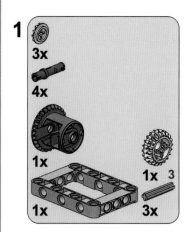

3x
4x
1x
1x   1x   3
3x

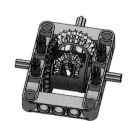

2

3
2x   8x
2x   2x

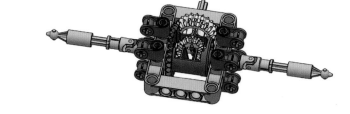

3

3
4x
2x   4x

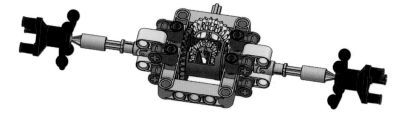

4

3
4x
4x

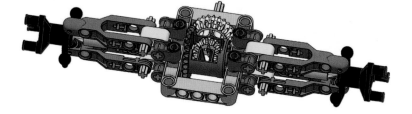

5

12x
3   4x
4x   4x   2x

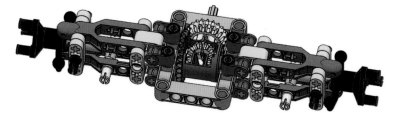

6

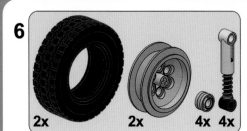

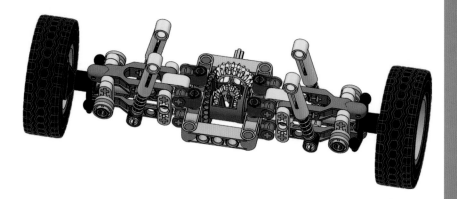

a floating axle with four links

This is a complex yet robust design with large travel. The instruction includes a partial body frame that can be easily extended to add another axle.

1

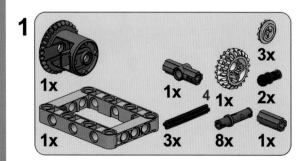

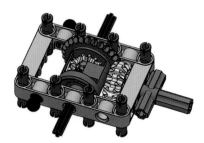

an independent suspension

This is a typical independent suspension. It's wide but provides good overall performance.

1

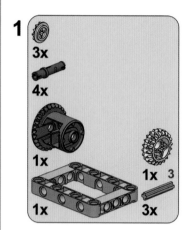

3x

4x

1x

1x

1x 3

3x

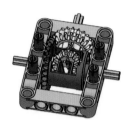

2

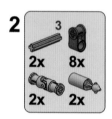

3

2x 8x

2x 2x

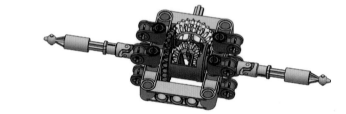

3

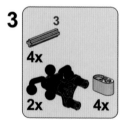

3

4x

2x 4x

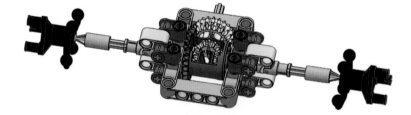

4

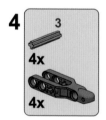

3

4x

4x

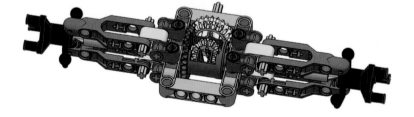

5

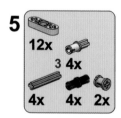

12x

3 4x

4x 4x 2x

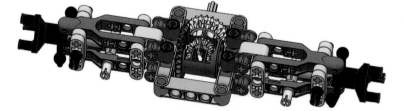

6

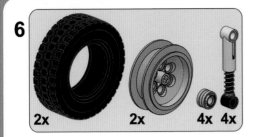

2x   2x   4x   4x

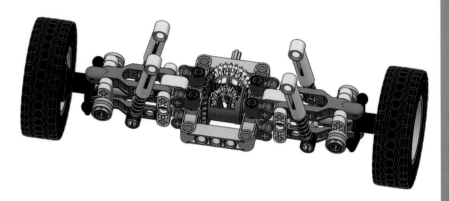

a floating axle with four links

This is a complex yet robust design with large travel. The instruction includes a partial body frame that can be easily extended to add another axle.

1

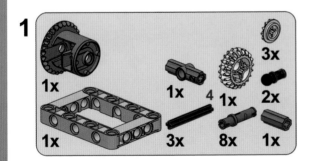

1x

1x   1x   4   1x   2x

1x   3x   8x   1x

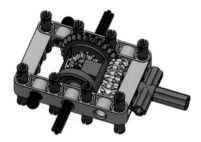

2

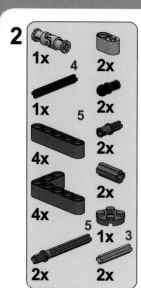

1x 4
1x 5
4x
4x
5
2x

2x
2x
2x
2x
1x 3
2x

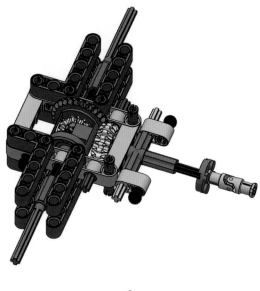

3

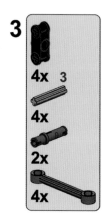

4x 3
4x
2x
4x

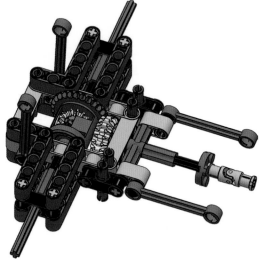

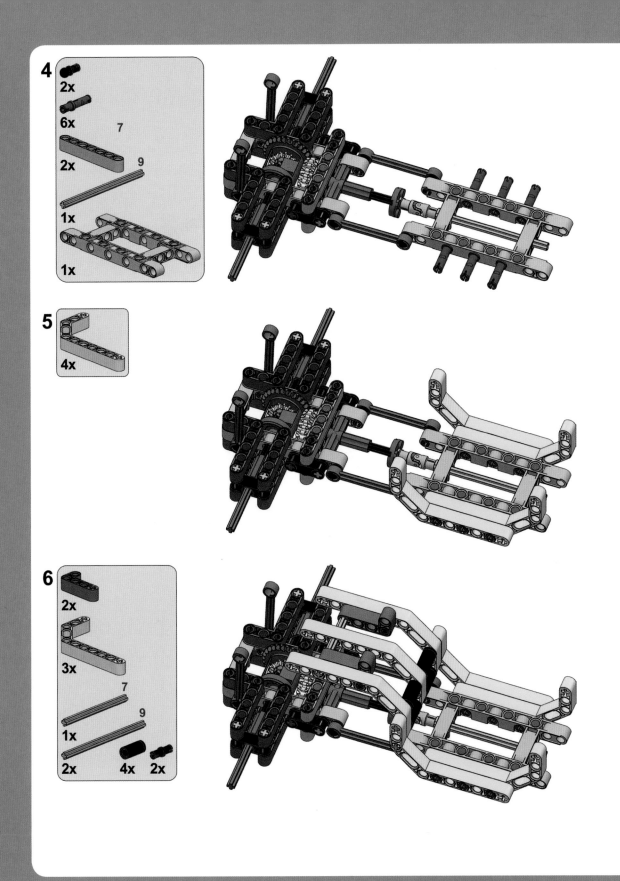

4
2x
6x
7
2x
9
1x
1x

5
4x

6
2x
3x
7
9
1x
2x   4x   2x

7

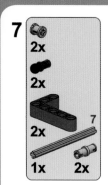

2x
2x
2x   7
1x   2x

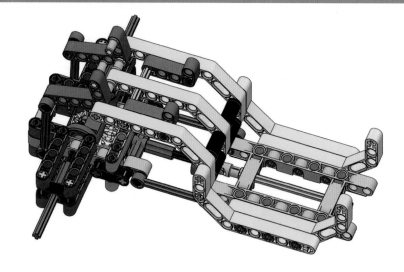

8

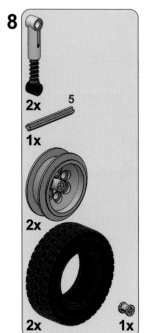

2x
1x   5
2x
2x
2x   1x

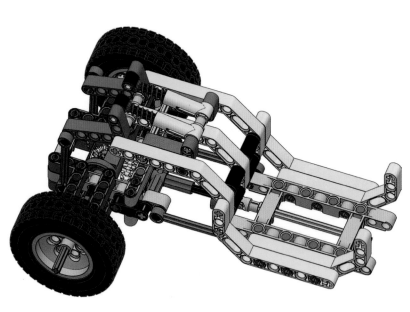

steered and suspended axles

Here's a look at some building instructions for axles that are suspended but can also be steered. These are commonly used for the front axle of real-wheel-drive cars.

a pendular steered axle

A simple design focused on small size. The red bricks simulate the chassis. Note that you can remove the shock absorbers if your vehicle's other axles make it stable enough.

1
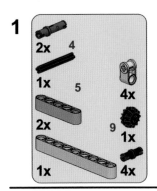
2x   4
1x   5
4x
2x   9
1x
1x   4x

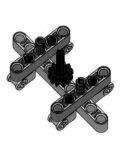

2
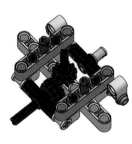
1x   3
2x
2x   1x
2x   4   2
1x   2x

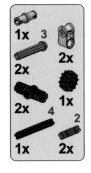

3
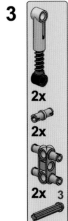
2x
2x
2x   3
2x

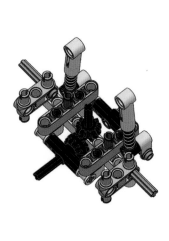

4
2x
1x   9
1x
1x   9
1x

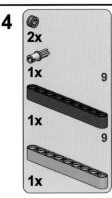

5
6x
2x
1x
2x   2x

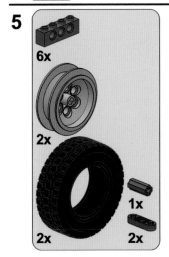
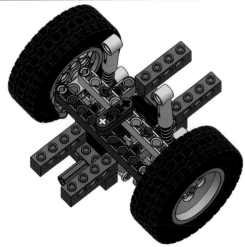

an independent steered axle

This design uses a number of specialized pieces to create the narrowest independent suspension possible. It's well suited for small, light vehicles.

1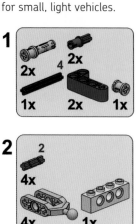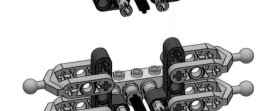

2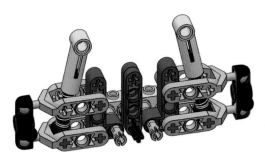

3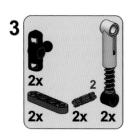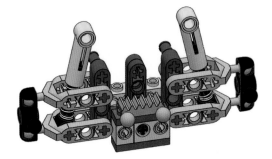

4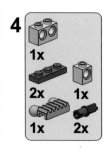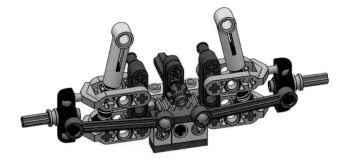

5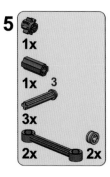

6

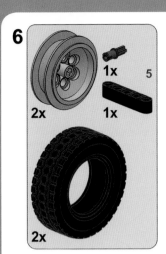

2x **1x** 5

1x

2x

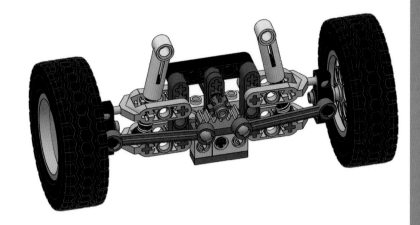

driven, steered, and suspended axles

Here are building instructions for the most complicated category of axles.

an independent axle

This axle is just slightly more complicated than the version without steering.

NOTE There is an older version of this suspension using different (older) pieces in the 8880 Super Car set.

1

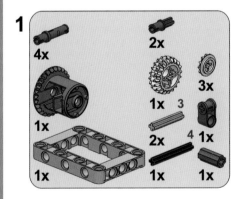

4x **2x**

1x 3 **3x**

1x **1x**

1x **2x** 4 **1x**

1x **1x** **1x**

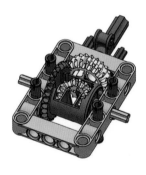

2

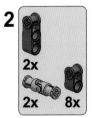

2x

2x **8x**

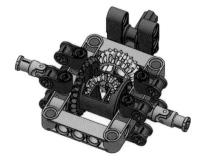

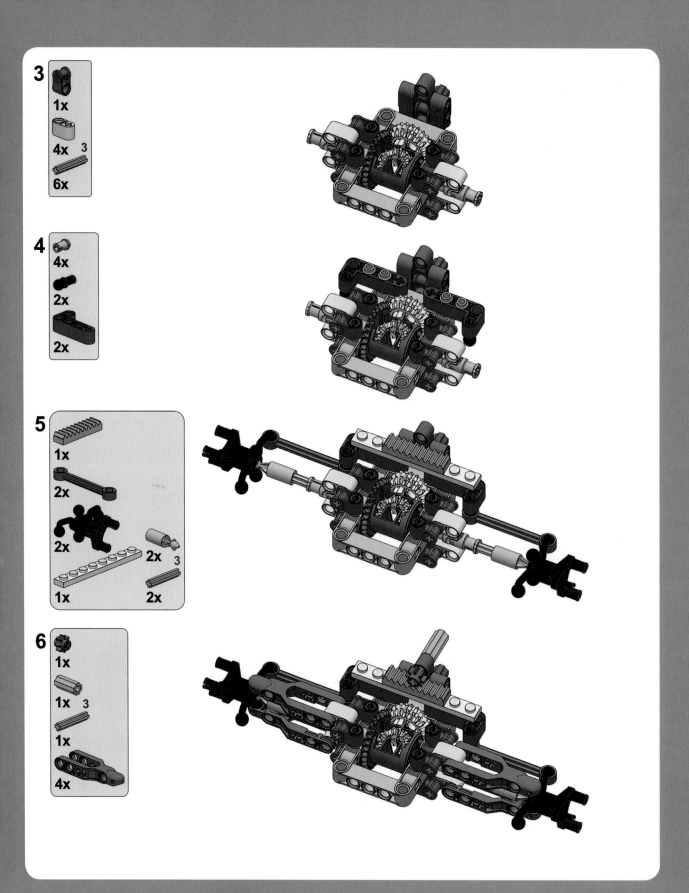

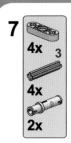

4x
3
4x
2x

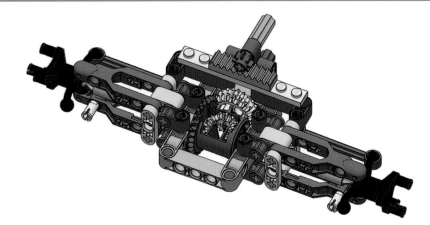

8

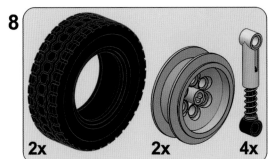

2x   2x   4x

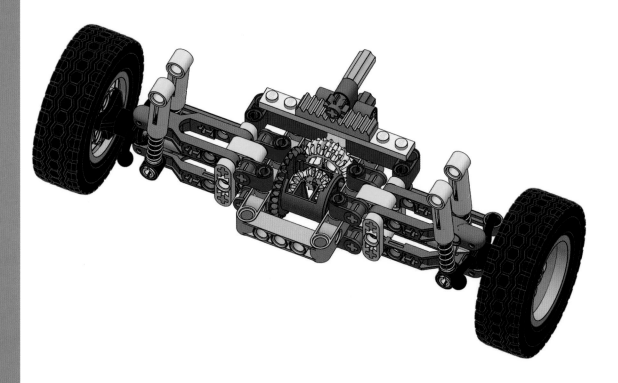

a heavy-duty pendular portal axle

This is a complex and extremely robust suspension designed for very rough terrain. It includes knob gears instead of a differential, and it consists mostly of basic studless pieces.

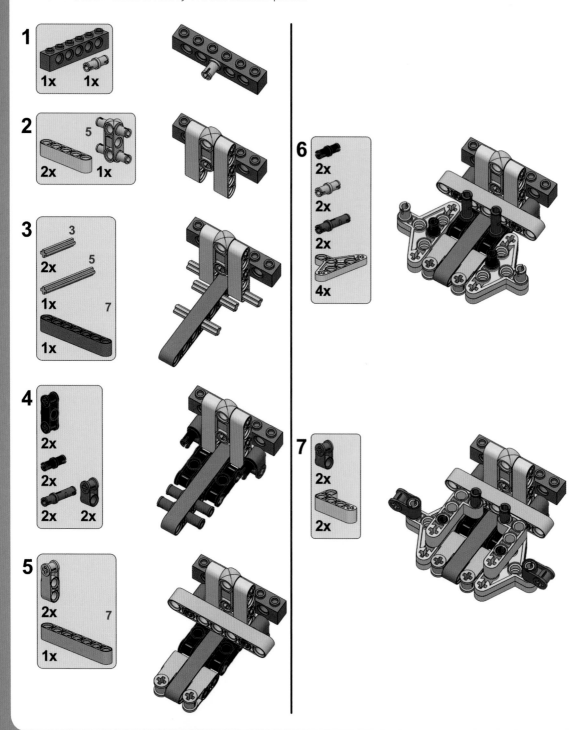

1
1x   1x

2
5
2x   1x

3
3
2x
5
1x
7
1x

4
2x
2x
2x   2x

5
2x
7
1x

6
2x
2x
2x
4x

7
2x
2x

8

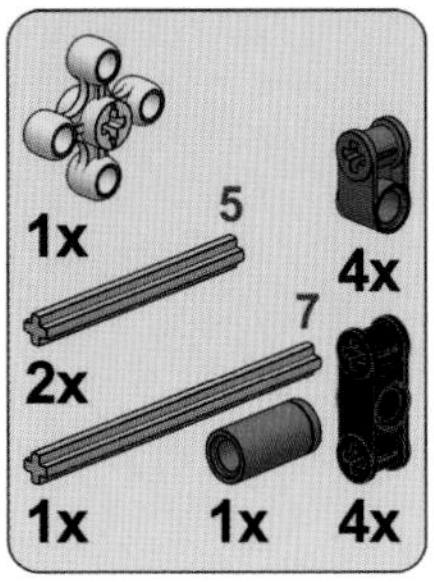

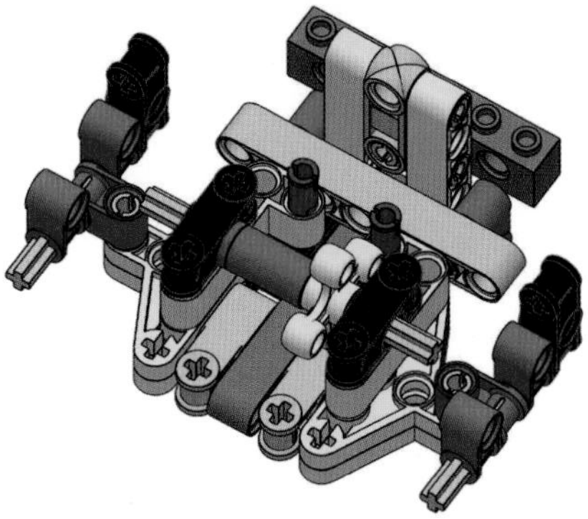

1x
5
2x
7
1x 1x
4x
4x

9

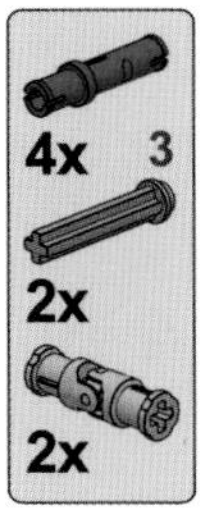

4x 3
2x
2x

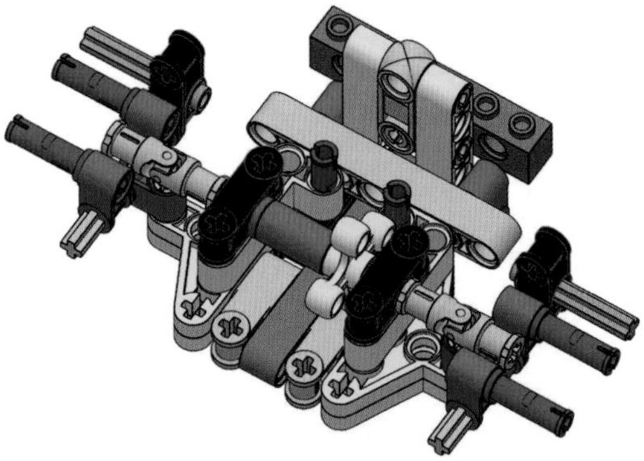

10

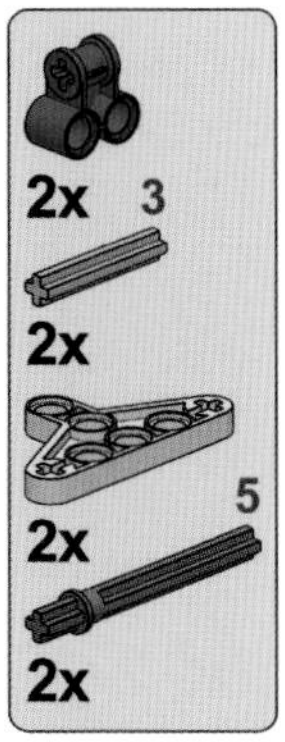

2x 3
2x
2x 5
2x

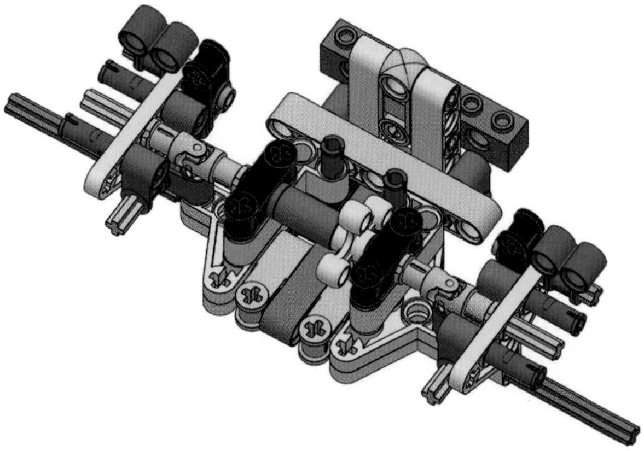

11

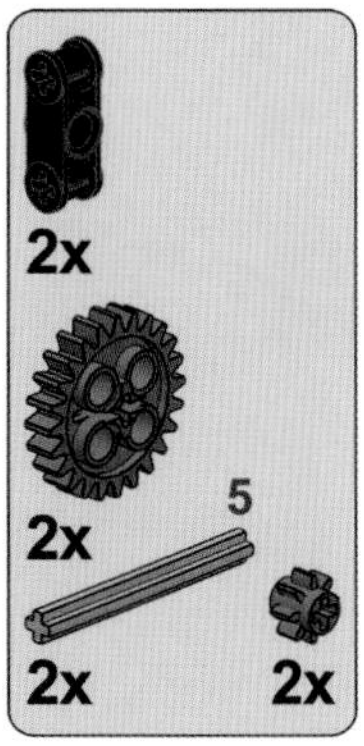

2x
2x 5
2x 2x

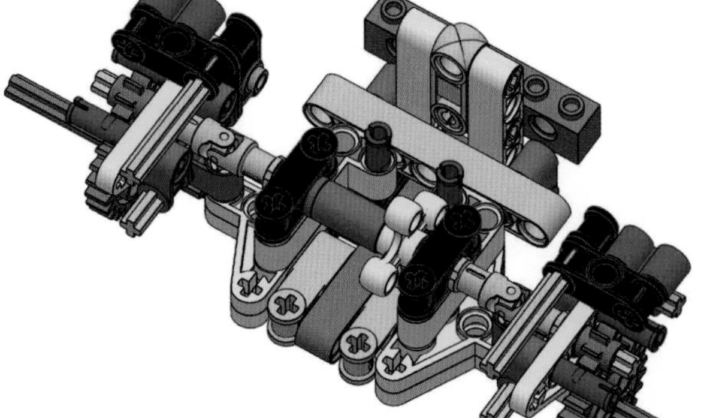

12

2x
2x   6
2x   7
1x   2x

13

2x
4x   3
1x   5
1x

14

2x
1x
1x   6
1x   3x

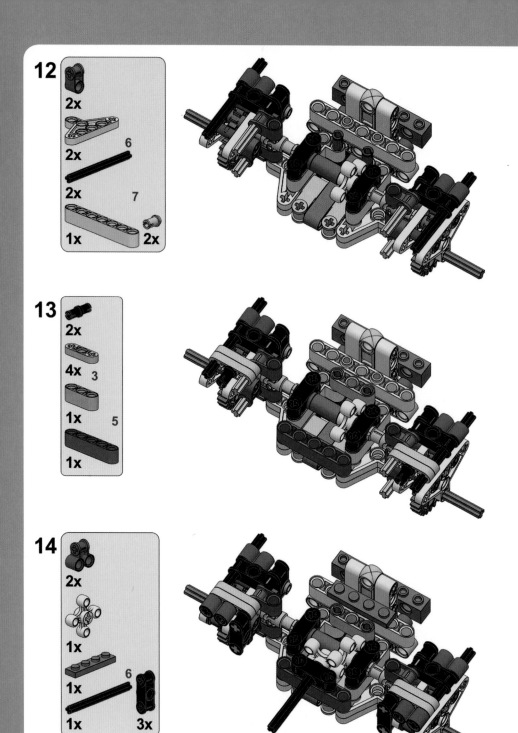

15

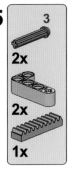

2x
3

2x

1x

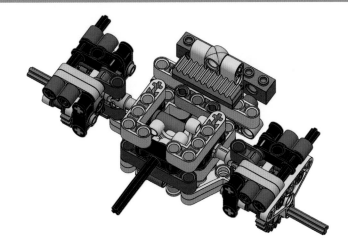

16

2x

2x

2x
5

1x
5

10x   2x

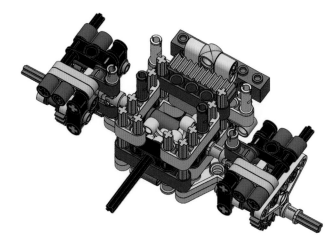

17

2x

2x   3

2x

4x

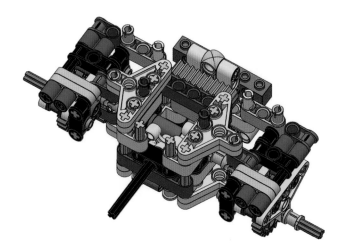

18

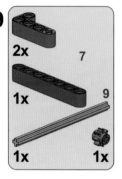

3x
4x
6x

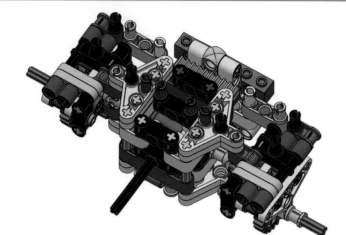

19

2x   7
1x   9
1x
1x

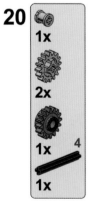

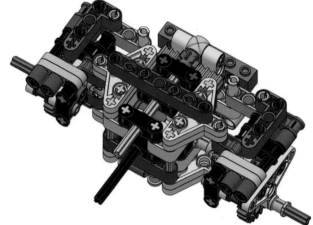

20

1x
2x
1x   4
1x

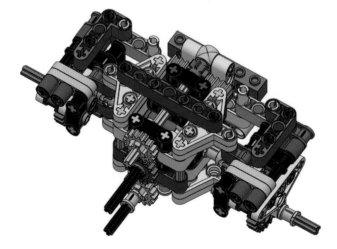

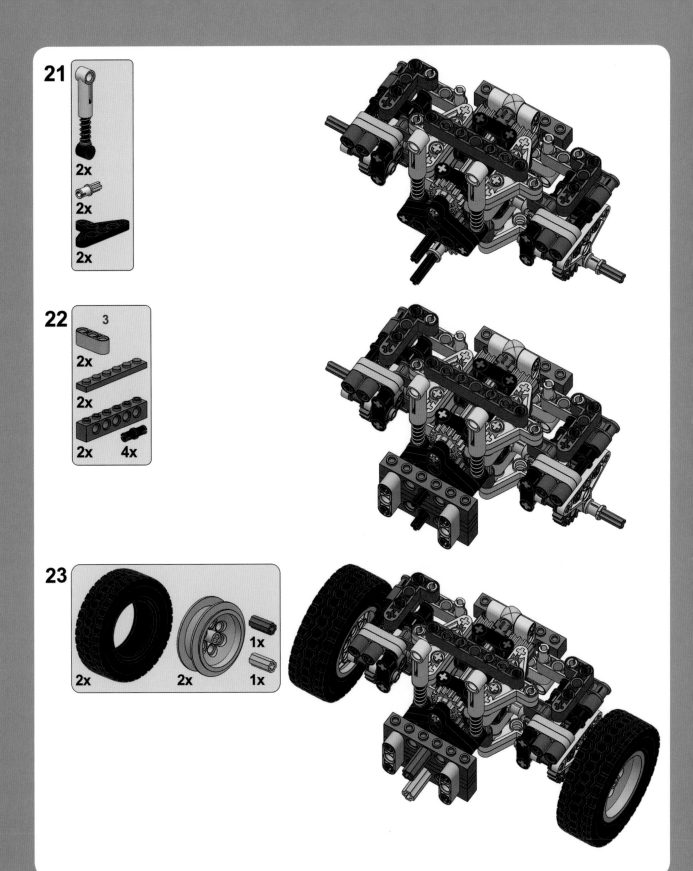

21

2x
2x
2x

22

3
2x
2x
2x   4x

23

2x   2x   1x
         1x

a pendular axle with a worm gear

This is a compact suspension that uses the middle differential variant and a worm gear. This makes it well suited for use with motors that require substantial gear reduction. At the same time, it generates large backlash because of the two 8-tooth gears meshed with one another.

1

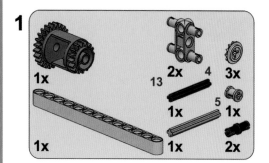

1x

13 **2x** 4 **3x**

1x 5 **1x**

1x **1x** **2x**

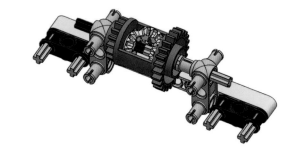

2

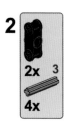

2x 3

4x

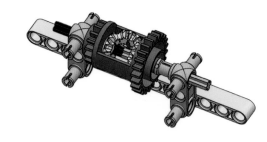

3

2x

7

2x

13

1x **2x**

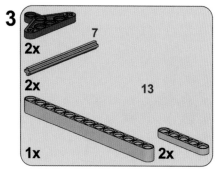

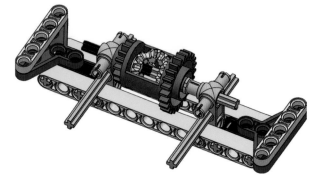

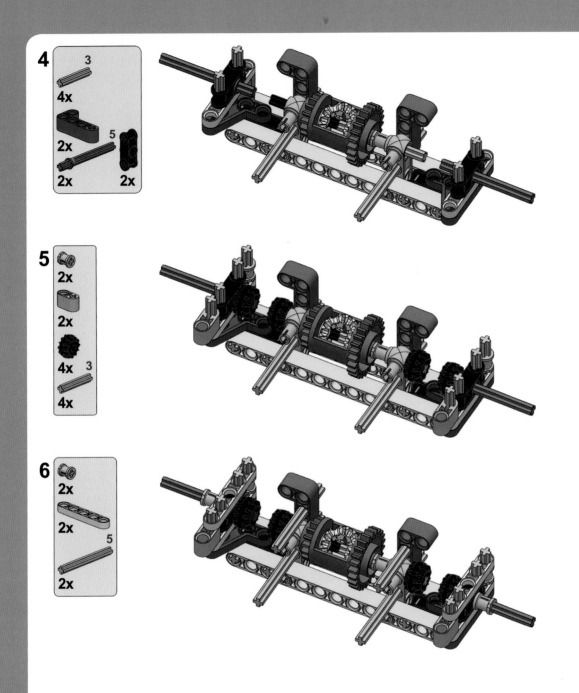

4

3
4x

2x

5

2x

2x

5

2x

2x

4x
3

4x

6

2x

2x

5

2x

7

2x
2x
2x
5
2x   2x

8

4x
4x
2x
4x

9

7
1x   11
2x

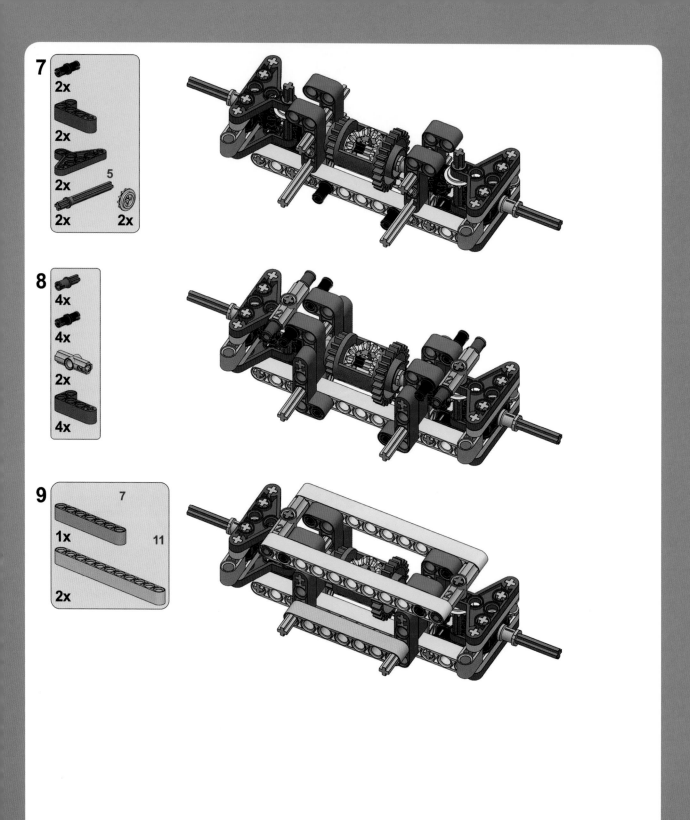

10

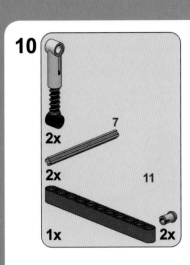

2x

2x 7

11

1x 2x

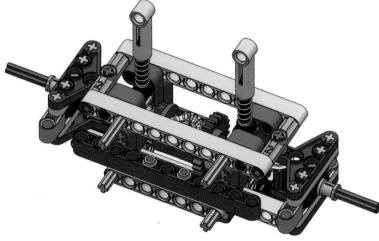

11

2x

4x

1x

1x 5 1x

1x 2x

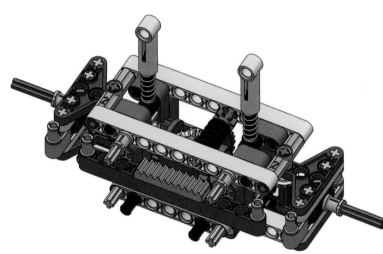

12

1x

1x 3

2x

2x 10

1x 1x 1x

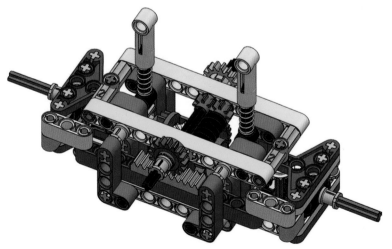

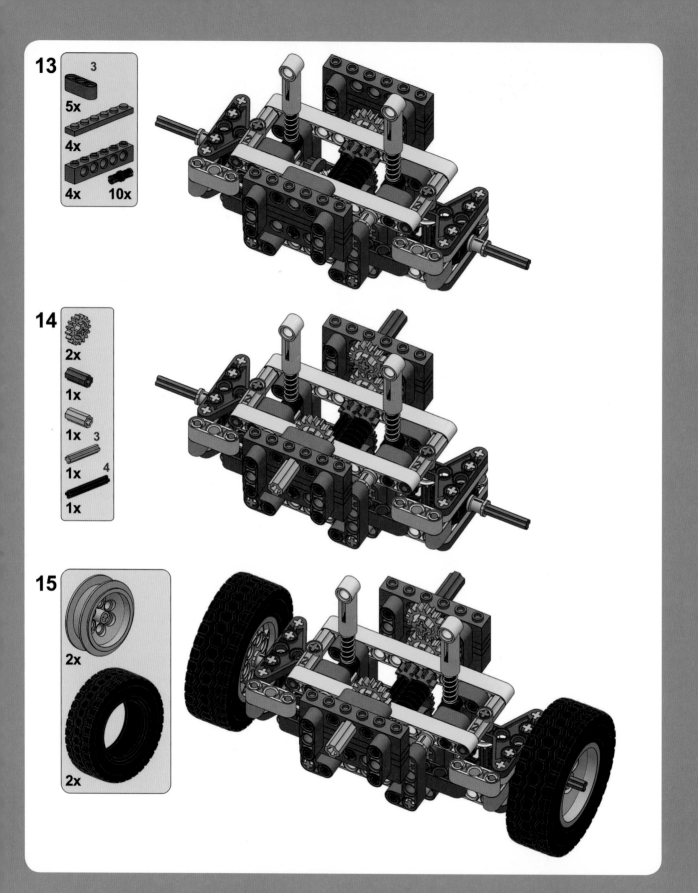

tracked vehicles and suspensions

Tracked vehicles are superior to wheeled vehicles for covering rough terrain. In a manner of speaking, tracks allow tanks and construction vehicles to "carry their own road" wherever they go. To create tracked LEGO vehicles, we have two options: rubber tracks and hard plastic tracks, each with a different set of advantages.

rubber tracks

LEGO's rubber tracks are made of a single, solid loop of rubber. LEGO produced seven rubber track variants, three of which are obsolete and difficult to find. The remaining four are quite similar to each other, and one variant dominates in terms of popularity (see Figure 18-1).

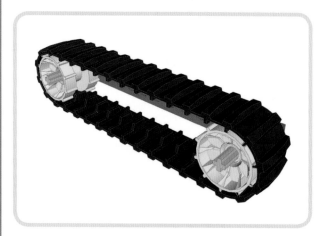

Figure 18-1: A large Technic tread and two Technic tread hubs

This track has 34 segments and is a little less than 3 studs wide. With its deep tread, the rubber provides excellent traction. The loop must be driven with a special type of sprocket wheel called a *tread hub*; the track requires two hubs 13 studs apart to be fully stretched, as shown in Figure 18-1. Tread hubs have a diameter of 3 studs, and their width is just a little bit less. They come in a variety of colors, and they use pin holes. In order to make your sprocket gears rotate with an axle, you must lock them with 16-tooth gears, as shown in Figure 18-2. You'll need two 16-tooth gears per hub—one on each side—or, to save space, you can use a single gear on one side and a bush on the other.

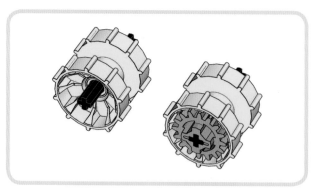

Figure 18-2: Two tread hubs: one empty (left) and one with a 16-tooth gear inserted (right). Since the hub is less than 3 studs wide, the gear sticks out slightly.

Advantages of rubber tracks:

* They are a single, unbreakable loop.
* They provide superb traction.
* They create minimal noise when driving.

Disadvantages of rubber tracks:

* Their length is limited and fixed.
* Their sprocket wheels are available in only one size.
* Rubber becomes less and less elastic over time.

hard plastic tracks

Hard plastic tracks (also known as *solid* tracks) are individual plastic links connected with one another. Their length can be easily adjusted, and they come in two versions: an older (and smaller) one and a newer (and bigger) one, both shown in Figure 18-3. Figure 18-4 shows a vehicle using the new plastic track type.

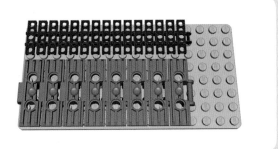

Figure 18-3: The older 15-link-long track and the newer 8-link-long track are both 13 studs long.

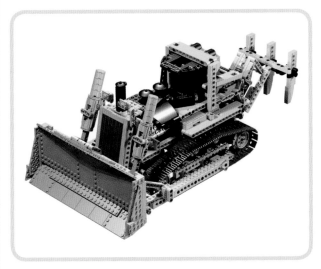

Figure 18-4: The newer type of solid track was introduced in the famous 8275 set.

Neither type of hard plastic track measures a whole number of studs in width. Instead, the tracks are slightly narrower, which prevents them from abrading the structure around them as they rotate. The older tread type is slightly less than 3 studs wide, and the newer one is slightly less than 5 studs wide. The length of tracks is a little difficult to compare, as no link is an equal number of studs long either; however, a 15-link-long section of older track is equal to an 8-link-long section of new track, and those lengths are both equal to 13 studs, as shown in Figure 18-3. A single link of the newer type is thus equal to 1.875 links of the older type. A link of the new track is 1.625 studs long, while the older link is 0.867 studs long.

The older tracks come primarily in black, and they are similar in construction to LEGO chains, as you can see from their links in Figure 18-5. This means that any gear that works well with a chain can be our sprocket wheel for a tracked vehicle. As shown in Figure 18-6, a single link occupies two teeth on a gear.

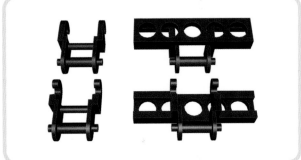

Figure 18-5: Regular LEGO chain links (left) and older-type track links (right). The older track links are just modified chain links.

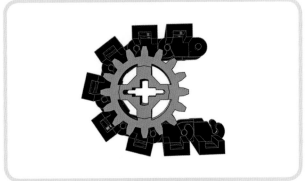

Figure 18-6: A section of older track wrapped around a 16-tooth gear

Five types of gears can be used as sprocket wheels for the older tracks (see Figure 7-5 on page 72). Other gears just aren't suitable because of the shape of their teeth or simply because of their small diameter.

The small openings in the older tracks can hold a plate, a tile (as shown in Figure 18-7), or even a brick that is at least 4 studs long. While bricks aren't typically used because they fall off too easily, plates and tiles can make the tracks wider and improve their appearance.

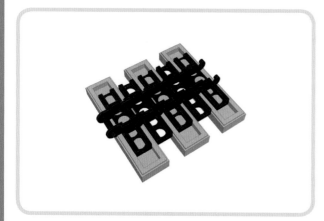

Figure 18-7: A section of older track with tiles added. Note that only every other link can have a piece inserted into it.

Figure 18-8 shows my model of a Liebherr R944C excavator, which combined two types of gears to keep the tracks in place. I used 24-tooth gears at the ends of the tracks and 16-tooth gears to give shape to the tracks' upper sections.

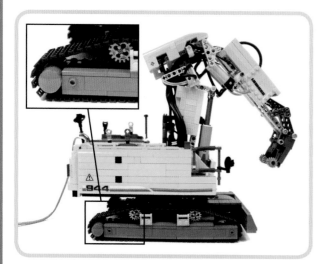

Figure 18-8: A model of a Liebherr R944C, using two types of gears

The newer tracks are made of massive links that come primarily in dark grey; black and metallic silver versions are available as well. Each link comes with two pin holes, which allow for modification (see Figure 18-9).

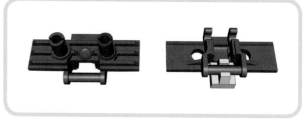

Figure 18-9: Adding a pin to a track allows us to attach bricks or tiles

The new solid tracks can't be driven by regular Technic gears; instead, they use special sprocket wheels. There are two options: a big wheel and a small one (both shown in Figure 18-10). The big sprocket wheel can have up to 10 links wrapped around it, is almost 2 studs thick, and comes primarily in yellow, with orange and black available, too. The small one can have up to 6 links wrapped around it, is 1 stud thick, and comes in black and pearl grey.

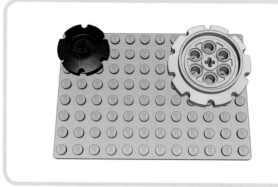

Figure 18-10: Sprocket wheels for the newer track type

The pin holes on top of the newer links can be used to attach Technic bricks (as shown in Figure 18-11) or beams (as shown in Figure 18-12) to them, making them wider and suitable for driving in snow. Both bricks and beams can be attached to every link using two half or three-quarter pins, with the latter ones being less likely to fall off. It is also possible to weave a regular rubber band into the pin holes, improving the traction of the tracks and reducing the noise they create while driving.

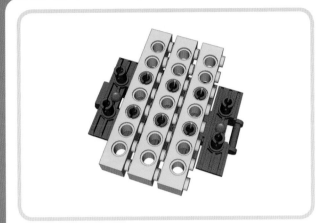

Figure 18-11: Section of the newer track with bricks attached

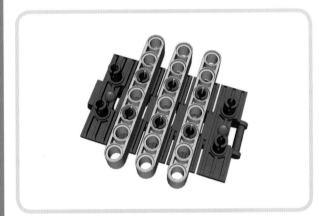

Figure 18-12: Section of the newer track with beams attached

The two solid track types differ in how much they can be stretched; the older type is more elastic but, at the same time, more fragile and prone to break. The newer type is much sturdier but very rigid, and as a result, it's difficult to obtain optimum tension with it. If your tread is too loose or too tight, it will affect how a vehicle drives. The rule of thumb is to tighten the track as much as possible and then give it at least half of a link of play.

Advantages of solid tracks:

* Their length is adjustable.
* They look more realistic than rubber tracks.
* They can be driven by a wider selection of sprocket wheels.

Disadvantages of solid tracks:

* They have poor traction.
* They're prone to coming apart (especially the older type).
* It's difficult to obtain optimum tension (especially with the newer type).
* They're noisy while driving (especially the newer type).

tracked wheel systems

Tracks greatly improve a vehicle's off-road performance, especially on mud, snow, or other unreliable surfaces. But how well a vehicle moves on its tracks depends largely on its wheels.

Strange as it may seem, wheels are no less important for tracked vehicles than they are for a car or truck. Firstly, they provide power to the tracks and keep them from falling off. Secondly, they can be suspended in order to improve the *flotation* of the vehicle, which describes how well the suspension handles obstacles. A suspension that adapts well to rough terrain provides good flotation, reducing the shock transferred to the vehicle as it moves.

NOTE The first tanks ever built provide a good example of just how important suspension is. Because these tanks lacked any kind of suspension, the crewmen of such tanks would often be knocked unconscious by shocks while traversing trenches.

Let's discuss the basic wheel systems. The simplest wheel system consists of two *sprocket wheels* per track, as shown in Figure 18-13. Usually about half of such a wheel comes in contact with the track, more than any other wheel in the system—which is why it's important that these wheels drive the tracks. Usually only one sprocket wheel is actually

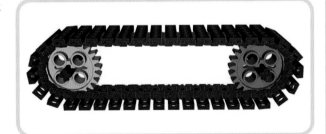

Figure 18-13: A track with two sprocket wheels: an idle one (grey) and a driven one (red)

driven, and it's often the rear one because it's convenient to have propulsion systems at the back of the vehicle. But it doesn't really matter which sprocket wheel is driven, as the track works like a chain and transfers the drive to the other wheel.

The second function of the sprocket wheels is to maintain the track's tension, which is particularly important as the vehicle moves over obstacles. Sprocket wheels can be suspended on an elastic element to maintain this tension. A loss of tension can cause the track to slip or even separate.

But with the basic two-wheel-per-track system, it would be difficult to add any suspension. We could suspend the nondriven sprocket relatively easily, but suspending the driven one would be much more challenging. This is why *road wheels* were invented.

A more advanced wheel system includes road wheels at the bottom of the vehicle (shown in blue in Figure 18-14). Road wheels can be used in any number, they are not driven, and they can be easily suspended. They are usually located closer to the ground than sprocket wheels, and they support the weight of the vehicle. Some vehicles come with sprocket and road wheels on the same level, making the road wheels difficult to suspend but increasing the total area of contact between the track and the terrain. Real tracked vehicles have been built both with many small road wheels (as shown in Figure 18-15) or with a few big ones. As a kind of compromise between the two extremes, modern tanks usually have six or seven road wheels per track that are just over half as big as the sprocket wheels.

The most complex wheel systems also include *return rollers* (shown in yellow in Figure 18-16). They are neither driven nor suspended, and their only function is to support the upper portion of the track. Return rollers can have minimal contact with the track and, in fact, don't even have to rotate—it's enough if the track can slide over them. As tracks are always more or less loose, vehicles with long tracks usually need at least two return rollers. It is also possible to use road wheels large enough to function as return rollers, as shown in Figure 18-17.

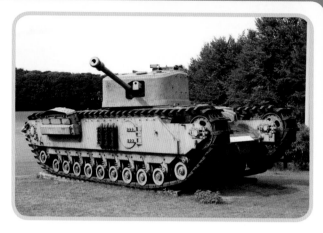

Figure 18-15: With 11 road wheels per track, the British Churchill tank is an extreme example of a design that includes many small road wheels.

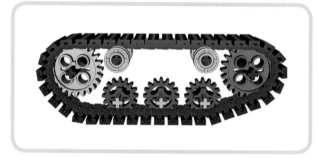

Figure 18-16: A track with two sprocket wheels, three road wheels, and two return rollers

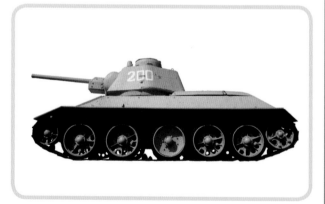

Figure 18-17: Soviet tanks from the World War II era—such as this T34—used road wheels so big that they had contact with both the lower and upper portion of the track, thus eliminating the need for return rollers.

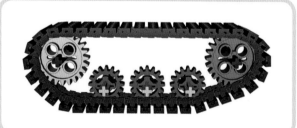

Figure 18-14: A track with two sprocket wheels and three road wheels

A good example of a modern wheel system is the one used on the classic Sherman tank. It includes two large sprocket wheels, six smaller road wheels, and two return rollers per track (see Figure 18-18). Note that the forward sprocket is driven and the rear one is idle.

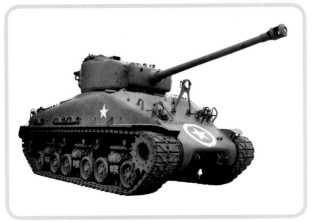

Figure 18-18: The classic Sherman tank used a wheel system that included return rollers.

Now that you know the types of wheels used in tracked vehicles, we can move on to the suspension systems.

suspension systems

The primary function of a suspension system is to increase stability and reduce the shock transferred to the vehicle. Its secondary function is to prevent the tracks from falling off. A suspension system achieves this function by keeping road wheels in close contact with the tracks regardless of the shape of the ground. The vast majority of tracked vehicles have suspension only on the road wheels, largely for simplicity's sake. All the suspension systems described here are designed for road wheels but can be used with sprocket wheels as well.

NOTE The type of LEGO track you use doesn't affect the suspension; the track determines only the type of sprocket wheels you can use. The examples of suspensions in this chapter show variants for both LEGO track types to demonstrate how a given suspension works with various wheels.

bogies

A bogie is the simplest type of tracked suspension. It is simply a beam that has one road wheel on either end; this beam freely rotates around a central axle connected to the vehicle, as shown in Figure 18-19. As the road wheels on the bogie go up and down, only half of their travel is transferred to the bogie's central axle—for example, when a wheel moves upward by 2 studs, the axle will only move upward by 1, as shown in Figure 18-20. So bogies provide reasonably good flotation, but they don't reduce shock.

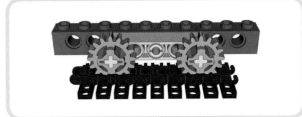

Figure 18-19: The yellow beam rotates around the central pin, creating a bogie with two road wheels.

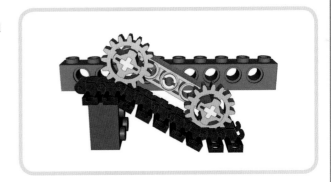

Figure 18-20: In this example, one road wheel is raised by 2 studs, but the bogie's central axle (and thus the vehicle) is raised only by 1 stud.

NOTE The basic principle of bogies is that only 50 percent of the road wheels' vertical travel is transferred to the vehicle. But note that this principle is true only if the obstacle is shorter than the length of the entire bogie—that is, shorter than the span of two road wheels.

Figure 18-21 shows an example of a bogie for the newer LEGO track type. The newer tracks are larger and usually used with larger and heavier vehicles, which is why this bogie variant is reinforced on the front and back sides (and is therefore sturdier).

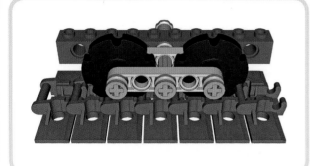

Figure 18-21: A reinforced bogie for the new LEGO track type

trailing arms suspension with shock absorbers

Trailing arms are used in more advanced suspension systems, where each road wheel is located on the end of an arm and supported against the weight of the vehicle by a shock absorber (or another elastic element), as shown in Figure 18-22. As most tracked vehicles usually have relatively low profiles, 6.5L shock absorbers are better suited to most tracked vehicles than their longer variants.

Trailing arm suspensions are sensitive to the direction of the tracks' rotation, and tracks always rotate more freely in one direction than the reverse. The arms are located in front of the road wheel.

There are a number of possible variants for this suspension system, depending on how much load each road wheel has to handle, how much space you can use, and what suspension travel and hardness you want to achieve. Figures 18-22 through 18-24 show some common variations.

NOTE The first and last road wheels in a track usually handle more load than the middle ones. It is therefore a good idea to use harder shock absorbers for these wheels than for the middle wheels. The weight distribution of the vehicle (front-heavy, center-heavy, or rear-heavy) should also be considered.

The setup in Figure 18-23 works only with 24-tooth gears and isn't that soft but takes little vertical space, which is helpful when you need the road wheels to be very close to each other.

Figure 18-24 shows another compact setup that works with all types of wheels, including those for the newer track system. It allows a lower overall profile, but it needs the road wheels to be spaced farther apart.

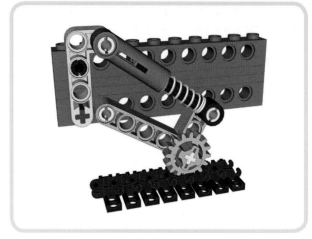

Figure 18-22: A simple trailing arm with a shock absorber

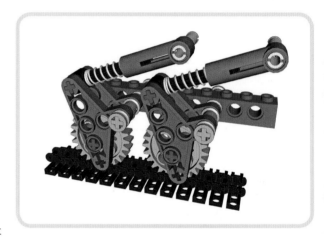

Figure 18-23: A more complex trailing arm system that works with 24-tooth gears

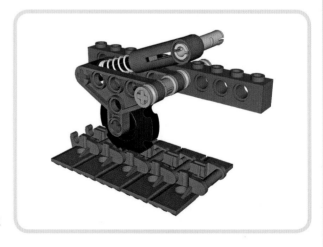

Figure 18-24: Another compact trailing arm setup

trailing arm suspensions with torsion bars

Shock absorbers are efficient but large; their length can force us to build our vehicles taller than we would otherwise need to. Thankfully, there's a very attractive alternative when building a trailing arm suspension: torsion bars.

A torsion bar is a long, slightly elastic element, positioned perpendicular to a vehicle's hull. One end of the bar is locked to the chassis so that it can't rotate. The other end is attached to a trailing arm with a road wheel on the other end, and it rotates together with the arm. So as the road wheel goes up, the arm twists the bar around its axis, as shown in Figure 18-25. And the great news is that all LEGO axles (except for the very short ones) are elastic enough to function as torsion bars.

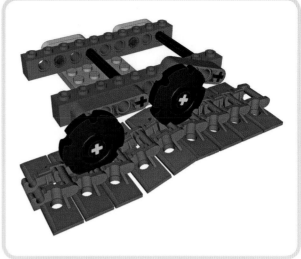

Figure 18-26: A more complex torsion-bar suspension

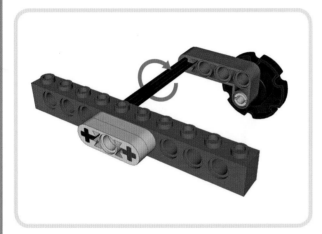

Figure 18-25: The basic scheme of a torsion bar

In the figure, the black 8L axle is functioning as a torsion bar; one end is locked into the chassis (represented by the red brick), and the other end is locked into the trailing arm (represented by the dark grey beam). Now, if the road wheel at the end of the arm meets an obstacle that makes it go up, the trailing arm will oscillate around the axle, making it twist a little. Once the obstacle is passed, the axle will untwist, returning the arm and the wheel to the initial position. Of course, in a real vehicle, the torsion bar needs to be supported.

Figure 18-26 shows a more complex example of the torsion-bar suspension in action, including such a support. Note that the 8L axles go through two bricks, but they are locked only with the one closer to the middle of the hull. They can freely rotate inside the outer brick, which is used only to support them.

The torsion-bar suspension requires only common pieces, and its hardness can be adjusted by using shorter or longer axles or by simply changing the point at which the axles are locked to the chassis (the closer to the trailing arm, the harder the suspension). Twisting LEGO axles may seem risky, but they are surprisingly resistant to damage. I have used 8L axles as torsion bars in a model with a total weight of around 3.5 kg, where each torsion bar handled an average load of almost 0.25 kg and a much greater load when negotiating obstacles. Even after the model went through a lot of tests on rough terrain, the axles were in pristine condition.

Unlike shock absorbers, this kind of suspension also has the advantage of using minimal space inside the tracks. Its disadvantages are that it takes 1 stud of vertical space at the bottom of the hull (as shown in Figure 18-27) and that this space is so densely filled with axles that it's usually impossible to use it for anything else. A torsion-bar suspension also doesn't work well for lightweight models. If the average load per road wheel is less than 100 g, the effect of this suspension is barely noticeable.

In the example in Figure 18-27, only 1 stud of vertical space inside the hull is taken by the suspension system, but it is taken quite completely. Note that the bars on each side are separate axles—in this case, 7 studs long each. It is possible to use a single axle that traverses the whole hull as long as it's locked securely in the middle so that twisting one of its ends doesn't affect the other end.

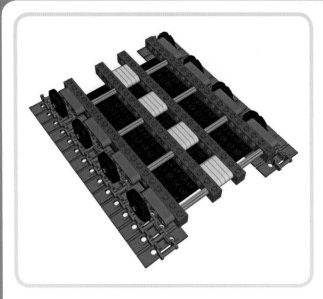

Figure 18-27: A hull floor of a vehicle with torsion-bar suspension

experimenting with road wheels

Early tracked vehicles were built with road wheels of solid metal. Later, engineers observed that vibrations between the tracks and the vehicles could be reduced by putting rubber rims over the road wheels. Today, rubber rims are considered standard for real-life tracked vehicles. Note that these rims are different from conventional tires: They are made of solid rubber, they're thin, and they have no tread.

There is an easy way to re-create a road wheel with a rubber rim using LEGO pieces so that it looks accurate: You can use a wedge belt wheel with a special solid tire (#70162), as shown in Figure 18-28.

We can use a pair of wedge belt wheels to create a single road wheel that braces the track from two sides, as shown in Figure 18-29. Wedge belt wheels look more accurate while modeling some tracked vehicles, and they also allow you to build compact suspensions, as shown in Figure 18-30. (LEGO models aren't heavy enough to effectively compress solid rubber, so the shock absorption effect achieved with these tires alone is minuscule.)

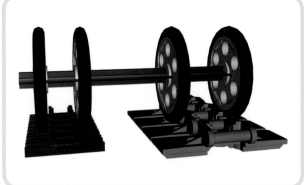

Figure 18-29: A pair of wedge belt wheels 1 stud apart can firmly secure the older type of track. If they are 2 studs apart, they can do the same with the newer type of track.

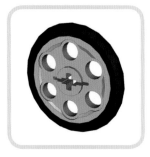

Figure 18-28: A belt wheel with a tire. The tire is solid rubber and very easy to put on and take off.

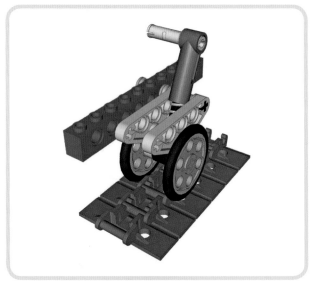

Figure 18-30: This suspension, which uses a trailing arm and a shock absorber, takes advantage of double road wheels to position the absorber as low as possible. With a central road wheel, the shock absorber would have to be moved to the outer side or be located much higher.

My model of a Soviet T-72M tank, shown in Figure 18-31, employed yet another approach: The wedge belt wheels with tires were simply inserted into the central portion of the track, and they held it in place surprisingly well. At the same time, they were all suspended on torsion bars.

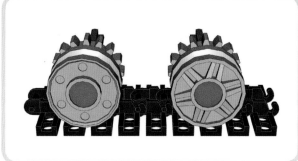

Figure 18-33: Concealing 16-tooth gears behind 18×8 mm wheels (#56902). As shown here, the two sides of these wheels look different and can be used together to create an interesting aesthetic effect.

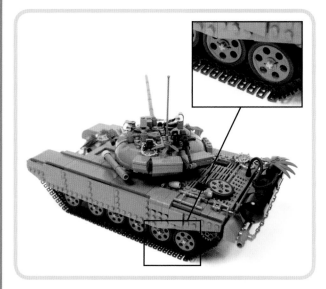

Figure 18-31: A model tank using wedge belt wheels with tires, suspended on torsion bars

Another interesting thing about wedge belt wheels is that without the tire, they have a diameter that perfectly matches that of certain sprocket wheels. They can be used to conceal colorful sprocket wheels for aesthetic effect, as shown in Figures 18-32 through 18-34.

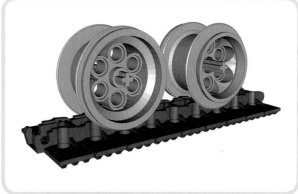

Figure 18-34: The newer type of track works fairly well with 49.6×28 VR wheels (#6595). These wheels also have two sides that look different, and their size and appearance make them very suitable for large models.

If you're curious about how we can power tracked vehicles like tanks and bulldozers, skip to "Subtractors" on page 336, where you'll learn the methods of steering tracked vehicles and independently driving each track.

custom heavy-duty tracks

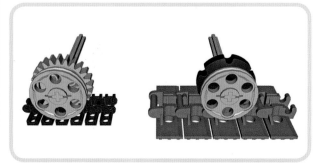

Figure 18-32: The diameter of a wedge belt wheel matches the diameter of a 24-tooth gear meshed with the central protrusion of the older track (left) or the diameter of a smaller sprocket wheel meshed with the central protrusion of the newer track (right). Thus, the wedge belt wheels can be used to conceal the real road wheels and improve aesthetics.

Ready-made LEGO tracks are great, but you might eventually discover that they're too narrow for your model or too fragile for outdoor use. That's when you should consider

custom-built, heavy-duty tracks, like the one in Figure 18-35. Although heavy and expensive to make, they're also extremely durable and impressive looking.

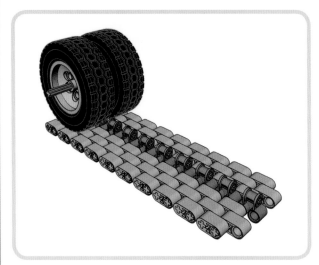

Figure 18-35: A custom, 7-stud-wide track with central guide teeth and two sprockets

Custom tracks are 1 stud thick and can be anywhere from 3 to 12 studs wide. The structure of the track is simple, consisting of transverse axles—whose length determine the width of the track—that are connected using 2L beams with one pin hole and one axle hole, all in the same orientation (in Figure 18-35, the axle hole is always on the left; the pin hole is always on the right).

The adjacent rows of beams overlap by 1 stud to keep the track together. This results in a structure that resembles a metal watch band, which is strong but flexible. Maintaining the orientation of all the beams in the track ensures that each beam is locked only to a single axle and can pivot around the second. This keeps the track flexible so each beam can rotate relative to the next one.

Special connectors that protrude by 1 stud are added in the middle of the track to act as guide teeth and prevent the wheels from coming off. It's easy to build the guide teeth closer to the side or even to add more than one row of teeth.

Custom tracks are unsuitable for tireless wheels for obvious reasons. A wheel with a simple road (not a balloon) tire will provide the traction necessary to move the track. And the bigger the wheel, the better, because the contact area with the track increases. I've tested these tracks and this propulsion method in multiple models—some particularly

fast and some particularly heavy (see Figure 18-36)—and the traction-based propulsion worked every time. If you experience any problems, you can experiment with tires of various sizes and treads: The 62.4×20 wheels, shown in Figure 18-35, are my favorites.

These custom tracks are durable and can handle asphalt, pavement, rock, or dirt without serious damage. They'll get a little scratched on the outer side, but the damage is usually minor. Figure 18-37 shows an example of my most worn track.

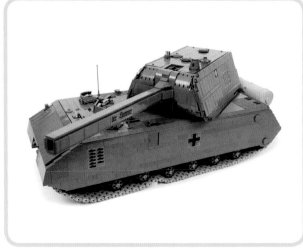

Figure 18-36: My massive model of the Maus tank moves on two custom tracks; each is 9 studs wide. They handle the enormous weight of the model (almost 6 kg) effortlessly.

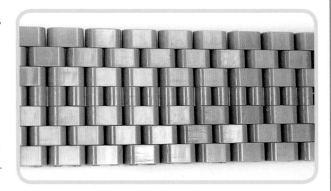

Figure 18-37: A section of the outer side of my most heavily worked track. It's been used for several days at high speeds, with heavy loads, and on all kinds of surfaces, even rocks. Some scratches are visible, but they're all superficial.

Consider the following when you're planning to use a custom track:

* The price and workload needed are considerable; a 7-stud-wide track can cost around $100 per meter depending on the color.
* The most common and cheapest beam colors are light grey, dark grey, and black. Consider the color of the axles as well because they'll show on the track's sides. Because tracks with central guide teeth are usually an odd stud width, the axles that fit will likely be light grey, forcing you to use light grey tracks.
* It's difficult and time-consuming to change the width of an already existing track, but shortening or extending a track is pretty straightforward.
* Because a track's width is equal to a full number of studs, it may rub against the hull or fenders of your vehicle if the tracks are partially covered. This can produce unwanted friction. In my Maus model, I used panels instead of full bricks, with the hollow sides facing the track to avoid contact; this created a tiny gap on each side of the track.
* The tracks maintain a good grip on horizontal surfaces, but they don't handle inclines well. A possible solution that works well on smooth, hard surfaces is to add rubber axle joints (see Figure 18-38) to the tracks, but these are expensive and weaker, and are more prone to wear than the plastic beams. Also, because they fit flush with the track, they won't work well on snow or dirt. Another solution that is particularly good for snow and dirt is to add connectors that face outward (see Figure 18-39) and can dig into the underlying surface. But this solution will not work well on hard, smooth surfaces, and it will make the track less flexible because it won't be able to bend inward.

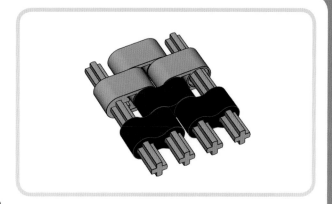

Figure 18-38: Rubber axle joiners (black) are the same size as 2L beams (light grey) and can be combined with them to add traction on smooth surfaces. It's even possible to build a completely rubber track, but it would be less durable and more expensive.

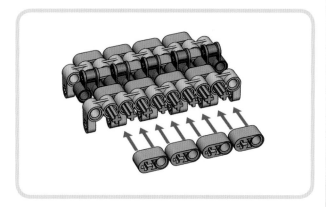

Figure 18-39: The addition of connectors that face outward (yellow) can increase traction in snow, but it will decrease flexibility.

a custom heavy-duty track

1
10x
7
20x

2
10x

3
10x

4
10x

5
10x

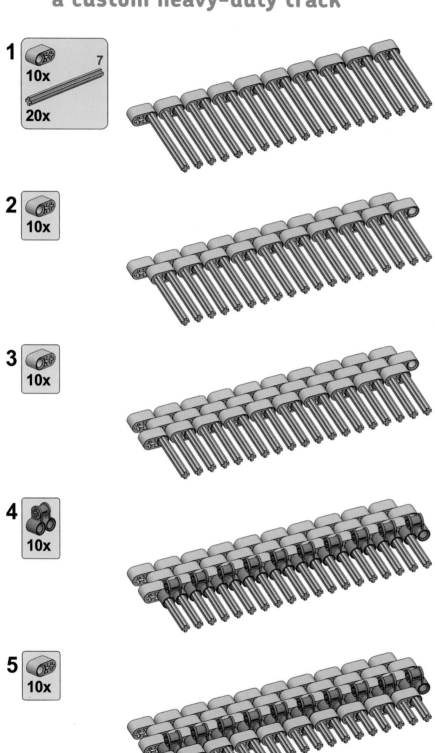

6

10x

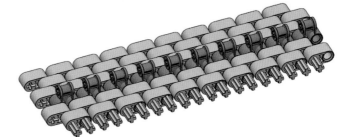

7

10x

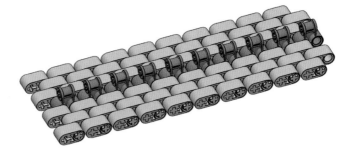

8

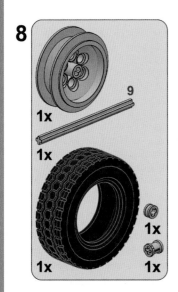

1x

9

1x

1x

1x

1x

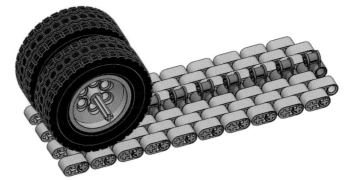

9

1x

1x

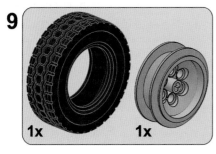

19

transmissions

Just like their real-life counterparts, LEGO transmissions are mechanisms capable of changing their internal gear ratio. They can increase gear reduction in the drivetrain when more torque is needed and decrease it when speed is of greater importance. It's the same principle at play when shifting gears in a car or in a bicycle, and this ability makes LEGO electric motors much more versatile.

A typical transmission has a number of fixed gear ratios, one of which can be selected at a time. Such a gear ratio is often simply called a *speed* or a *gear*: We can shift to lower gear (increasing the gear reduction) or to higher gear (decreasing the gear reduction). Therefore, a transmission must have at least 2 gears (as shown in Figure 19-1), while some of the most complex ones can have more than 10. Depending on their number of gear ratios, we call them 2-speed transmissions, 3-speed transmissions, and so on.

A transmission usually has a single input and a single output; the input is connected to the drive motor, and the output is connected to the final drive (wheels or tracks). A typical transmission also houses a number of gears, and each speed uses only a few of them. In other words, while some of the gears are used to transfer the drive and affect the current gear ratio, other gears just rotate unused. This

makes them work like idler gears: driven but idle. In transmissions, they are called *dead* gears, and the fewer their number, the more efficient the transmission, as they add weight and therefore friction.

Lastly, we'll consider a special type of transmission called a *distribution* or *split transmission*. This type of transmission has one input but several outputs. Such a transmission allows several mechanisms to be driven by a single motor without interfering with each other, as only one mechanism is driven at a time. We will discuss this particular type of transmission at the end of this chapter; for now, let's focus on the simpler ones.

types of transmissions

When it comes to transmissions, we can organize our models into several categories. Firstly and most importantly, a transmission can be *synchronized* or *nonsynchronized*. This refers to how easy it is to make gears mesh while shifting gears. Whenever a gear is shifted, one pair of gears has to *disengage*, and another pair has to *engage*. In synchronized transmissions, gears can engage at any speed and any position; in nonsynchronized transmissions, engagement is a matter of making the gears' teeth meet properly, which can succeed or fail, depending on the gears' positions and on the difference of their speeds. If gears fail to engage properly, they grind their teeth, and we have to try to shift the gear again. We can assume that gears will always engage in synchronized transmissions; in nonsynchronized ones, successful shifting is a matter of the shape of the gears' teeth, the speed of shifting, and a degree of luck. Some types of gears mesh more easily than others in nonsynchronized transmissions. For example, double-bevel gears, because they are beveled, engage more easily than typical spur gears. Naturally, it's

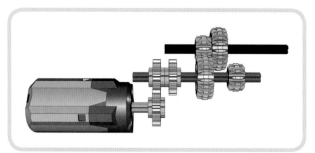

Figure 19-1: The inside of a simple 2-speed transmission. Consider what happens if we move the red axle 1 stud to the left and the green gears disengage and blue gears engage, changing the gear ratio between the motor and the output axle.

much easier to shift a nonsynchronized transmission while its input is stopped; in a synchronized transmission, it makes no difference.

Secondly, transmissions can be categorized as sequential or regular. *Sequential* (or *linear*) transmissions can only be shifted from one gear to the next closest one. That is, they can be shifted from 2nd to 3rd gear, but they can't be shifted from 2nd to 4th gear directly; instead, they have to shift from 2nd to 3rd and then to 4th. *Regular* (or *nonlinear*) transmissions, on the other hand, are not bound by this restriction, and they often use elaborate shift sticks, like the one in Figure 19-2. They can shift even from 10th to 1st gear directly, even though it may be dangerous to change the gear ratio so much so quickly. In real life, sequential transmissions are common in bicycles and motorbikes, while regular ones are found in cars.

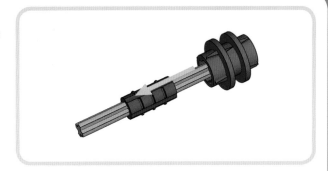

Figure 19-3: The transmission driving ring (red) must be placed over an axle joiner (blue). The axle joiner connects two axles that each go 1 stud deep inside it.

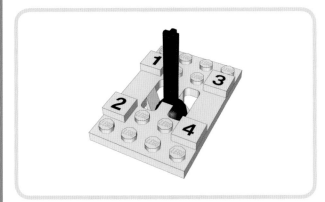

Figure 19-2: The unique shift stick from the 8880 set, the first LEGO set with a nonlinear and synchronized transmission. The transmission has 4 speeds, and the stick can move in an H pattern, allowing it to shift from one gear to any other.

how LEGO transmission driving rings work

Building a synchronized transmission with regular pieces is quite difficult, but LEGO has developed a special piece just for this task. It's called a transmission driving ring and is shown in Figure 19-3.

Once the transmission driving ring is placed on an axle joiner, the two pieces will rotate together; at the same time, the ring can slide forward or backward along the joiner. You can use a ribbed joiner if you want the ring to need some force to slide, thus preventing it from sliding accidentally, or a smooth joiner if you want it to slide easily (see Figure 19-4). Figure 19-5 shows what happens when you put two 16-tooth gears with clutches on the axle next to the ring. The gears rotate freely on the axle unless they're engaged by the driving ring that slides into them.

The easiest way to control the transmission driving ring is to use another special piece called the transmission changeover catch, shown in Figure 19-6. It was developed specifically to move the ring back and forth, engaging and disengaging it with the adjacent gears. The catch should be located above the ring on a separate transverse axle.

Figure 19-7 shows a very simple 2-speed transmission that uses a driving ring controlled with a catch. If you engage the ring with the gear to its left (as shown in the middle), the resulting gear ratio will be 3:1. If you engage the ring with the gear to its right (as shown on the bottom), the resulting gear ratio will be 1:1. The key to understanding how this mechanism works is to remember that 16-tooth gears with clutches rotate freely on axles unless they're engaged with the driving ring. Therefore, they can be used to transmit drive over the axle they sit on without driving that axle or any other gears on it.

The main advantage of the transmission driving ring is that it can engage at any moment, at any speed, and without needing to stop the input axle. The main disadvantage is that it works only with 16-tooth gears, so additional gears are needed just to achieve various gear ratios, resulting in a number of dead gears.

WARNING The transmission driving ring is also a torque-sensitive piece; it can disengage itself or even get physically damaged if a large torque is applied to it. This makes nonsynchronized transmissions a more common choice for high-torque applications.

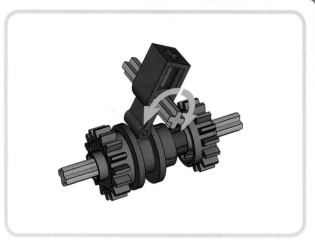

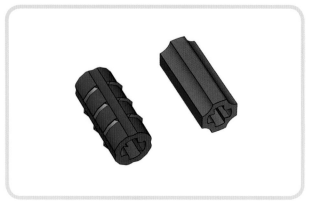

Figure 19-4: A ribbed 2L axle joiner (blue) and a smooth 2L axle joiner (green) both work with a driving ring; the smooth joiner makes operating the driving ring easier, which may be helpful in remotely shifted transmissions.

Figure 19-6: The transmission driving ring and the transmission changeover catch. Note that the catch rotates together with the axle it sits on, but it can slide along it freely. Some transmissions use this property to let a single catch control several adjacent rings. To see an animation of this process, visit http://bricksafe.com/files/blakbird/Technicopedia/animations/driving.gif.

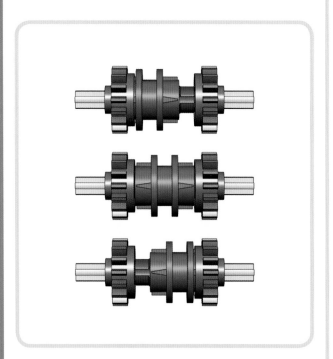

Figure 19-5: The three positions possible for a transmission driving ring are engaged with left gear (top), neutral (middle, no gears engaged), and engaged with right gear (bottom). Note that only engaged gears rotate in unison with the axle.

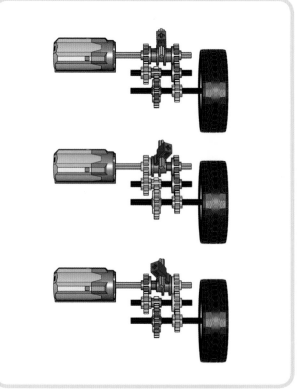

Figure 19-7: A simple 2-speed synchronized transmission set in neutral gear (top), low gear (middle), and high gear (bottom)

If you want to experiment with complex synchronized transmissions, it's difficult to go beyond four speeds without using an extension driving ring, shown in Figure 19-8. It works like an overlay for the regular transmission driving ring, allowing it to engage placed gears 1 stud away from it, as shown in Figure 19-9.

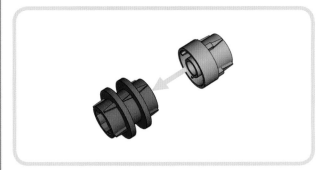

Figure 19-8: The extension driving ring (light grey) can be placed over the transmission driving ring (red) to extend it by 1 stud. Note that there is a large backlash between the driving ring and the gear it engages through extension.

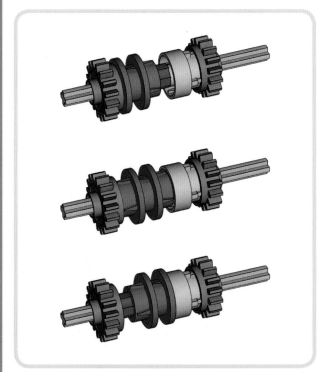

Figure 19-9: The driving ring engaging a gear directly (top), disengaging (middle), and engaging a gear via the extension (bottom). Note that the extension doesn't slide with the driving ring but acts like a part of the gear and rotates together with it.

Because it's 2 studs long, the driving ring is poorly suited for studless constructions, which favor pieces in odd lengths. That's the reason LEGO introduced a newer variant of the transmission driving ring in 2015, shown in Figure 19-10, which is 3 studs long instead of 2. Other than that, it's nearly identical to the earlier ring. With it came two new 3L axle joiners: a smooth one and a ribbed one (also in Figure 19-10) and a double-sided 16-tooth gear with a clutch (see Figure 19-11). Note that the 3L axle joiner has 1-stud-deep axle holes on either end and a solid 1-stud-long section in the middle.

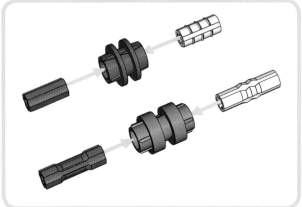

Figure 19-10: The old 2L (red) driving ring is meant to work with 2L axle joiners and the new 3L (dark grey) driving ring is meant to work with 3L axle joiners. You can swap the joiners, but the rings won't work well with the wrong joiners. Note that both 2L and 3L axle joiners come in two variants: smooth (red, left) and ribbed (white, right).

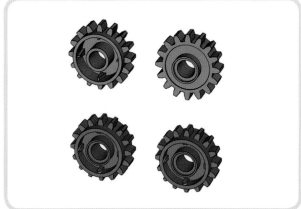

Figure 19-11: The old 16-tooth clutch gears (top) have one side with a clutch (top left) and one without a clutch (top right). The new 16-tooth clutch gears (bottom) have two identical sides with a clutch.

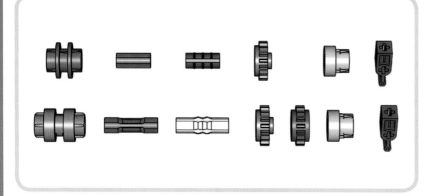

Figure 19-12: Two types of driving rings (2L on top, 3L on bottom) along with all the pieces they're compatible with. Notably, the 2L driving ring won't engage with double-sided 16-tooth gears with a clutch.

The new pieces are very similar to the old ones and were created to make things easier rather than to create new possibilities. The new 16-tooth gear with clutch no longer has a "right" and "wrong" side, for example. It will work no matter which side is facing the driving ring, whereas the older gear was a common source of building errors. Similarly, the 3L driving ring doesn't make new transmission designs possible; it's just much simpler to use with studless constructions (whereas the 2L driving ring is better suited for studded constructions). Note that the shape of the 3L ring's teeth is different from that of the 2L ring and appears to be optimized to lower the risk of disengaging under stress.

However, there's an interesting distinction between the rings: The 3L ring works with old 16-tooth gears, but the 2L ring can't work with the new 16-tooth gears. It simply won't engage with them. Figure 19-12 shows pieces compatible with each ring type.

transmission designs

This section lists a number of designs for complete transmissions. For each design, there is the type of transmission, a short description, and a scheme showing which gears are active at which speed. Building instructions for selected transmissions appear at the end of the chapter.

The following colors are used to mark pieces: green for the input axle, red for the output axle, and light blue for the active gears. The changeover catches are removed for clarity.

Keep in mind that it's also possible to combine two or more transmissions of any type by making one transmission's output another one's input. The number of speeds will

be effectively multiplied: For example, a 2-speed transmission combined with a 4-speed one will produce 8 speeds.

Some builders like to include a reverse gear in their transmissions. This is accurate in relation to real transmission systems but redundant when used with an electric motor that can be reversed at any moment. I have omitted such designs on purpose because I think they waste a potentially useful speed for no good reason.

Many builders consider a sequential synchronized transmission the best variant of all because it can be easily shifted *remotely*. While beyond the scope of this book, such a transmission relies on a control mechanism that is independent of the actual transmission and that can be used with many of the designs shown below. For ideas on creating remote-controlled transmissions, check out the website of Sheepo, one of the best LEGO transmission builders: *http://www.sheepo.es/*.

2-speed synchronized transmission

Type: sequential, synchronized

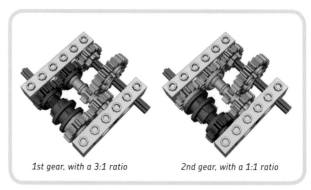

1st gear, with a 3:1 ratio   2nd gear, with a 1:1 ratio

This is the simplest synchronized transmission possible. (Building instructions are on page 311.)

2-speed linear heavy-duty transmission

Type: sequential, nonsynchronized

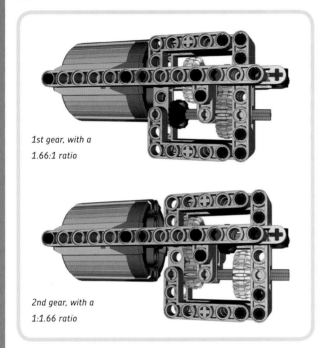

1st gear, with a 1.66:1 ratio

2nd gear, with a 1:1.66 ratio

A transmission designed specifically to handle high torque, shown here with the PF XL motor. Gears are shifted by sliding part of the transmission together with the motor attached to it. This makes the transmission simpler and reduces the number of gears.

Building instructions are on page 312.

2-speed RC motor transmission

Type: sequential, synchronized

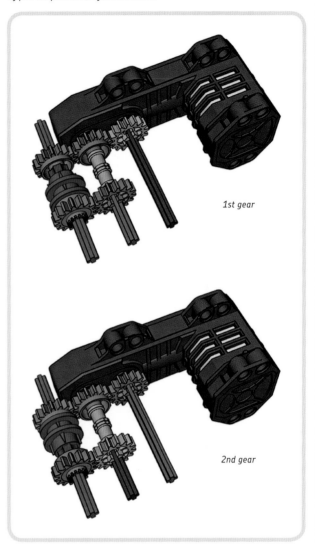

1st gear

2nd gear

This unusual transmission can be built with one or two RC motors. LEGO RC motors have two outputs instead of one, with the outer output having 26 percent more torque and less speed than the inner output. This transmission is connected to both of the motor's outputs at the same time, allowing us to select which one drives it. This allows us to make use of the difference in the outputs' properties, even though the gear ratio of the transmission itself is 1:1 at both speeds.

Building instructions are on page 314.

2-speed orbital transmission

Type: sequential, synchronized

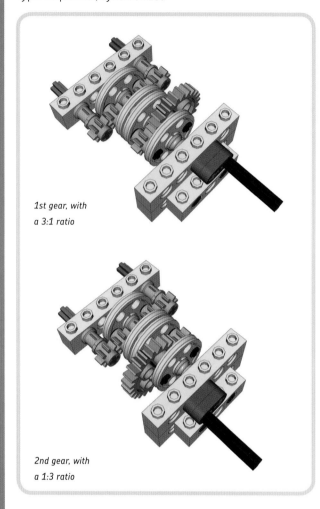

1st gear, with a 3:1 ratio

2nd gear, with a 1:3 ratio

2-speed ratchet transmission

Type: sequential, synchronized

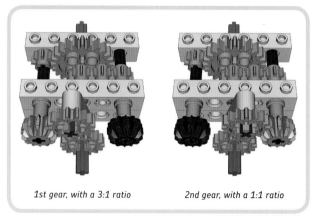

1st gear, with a 3:1 ratio   *2nd gear, with a 1:1 ratio*

This transmission uses a ratchet to shift gears. It shifts when the direction of the motor that drives it changes. It's small, simple, and synchronized without the use of the transmission driving ring. It can handle significant torque, but its output always rotates in the same direction, regardless of its input direction. So when it's used in a car, it makes the car drive only forward or only backward.

The transmission works like this: The direction of the input tilts the ratchet left or right. A 16-tooth gear on top of the transmission meshes with one of two 12-tooth double-bevel gears when the ratchet is tilted. The 16-tooth gear sits on an axle pin with friction, and the resistance created this way makes the ratchet press hard against the 12-tooth double-bevel gears. The greater torque is handled by the transmission. The greater the resistance on the ratchet, the harder it presses, meshing its top gear more effectively. There is, of course, a limit to how much torque can be handled.

Building instructions are on page 317.

This transmission is placed between two gears and shifted by rotating it 180 degrees. In this example, rotation is done with a dark grey crank that should be blocked once rotated. You can use a worm gear to rotate and then block the transmission. The transmission is synchronized without using the transmission driving ring and provides a vast difference in gear ratios. Additionally, it has no dead gears.

Note the half bushes used to create a gap between the transmission and the bricks on its sides. The gap is intended to prevent the 4L axles on the sides of the transmission from getting into the holes in the bricks and blocking the transmission.

Building instructions are on page 316.

3-speed linear transmission

Type: sequential, nonsynchronized

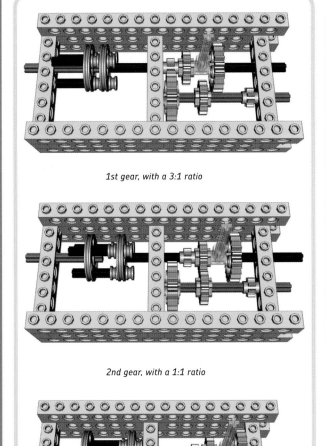

1st gear, with a 3:1 ratio

2nd gear, with a 1:1 ratio

3rd gear, with a 1:3 ratio

4-speed double-lever transmission

Type: regular, nonsynchronized

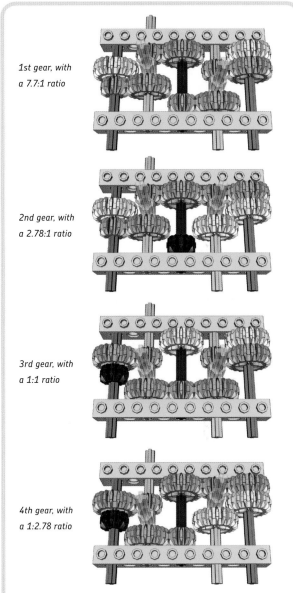

1st gear, with a 7.7:1 ratio

2nd gear, with a 2.78:1 ratio

3rd gear, with a 1:1 ratio

4th gear, with a 1:2.78 ratio

This transmission is simple but large. It uses an extendable driveshaft to make the input driven and movable at the same time. The control lever is shown semitransparent for clarity.

Building instructions are on page 318.

This regular transmission is strong and useful. It's very simple and relatively small, but it has two control levers, which is challenging when it comes to remote control. It consists of three shafts connecting input and output: one fixed and two that can slide by 1 stud. Due to its simplicity, no building instructions are provided, just the schemes of its speeds. The control levers are shown semitransparent for clarity.

4-speed synchronized transmission

Type: regular, synchronized

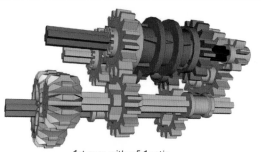

1st gear, with a 5:1 ratio

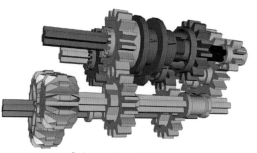

2nd gear, with a 3:1 ratio

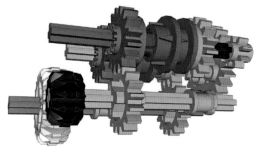

3rd gear, with a 1.66:1 ratio

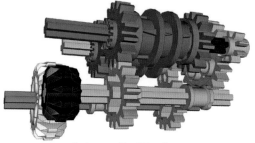

4th gear, with a 1:1 ratio

NOTE The structural parts and the control levers have been removed for clarity.

This synchronized transmission, shown in Figures 19-13 to 19-15, has two transmission driving rings, only one of which should be engaged at a time. Relatively small and providing a large difference in gear ratios, it can be controlled by a single lever moving in an H pattern or by two levers, one for each driving ring. It has a lot of dead and idler gears.

Building instructions are on page 320.

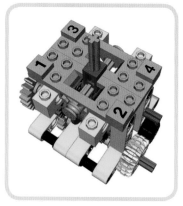

Figure 19-13: The 4-speed synchronized transmission with a single control lever moving in an H pattern. Note the special so-called "changeover plates" (light grey) used to control the shifting lever's movement and to support the axle it moves along.

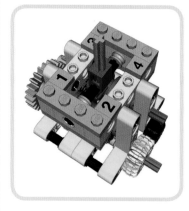

Figure 19-14: The 4-speed synchronized transmission with a single control lever moving in an H pattern. The lever is housed and supported by common LEGO pieces.

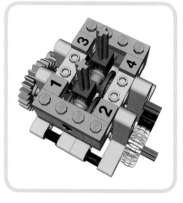

Figure 19-15: The 4-speed synchronized transmission with two control levers, each controlling a single transmission driving ring. Note that both rings can't be engaged at the same time: One has to be set in neutral position before the other one is engaged.

4-speed sequential RC synchronized transmission

Type: sequential, synchronized

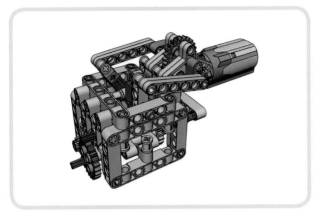

This variation of the regular 4-speed synchronized transmission includes a control mechanism that uses a single motor. This effectively turns it into a sequential transmission that can be shifted remotely and shifts in an endless loop from 1st to 4th gear and back again. For example, if you start at 1st and continue shifting up, you'll go through 2nd, 3rd, and 4th gears and then back to 1st again. If you start at 1st and continue shifting down, you'll go through 4th, 3rd, and 2nd gears and then back to 1st again. Because one of the two driving rings is always engaged, this transmission has no neutral gear.

This 4-speed synchronized transmission is heavily reinforced and can withstand significant torque due to the use of a worm gear, which keeps the driving rings engaged. In fact, it's the most complete and practical transmission you'll find in this book. Once I developed it, I pretty much stopped using any other designs.

But there's one crucial requirement for using this transmission: For the transmission to shift, one driving ring must disengage and the other must engage. If both rings become engaged accidentally, the transmission will lock up. To avoid such an incident, use your ear while shifting: The driving rings produce a distinctive "click" sound while shifting. Therefore, you need to hear two clicks to know that the transmission has shifted properly. This is why it is not recommended to use this transmission with smooth axle joiners inside the rings, as that will eliminate any sounds while shifting.

This design was optimized for the new, 3L driving rings, but it can be easily converted for use with the older versions by adding half-stud-thick beams on the sides. Note that the blue axle marks the input and the red axle marks the output.

Building instructions are on page 321.

5-speed linear transmission

Type: sequential, nonsynchronized

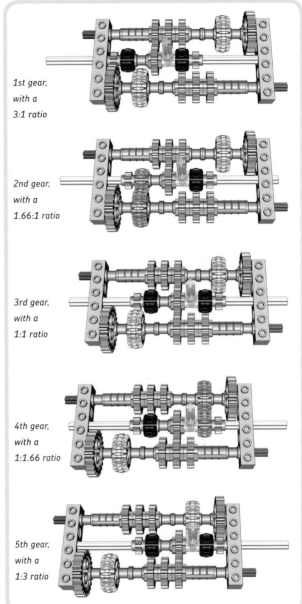

1st gear, with a 3:1 ratio

2nd gear, with a 1.66:1 ratio

3rd gear, with a 1:1 ratio

4th gear, with a 1:1.66 ratio

5th gear, with a 1:3 ratio

This transmission has one central shaft that can slide by 4 studs. Its disadvantage is that the central shaft makes use of a rare 16L axle, which can bend and disengage gears under high torque. Due to its simplicity, no building instructions are provided here, just the schemes of its speeds. The control lever is shown semitransparent for clarity.

10-speed synchronized transmission

Type: regular, synchronized

NOTE This is the bottom view with the structural parts and the control levers removed for clarity.

This transmission has a 4-speed design that's expanded further with the use of extension transmission driving rings.

If you study it closely, you'll notice that it can be expanded beyond 10 speeds by adding another pair of extensions and then four regular transmission driving rings. You can continue to expand it beyond this point by again adding two extension driving rings and so on. There's no limit to how many speeds can be added this way, except that the number of dead gears in the transmission increases quickly and a 14-speed version generates enough resistance to stall a PF XL motor. (Building instructions are on page 326.)

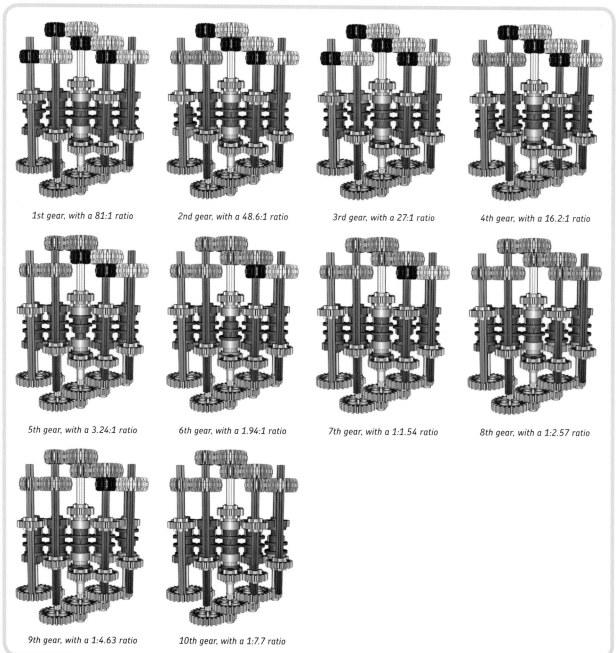

1st gear, with a 81:1 ratio   *2nd gear, with a 48.6:1 ratio*   *3rd gear, with a 27:1 ratio*   *4th gear, with a 16.2:1 ratio*

5th gear, with a 3.24:1 ratio   *6th gear, with a 1.94:1 ratio*   *7th gear, with a 1:1.54 ratio*   *8th gear, with a 1:2.57 ratio*

9th gear, with a 1:4.63 ratio   *10th gear, with a 1:7.7 ratio*

continuously variable transmission

Type: sequential, synchronized

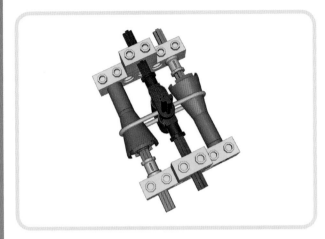

The continuously variable transmission (CVT) is a special type of a transmission. It doesn't have a definite number of speeds with fixed gear ratios. Instead, it has a minimum and maximum ratio, and it can be shifted continuously between them.

Real-life CVTs are very useful, but at the same time, they are very complex and often based on hydraulics or magnets. The easiest way to build a CVT with LEGO pieces is by using cones and a rubber band.

As you see, the transmission consists of input and output shafts with opposing cones connected by a rubber band. The band can be moved left or right so that it's wrapped around the broader portion of one cone and the narrower portion of the other. The circumference of the each cone is 22 mm at its narrowest and 50 mm at its broadest, which corresponds to a 1:2.27 ratio. This transmission can therefore be shifted smoothly between ratios 1:2.27 and 2.27:1.

The transmission can't handle much torque, and the tension of the rubber band has to be adjusted carefully in order for it to work properly. Too little tension will make the rubber band slip; too much tension can displace the cones. The original LEGO rubber bands work best as they are sticky and have a round profile; they come in many variants of different lengths that can work better or worse depending on the distance between the shafts in the transmission. Also note that the control lever module is mounted between two 1×2 bricks with axle holes. Axle holes not only keep the control lever straight. They also add some resistance so that it takes force to move the lever and thus the lever can't be moved by the rubber band's tension.

Building instructions are on page 331.

distribution transmissions

One type of transmission's primary function isn't to change gear ratios but to change which output is driven at the moment. This transmission, the distribution transmission, can be synchronized or not, depending on whether transmission driving rings are used. Distribution transmissions are very useful whenever there is a need for one motor to control one of many functions at a time, and they are quite popular in LEGO Technic sets.

In most cases, the distribution transmissions themselves are fairly simple; it's transferring the drive from them to several receiving mechanisms that can be tricky. Figures 19-16 to 19-20 present a few examples of such transmissions with various numbers of outputs, shown without housing for clarity. Note that the examples have a 1:1 ratio on all outputs for simplicity, but it's possible to create various ratios on various outputs.

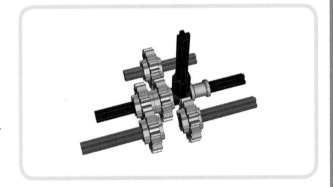

Figure 19-16: A nonsynchronized distribution transmission with two outputs

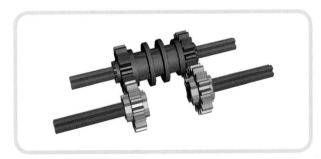

Figure 19-17: A synchronized distribution transmission with two outputs

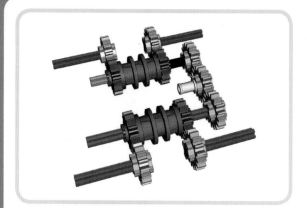

Figure 19-18: A synchronized distribution transmission with four outputs

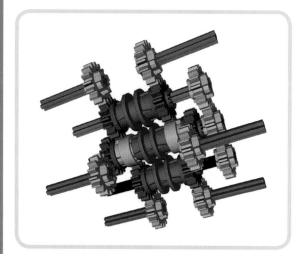

Figure 19-19: A synchronized distribution transmission with six outputs

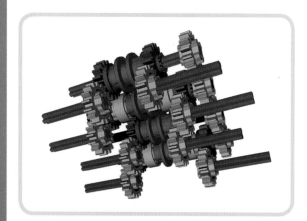

Figure 19-20: A synchronized distribution transmission with eight outputs

a 2-speed synchronized transmission

1

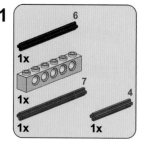

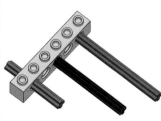

6
1x
7
1x
1x   1x   4

2

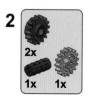

2x
1x   1x

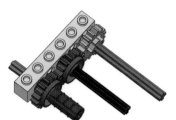

3

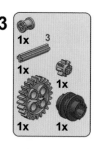

1x
3
1x
1x
1x   1x

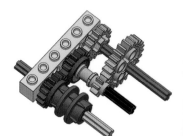

4

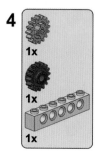

1x
1x
1x

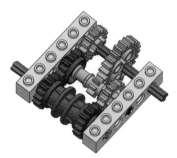

a 2-speed linear heavy-duty transmission

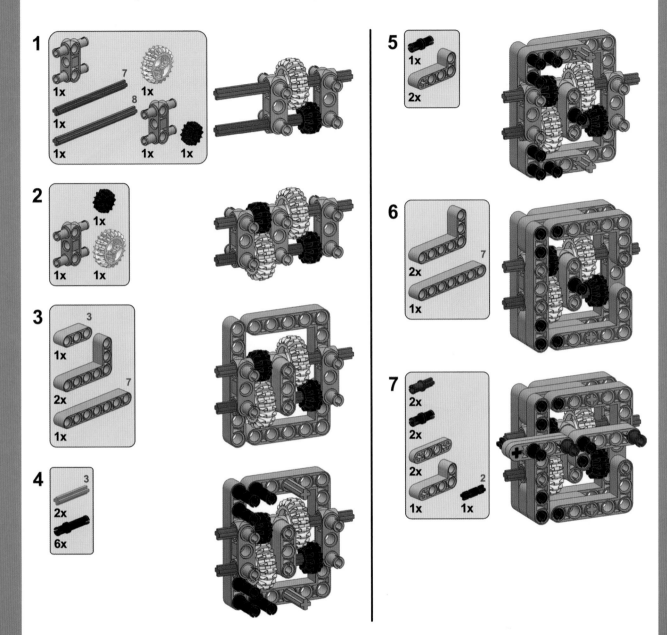

1
1x
7 1x
8
1x
1x 1x 1x

2
1x
1x 1x

3
3
1x
7
2x
1x

4
3
2x
6x

5
1x
2x

6
2x
7
1x

7
2x
2x
2x
2x
2
1x 1x

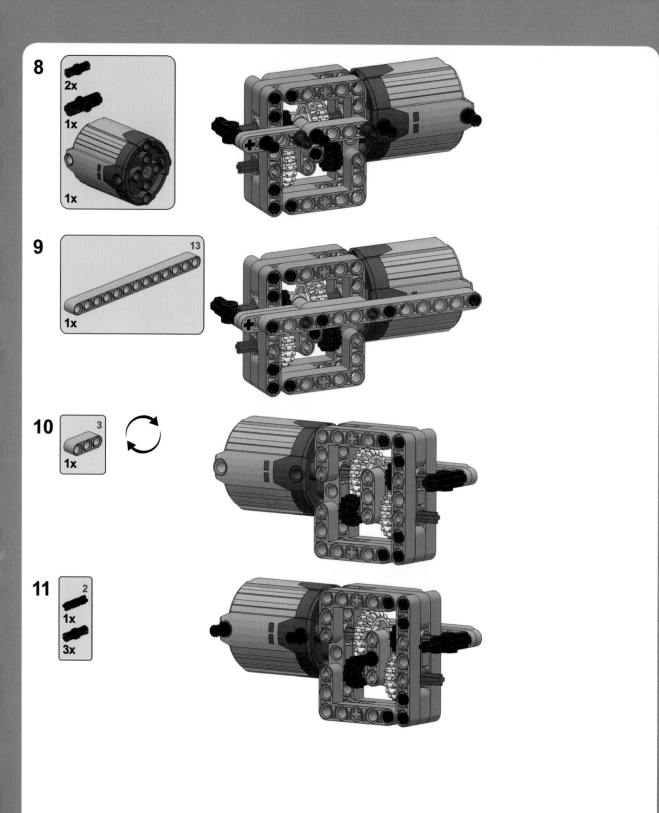

12

2x
2x
2x
1x

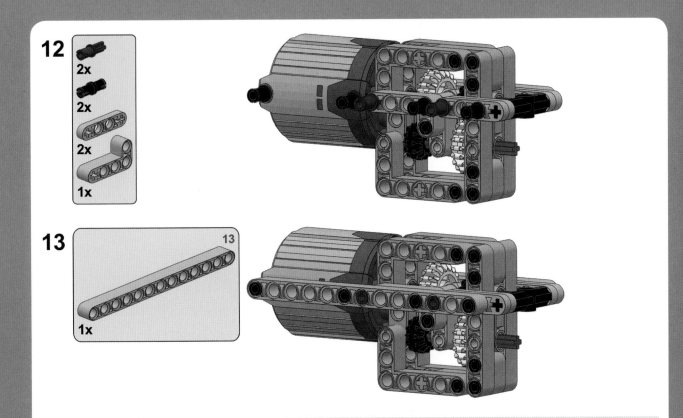

13

13

1x

a 2-speed RC motor transmission

1

5
6
10

1x
1x
2x

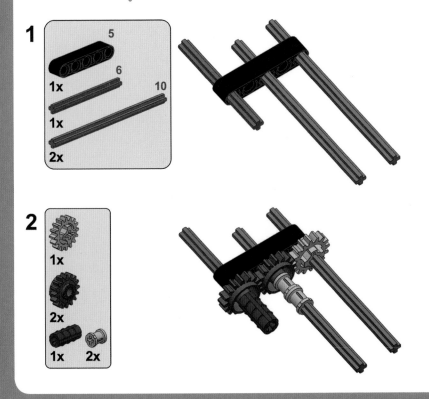

2

1x
2x
1x   2x

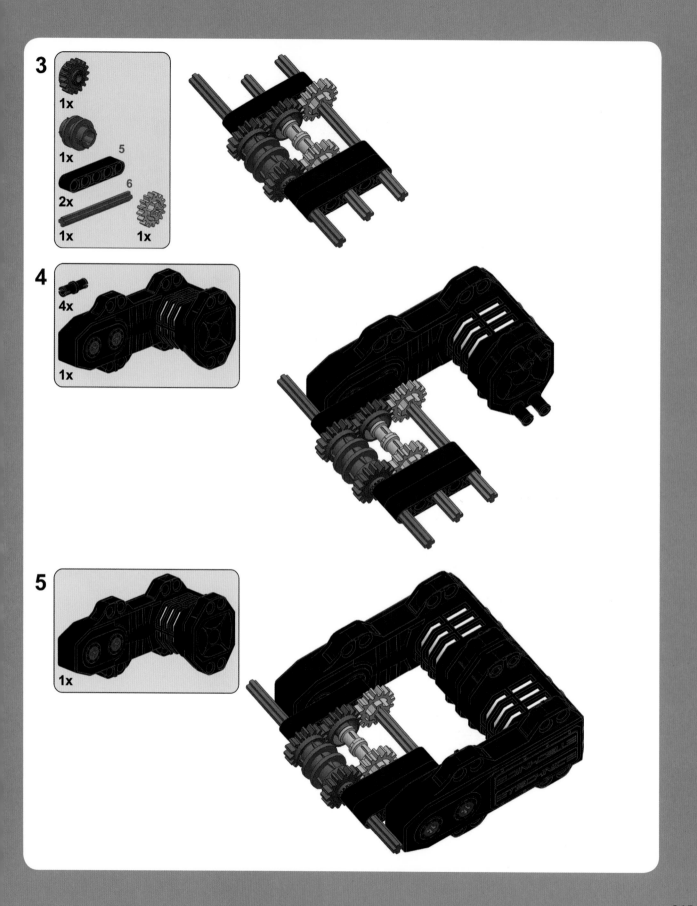

a 2-speed orbital transmission

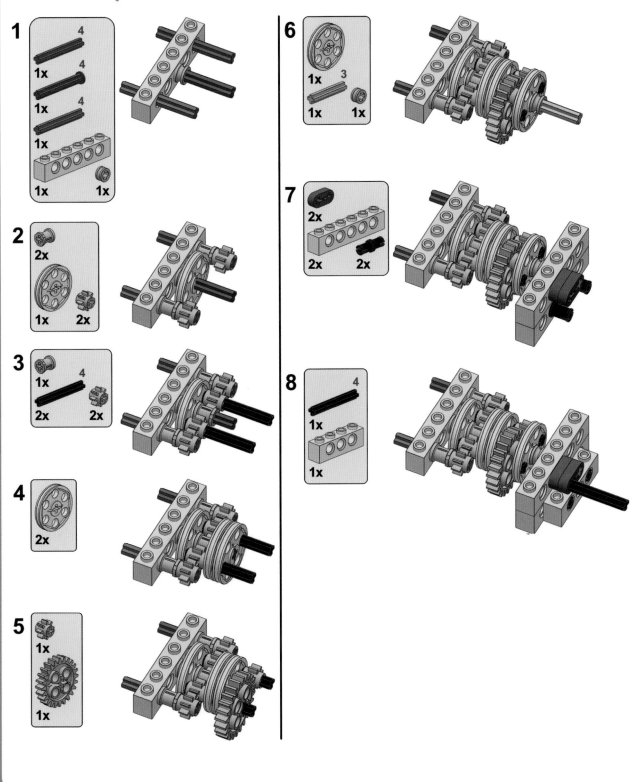

1
4
1x
4
1x
4
1x
1x   1x

2
2x
1x   2x

3
1x
4
2x   2x

4
2x

5
1x
1x

6
1x
3
1x   1x

7
2x
2x   2x

8
4
1x
1x

a 2-speed ratchet transmission

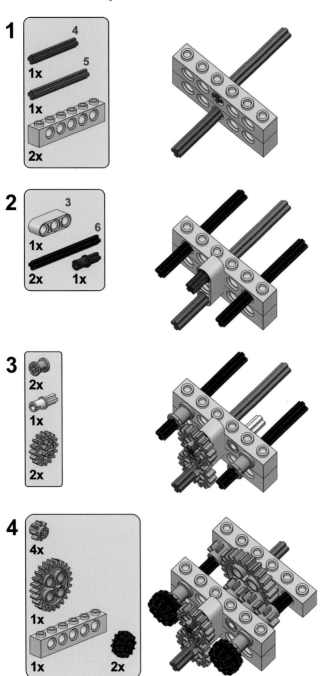

1

4
1x

5
1x

2x

2

3
1x

6
2x   1x

3

2x

1x

2x

4

4x

1x

1x   2x

a 3-speed linear transmission

1

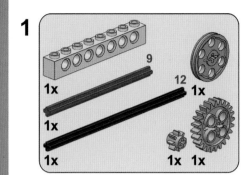

9
12

1x
1x
1x
1x
1x
1x

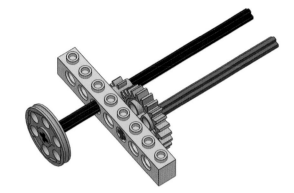

2

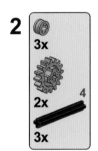

3x
2x
4
3x

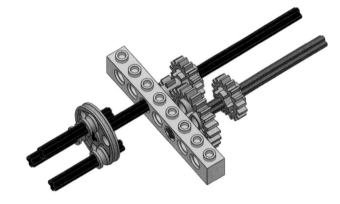

3

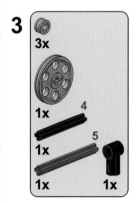

3x
1x
4
1x
5
1x
1x

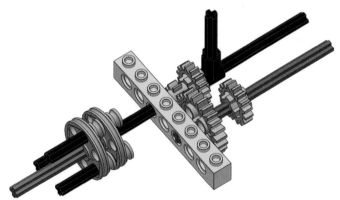

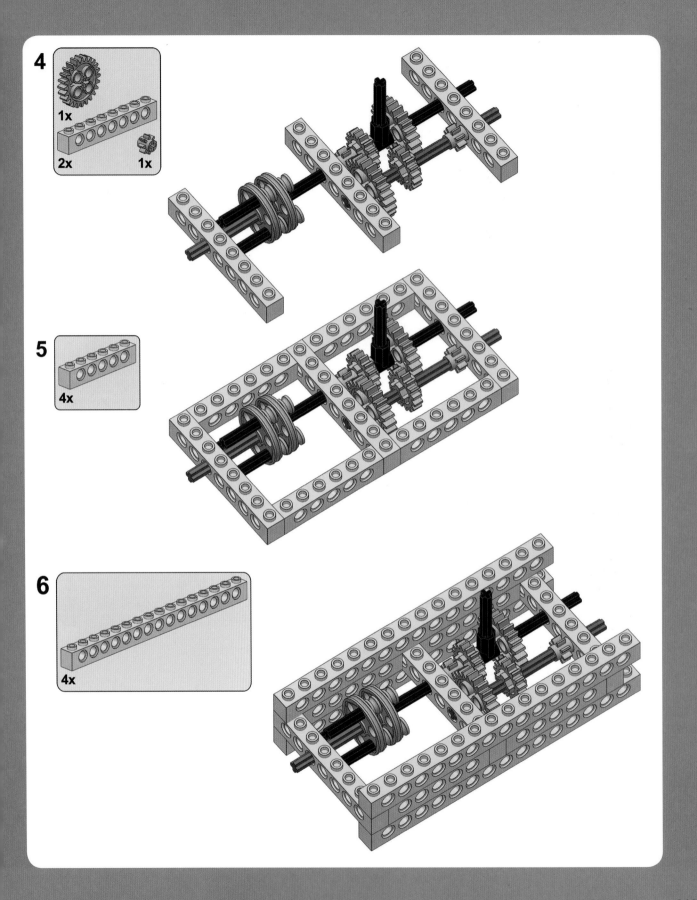

4

1x

2x   1x

5

4x

6

4x

a 4-speed synchronized transmission

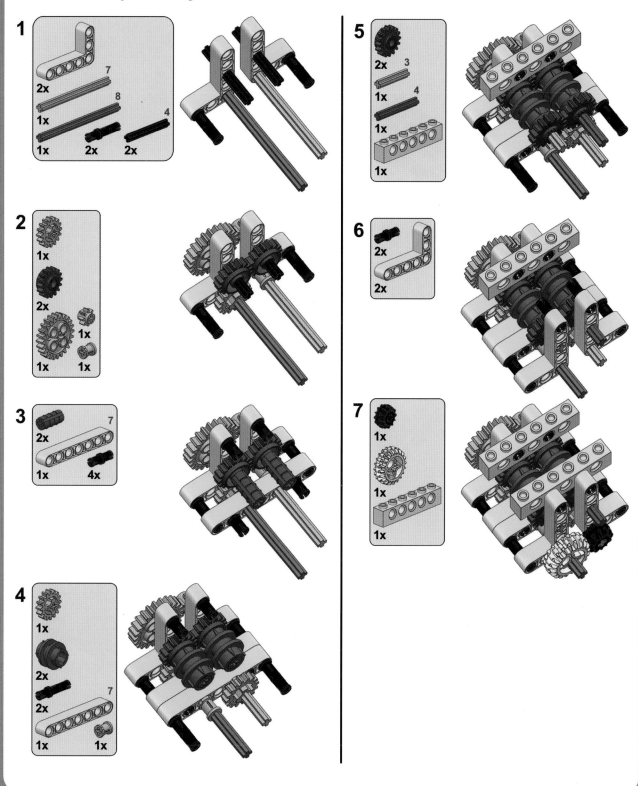

1
2x
7
1x
8
1x
4
2x
2x

2
1x
2x
1x
1x
1x

3
2x
7
1x
4x

4
1x
2x
2x
7
1x
1x

5
2x
3
1x
4
1x
1x

6
2x
2x

7
1x
1x
1x

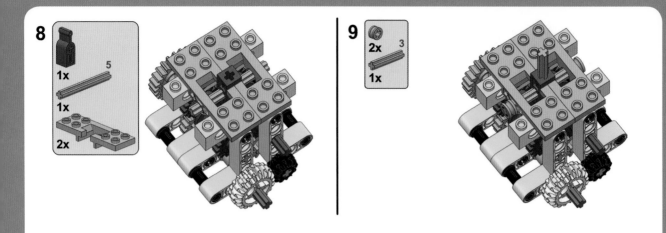

8 1x 5 1x 2x

9 2x 3 1x

a 4-speed sequential RC synchronized transmission

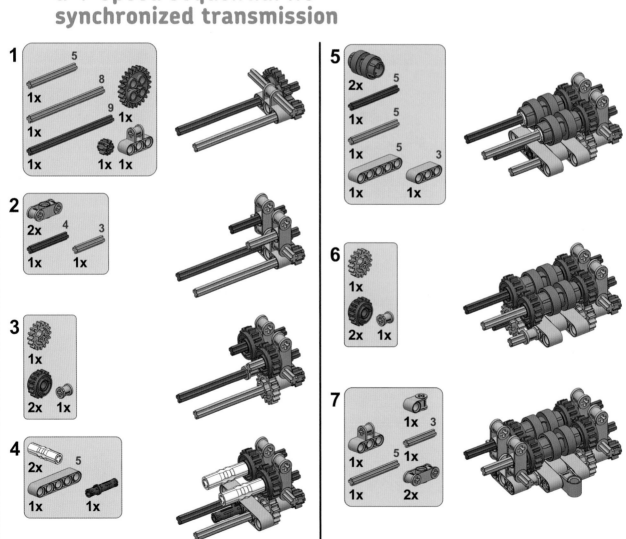

1 5 8 1x 1x 9 1x 1x 1x 1x

2 2x 4 3 1x 1x

3 1x 2x 1x

4 2x 5 1x 1x

5 2x 5 1x 5 1x 5 3 1x 1x

6 1x 2x 1x

7 1x 3 1x 5 1x 1x 2x

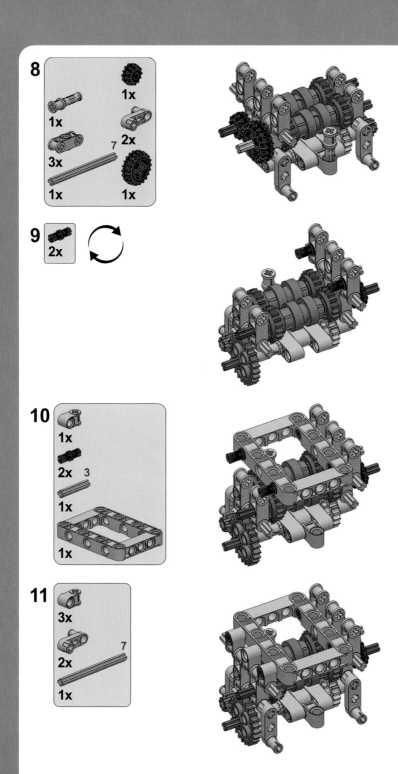

12

1x
1x
1x

12

1x

13

1x
1x

14

2x
2x
2x
2x

3

15

2x
1x

5

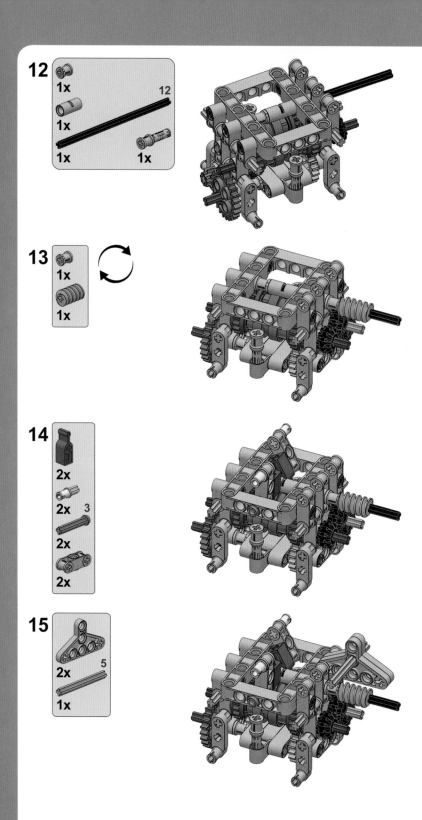

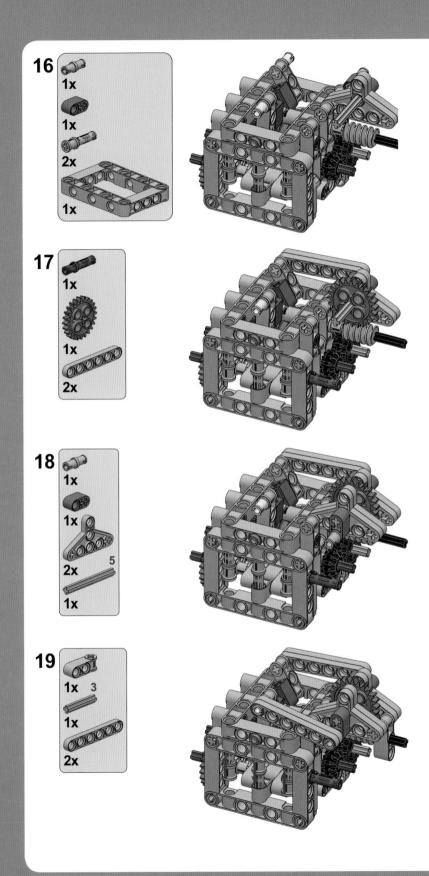

16

1x
1x
2x
1x

17

1x
1x
2x

18

1x
1x
2x 5
1x

19

1x 3
1x
2x

20
1x

21
2x
1x

22
1x
7
1x
1x

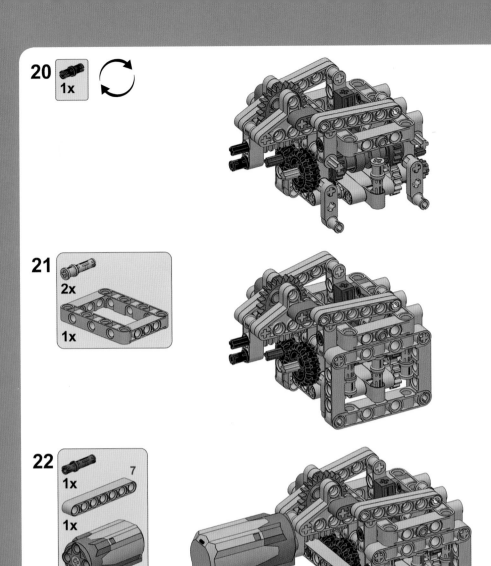

a 10-speed synchronized transmission

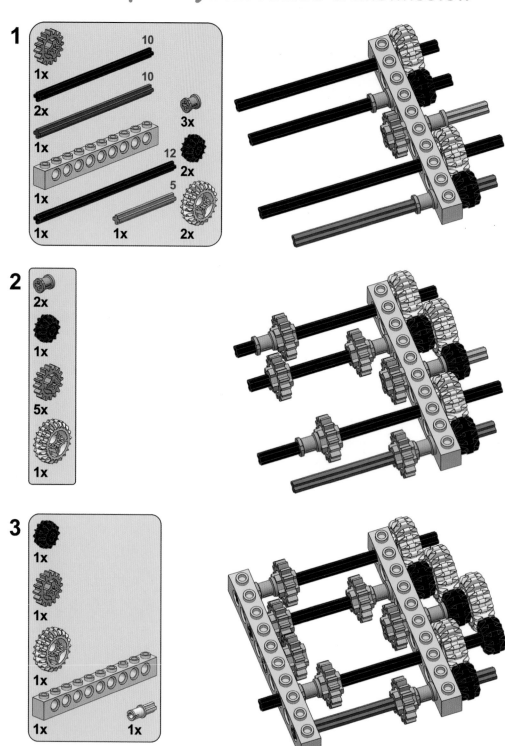

1
10
1x
10
2x
1x
3x
12
2x
5
1x
1x
2x

2
2x
1x
5x
1x

3
1x
1x
1x
1x
1x

4

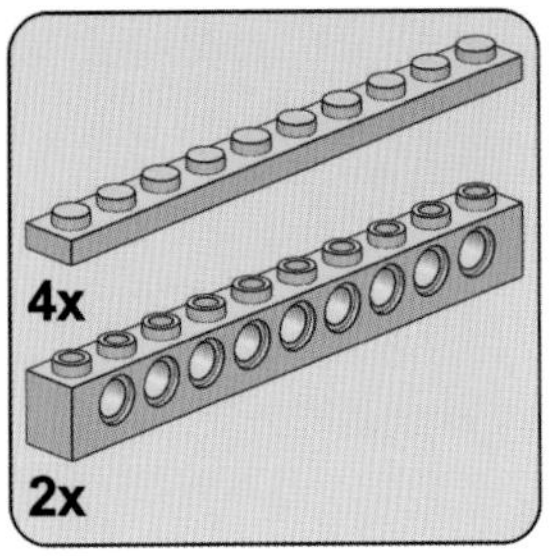

4x

2x

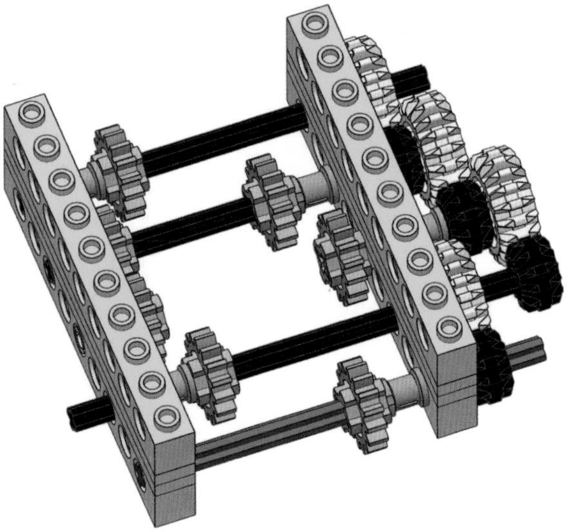

5

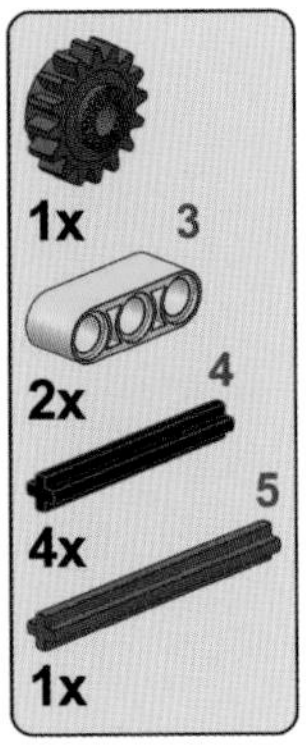

1x

3

2x

4

4x

5

1x

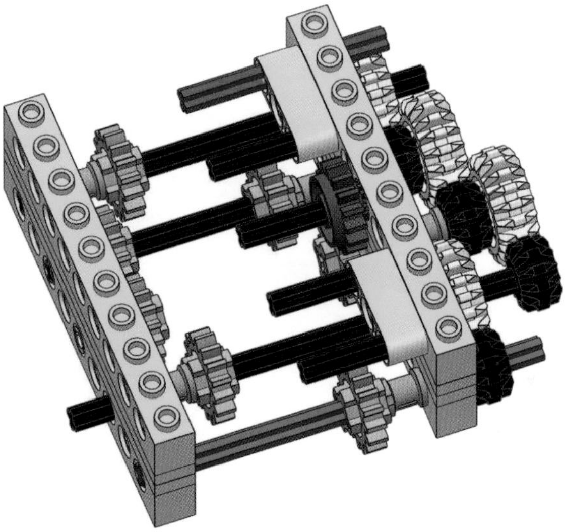

6

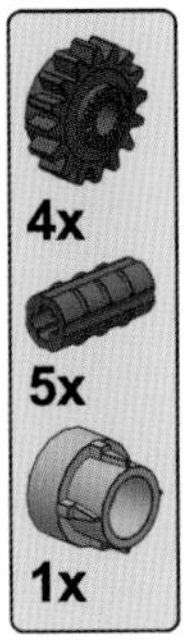

4x

5x

1x

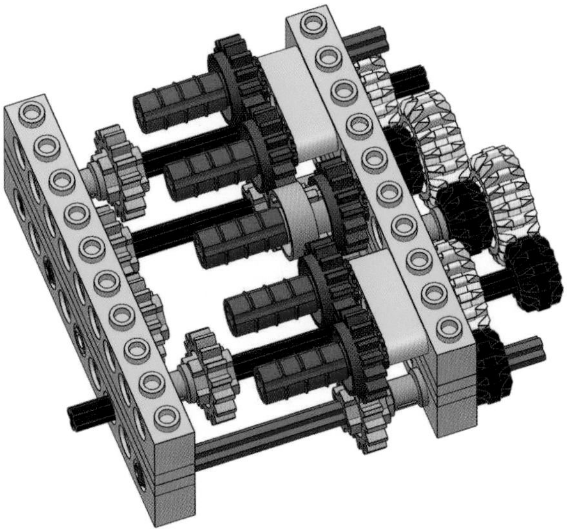

7

5x

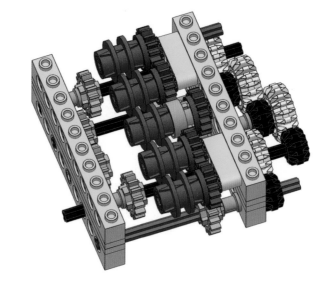

8

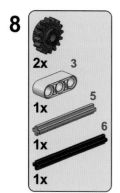

2x 3

1x 5

1x 6

1x

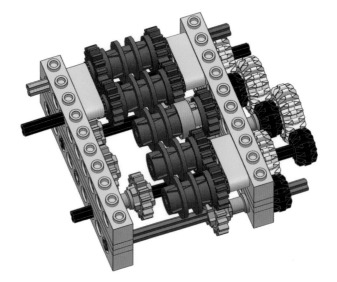

9

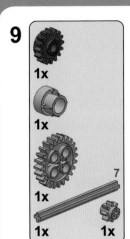

1x

1x

1x

7

1x   1x

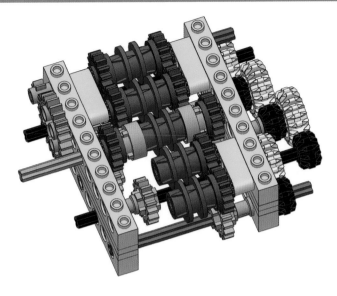

10

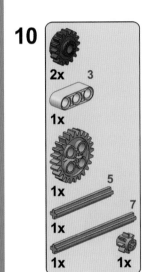

2x   3

1x

1x

5

1x

7

1x   1x

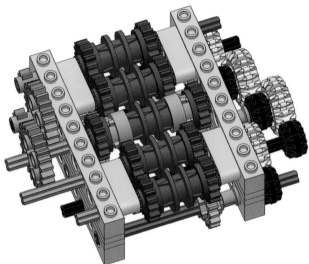

11

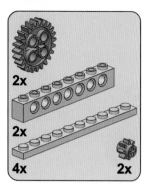

2x
2x
4x 2x

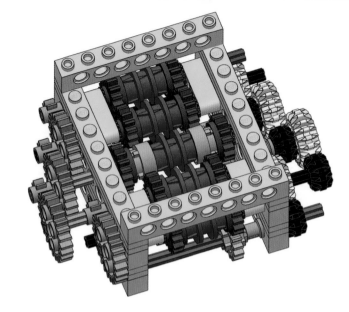

12

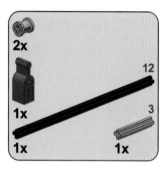

2x
1x
1x

12

3

1x

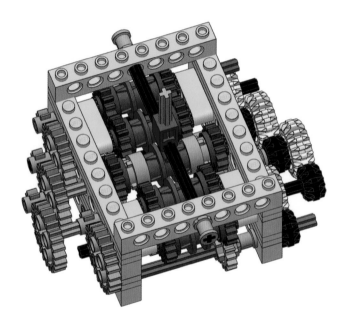

a continuously variable transmission

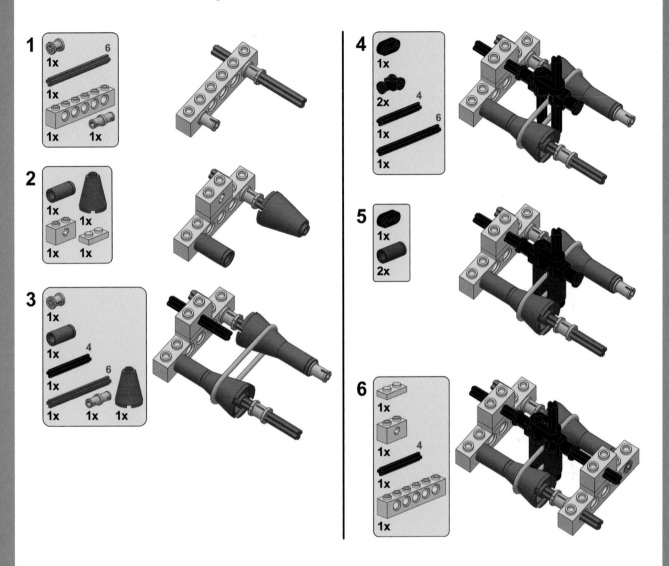

1

1x 6
1x
1x 1x

2

1x 1x
1x 1x

3

1x
1x 4
1x 6
1x 1x 1x

4

1x
2x 4
1x 6
1x

5

1x
2x

6

1x
1x 4
1x
1x

20

adders and subtractors

Adders and subtractors are mechanisms used to couple two or more motors together. Coupled motors are usually used to control a single function, most often the propulsion of a vehicle. They can work together (in an adder) or against each other (in a subtractor). Both mechanisms make use of differentials, and both are examples of advanced mechanics. The way subtractors work is particularly fascinating.

You'll find that using adders is a great way to give your motor even more power. Subtractors will be most useful when building tanks and construction vehicles, as these mechanisms have two outputs perfectly suited for controlling two treads.

hard-coupling

But first, let's consider a simpler way of coupling motors, one that forces two motors to run at the same speed. Making such a connection is called *hard-coupling* (see Figure 20-1).

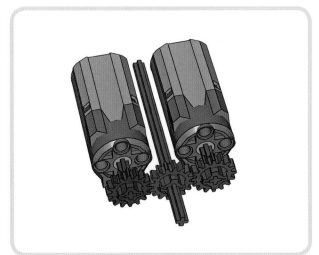

Figure 20-1: Two hard-coupled motors with a single output, shown in red

Forcibly slowing or speeding up a motor can be harmful and may permanently degrade its performance. Still, hard-coupling isn't that different from a LEGO motor's regular use, where motors are slowed down by a load or sped up by a vehicle rolling downhill. Hard-coupling two or more motors of the same type is a fairly low-risk way to increase your model's power. But what if we want to couple motors of different types or if we find hard-coupling too risky? This is where adders come in.

NOTE The performance of identical electric motors can vary, making their speeds differ by a few percent. One reason is that every motor includes moving parts that are prone to wear. Another is that the precision of the production process that makes motors can vary between batches.

coupling motors with adders

Adders couple two motors to work as one; in doing so, adders sum the motors' individual torques. As a result of this coupling, the output will be the average of the two motors' rotational speeds. This means that we can use two coupled PF Medium motors in cases where one Medium motor is too weak and an XL motor is too large.

summing torque with an adder

An adder makes use of a differential in order to equalize the differences between two or more inputs and to drive a single output. A differential has three elements that can be used as inputs or outputs: the two axles that come out of it and the case of the differential itself, as shown in Figure 20-2.

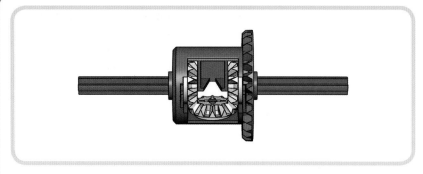

Figure 20-2: A differential that includes two axles (green and blue) and the differential case (red)

A differential consists of a housing with three bevel gears inside, two of which are set on two axles that enter it from opposite sides. The third gear is connected to the housing only. The first two gears are called *spider gears* or *side gears*, and the gear fixed to the housing is called a *planet gear*.

When a differential is used to couple motors, any difference between inputs will be equalized by the system of the differential's inner gears. The output will be driven by the sum of the inputs' torques and the average of their speeds. Figures 20-3 through 20-6 show some examples of two motors coupled with an adder in various ways. The biggest distinction among these variations is the use of different differentials. The motors' inputs are blue and green, and the adder's output is red.

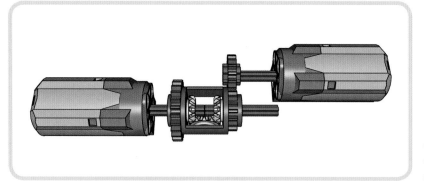

Figure 20-3: Two PF Medium motors are driving the differential case (blue) and one of the axles (green). The other axle (red) is the output.

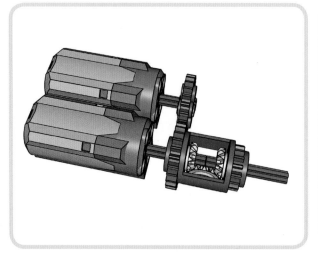

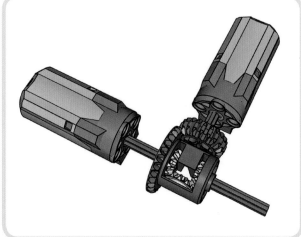

Figure 20-4: The same setup as in Figure 20-3 but with the motors placed side by side

Figure 20-5: An adder using the latest differential variant

20

adders and subtractors

Adders and subtractors are mechanisms used to couple two or more motors together. Coupled motors are usually used to control a single function, most often the propulsion of a vehicle. They can work together (in an adder) or against each other (in a subtractor). Both mechanisms make use of differentials, and both are examples of advanced mechanics. The way subtractors work is particularly fascinating.

You'll find that using adders is a great way to give your motor even more power. Subtractors will be most useful when building tanks and construction vehicles, as these mechanisms have two outputs perfectly suited for controlling two treads.

hard-coupling

But first, let's consider a simpler way of coupling motors, one that forces two motors to run at the same speed. Making such a connection is called *hard-coupling* (see Figure 20-1).

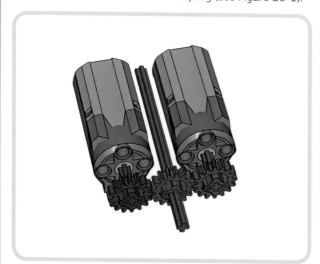

Figure 20-1: Two hard-coupled motors with a single output, shown in red

Forcibly slowing or speeding up a motor can be harmful and may permanently degrade its performance. Still, hard-coupling isn't that different from a LEGO motor's regular use, where motors are slowed down by a load or sped up by a vehicle rolling downhill. Hard-coupling two or more motors of the same type is a fairly low-risk way to increase your model's power. But what if we want to couple motors of different types or if we find hard-coupling too risky? This is where adders come in.

NOTE The performance of identical electric motors can vary, making their speeds differ by a few percent. One reason is that every motor includes moving parts that are prone to wear. Another is that the precision of the production process that makes motors can vary between batches.

coupling motors with adders

Adders couple two motors to work as one; in doing so, adders sum the motors' individual torques. As a result of this coupling, the output will be the average of the two motors' rotational speeds. This means that we can use two coupled PF Medium motors in cases where one Medium motor is too weak and an XL motor is too large.

summing torque with an adder

An adder makes use of a differential in order to equalize the differences between two or more inputs and to drive a single output. A differential has three elements that can be used as inputs or outputs: the two axles that come out of it and the case of the differential itself, as shown in Figure 20-2.

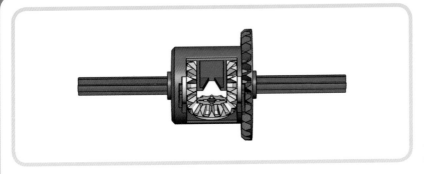

Figure 20-2: A differential that includes two axles (green and blue) and the differential case (red)

A differential consists of a housing with three bevel gears inside, two of which are set on two axles that enter it from opposite sides. The third gear is connected to the housing only. The first two gears are called *spider gears* or *side gears*, and the gear fixed to the housing is called a *planet gear*.

When a differential is used to couple motors, any difference between inputs will be equalized by the system of the differential's inner gears. The output will be driven by the sum of the inputs' torques and the average of their speeds. Figures 20-3 through 20-6 show some examples of two motors coupled with an adder in various ways. The biggest distinction among these variations is the use of different differentials. The motors' inputs are blue and green, and the adder's output is red.

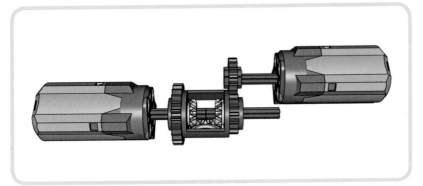

Figure 20-3: Two PF Medium motors are driving the differential case (blue) and one of the axles (green). The other axle (red) is the output.

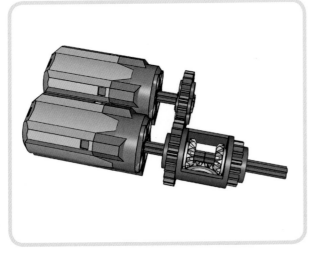

Figure 20-4: The same setup as in Figure 20-3 but with the motors placed side by side

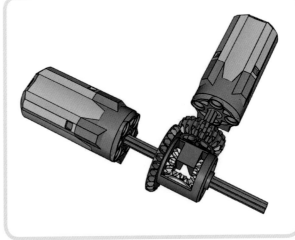

Figure 20-5: An adder using the latest differential variant

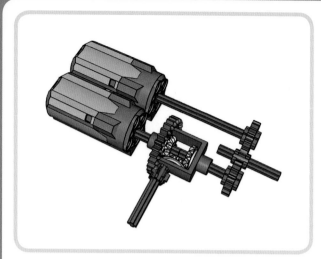

Figure 20-6: An adder using the oldest differential variant

NOTE When using adders, always try to have similar gear ratios between the motors and the adder. Differences in gear ratios will make the motors share the load unevenly, with one motor working harder than the other. The gear ratio immediately after the adder (that is, between the adder and the mechanism it drives) does not affect the load distribution.

You already know that an adder sums the torques of its inputs and averages their speeds, but let's express these relationships mathematically. If we have one motor, $motor_1$, and another motor, $motor_2$, then the adder's *torque* is equal to

$$torque(motor_1) + torque(motor_2)$$

and if n is the total number of motors, the adder's *speed* is equal to

$$\frac{speed(motor_1) + speed(motor_2) + ... + speed(motor_n)}{n}$$

One important consideration when building adders is the direction each input rotates. Coupled motors are usually powered from the same source, resulting in an identical direction of rotation. But depending on whether the inputs' directions match, the two motors can work together or against each other. The latter case is obviously undesirable, as it results in decreased torque and speed.

All the examples shown above have motors running in the same direction; however, in some cases, it's convenient to have the motors oriented so that they run in opposite directions. For the adder to work properly in such a case, we need to reverse the direction of one motor, either by powering it from a power source with the opposite polarity or by connecting it to a shared power source through a switch (shown in Figure 20-7). With older 9V motors, you can reverse the polarity of a motor by simply rotating its wire connector 90 degrees.

Figure 20-8 shows two examples of adders that need one of their motors reversed.

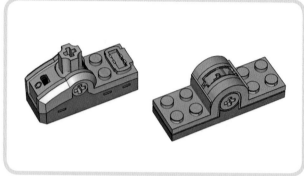

Figure 20-7: A Power Functions switch (left) and a 9V system switch (right)

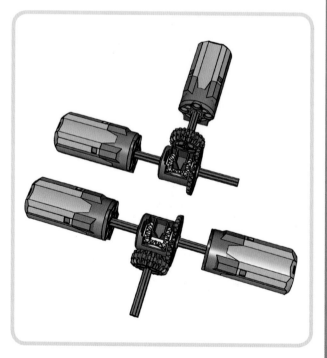

Figure 20-8: These two adders won't work properly unless we change one motor's rotational direction.

adding more than two motors

In most cases, coupling two motors will give us enough torque, but what if we want even more torque? We can use an adder to couple more than two motors, but unfortunately the mechanism's size and complexity will increase dramatically, since every motor beyond two requires one more differential (see Figure 20-9).

Each differential other than the first one has one input already taken, as it's connected to the previous differential (the second differential is connected to the first one, the third to the second one, and so on). Thus, we are left with only one free input, and we can add only one motor for each differential. Unfortunately, the resulting high torque makes chaining adders in this way fairly risky.

When more than two motors need to be coupled, it's usually a better choice to use motors of the same type and hard-couple them. This is true not only because the coupling takes less space but also because with more motors, there is more torque to transfer and differentials are not fit for handling high torque. Hard-coupling with knobs (shown in Figure 20-10) is a reasonable alternative.

subtractors

Subtractors combine the power of two motors in a more complex way. Each subtractor has two inputs and two outputs and also uses two differentials. Rotating one input of a subtractor makes both outputs rotate in the same direction; rotating the other input makes the outputs rotate in opposite directions. Both inputs can be rotated at once, making the outputs rotate at different speeds.

It's easier to understand how a subtractor works when thinking of its most common use: driving tracked vehicles. A typical tracked vehicle has two tracks: left and right, as shown in Figure 20-11. When both tracks rotate in the same direction, the vehicle moves forward or backward along a straight line. When the tracks rotate in opposite directions, the vehicle turns in place. When the tracks rotate in the same direction at different speeds, the vehicle makes a wide turn, as a car would, and the greater the difference between motor speeds, the tighter the turn.

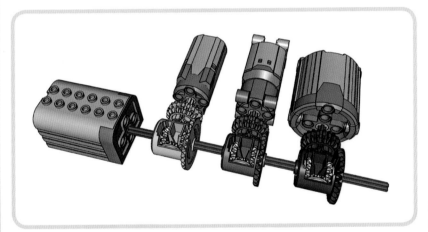

Figure 20-9: It takes three differentials to couple four motors in this chain of adders.

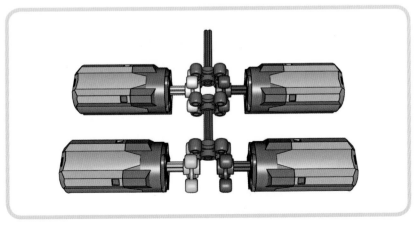

Figure 20-10: These four motors are hard-coupled with knobs, making them more torque resistant than differentials.

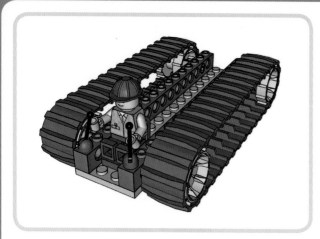

Figure 20-11: A simple tracked vehicle

With tracked vehicles, we can assume that one of the subtractor's input motors is for driving and the other is for turning. Let's call these motors *D* and *T*, respectively, and note that *D* is usually faster than *T*. If only *D* is running, both tracks (that is, both *outputs*) rotate in the same direction, making the vehicle drive straight. If only *T* is rotating, both tracks rotate in opposite directions, making the vehicle turn in place.

Now, an interesting thing happens when both *D* and *T* are running at the same time: One track gets accelerated by the turning motor (*D* + *T* speed), while the other gets slowed down by it (*D* – *T* speed). This effectively causes the vehicle to make a turn, the sharpness of which depends strictly on how different the speeds of *D* and *T* are. Figure 20-12 shows how *D* and *T* affect the motion of a vehicle.

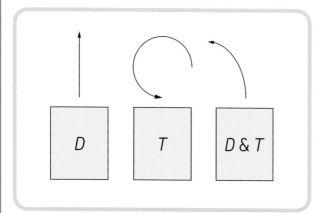

Figure 20-12: The path of a tracked vehicle with subtractors' inputs being driven. D represents the driving motor (faster), and T represents the turning motor (slower).

By adjusting our inputs' speeds, we can achieve any combination of the tracks' speeds: Each track can be stopped or can rotate forward or backward at a speed ranging from almost zero to the sum of the speeds of both inputs.

Note that the relationship between the motors' maximum speeds affects the way the subtractor works. For example, let's say we have a vehicle driving straight at full speed and we start turning at full speed. There are three possibilities:

* If the speed of *D* is *greater* than that of *T*, neither track will be stopped or reversed; one track will slow down, and the other will accelerate. The vehicle will start turning along an arc while continuing to drive in the same direction.
* If the speed of *D* is *equal* to that of *T*, one track will stop, and the other will accelerate; the vehicle will start turning almost in place, with the stopped track being the center of the turn.
* If the speed of *D* is *less* than that of *T*, one track will be reversed, and the other will accelerate; the vehicle will start turning almost in place, with the center of the turn located between the tracks at a point proportional to their speeds (closer to the slower track, farther from the faster one).

The difference between the maximum speeds of *D* and *T* is a crucial consideration when selecting motors and gear ratios to drive the subtractor. Usually, the first of the three cases listed above (with the faster drive motor and the slower steering motor) is the most realistic and convenient case: A vehicle that goes straight faster than it turns is easy to control and behaves real tracked vehicles do.

Also, the turning input's speed is very important when a vehicle is turning in place. The tracks rotate in different directions, so the difference between the two tracks' speeds is equal to twice the turning input's speed. Applying too much turning speed will make our vehicle look like a carousel rather than, say, a tank. Additionally, turning in place involves significant friction, as the tracks scrub the ground over a large area. Therefore, it's a good idea to use gear reduction on the turning input, sacrificing speed for torque.

why use a subtractor?

As you might imagine, a tracked vehicle can be driven with two separate motors as well: one motor driving the left track and the other driving the right track. Using a subtractor takes two motors, too, but has several advantages:

better control   A vehicle with a subtractor can drive in a perfectly straight line, while a vehicle with two separate motors is sensitive to differences between the motors' speeds and to its own weight distribution, which can weigh down the motors unevenly.

lower power consumption   In a subtractor, one motor is for driving, and the other is for turning; therefore, we can use two different types of motors together. Driving tracks separately, on the other hand, requires two identical motors, and two strong motors have a higher total power consumption than one strong motor and one weak one.

more mechanisms   Connecting another mechanism (a replica piston engine or a rotating fan in the engine bay, for example) to the drivetrain is easy with a subtractor, as it has one motor used specifically to drive. When two separate motors are used, connecting a mechanism to both of them is impossible, and connecting a second function to one motor can slow it down, resulting in a mismatch in speed.

better remote control   Without a subtractor, you need the Power Functions remote with speed control dials to make the vehicle turn in an arc. The regular Power Functions remote will only be able to make the vehicle drive straight or turn in place.

The advantages of a subtractor are somewhat diminished if you have the Power Functions remote control with speed dials, which enables a driver to control the speed of each track independently. Subtractors also have some disadvantages, which should be taken into account at all times. First, a subtractor is relatively large and complex, requires plenty of parts, and adds to the vehicle's weight. Second, a subtractor relies on differentials, which can be damaged by high torque. My experience shows that using a subtractor to drive a vehicle heavier than 3 kg involves a serious risk of breaking the bevel gears inside the differentials, regardless of the gear ratio between the subtractor and the sprocket wheels. The other disadvantage to subtractors is that they don't give you the power benefit of having two drive motors.

longitudinal subtractor

A longitudinal subtractor's elongated, narrow shape makes it a good choice for tracked vehicles that have long, narrow hulls between their tracks. Figure 20-13 shows the driving input (*D*) in blue, the steering input (*T*) in green, the outputs in red, and the sprocket wheels driving the tracks in yellow.

Notice that each motor drives both differentials at once. The PF XL motor drives with a 1:1 gear ratio. The PF Medium motor turns with a 9:1 gear ratio. That ratio makes the turning input's speed slower than the driving input's speed, even though the Medium motor's rotational speed is faster than the XL's. The driving input rotates at 146 rpm

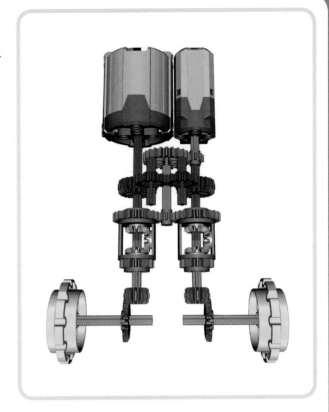

Figure 20-13: A longitudinal subtractor

(the normal speed of the XL motor), and the turning input rotates at 30.6 RPM (that is, the speed of the Medium motor reduced by a factor of 9).

Obviously, a subtractor can work with different combinations of motors and gear ratios; the one shown here exemplifies this and is the most efficient combination for most uses. If you use the right gear ratio at the sprocket wheel, you can easily use a single XL motor to drive a 2 kg vehicle. However, a vehicle's efficiency at heavier weights depends greatly on the type of surface the model is driving over. To achieve more power for heavier vehicles, you can connect more than a single motor to the driving input, for example, by using an adder.

The following are instructions for building this subtractor inside a studfull structure. Note that many details can be changed as needed, including the types and number of motors and the gear ratio of the inputs and outputs. You'll want to replace the bevel gears on the outputs with knobs if you're building a heavy vehicle.

a longitudinal subtractor

1

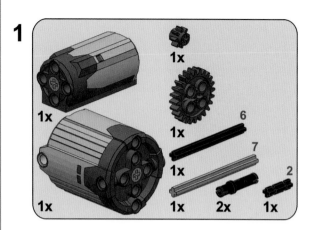

1x
1x
1x
1x

1x
1x
6
1x
7
1x
2x
2
1x

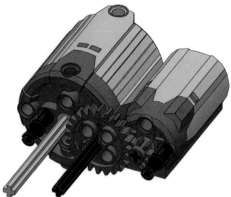

2

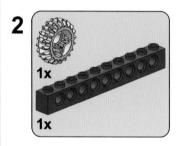

1x
1x

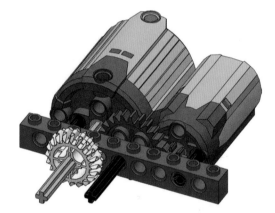

3

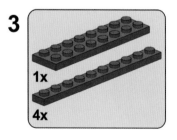

1x
4x

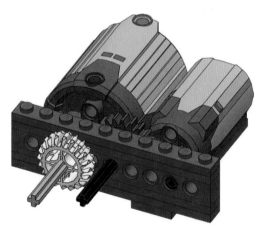

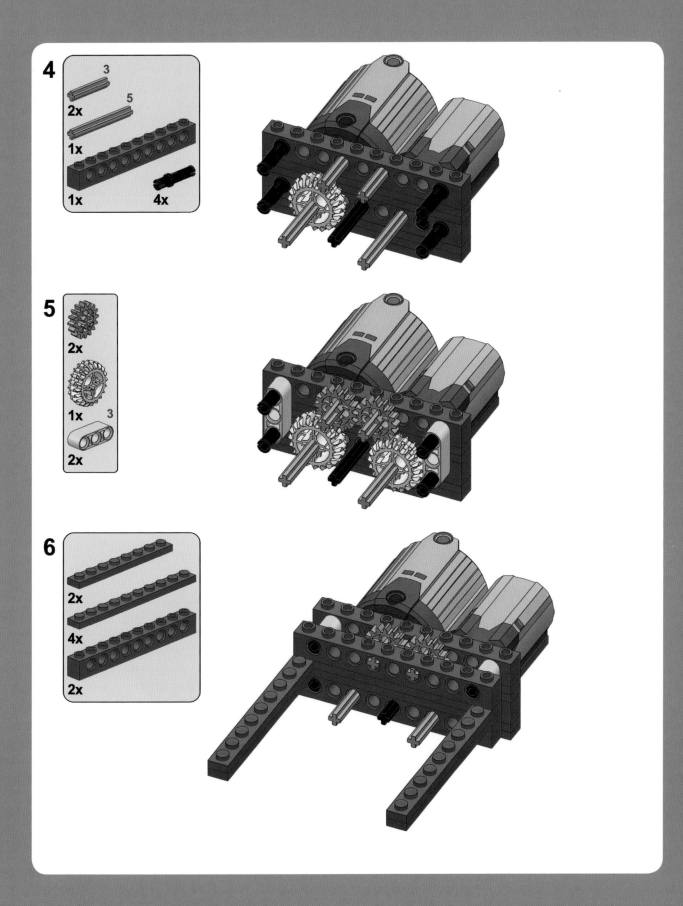

4

3
2x
5
1x
1x   4x

5

2x
1x   3
2x

6

2x
4x
2x

7

1x

4x

2x

8

2x

1x

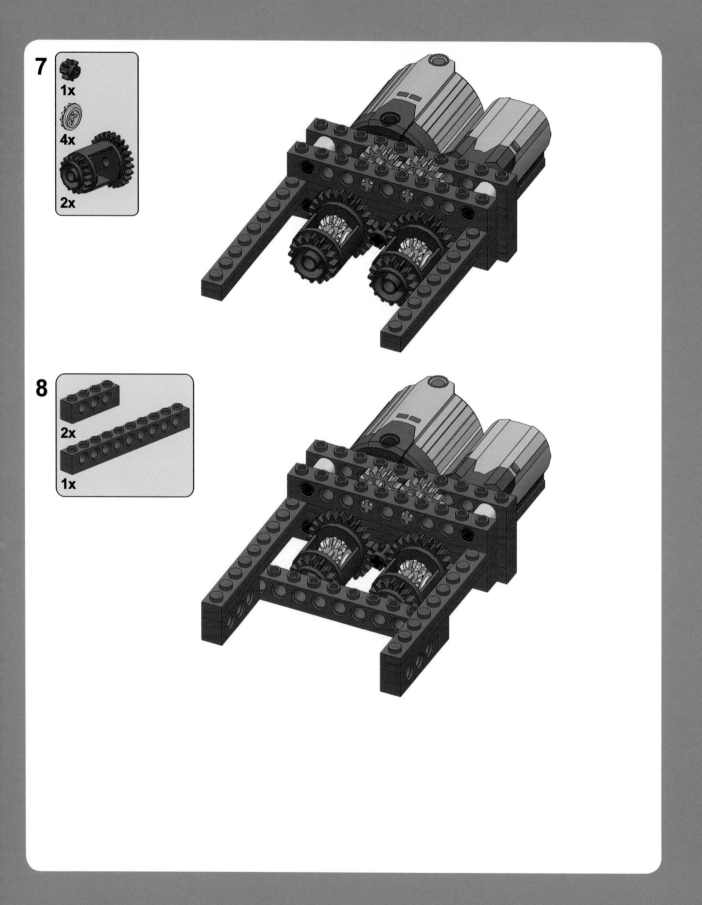

9

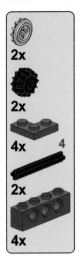

2x

2x

4x   4

2x

4x

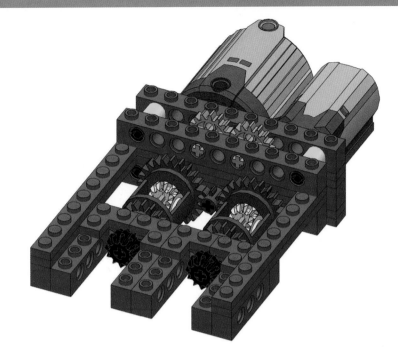

10

2x   7

2x

1x

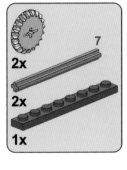

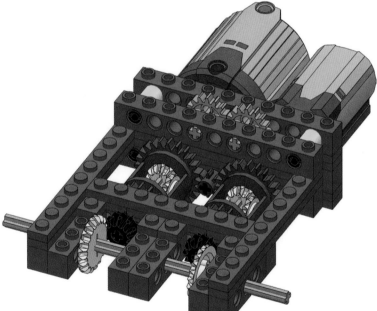

11

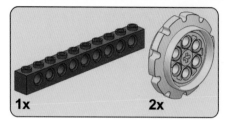

1x   2x

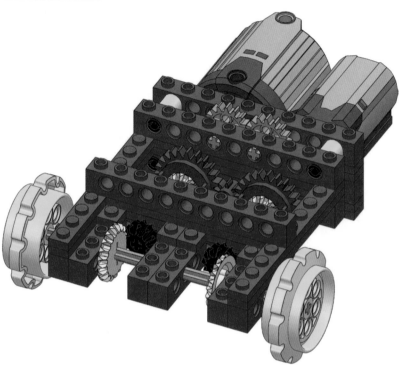

transverse subtractor

This subtractor is smaller and a little less complex than the longitudinal one. Figure 20-14 shows an example of this subtractor with two outputs (shown in red), the driving input (blue), and the turning input (green). Note that we can use the outputs coming from the other differential just as well, and it will work, but the inputs' roles will be swapped: The turning input will become the driving input, and the driving input will become the turning input.

The transverse subtractor differs from the longitudinal version in several ways. Each motor drives a single differential, and two sets of gears connect the two differentials. One set has an even number of gears, and the other an odd number.

The important thing is that both sets have a 1:1 ratio. Therefore, when using this subtractor with two different motors, it's crucial to make sure that the stronger motor doesn't drive the weaker one—a gear reduction at the weaker motor should prevent this.

This configuration offers more room for experimentation than the longitudinal subtractor does. For instance, we can relocate the motors if we drive the differentials with worm gears, preventing the problem of one motor driving another, as shown in Figure 20-15.

Finally, it is possible to build a fully studless variant of this subtractor using the new 28-tooth differentials (see Figure 20-16). It looks very different, but it works just the same.

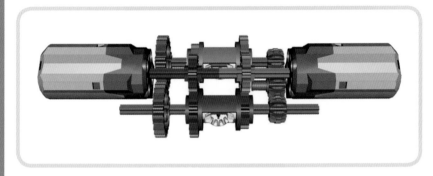

Figure 20-14: A transverse subtractor

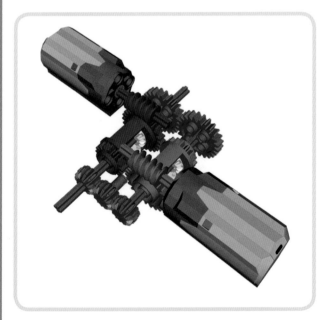

Figure 20-15: A transverse subtractor with worm gears

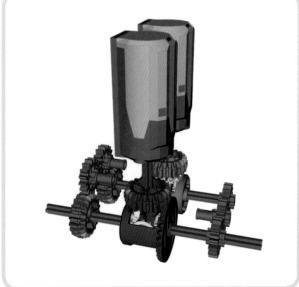

Figure 20-16: A transverse subtractor with the latest differential variants

a transverse subtractor

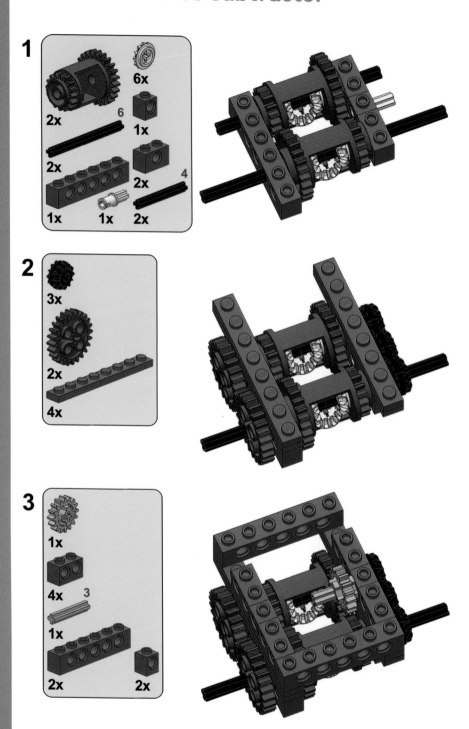

1

2x 6

2x

1x 6x

1x

2x

1x 1x 2x 4

2

3x

2x

4x

3

1x

4x 3

1x

2x 2x

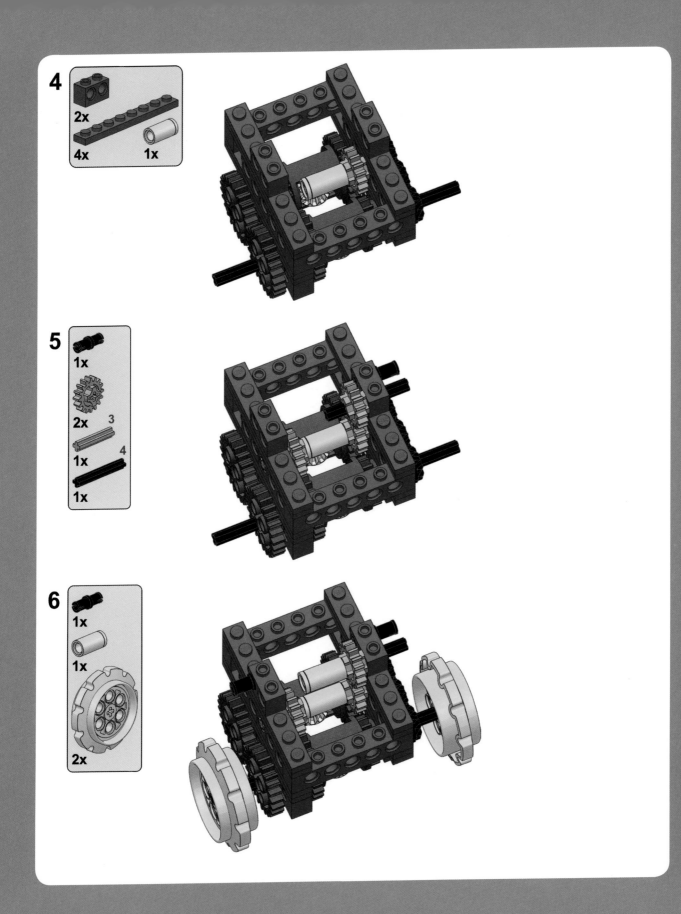

4

2x
4x   1x

5

1x
2x   3
1x   4
1x

6

1x
1x
2x

7

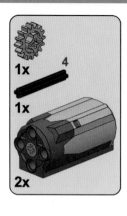

1x 4
1x
2x

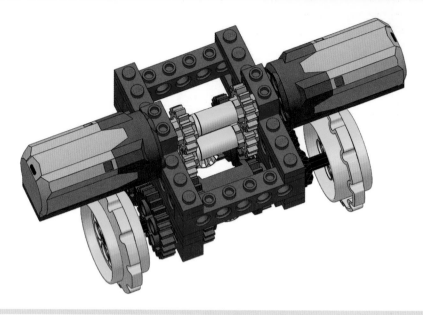

---

a studless transverse subtractor

1

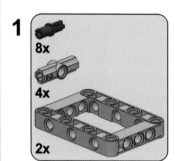

8x
4x
2x

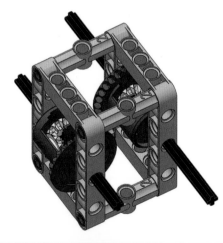

2

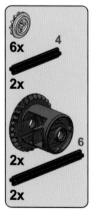

6x 4
2x
2x 6
2x
2x

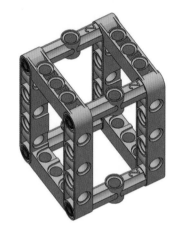

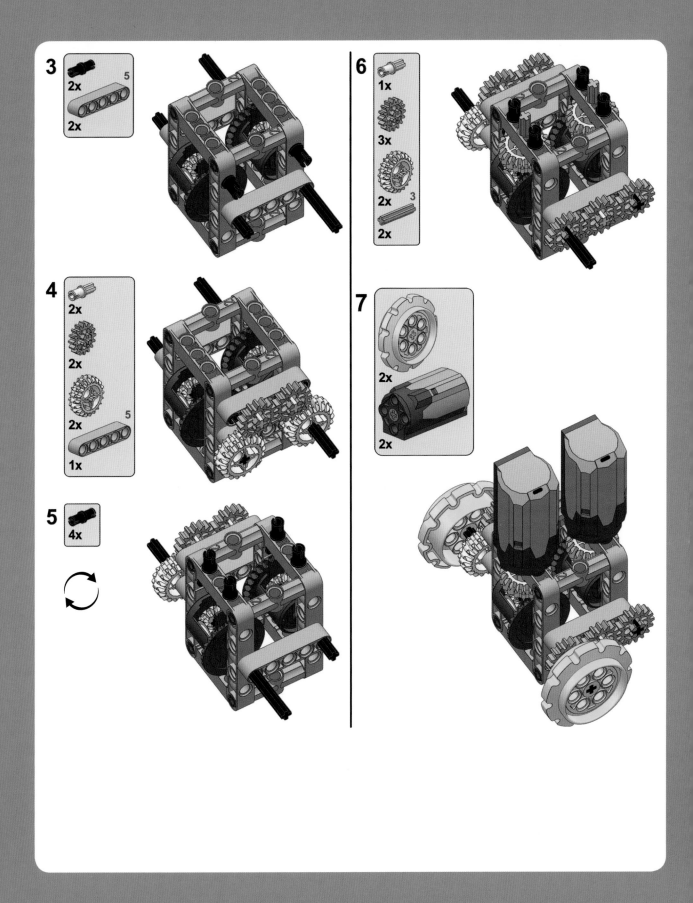

21

planetary gearing

Planetary gearing, also known as *epicyclic gearing*, is an unusual-looking system of gears that allows you to significantly change the gear ratio within a limited space. It's very common in the real world; you can find it in bicycles, car transmissions, differentials, all kinds of toys, and even mechanical pencil sharpeners.

A planetary gear system, as shown in Figure 21-1, consists of four elements:

* A single gear in the center called the *sun gear*.
* Two or more gears called *planet gears* that rotate around the sun gear.
* An element called a *carrier* that holds the planet gears together. The carrier is mounted on the sun gear's axle and can rotate independently of it. The planet gears, while attached to the carrier, can also rotate independently of it. (A planetary gear system without a carrier is called a *free planet drive*.)
* An outer ring with teeth on the inside, meshed with planet gears, called an *annular gear*, *annulus*, or *ring gear*.

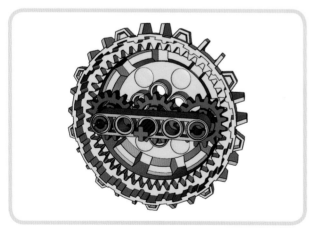

Figure 21-1: A working LEGO planetary gear system with a sun gear (red), two planet gears (blue), a carrier (light grey), and an annular gear (yellow)

Note that the planet gears simply act as idlers and thus don't affect the ratio of the whole gearing. For simplicity, you can consider them part of the carrier. In fact, an entire series of planet gears can be located on the carrier and they will still act as idlers.

For the gearing to work, two parts must be free to move, and the third part must be fixed. That means there are three planetary gearing variants, all of which are commonly found in the real world:

* Rotating sun and carrier with a fixed annular gear
* Rotating sun, a fixed carrier, and a rotating annular gear
* Fixed sun, a rotating carrier, and an annular gear

Any of these three parts can act as input or output, and the third acts as an idler, joining the other two. This is how automatic transmissions work: They change their gear ratio by locking one of these three elements and releasing the other two. Unfortunately, few LEGO pieces can be used as annular gears, although compatible gears are simple to make using 3D printing—we'll cover that in the next chapter. In this chapter, we'll only discuss solutions that are possible using original LEGO parts.

LEGO annular gears

Although the LEGO Group often uses planetary gearing for gear reduction *inside* the housing of its electrical motors, it's extremely rare in other applications. The reason is that the essential part of planetary gearing is the annular gear, and only three LEGO elements can practically act as an annular gear (see Figure 21-2): the type 1 and type 2 large Technic turntables (24 inner teeth) and the #64712 wheel (48 inner teeth). The Hailfire Droid wheel can also act as an annular gear, but it's so impractical and rare that we'll ignore it here.

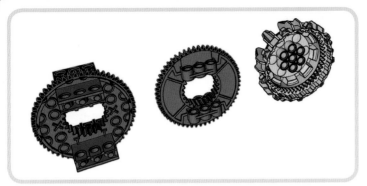

Driving any annular gear directly—that is, without using the planet gears—results in a standard gear ratio that is less than what planetary gearing can provide. For example, driving a large turntable from the inside directly with an 8-tooth gear results in a 3:1 (24:8) gear ratio, whereas planetary gearing that uses 8-tooth gears results in a 4:1 gear ratio.

Figure 21-2: LEGO elements suitable for use as the annular gear (left to right): type 1 large turntable (24 inner teeth), type 2 large turntable (24 inner teeth), and #64712 wheel (48 inner teeth)

a planetary gear system with a turntable

Both large turntables offer only one option for planetary gearing: three 8-tooth gears inside with one acting as the sun gear and two acting as planet gears connected by a carrier. To make things even trickier, each turntable consists of two parts: a top and a bottom, which rotate freely around a fixed center. But the inner teeth are part of the bottom, and there's no simple way to lock the bottom with the top, which means you can't make the top act as the annular gear. Therefore, you can't use the turntable as the output. Instead, the best option is to make the turntable the fixed element of the gearing, connect a motor as the input, and use the carrier as the output. The following instructions demonstrate how to do this. Note that in this solution, the motor and annular gear are locked and fixed, and the blue axle is the output. This gearing provides a 4:1 gear reduction.

1

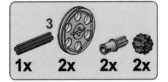
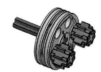

2

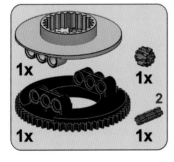
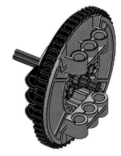

3

4x

1x

4

4x

2x

2x

5

7

1x

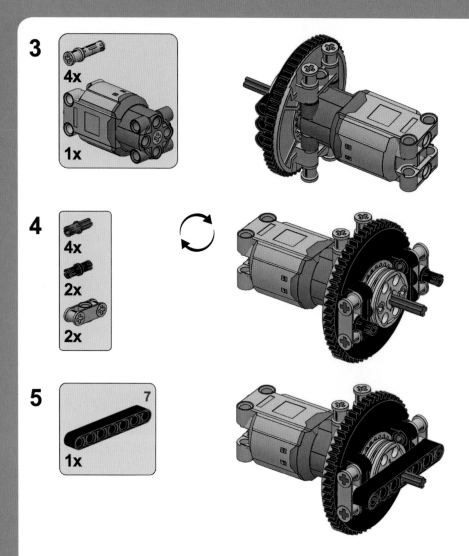

a planetary gear system with the #64712 wheel

The #64712 wheel is an unusual element. Originally created for the Power Miners series as part of a mining drill, it's been used as a regular wheel or decorative element in many sets since then, making it fairly common. It has 48 inner teeth, and unlike the turntables, it's a fixed and single-piece element. Unfortunately, its outer rim doesn't connect to any LEGO pieces, so it can only be connected using the seven pin holes inside it.

Although the size of the #64712 wheel element and the pin holes allow for more experimentation than do the turntables, the simplest option is still to make the wheel fixed and use the carrier as the output. The following instructions demonstrate how to do that using three 16-tooth gears with the blue axle as the output. This gearing also provides a 4:1 gear ratio.

1

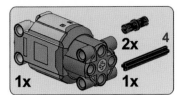
2x 4
1x 1x

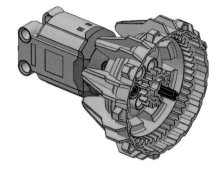

2

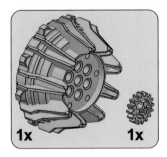
1x 1x

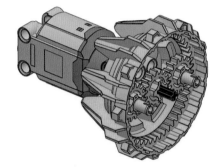

3

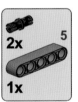
2x
2x

4

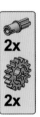
2x 5
1x

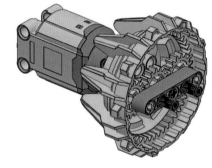

5

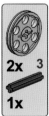
2x 3
1x

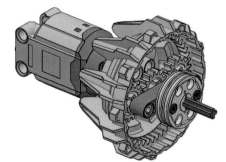

gear ratio and planetary gearing

So how do you calculate the gear ratio of a planetary gearing? The answer isn't simple: There's a separate equation for each of the three fixed and rotating element variants mentioned earlier. However, the number of teeth of the sun and the annular gears is all that matters.

If you assume that the sun gear is always the input, that T_s is the number of the sun gear's teeth, and that T_a is the number of the annular gear's teeth, then:

* For a rotating sun, a rotating carrier, and fixed annular gear, the ratio is equal to $1 + T_a / T_s$: 1.
* For a rotating sun, a fixed carrier, and a rotating annular gear, the ratio is equal to T_a / T_s: 1.

Both building instructions that result in the 4:1 gear ratio (shown earlier) rely on the first equation. Let's examine why the ratio of both is equal to 4:1:

* For the turntable: 1 + 24 / 8 = 1 + 3 = 4. Thus, the ratio is equal to 4:1.
* For the #64712 wheel: 1 + 48 / 16 = 1 + 3 = 4. Thus, the ratio is, again, equal to 4:1.

Planetary gearing is more effective with small sun gears and larger planet gears. To see the extent of this effectiveness, let's imagine we somehow overcame the practical difficulties of using a Hailfire Droid wheel as the fixed annular gear, and we found some planet gears (maybe they were 3D printed) that allowed us to use an 8-tooth gear as the sun gear again. The ratio of such a theoretical gearing would be equal to 1 + 168/8 = 1 + 21 = 22, resulting in a 22:1 ratio. (In real life, there are planetary gearings capable of achieving a 1000:1 ratio in a single stage!)

advantages of planetary gearing

What are the advantages of the planetary gearing, considering that it's difficult to achieve a gear ratio larger than 4:1 with common LEGO pieces? Consider the following benefits:

* Input and output axles are aligned end to end (or *coaxial*), which is very convenient. It means that we can install planetary gearing between any two axles: One would be the planetary gearing's input and the other its output.
* The direction of the output and input axles' rotation is the same; only the gear ratio is different, unless the carrier is fixed, in which case the direction is reversed.
* Planetary gearing usually has a large diameter, at least equal to the annular gear's diameter, but it's always very short. The turntable solution is only 3 studs long!
* The entire gearing is very robust and exceptionally well suited for high-torque applications because all axles are parallel, no bevel gears are used, the torque from the sun gear is evenly distributed between two or more planet gears, and the whole gearing is braced by the annular gear.
* The gearing is highly effective because it transfers the torque to multiple gears, all of which are parallel to each other.

In everyday use, the main advantage of planetary gearing is that it just keeps things simple. It doesn't require the output axle to be located next to or at an angle to the input axle, which is why it's so well suited as internal gearing for LEGO motors. And it's more effective than alternative solutions—although a worm gear, for instance, will deliver higher gear reduction, it does so at the price of higher friction, and its output axle must be set adjacent to the worm gear and at a right angle to it.

22

3D printing

As 3D printing technology becomes more widespread and affordable, it's natural for LEGO builders to consider its usefulness. At the moment, the quality of 3D-printed elements still isn't on par with original LEGO pieces, and the printing costs are too high to allow for mass production. So instead of merely copying pieces that have already been manufactured by LEGO, I'll explore printing elements to complement existing LEGO pieces. At its current level of development, 3D printing makes it possible to create small quantities of highly specialized elements that fit together with original LEGO pieces but are new elements—pieces that LEGO doesn't make—and therefore open up new possibilities.

What might builders want to build? For example, you can create a gear wheel that is similar to the normal LEGO design but differs in size and in number of teeth. Such elements, shown in Figures 22-1 and 22-2, aren't copies but completely new pieces that can be combined in new ways and—in the case of gear wheels—create new gear ratios.

in the land of unlimited possibilities

3D printing can be an incredible boon to the LEGO Technic builder. The possibilities are nearly limitless, and it's easy to let your imagination run wild! But this mind-set can result in impractical designs, too. You must consider strength and rigidity as well as the practical limitations of 3D printing. Let's start by discussing 3D elements that follow the design principles of traditional LEGO pieces and keep the "custom" part to a minimum. LEGO could start making these pieces tomorrow if it chose to.

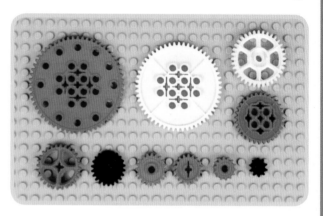

Figure 22-1: 3D-printed LEGO-compatible gears by Efferman

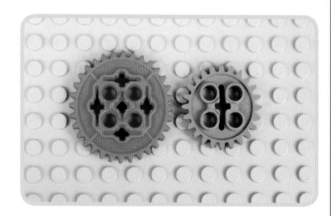

Figure 22-2: The gear by Efferman (left) follows the design of a LEGO gear (right) but allows builders to work with sizes LEGO doesn't provided.

3D DESIGNERS

All custom elements shown in this chapter are printed by Shapeways and are created by three designers:

* Efferman: *http://www.shapeways.com/designer/efferman/*
* SevenStuds: *http://www.shapeways.com/designer/sevenstuds/*
* stop4stuff: *http://www.shapeways.com/designer/stop4stuff/*

3D printing is still something of an art, and new designers and artists are always pushing the boundaries of creative problem solving. Elements printed by other vendors will behave differently, so it's best to read reviews by LEGO builders who use particular vendors and check out the Resources page at *https://www.nostarch.com/technicbuilder2/* for links to recommended vendors.

modifying existing designs

The first category of 3D-printed LEGO designs is elements that are just slight modifications of existing LEGO pieces. Figures 22-3 to 22-6 demonstrate that you can make entirely new things possible by slightly modifying the size of common LEGO pieces or by changing some angles and adding a bit here or there.

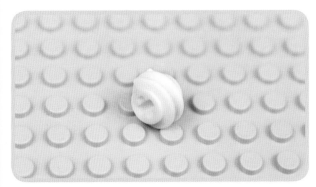

Figure 22-3: This worm gear by Efferman is a great example of a slight but useful modification of an original LEGO piece: it's half as long as LEGO worm gears, and it's profiled to fit double-bevel gears.

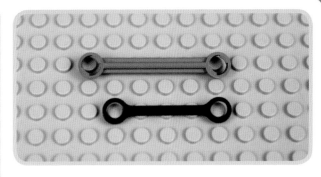

Figure 22-4: LEGO makes 5- and 6-stud steering arms but only 6-stud steering links (top). That's where a custom 5-stud steering link by Efferman (bottom) can come in handy.

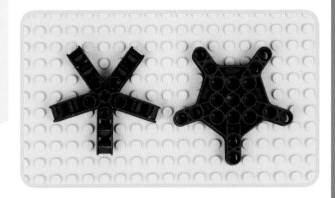

Figure 22-5: LEGO doesn't make 5-sided connectors. So if you're building, for example, a helicopter model with a 5-blade rotor, you might want to consider custom connectors like these by Efferman (left) and SevenStuds (right).

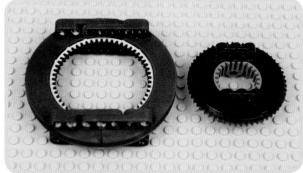

Figure 22-6: This 11-stud-wide turntable by Efferman (left) is essentially a bigger version of the regular 7-stud-wide LEGO Technic turntable (right). The design was printed in three separate pieces (a bottom plate and the top in two halves) and then joined together, whereas the LEGO version consists of two pieces (bottom and top). The gear's white sections are where the plastic has been filed to make the parts fit together better.

complementary LEGO pieces

You can also create counterparts to go with traditional LEGO pieces. For example, differentials and hubcaps are shown in Figures 22-7 to 22-10. These play the same role as already manufactured pieces, but they're miniaturized or specialized, in the case of differentials, and modeled after specific cars, in the case of hubcaps.

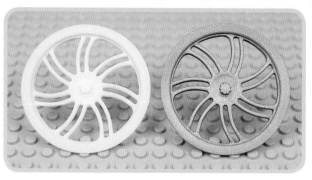

Figure 22-9: The Pagani Huayra hubcaps by SevenStuds are made to fit LEGO Technic Racing Medium rims. The printing is done in pure white plastic (left). Applying the Metallic Steel Revell paint makes the grainy surface more noticeable (right). The two caps are mirrored copies of each other, just like the left and right hubcaps on a real car.

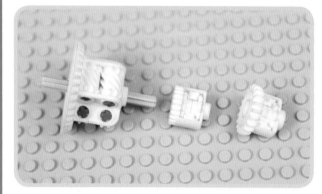

Figure 22-7: Custom differentials by Efferman. On the left is a Torsen (torque-sensitive) differential with helical gears. The other two are regular differentials miniaturized to fit in smaller bracings.

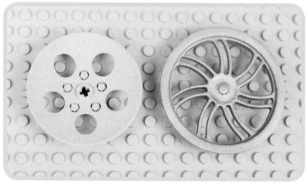

Figure 22-10: The Lamborghini Countach hubcap by Efferman (left) and the Pagani Huayra hubcap by SevenStuds (right). The Countach cap has a Metallic Plastic finish applied by Shapeways, which looks a bit flaky, and the Huayra cap has been hand painted with Revell paint.

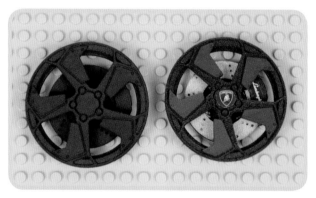

Figure 22-8: The Lamborghini Reventon hubcap by SevenStuds is made to fit LEGO Technic Racing Medium rims. It comes straight from the printer with a black finish (left), and you can apply paint and custom stickers to make it look authentic (right).

third-party adapters

You can also create adapters that allow you to connect LEGO elements to other objects. For example, you can make GoPro camera mounts (see Figure 22-11) or screws for RC wheels. You can even make a cap that connects to a regular soda bottle, allowing you to create a custom airtank, as shown in Figure 22-12.

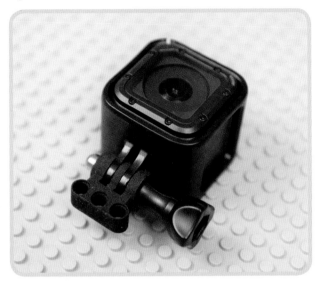

Figure 22-11: This simple custom connector by SevenStuds connects to a GoPro camera mount. It's a great example of a custom element that's small, simple, and cheap yet extremely useful.

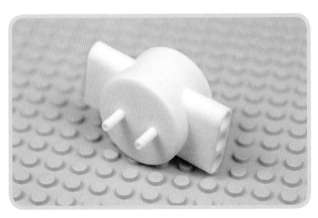

Figure 22-12: This unusual element by stop4stuff is a bottle cap that connects to pins and has two ports for LEGO pneumatic hoses. It allows you to easily use a regular bottle as a custom airtank or as a pressure pump for LEGO pneumatics.

specialized real-world designs

Additionally, there are highly specialized elements that replicate real-world mechanical solutions. These elements introduce certain designs that LEGO chose to omit, such as helical gears (see Figure 22-13), realistic boat propellers (see Figure 22-14), and shock absorbers designed to be stretched rather than compressed (see Figures 22-15 and 22-16).

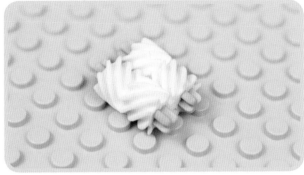

Figure 22-13: These small helical gears by Efferman present a real-world design that is missing from the LEGO world. They are superior to the spur and bevel gears that LEGO makes because their teeth engage gradually. They work smoothly and quietly, and are well suited for high-load applications. By using a combination of "left" and "right" helical gear pieces, you can create double helical gears, as shown here, which perform even better.

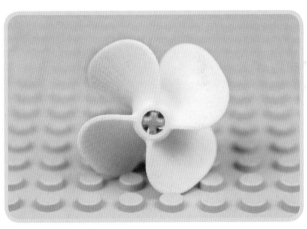

Figure 22-14: This 5-stud-wide propeller by Efferman is modeled after propellers on modern boats. Its efficient profile allows it to outperform similarly sized LEGO propellers.

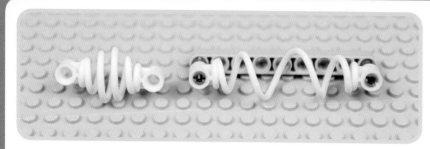

Figure 22-15: Plastic used for printing is less dense and thus more elastic than the plastic used in LEGO pieces—a property Efferman used to its advantage when creating this custom spring. It's very soft and easily stretched but prone to fatigue, and its shape can be altered by prolonged stress.

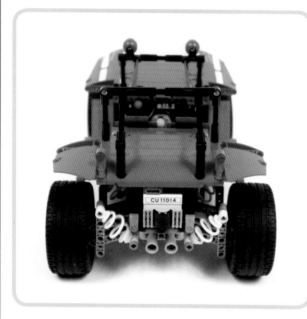

Figure 22-16: A simple buggy I built to test Efferman's springs. Note the unusual rear suspension design: The springs need to be stretched, not compressed like LEGO shock absorbers. The suspension proved very soft and responsive, but its load capacity was limited.

the downsides of 3D printing

You now have some idea of what you can create with 3D-printing technology and for what purpose. But how do the custom elements compare to the original LEGO pieces? Enthusiasts of 3D printing like to boast that the two are equivalent, but in my experience, this is still far from being true. The 3D-printed elements can be surprisingly high quality, and the technology is likely to continue to improve; however, because their manufacturing process differs drastically from that of the LEGO pieces, so do their properties.

3D-printed elements have some serious drawbacks, described here in detail.

difficult to fit with LEGO pieces

Although the dimensions of the LEGO pieces are well-known, it's not easy to transfer them to 3D-printed elements due to 3D-printing tolerances. Because elements are printed individually, one after another, they are sensitive to changes, such as in temperature or humidity, during the printing process. Professional vendors usually print in a carefully controlled environment, but even so, several copies of the same element made on one printer may have slight variations, and the same design printed by another printer can produce very different results. The printing process also involves hot plastic, which shrinks a little as it cools. The dimensions can be further changed by polishing a piece or applying a finish.

Some LEGO standards have a lower tolerance than others: For example, it's usually easy to correctly print a pin hole, but an axle hole is notoriously difficult to get right, even for experienced designers. Consider the boat propeller in Figure 22-14: I actually had to hammer a LEGO axle into it.

difficult to fit with each other

A file is a 3D printer's best friend, not only for fitting custom elements with LEGO pieces, but also for fitting them with each other. In my experience, basically any multipart custom element, such as the large turntable in Figure 22-6 and the Torsen differential in Figure 22-7, requires a healthy dose of filing just to start working, even though they were specifically designed to fit each other and were made by the same printer. The surface of custom elements is grainy and porous, so it generates some friction when it comes in contact with smooth LEGO pieces and even more friction when it comes in contact with other custom elements.

grainy, rough, and ugly

LEGO pieces are so smooth, you can see your own reflection in them. Custom 3D-printed elements, as noted above, are grainy and porous, and their rough surface becomes clearly visible when coated in paint, especially a shiny paint (see Figure 22-10). You can instantly distinguish custom elements from LEGO pieces by touch, and the printed pieces look ugly in any color other than pure white. Certain vendors, such as Shapeways, print in premium materials, such as nylon, which is smoother and less porous than plastic, but those elements come at an additional cost and still have some printing marks on the surface (see Figure 22-17).

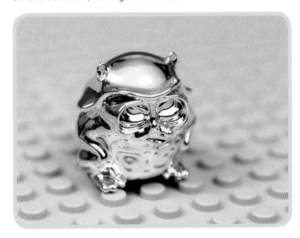

Figure 22-17: This small hamster figurine by SevenStuds was printed by Shapeways in nylon at an "extreme detail" level and cost nearly €25. Although it was manufactured with the highest possible quality, the figurine's surface retained some printing marks. It was then custom chromed by Chrome Block City six times to make it perfectly smooth.

prone to wear

The custom elements are generally impressively hard, especially given that they weigh so little. But the plastic they're made of is less dense than the plastic in LEGO pieces, simply because of the different manufacturing process. With 3D printing, plastic is added bit by bit, whereas LEGO pieces are made by injecting plastic into molds under pressure. The 3D-printing process makes custom elements brittle and prone to signs of early wear. Consider the wheels in Figure 22-18, both of which are made from plastic: The custom wheel, being less dense, wears down very fast, while the LEGO wheel shows hardly any visible wear. The difference is even more apparent because the custom wheel is printed in

white plastic coated in black, and as it wears down, the coat starts to rub away. In contrast, the LEGO wheel is cast in black plastic, so there is nothing to rub away.

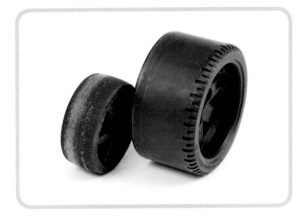

Figure 22-18: 3D-printed parts may not stand up to nearly as much wear and tear as regular LEGO pieces. A custom drifting wheel by SevenStuds (left) is shown after roughly one hour of use next to a LEGO 68.8 mm solid plastic wheel (right) after roughly three months of use.

sensitive to water

3D-printed plastic is not watertight. It's not exactly leaky, but water will seep through its porous structure. To make matters worse, the colored finishes that Shapeways applies use a water-based dye; as a result, prolonged exposure to water can make the color come off the custom elements. In addition, pure white elements without any finish can be yellowed by contact with human skin.

almost impossible to chrome

The process of custom chroming, which I'll discuss fully in Chapter 25, involves baking pieces at 80°C (176°F). For many 3D-printing materials, including those printed by Shapeways, that temperature is dangerously close to their melting point. Because of the low density and porosity of the 3D-printed plastic, a certain amount of air is trapped inside custom elements, and this air is exuded during the baking process, ruining the chrome film on the element's surface. When experimenting with chroming a 3D-printed figurine, shown in Figure 22-17, it took *six* repetitions of the chroming process to get its surface smooth. For a larger element with a greater volume of air inside, this would probably still be insufficient to produce a smooth surface.

expensive to make

When printing with your own 3D printer, you're limited by its dimensions and the amount of plastic available to you. When using a vendor to print, you're not limited but are charged for these two factors, which are called *machine space* and *material volume*, respectively. To make a long story short, the larger the printed item, the more expensive it is. In fact, I was forced to abandon a number of projects because of the printing costs alone, even for relatively thin or small elements such as custom rotor blades and paddle wheels. There are ways to minimize the material volume, but there is no escaping the machine space cost. It can be 10 times more expensive to create a custom 3D-printed element than to use a LEGO piece, even a rare one.

getting started with 3D printing

With the knowledge you now have of some of the possibilities and drawbacks of 3D printing, let's consider how to do it. To get started, you have two options: buy your own desktop 3D printer or print with a vendor.

printing your own

The first option, printing your own elements, is definitely more difficult than the second option, because it's up to you to learn to work with the printer you've purchased and the risk of failure when creating your first elements is high. But this approach is more cost-effective in the long run if you intend to print often. Also, it has the added benefit that printed elements are available to you instantly. Because many new printers are released every year, any review that I would have included in this book would have quickly become outdated. It's best to read reviews of new printers as they pop up on the market and ask for advice among the members of 3D-design communities. A good place to start is at Thingiverse (*http://www.thingiverse.com/*), which focuses on helping beginners.

working with a vendor

The second option, working with a vendor, is much simpler and is initially cheaper: You submit your own design or buy someone else's, and a specialized vendor prints it for you. It's a better option if you just want to see whether 3D printing is suitable for you or if you want to test a few elements now and then. The vendor provides the hardware, handles the printing process, and ships the resulting elements to you. The pros include a low risk of failure (the vendor ensures that printing goes smoothly, and commercially available designs are usually well tested), low startup costs (no hardware investment and no maintenance), and exceptional ease of use (ordering elements is no different from regular online shopping, and the products are shipped to you). The cons are long waiting times (popular vendors' factory queues can span up to several weeks plus shipping time) and higher costs over the long run (vendor's fee plus designer's fee if you buy someone else's design).

Note that at the time of this writing, vendors still have a technological advantage: The printing technology they use (laser sintering) is not yet available for desktop printers. Several vendors are worth considering. The dominant one is Shapeways (*http://www.shapeways.com/*), which has factories in Queens, Seattle, and Eindhoven, making its services easily available in the United States and Europe. Shapeways is known for its excellent customer service and its popularity with designers, which translates into a wide range of commercially available designs. However, its popularity means long wait times. Shapeways is also one of the few vendors that offers finishes for printed elements.

Alternative vendors based in Europe include i.materialise (*http://www.i.materialise.com/*), which offers printing in multiple materials, finishes, and online shopping by design; MeltWerk (*http://www.meltwerk.com/*), which is known for its low prices but doesn't sell any designs; and Sculpteo (*http://www.sculpteo.com/*), which offers high quality at high prices.

PART V

models

23

form vs. function

Builders are usually inspired to create their own models for two reasons: the desire to model a real-life object (like a favorite car or truck) or the desire to model a real-life mechanism or function (for example, a 4×4 drive or a pneumatic system). If you're inspired by mechanisms, just look for models that could include one. When you decide to build a model, you'll want to start by asking yourself three questions:

1. Can I make it work well?

2. Can I make it look good?

3. Can I find sufficient reference material to accurately model this object?

Finding a balance between the aesthetics and functionality of the model is an extremely sensitive task, and it often helps to decide which is more important to you before you start building. As you build and rebuild your models, you'll likely reexamine your priorities. It's best to accept one of two options before you even start building: *I can compromise the look in favor of functionality*, or *I can compromise functionality in favor of the look*.

Looking at the silhouette of the object you want to model may also help in the early stages. Bear in mind that most LEGO pieces fit well within straight lines, right angles, and rectangular shapes. This makes trucks much easier to build than motorbikes, for example. You can, of course, use flexible axles and Technic panels to model curved, flowing shapes, but the resulting aesthetic is generally poorly received outside the Technic community and sometimes within it, as well.

cars

Your typical car is challenging to model because of the limited space it provides for electric and mechanical components (see Figure 23-1). Big elements, such as power supplies, IR receivers, and motors, are difficult to incorporate into a car.

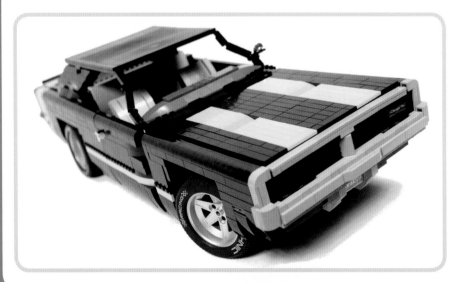

Figure 23-1: My 1969 Dodge Charger model appears to have a massive hood with plenty of space beneath it. However, since I decided to model the car's huge engine, almost none of this space was available for mechanical components, and I was barely able to fit a mechanism to lift the distinctive grille that reveals the car's headlamps. Most of the electric components ended up in the trunk.

In most cases, the only spaces available for those elements are the cabin floor, the central space between the seats, the trunk, and the space normally taken by the engine (if you choose not to include a replica of the engine in your MOC). You can also build a motor-free model, with all the functions activated manually, in the spirit of many LEGO sets.

Space constraints become even more challenging with sports cars, which are slung low to the ground and often have open tops, exposing any mechanism installed in the cabin. Cars of this type often use wide tires and independent suspensions, which can result in width issues if you decide to include both in your model. Finally, as sports cars' engines are particularly huge, choosing between a front-engine and central-engine car greatly affects the amount of space available in the front and in the rear, as well as the silhouette of the model. Figure 23-2 shows an extreme example of this, comparing a front-engine Dodge Viper and a rear-engine Pagani Zonda. Note how the silhouettes of the cars differ—the Viper's cabin is moved far back, adjacent to the rear wheels, while the Zonda's cabin starts just behind the front wheels. Both cars, although similar in many respects, offer different challenges and opportunities to a model builder.

Off-road cars, such as SUVs, have taller silhouettes and offer more space, especially in the chassis, but they also have more complex and space-consuming drivetrains and suspension systems. Their engines are usually under the hood, as in the Jeep Wrangler Rubicon shown in Figure 23-3. And many SUVs have hard-top bodies, making it possible to use some of the cabin's internal space (but also making the car more top-heavy).

Finally, there are cars such as buggies and truggies, whose bodies are built primarily with pipes and whose internal elements are exposed, as shown in Figure 23-4. There are many ways to install elements of the Power Functions system, such as motors and battery boxes, in these cars so as to mimic the original cars' fuel tanks and other parts.

trucks

Trucks have many qualities that make them easy to model, and they are one of the favorite themes of model builders. They are technically simple to build, and they offer plenty of space for internal components and many possibilities for experimenting with aesthetics. They are also often large enough to conceal even very complex mechanisms—for example, my tow truck model housed 17 motors.

Trucks can be divided into two categories with different appearances and different amounts of space available: longnose (or US) trucks and cab-over-engine (or European) trucks. Longnose trucks, which are designed to travel over longer distances, have a hood (or bonnet) with the engine in front of the cabin. They often have a sleeper module behind the cabin—that is, a simple structure adjacent to the cabin, where the driver can sleep or relax (see Figure 23-5). The cab-over-engine variant is generally smaller and more compact with, naturally, a simple cabin over the engine. European-style trucks have no hoods, and the optional resting space for the driver is located inside the rear part of the cabin rather than in a separate body module.

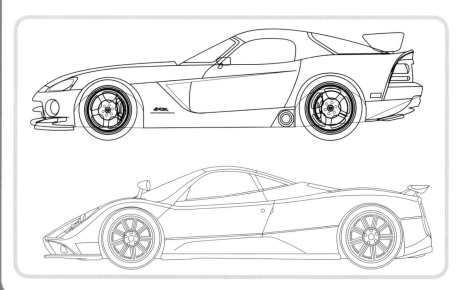

Figure 23-2: The Dodge Viper (top) and Pagani Zonda (bottom) are two sports cars with different engine locations.

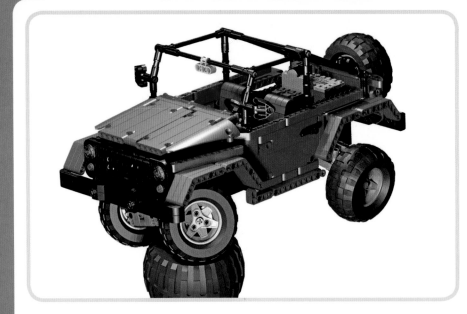

Figure 23-3: My model of the Jeep Wrangler Rubicon, which is a small open-top car, had motors under the hood and had the battery and IR receiver in the trunk. This way it had a good weight distribution and plenty of space left for some decorative elements in the cabin interior, including seats and the steering wheel.

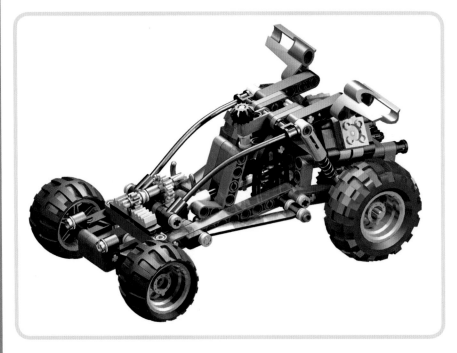

Figure 23-4: The 8296 set features a simple dune buggy with a typical pipebuilt body.

Note that trucks of both categories usually have *air deflectors* on top of the cabin. In longnose trucks, however, the sleeper modules may have their own extensive air deflectors that direct the air flow between the cabin and the trailer. With cab-over-engine trucks, the deflectors appear only on the cabin and may be quite tall to compensate for the difference in height between the cabin and the trailer, as shown in Figure 23-6.

Longnose trucks definitely have more advantages for model builders: They offer more internal space, especially with the addition of a sleeper module, and there are more ways to experiment with their aesthetics. Note that in the trucks with no hood—longnose and cab-over-engine alike—the engine is accessed by lifting up the cabin, which tilts forward. This is difficult to include in a model, and engines are often omitted completely from the models of

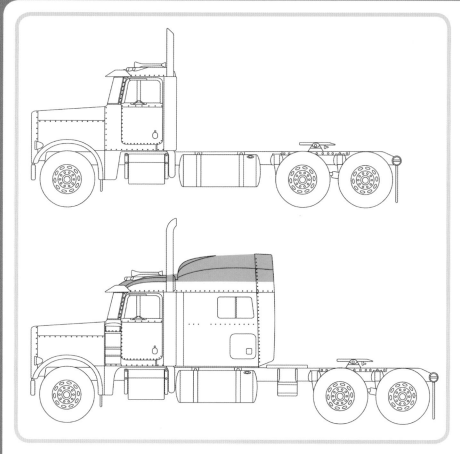

Figure 23-5: The longnose Peterbilt truck, shown without the sleeper module (top) and with sleeper module (bottom). The air deflector is marked with orange.

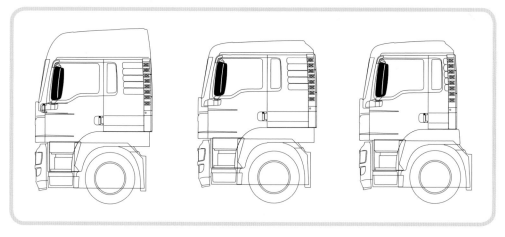

Figure 23-6: Three cabin variants of the same European MAN TGS truck (from left to right): with tall airfoil and resting space, with low airfoil and resting space, with low airfoil and no resting space

cab-over-engine trucks, especially since engines use space that is best suited for the steering system. Trucks with hoods, on the other hand, can have working hoods with replicas of the engine beneath, and this still leaves plenty of space below the cabin for steering mechanisms. As Figure 23-7 shows, the space under the hood can be used to create a fairly complex engine replica, as well as to house some electric components.

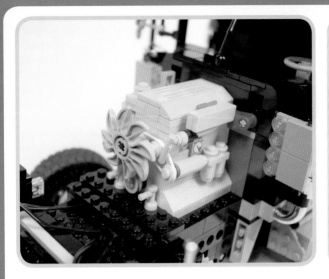

Figure 23-7: The hood of my tow truck model housed a replica of the original Caterpillar engine and a Power Functions battery, located between the engine and the front of the cabin. The red connector piece adjacent to the engine functioned as the model's master power switch.

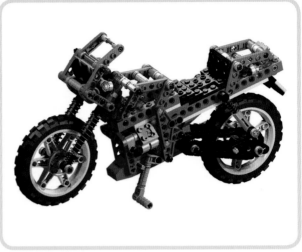

Figure 23-8: The 8422 set features a typical motorcycle with a suspension system and a piston engine connected to the real wheel. Note that even though the model uses one of the largest LEGO wheels in existence, it's still rather small.

motorcycles

Motorcycles, like the one shown in Figure 23-8, are very challenging to model for a number of reasons—the most important one being the fact that they have only two wheels. In order to stand on its own, a model requires at least three wheels (or wide, flat tires). To enable a motorcycle model to stand on its own, you can add a small, unobtrusive wheel or a full sidecar. Sidecars have the advantage of offering plenty of internal space near the bike's rear wheel, so they can be used to house a propulsion motor. Another alternative is to build a trike or a quad, which is something like a four-wheeled bike.

Other difficulties you may encounter while building bikes include motorizing the steering system, the limited variety and size of matching LEGO wheels, and the overall small size and exposed body, which make it difficult to install any large electric components. All in all, motorcycles are aesthetically interesting models to build but difficult ones to motorize. Among the LEGO sets, as well as among MOCs, most motorcycles have only basic functions, such as a suspension system and drivetrain with a replica of an engine, while motorized models are a rarity. For an example of a motorized model, see Figure 23-9.

tracked vehicles

Tracked vehicles are a diverse group, but they are almost always fairly easy to model. First of all, the use of the tracks eliminates the need for any complex steering system (unless we decide to use a subtractor). Secondly, the suspension system is located either on the sides or on the bottom of the hull, taking little or no space inside the model, as shown in Figure 23-10. In fact, the hull of most tracked vehicles is a simple box with tracks on its sides and plenty of space inside, and it also functions as a body frame.

Tanks have large hulls whose space can be arranged in several ways. After building plenty of tank models, I have developed a reliable arrangement: The propulsion motors go in the lower-rear part of the hull, with IR receivers on top of them. For modern tanks with large turrets, the receivers have to be moved to the very rear end of the hull to avoid being blotted out. The central part of the hull can house the power supply with the turret rotation mechanism on top of it. The front part can be used for the power supply as well, but not for the IR receivers, as the models are typically controlled from behind. The turret itself can house the gun control

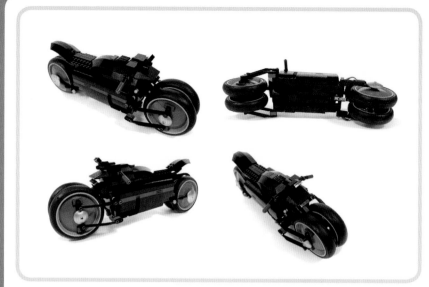

Figure 23-9: The Dodge Tomahawk concept motorcycle comes with double front and rear wheels, thus providing four fulcrums rather than two. I built a motorized model of this bike to prove that it could be motorized and drive stably; however, it couldn't turn because it was too small to house a steering system and a propulsion system at the same time.

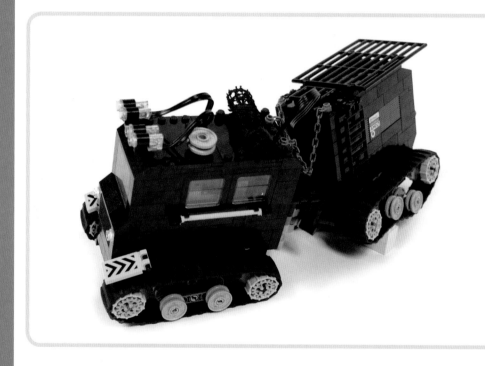

Figure 23-10: The Swedish Hagglunds BV 206 personnel carrier consisted of two parts connected by an articulated joint. This very tiny model housed one steering and two propulsion motors, a battery, and an IR receiver, while its simple suspension was located entirely within the tracks.

mechanism, but it's also a good, well-exposed place for the IR receivers if it's tall enough to house them. See examples of tanks I have modeled in Figures 23-11 and 23-12.

You might also want to model half-track vehicles, which have regular steered front wheels and tracks replacing the rear wheels, as shown in Figure 23-13. This rare combination is used almost exclusively in military vehicles, such as trucks and armored personnel carriers. Most of the vehicle, including the cabin, the front axle, and the engine bay, needs no alteration from a wheeled version, while the tracks need no steering system, as steering is provided by the front wheels. Some of the heaviest historical half-tracks, however, included a braking system that slowed one of the tracks while turning to improve handling of the vehicle.

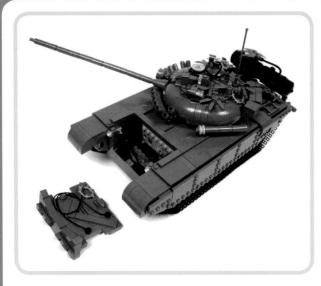

Figure 23-11: My T-72M tank model was small and low, with an angled glacis plate that left very little space in the front of the hull. The very front of the hull housed only some wires, and the glacis plate was removed to access the battery.

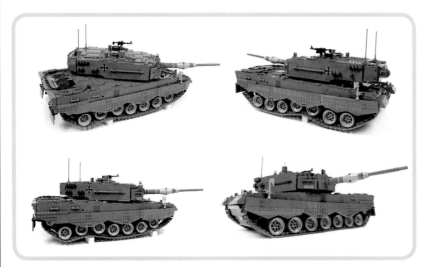

Figure 23-12: My model of the Leopard 2A4 tank was large and heavy. I used four XL motors for propulsion, powered from two battery boxes located in the middle of the hull. It wasn't fast, but it had plenty of torque and handled obstacles extremely well for its weight.

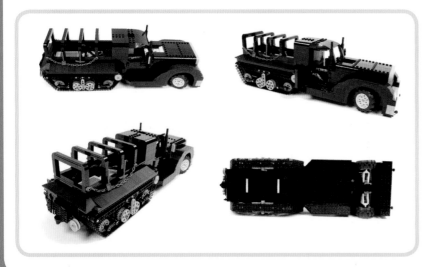

Figure 23-13: My model of a half-track truck. Vehicles of this type are driven by tracks and steered by front wheels.

aircraft

Modeling aircraft offers plenty of intriguing possibilities and challenges. Such vehicles can be motorized to have rotating propellers or turbines. They can also have working ailerons, elevators, and rudders, as well as retractable gears and flashing position lights. But LEGO aircraft can't fly.

NOTE Building a 100 percent LEGO plane or helicopter capable of flying is physically impossible because of the weight of LEGO pieces and the limited power of LEGO motors. Additionally, an aircraft built exclusively with LEGO pieces would have difficulties with balance and with achieving an aerodynamic profile.

Any aircraft you model can be made even more impressive when installed on a boom that can lift it up and move it around, imitating free flight. The 8485 set includes such a model, shown in Figure 23-14.

planes

One of the main challenges involved in building a model of a plane is the shape of its hull. A plane hull's cross section is more or less circular. You can model it with studfull pieces using curved slopes, or you can just mark some edges of the hull with flexible axles. The wings and tail can be modeled with slopes, plates, and tiles, or with axles or even bricks and beams if you mark only the edges, as Figure 23-15 shows.

Minifigure-scale planes can use the ready-made tails, noses, and hull sections that can be found in regular LEGO sets.

Your model can also take advantage of one of the large number of ready-made LEGO propellers, shown in Figure 23-16. These propellers can work in air as well as in water, and when motorized, some of them can generate thrust that is noticeable, though still insufficient for flying.

With jet engines, it's relatively easy to create mock-ups of turbines that can rotate. Figure 23-17 shows a simple example of a mock-up built around a 4-stud-long bar. You can also use LEGO LEDs with translucent red or translucent orange pieces to illuminate the engine's nozzle. Installing a small LEGO propeller inside a duct with a round cross section can generate more thrust than when the same propeller works outside the duct.

helicopters

Helicopters are generally easier to model than planes. They have dense hulls, tiny wings or no wings at all, and a single boom with a tail rotor. They offer plenty of internal space and often include more functions than planes do: Some helicopters come with winches to lift loads off the ground, some come with retractable gear, and even the simplest helicopters have large rotating blades that look impressive when motorized.

When it comes to modeling a helicopter, the primary challenges are the windscreen, which has a complex shape in some machines, and the rotors. A typical helicopter comes with a single main rotor with two to six blades and a single

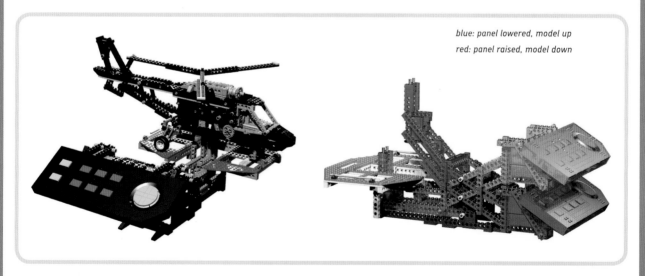

blue: panel lowered, model up
red: panel raised, model down

Figure 23-14: The 8485 Control Center II set features a large helicopter on a simple boom (left). By manually lowering the control panel (right), which acts as the helicopter's counterbalance on the boom, we can lift the model up and simulate the movement of free flight—for example, the tilting of the hull.

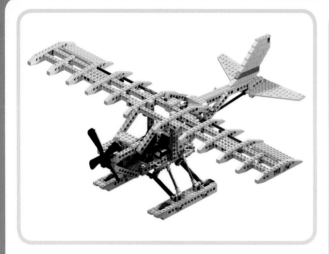

Figure 23-15: The 8855 Prop Plane set is a fairly typical example of a Technic plane. It has no motors and just basic functions, with parts such as ailerons and elevators controlled by a single yoke.

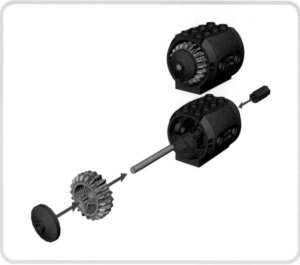

Figure 23-17: One of many ways to build a small mock-up of a turbine engine with just a few LEGO pieces. The axle joiner (blue) allows us to connect the central bar to a regular axle and thus motorize the "turbine."

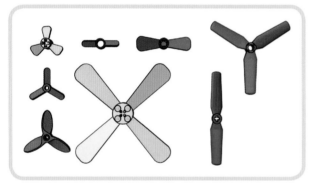

Figure 23-16: The LEGO ready-made propellers with pin holes (red) and axle holes (yellow), along with the #2952 propeller (blue), which can be used in pairs to create a 1-stud-thick, four-bladed propeller

tail rotor with two to four blades. Figure 23-18 provides an example of a helicopter with a six-bladed main rotor, which helps the aircraft handle its weight. Some helicopters, such as the Kamov Ka-50 Hokum, come with two main rotors and no tail rotor. The two rotors rotate in opposite directions, and if they are coaxial—which is not always the case, as Figure 23-19 shows—modeling them can be an interesting technical challenge.

The tail rotor is usually located on one side of the tail fin. In some helicopters, however, it is mounted inside an opening in the fin. Such a design, shown in Figure 23-20, is called a *fantail*, and rotors used in it are smaller and have

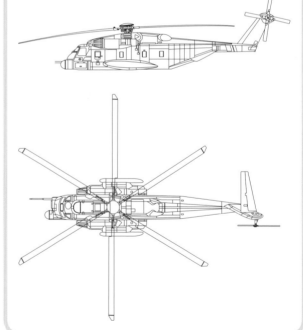

Figure 23-18: The Sikorsky MH-53 Pave Low is a massive military transport helicopter. Its six-bladed main rotor helps to handle its weight, which can reach 21 tons when the chopper fully loaded.

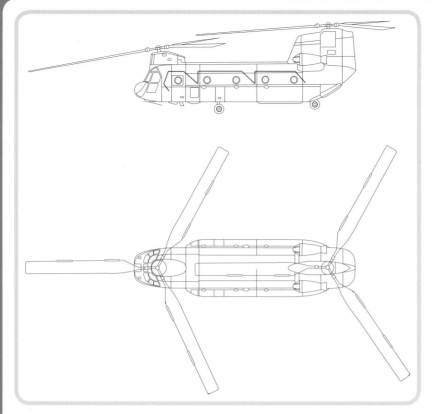

Figure 23-19: The Boeing CH-47 Chinook also comes with two main rotors, located at opposite ends of the hull and at different heights. Such an arrangement is called a tandem.

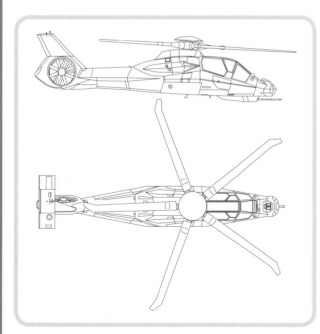

Figure 23-20: The Boeing Sikorsky RAH-66 Comanche was designed to be an advanced reconnaissance and attack helicopter. It used a fantail instead of a typical rear rotor, and the complex shape of its hull resulted from incorporating stealth technologies.

between 8 and 18 blades. It's very difficult to properly model a fantail because there is no easy way to mount and drive a LEGO rotor inside it.

The real main rotor head of any helicopter is an advanced mechanism, allowing adjustments to the pitch of its individual blades or all blades together to weather conditions. This enables the vehicle to perform complex movements, such as flying backward or sideways. A simple mechanical solution allowing the rotor to tilt forward and backward or left and right is shown in Figure 23-21. Tilting the rotor in multiple planes is also possible with the use of towballs and links, as shown in Figure 23-22.

The rotor itself consists of a rotor hub with blades attached around it. The blades can easily be built with plates and tiles or with ready-made pieces from the 9396 Helicopter set, though building the rotor hub to connect these blades can be more difficult. Figures 23-23 to 23-25 show example hubs, with short red plates noting blade placement.

Now that you've seen the possibilities and challenges of different vehicle types, it's up to you to choose what to model. Assuming that you have a model in mind ready to scale, proceed to Chapter 24, which explains how to model it accurately.

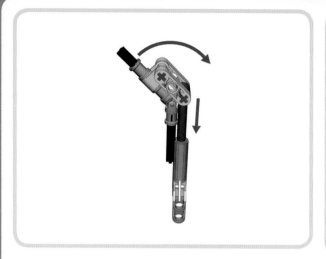

Figure 23-21: An example of a simple rotor-tilting mechanism. The black axles with a universal joint are the driveshaft, connecting the rotor on the top with a motor on the bottom. Retracting and extending the linear actuator changes the angle of the axle above the joint and thus of the whole rotor.

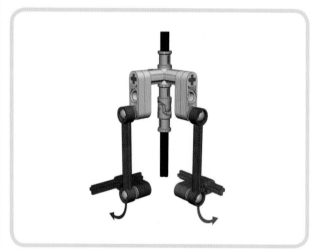

Figure 23-22: A mechanism for tilting a rotor in two planes. Rotating the green axle tilts the rotor in one plane—for example, forward and backward—while rotating the blue axle tilts the rotor in another plane—for example, left and right. Thanks to the use of links and towballs, both angles of the rotor can be changed simultaneously without interference.

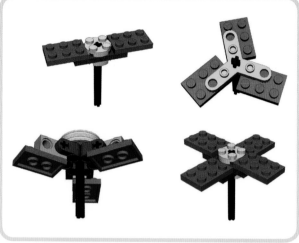

Figure 23-23: Simple hubs with two to four blades

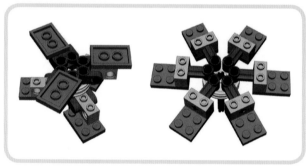

Figure 23-24: A six-bladed hub can be built by doubling the three-bladed version or by simply attaching the blades to a wedge belt wheel with pins so that the centrifugal force of the rotating rotor aligns them.

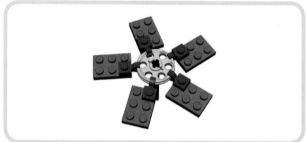

Figure 23-25: Finally, a hub with any number of blades can be built by attaching 1×1 plates with clips to the edge of a wedge belt wheel. This solution, invented by Polish builder Marcin "Mrutek" Rutkowski, results in a surprisingly robust setup, which can be made even stronger if you attach blades using two wedge belt wheels and two clips. You will, however, need to align the blades by hand, so a protractor may be useful.

24

scaling a model

Scaling is a fairly straightforward process requiring simple multiplication and division. To begin, we need two things: a *blueprint* of the original object and a *point of reference* that will determine the resulting size of our model.

blueprints

A blueprint is a technical drawing that typically includes a front, side, rear, and top view, as Figure 24-1 shows. We'll want to find blueprints whose views show the object at the same scale.

A proper blueprint shows only the important edges of the object, without any filling, shading, colors, or textures. Figure 24-2 shows the same object with and without the central perspective—that is, a "vanishing point." As you can see, perspective can distort the image and thus affect the measurements we take from it.

Where do you find blueprints? The best free source is *http://www.the-blueprints.com/*. If you can't find the blueprint you need there, you can check LEGO MOCs websites, like *http://www.brickshelf.com/* and *http://moc-pages.com/*, as some builders publish their MOCs along with the blueprints they used. If you plan to model construction equipment, such as

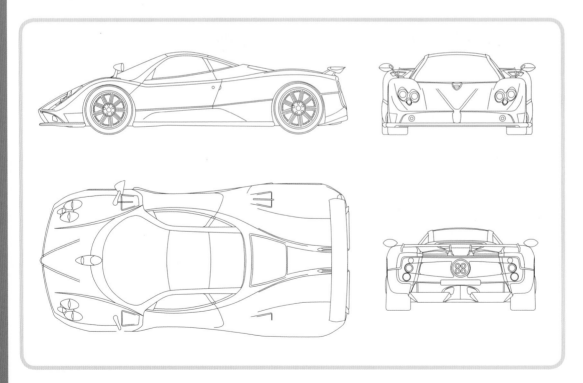

Figure 24-1: A typical blueprint showing the Pagani Zonda C12 F sports car

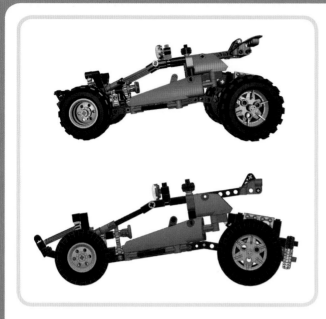

Figure 24-2: Side view of the same model with central perspective (top) and without central perspective (bottom)

excavators, dump trucks, and so on, you can check the website of the original machine's manufacturer. Many major manufacturers, such as Caterpillar, JCB, Komatsu, Liebherr, and Volvo, publish product brochures, usually as PDF files, that include a blueprint showing a machine's dimensions in at least two views. Alternatively, you can look for 3D models—some vehicles are popular with 3D artists, who often present their work on the Internet in a blueprint-like form. Model-building kits can also be a source of high-quality blueprints, as their instructions often include painting diagrams that look exactly like blueprints. For example, Revell offers many instructions for free (*http://www.revell.com/support/instructions.html*).

As a last resort, you can use photographs in place of a blueprint. The ideal set of photos shows the entire unobstructed vehicle from direct angles, preferably from a distance. The photos should obviously be as large, clean, and bright as possible, and they should be scaled to show the object at the same size from various angles. Figures 24-3 and 24-4 provide examples of unusable and usable photos, respectively.

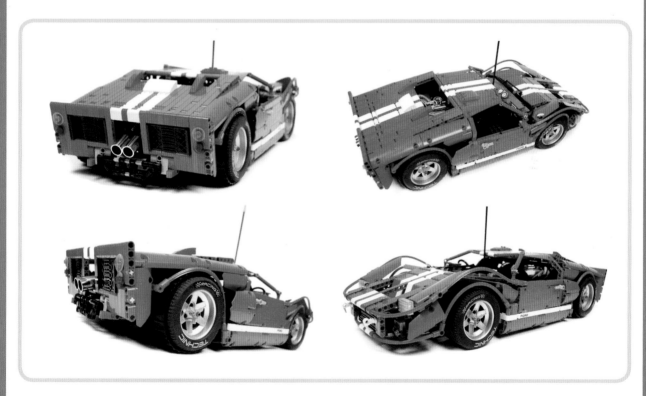

Figure 24-3: These photos can't be used in place of a blueprint. They show the object from mixed angles (for example, rear/side), and they are highly distorted by perspective, as a result of having been taken from a short distance.

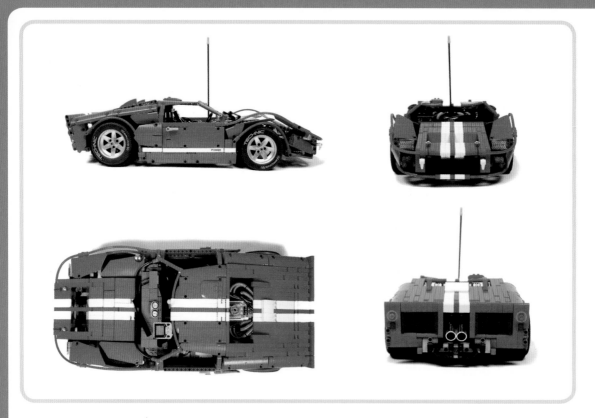

Figure 24-4: These photos are perfectly usable in place of a blueprint. They present the object from direct angles, and they are taken from far enough away that the images are not distorted.

points of reference

A *point of reference* is a constituent part that determines the size of a model. We use it to calculate how much smaller (or larger) than the original object the model has to be. Basically, we need some part in our model whose size can be compared with the size of its real counterpart. For wheeled vehicles, comparing wheels—or, more specifically, the diameter of tires—works best. Because LEGO wheels have a fixed size, we can easily scale the rest of our model to be the appropriate size.

The general rule of thumb for any build is to select the vehicle's most specialized part. Since we can't adjust the size of LEGO wheels, tracks, or propellers, we have to start with them as a reference point and then scale accordingly. Bear in mind other space constraints, like a vehicle's hull dimensions and your model's target functionality, as you work from your point of reference.

For tracked vehicles, we can use the width of the tracks as a reference point. This is an optimal reference point because a poor fit is usually more noticeable when it comes to track width than, for instance, the diameter of the sprocket wheels.

A helicopter model can be scaled using the ready-made LEGO propeller that will be used as the tail rotor. A jet plane model can be scaled using the cylindrical LEGO piece that will be used as the jet engine housing. And a boat can be scaled using a ready-made LEGO hull (these come in many variants, including watertight ones).

scaling

Let's assume we have a good blueprint of the vehicle we want to scale and we have chosen a LEGO wheel as our point of reference. Now we can begin the actual scaling. (Note that the following process works the same way regardless of the part we use as our reference point.)

We will be taking various measurements off the blueprint. We can do that directly in the blueprint file, measuring distances with a program such as GIMP or Windows Paint. When you open the file in Paint, for example, and draw a line, the dimensions of the line (in pixels) will be shown in the lower-right corner of the program window. By holding down the SHIFT key while drawing, you can make sure the line is perfectly horizontal or vertical. The other way to measure the blueprint is to print it out and simply use a ruler. Personally, I prefer this method, as it allows me to add notes to the printout, and it doesn't require using a computer every time I need to measure something. The notes on such a blueprint can become quite elaborate and include a great deal of information, as Figure 24-5 shows.

First, we have to determine the *scaling ratio*—the difference in dimensions between the blueprint and our model—which will allow us to calculate all of our model's target dimensions. We can do this by comparing the size of our point of reference—in this case, a LEGO wheel—with its counterpart on the blueprint.

Let's assume that we want to scale a Dodge Viper using a wheel from the 8448 Super Street Sensation set, which has a diameter of 10 studs. We begin by measuring the diameter of the wheel on a blueprint (indicated by the blue line in Figure 24-6), and the result is 28 mm. Now we divide the diameter of our LEGO wheel by the diameter of the wheel on the blueprint:

$$\frac{10 \text{ studs}}{28 \text{ mm}} = 0.357 \text{ studs/mm}$$

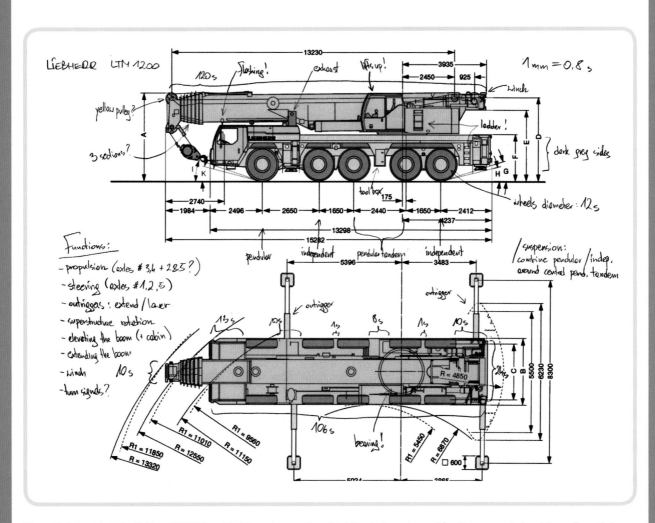

Figure 24-5: A printout of a Liebherr LTM1200 mobile telescopic crane blueprint. All basic dimensions and functions are marked, and the scaling ratio is noted in the upper-right corner. The blueprint comes from the manufacturer's product brochure.

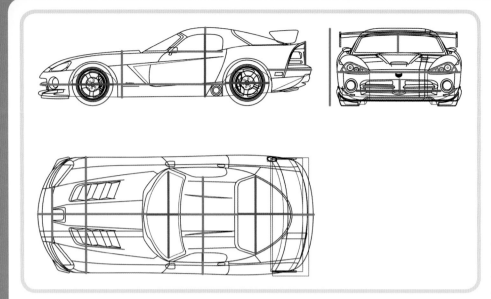

Figure 24-6: A Dodge Viper's blue-print with three views. Colored lines mark various dimensions that can be easily measured.

We can round this value to 0.36 studs/mm. This is our *scaling ratio*—it shows how many studs are equal to 1 mm on the blueprint:

$$1 \text{ mm} = 0.36 \text{ studs}$$

Now we can calculate any dimension of our LEGO model by measuring the corresponding dimension on the blueprint and multiplying it by the scaling ratio. For example, we can start with the width of the vehicle, which is 81 mm on the blueprint.

$$81 \text{ mm} \times 0.36 \text{ studs/mm} = 29.2 \text{ studs}$$

The width of my model should be 29 studs.
To summarize, we can calculate the scaling ratio, like so:

$$\text{Scaling Ratio} = \frac{\text{Dimension}_{\text{reference}}}{\text{Dimension}_{\text{blueprint}}}$$

And then we can use that ratio to calculate the model's width, height, and any other dimension we'd like, using this formula:

$$\text{Dimension}_{\text{model}} = \text{Dimension}_{\text{blueprint}} \times \text{Scaling Ratio}$$

Let's put the formula to work to see how wide the same model would have to be if I scaled it for smaller LEGO wheels (8 studs instead of 10 studs):

$$\text{Dimension}_{\text{reference}} = 8 \text{ studs}$$

$$\text{Dimension}_{\text{model}} = 81 \text{ mm} \times \left(\frac{8 \text{ studs}}{28 \text{ mm}} \right)$$
$$\approx 81 \text{ mm} \times 0.29 \text{ studs/mm}$$
$$\approx 23.49 \text{ studs}$$
$$\approx 23 \text{ studs}$$

And if I scaled for slightly bigger LEGO wheels:

$$\text{Dimension}_{\text{reference}} = 12 \text{ studs}$$

$$\text{Dimension}_{\text{model}} = 81 \text{ mm} \times \left(\frac{12 \text{ studs}}{28 \text{ mm}} \right)$$
$$\approx 81 \text{ mm} \times 0.43 \text{ studs/mm}$$
$$\approx 34.83 \text{ studs}$$
$$\approx 35 \text{ studs}$$

With the scaling ratio determined, we can proceed to take all the measurements we need from the blueprint. As Figure 24-6 shows, practically any object can be broken into a number of lines marking distances along the three basic dimensions: length, width, and depth.

For our Dodge Viper, the most important dimensions to calculate are the following:

* Total length, width, and height
* Height from the bottom of the body to the top of the cabin
* Height from the bottom of the side window to the top of the cabin
* Height from the bottom of the body to the top of the hood
* Length of the body behind the rear wheels
* Length of the body in front of the front wheels
* Distance between the front and rear wheels
* Length, width, and height of the windshield and all windows
* Length of the trunk and hood
* Length and width of the cabin roof
* Distance between the headlights
* Distance between the side window and the edge of the body
* Length and width of the front grille
* Height of the body's rear end above the bumper

Figures 24-7 to 24-9 show the most important dimensions of other types of vehicles.

Once you have your dimensions, it is possible to determine the *scale* of your model. To do this, we need to compare certain dimensions of the model with the dimensions of the original object using the same units. It's a good idea to check body width—it's one of the most important dimensions of any vehicle. Let's assume that I have built my Dodge Viper model 29 studs wide, as originally planned. Because 1 stud equals 8 mm, 29 studs equal 232 mm. According to Dodge, the body width of the real car is 1920 mm. Now, 1920 / 232 equals 8.276. We can round this number to 8, which makes 1:8 the scale of my Viper. In other words, my model is 8 times smaller than the real vehicle.

NOTE Before dividing, make sure you're using the same units for both dimensions.

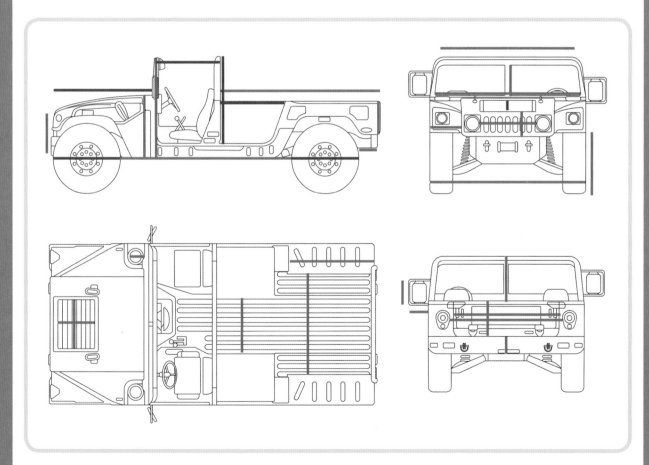

Figure 24-7: A blueprint of the Humvee with the core dimensions marked. The angular silhouette of this car is convenient for both measuring and modeling.

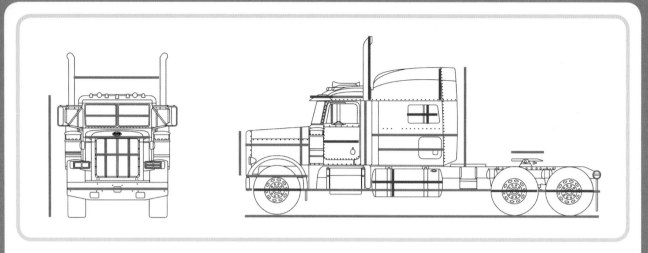

Figure 24-8: A blueprint of the Peterbilt 379 truck with the core dimensions marked. These include the dimensions of the airfoil, fifth wheel, hood, and side fuel tanks.

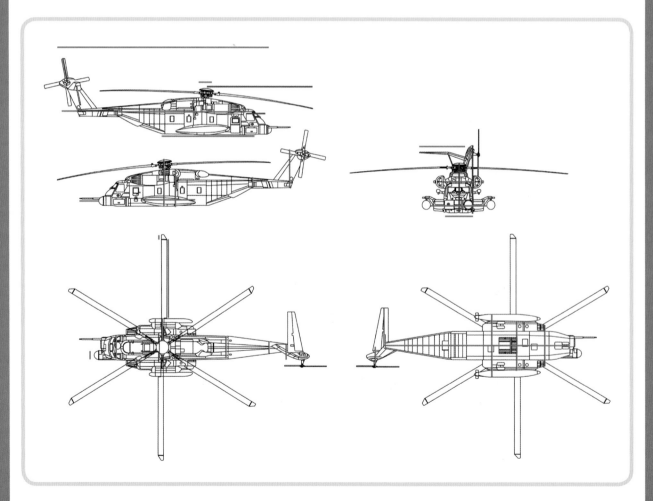

Figure 24-9: A blueprint of the Sikorsky MH-53 Pave Low helicopter with the core dimensions marked. These include the dimensions of the hull, tail boom, tail fin, both rotors, and main rotor hub.

Here is the formula for determining the scale of your models:

$$\text{Scale} = \frac{\text{Dimension}_{model}}{\text{Dimension}_{real}}$$

where

Dimension_{model} = the dimension on the model

Dimension_{real} = the same dimension on the real object

Sometimes you may want to build a model to an already determined scale. For example, you might want to build a model that matches the size of someone else's construction. Building a model to an already determined scale makes calculating the dimensions slightly more complicated. First, you need to know at least one dimension of the original object and compare it to the same dimension on the blueprint. Let's assume I want to build the 1920 mm wide Dodge Viper to a 1:12 scale. The width on the blueprint is 81 mm. We need to calculate the *blueprint ratio*, that is, the difference between the dimensions of the real car and those of the car on the blueprint. In this case, the ratio is 1920 / 81, which equals 23.7. We can round the result to 24 to get our blueprint ratio. The formula is as follows:

$$\text{Blueprint Ratio} = \frac{\text{Dimension}_{real}}{\text{Dimension}_{blueprint}}$$

Now we can proceed to calculate any dimension by measuring the part on the blueprint, multiplying it by the blueprint ratio, and then dividing it by the scale. For example, let's check to see what size wheels I'm going to need for my 1:12 model. The wheel's diameter on the blueprint is 28 mm. Therefore, we perform the following calculation:

$$\frac{28 \text{ mm} \times 24}{12} = 56 \text{ mm}$$

This means the diameter of the model's wheels should be 56 mm, which equals exactly 7 studs.

Given this information, we can calculate any dimension for a predetermined scale using the following formula:

$$\text{Dimension}_{model} = \text{Dimension}_{blueprint} \times \text{Blueprint Ratio} \times \text{Scale} \times \left(\frac{1 \text{ stud}}{8 \text{ mm}} \right)$$

Of course, the actual vehicle consists of more complex shapes than just those created by perpendicular lines, and these shapes need to be approximated with LEGO pieces. But by keeping our approximation within the core dimensions, we make sure the model has the right size, right angles, and right proportions. A model that has a few details awry but accurate proportions always looks better than a model with plenty of intricate details but the wrong proportions. Details can impress, of course, but they can't hide errors in the proportions of the model.

Now that we can calculate the important dimensions, the next chapter will focus on modeling and other details.

the modeling process

Now that you have your ideal model in mind and you've learned how to scale all dimensions of the object accurately, it's time to start building. This is where you start putting your plans to the test, figuring out all those little details.

size matters

While many builders are tempted to build big, and while size can indeed be an impressive feature of any LEGO construction, Technic models don't necessarily benefit from large size. Going big creates a number of problems that increase rapidly with size, including significant stress on many sensitive pieces and problems with the mobility, balance, and structural integrity of a model. One of my models was tall and very heavy, with a tracked chassis that I thought was strongly reinforced. When it reached a weight of 7 kg, the chassis was bending so much that it couldn't keep the body stable while moving. Even sturdy Technic bricks become quite elastic if the load exerted on them is large enough.

A good rule of thumb, especially for less experienced builders, is to *build as big as needed rather than as big as possible*. In other words, you should aim to make your model as small as possible. To estimate how small it can be, you have to consider the largest single-piece elements it's going to house, such as battery boxes, motors, and IR receivers. Tracked vehicles are a good example here—their box-shaped hulls need to be wide enough for two motors set either side by side (see Figure 25-1) or back-to-back (see Figure 25-2). If a narrower hull is used, wider elements—such as the power supply—must be set above the tracks.

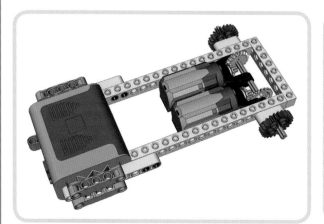

Figure 25-1: An 8-stud-wide hull with a 6-stud-wide internal space, large enough to house two PF Medium motors side by side, one driving the left sprocket wheel and the other driving the right sprocket wheel. A Power Functions battery box can also be housed inside if you make holes for it in the sides of the hull. The protruding parts of the battery box can be concealed inside the tracks.

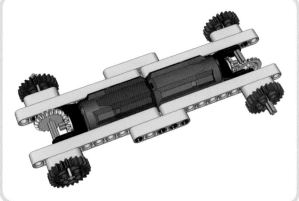

Figure 25-2: A 5-stud-wide hull with a 3-stud-wide internal space, large enough to house two PF Medium motors back-to-back. As the red and blue colors indicate, one motor drives the front right sprocket wheel, while the other drives the rear left one. The remaining two sprockets are idlers. Wider elements, such as the power supply, must be moved above the tracks where the hull is wider.

There are many creative ways in which you can fit large elements into a small model. For example, when building an excavator, you can try to fit small motors, such as PF Mediums, in the arm if it's massive enough, or you can install them between the tracks if the ground clearance allows (see Figure 25-3). You can also try to disguise the motors. One of the trucks I built could house motors only in its cargo hold. When I covered the motors up with plates, it looked like the cargo hold was gone. When I left the motors exposed, they looked like a load carried by the truck. Try to experiment—the more solutions you attempt, the closer you will be to finding the best one.

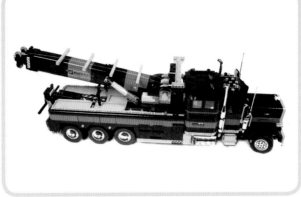

Figure 25-4: My tow truck model housed 17 motors and nearly 19 m of electrical wires, requiring ducts inside the body. Note that the mechanical and electrical parts are all enclosed within the body, with a few minor exceptions, such as the PF Medium motor, which is partially visible by the boom's winch, and the gears of the steering system, which are visible next to the front mudguard.

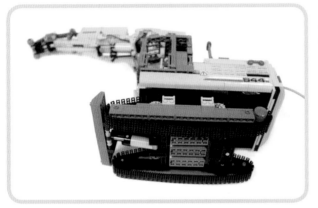

Figure 25-3: My model of the Liebherr R944C tunneling excavator housed more motors in the chassis than it did in the superstructure, at the cost of nearly zero ground clearance. With more space available inside the superstructure, I was able to take better care of its aesthetics.

The complexity of a model is another issue. Very complex models are always impressive, but they are also very difficult to build. My most complex model so far, the tow truck shown in Figure 25-4, housed 17 motors and nearly 19 m of electrical wires. To make it possible, I had to provide special isolated ducts inside its body specifically for wires. It's always a good idea to keep in mind that *complexity should be a result, not a goal in itself.*

Regardless of how confident you feel, it's good to gather some experience building reasonably small and simple models before trying something big and complex. With enough experience, you will notice that big and complex vehicles are often basically a sum of what you've done with smaller ones. For example, you might combine one model's suspension with another's gearbox. Bigger and more complex projects feel more rewarding when completed, but they are also more likely to fail.

wheels

Chapter 5 covers the technical specifications of LEGO wheels, so in this section, we'll discuss them purely in terms of aesthetics and realism. Most LEGO wheels have different proportions than wheels used in real vehicles—they are significantly wider. While this may not be a big problem for many types of models, it can become an issue for vehicles that have more than two wheels on a single axle, trucks being the primary example. The vast majority of trucks use double wheels on all rear axles. Models with single wheels, no matter how wide, just don't look accurate. For example, the 62.4×20 wheels, a favorite of LEGO truck builders, are 5 studs wide when doubled. That means that an axle with four wheels of this type needs a 10-stud-wide space just for the wheels alone. As Figure 25-5 shows, such an axle can't possibly get narrower than 16 studs, unless you abandon the differential.

As you can see in Figure 25-6, the width of the driven axle is one of the major factors affecting the size of the model. And things get even more difficult when there is a suspension system, especially an independent suspension that takes plenty of space between the chassis and the wheels.

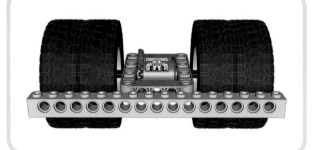

Figure 25-5: It's possible to build a driven axle with four 62.4×20 wheels that fits within a 16-stud width—but just barely.

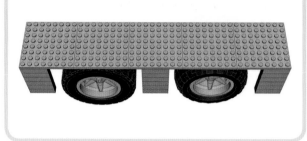

Figure 25-7: The Technic Racing wheel with a regular tire (left) and a balloon tire (right), viewed from the side and under a mudguard. The regular tire appears bigger because of its larger side surface, even though its diameter is actually slightly smaller than that of the balloon tire.

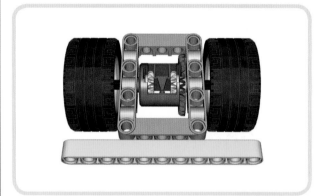

Figure 25-6: Small wheels are often wide, so it's difficult to use more than two per axle. These wheels, often used in small trucks, are 3 studs wide with just a 5.5-stud diameter. An axle with two of these is 11 studs wide, while an axle with four would be 17 studs wide.

Another important issue is the profile of the tire, which can be rectangular (as with regular tires) or round (as with so-called balloon tires). Even when diameter of a balloon tire is bigger than that of the regular one, its side surface is usually smaller because of its profile. Balloon tires look good fully exposed, but when viewed from the side, especially when enclosed within the body, they can actually appear smaller than regular tires, as Figure 25-7 demonstrates.

The final issue involving wheels is steering geometry. In most real cars, when the wheels are steered, they rotate around a pivot point—that is, a vertical axle that goes nearly through their center. As the wheel is turned left or right, its center stays in place, as shown in Figure 25-8. The only

LEGO wheels that follow this behavior are from the 8448 Super Street Sensation set, shown in Figure 25-9. The other wheels rotate around a pivot point that is near their side but far from their center. This means that their centers actually move around when they are turned, as shown in Figure 25-10. LEGO portal axles are most problematic when it comes to steering geometry due to the distance between the wheel and the pivot point (see Figure 25-11).

The crucial difference between the two behaviors is the amount of free space required around the wheel in order for it to turn. Wheels with "real" steering geometry require very little space, and they fit within very tight mudguards. Wheels with the LEGO steering geometry require much more space, as they move back and forth relative to the body when being turned. This means that *steered wheels in LEGO models need bigger mudguards than real steered wheels*.

The difference in the size of the mudguards can also affect the look of the LEGO model. LEGO mudguards are larger than those of the original vehicle, and the wheels appear smaller inside them. Figure 25-12 shows the difference.

As you can see, wheels require careful consideration during the modeling process. It's a common mistake to make them too small, which is more evident in a finished model than when they are too big. Many inexperienced builders produce otherwise well-designed models on wheels that are clearly too small. When in doubt, try to make your wheels too big rather than too small.

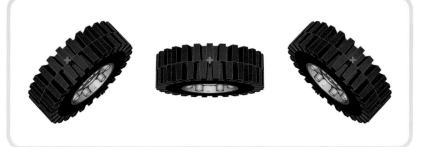

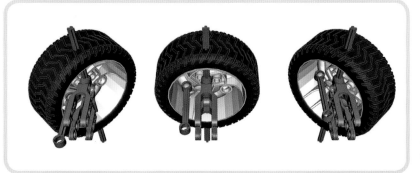

Figure 25-8: The steering geometry of a real vehicle's wheel: As the wheel is steered, it rotates around a pivot point going through its center, marked in this series of images by an imaginary red "axle."

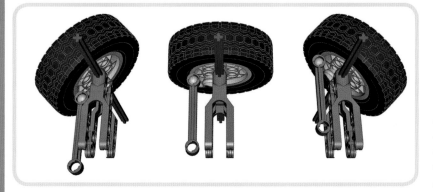

Figure 25-9: Of all existing LEGO wheels, only the 8448 set's wheels rotate around their centers when steered—and they are still a little off.

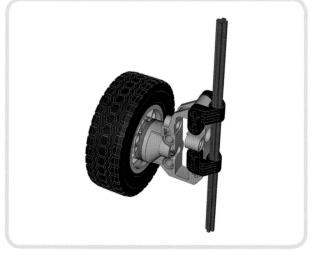

Figure 25-10: When steered, a typical LEGO wheel rotates around a pivot point that is often well outside it. It requires more free space around the wheel, and it also makes the front of the vehicle move while steering in place.

Figure 25-11: LEGO portal axles are worst in terms of steering geometry. Their pivot point is located between the chassis and the gear hub, quite far from the actual wheel.

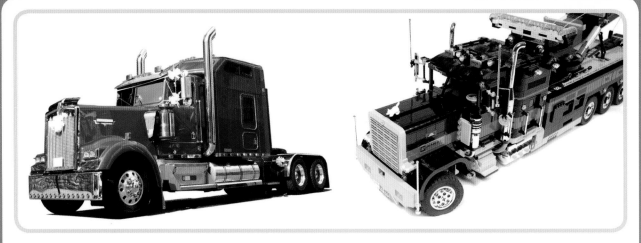

Figure 25-12: Because of their unrealistic steering geometry, LEGO wheels need more spacious mudguards than real wheels do. If the mudguards of my tow truck weren't sized up relative to the real ones, the wheels would collide with them.

other circular elements

Circular parts are quite tricky to model. You either have to use ready-made pieces, whose variety and availability are limited, or create complex structures of many small pieces, which are fragile and can disintegrate in an instant if sufficient stress is applied. Figures 25-13 and 25-14 show examples of such structures.

colors

Colors are a tricky issue when it comes to LEGO pieces. Typical Technic sets use a fairly limited palette, with yellow and red being dominant. When choosing a color, you are always limited by the availability of LEGO pieces in a particular color, and it only gets worse with bigger, more complex models that require more pieces to be visible from the outside.

Over the years, more than 150 LEGO colors have been developed, including speckle colors, glitter colors, semitransparent colors, chrome colors, and even a glow-in-the-dark color. Some of the colors have been discontinued, while new ones are added every now and then. Some colors are actually very difficult to tell apart, such as the very light bluish-grey color that dominates the Mindstorms NXT sets and regular white. In terms of the number of pieces they're used for, the top five LEGO colors are white, black, red, yellow, and blue.

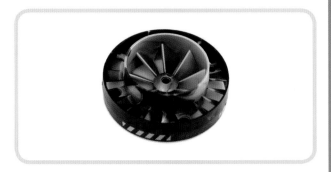

Figure 25-13: The 53983 turbine is an example of a singular circular piece that builders may find disappointing. Not only does it come with a pin hole instead an axle hole, which makes it difficult to drive, but also its inner and outer blades are set in opposite directions, making it useless as a propeller. Finally, the mixed colors appeal to few.

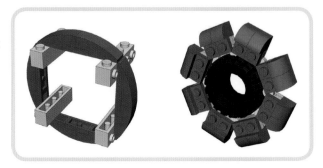

Figure 25-14: Two circular structures built with small basic pieces. One is built around bricks with studs on the side, and the second is built with hinge plates embracing a tire. Both are prone to disintegration if sufficient stress is applied.

When making use of colors in your models, remember that dividing a model into a few unicolored areas almost always produces a better effect than mixing colors. Due to the rectangular shape of most LEGO pieces, mixtures of variously colored pieces just don't look good and make details difficult to spot.

Building the inside of your model in black conceals gaps in your model's body. Dark colors also make your model appear larger. Keep in mind that it's quite common for LEGO builders to substitute certain colors for others when they can't match the actual vehicle exactly. The most common example is LEGO dark bluish grey, which builders often use in military models instead of khaki and olive, which have no LEGO counterparts.

Sometimes it's impossible to find a given LEGO piece in the color you desire, but few builders paint their pieces to remedy this issue. This is because painting rarely produces an effect even remotely close to a stock-colored LEGO piece and is often considered cheating in the community. But this isn't true when it comes to chrome; any LEGO piece looks excellent when chromed, yet there are fewer than 100 types of originally chromed pieces. Consequently, many builders try *custom-chroming* regular LEGO pieces. The resulting size of the piece is slightly increased by the thin chrome film, so chromed pieces are best used for purely decorative purposes rather than as mechanical elements. During custom-chroming, one part of the piece is usually attached to another piece and remains free of the film; this is the only visible difference between original and custom-chromed LEGO pieces (see Figure 25-15). The two largest sources of custom-chromed LEGO pieces are the ChromeBricks shop, at *http://www.bricklink.com/store/home.page?p=ChromeBricks*, and Chrome Block City, at *http://www.bricklink.com/store .asp?p=Aurimax*.

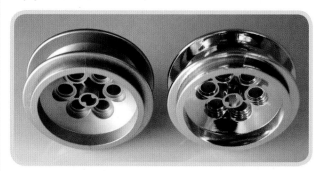

Figure 25-15: The 62.4×20 wheel in stock metallic silver (left) and custom chromed by Chrome Block City (right). Note that the inside of the custom-chromed piece's axle hole lacks chrome film and shows that the wheel was originally white.

devil in the details

When building LEGO models, we regularly have to build things smaller than our scale would indicate. It's very difficult to model details smaller than a single stud, and that means that a lot of approximation is involved. Approximating means that some elements of your model will only vaguely resemble the real ones. You have to make some of them bigger or smaller than they should be and discard some elements entirely. Some builders also resort to custom-made stickers to reproduce the tiniest details.

The barrels of tanks are a particularly good example of approximate building. They almost always consist of a number of sections with slightly different diameters, and it's difficult to find circular LEGO pieces whose differences in diameter are proportionally the same. Because of this, some parts of the barrel need to be built thinner or thicker, as shown in Figure 25-16. It's important to consider the impression each of these deviations will create. People expect a tank to look threatening, which it does with a thick barrel. I have built many tanks with barrels too thick, and not a single person noticed it. But when I built one with a barrel too thin, I received plenty of complaints about it.

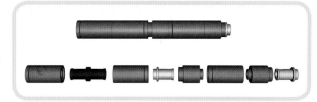

Figure 25-16: Two sections of my T-72M tank's barrel. They are made of slightly different pieces, but they have identical dimensions and a clearly visible notch between them. The resulting barrel, over 20 studs long, is surprisingly sturdy.

A good way to plan a model is to decide which of its features are most important and to try to retain or even exaggerate those features. If the original object you chose has distinctive big wheels, high ground clearance, or an elongated silhouette, exaggerating those features (within reason) can ensure that your model will be easily recognized. Bear in mind that it's easy to go over the top, as Figure 25-17 shows.

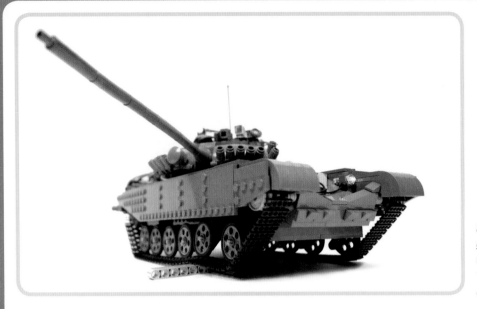

Figure 25-17: Exceptionally high ground clearance is one of the distinctive features of the real T-72M tank. This feature, however, has been exaggerated in my model.

When looking for distinctive features, always try to think in three dimensions. For example, I have built two models of the Scania trucks, whose distinctive feature is a massive front grille with large horizontal openings. The first model simply used black plates to mimic the openings, and it looked very flat when compared to the real truck. So in the second model, shown in Figures 25-18 and 25-19, I created 1-stud-deep openings closed with black plates, and this turned out much better.

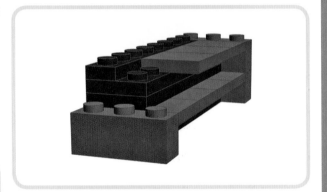

Figure 25-19: I created the openings in my Scania truck's grille using a mixture of plates and tiles. It was crucial to make the ledges between the openings as thin as possible; they are only 1 tile thick here.

building at odd angles

Both Technic and non-Technic connector pieces can be used to re-create complex angles. Certain vehicles, such as the armored personnel carrier shown in Figure 25-20, have bodies with almost no right angles. By building such models with plates and tiles joined by hinged connectors, shown in Figure 25-21, you can make them look good and weigh little. Some particularly challenging angles can be retained by using Technic connectors with ball joints; Figure 25-22 shows an example of this. Bionicle sets are a good source for these kinds of connectors.

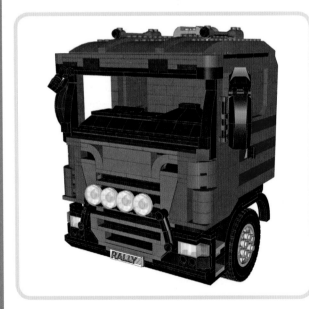

Figure 25-18: The cabin of my second model of the Scania truck with 1-stud-deep openings in its distinctive massive grille.

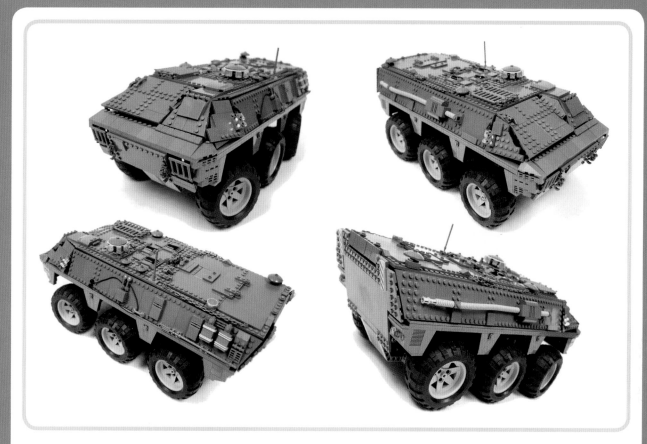

Figure 25-20: The Spanish BMR-2 is a typical armored personnel carrier, with a body made of surfaces connected at complex angles. My model had a body made of plates and tiles kept in place by a system of hinge plates.

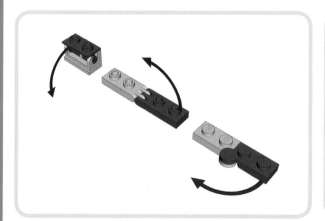

Figure 25-21: Various non-Technic connector pieces, in this case hinge bricks and plates, can keep other pieces oriented at unusual angles.

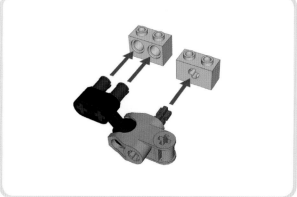

Figure 25-22: To re-create very complex angles, you may resort to joining certain Technic connectors by a ball joint. The connectors shown here can be combined with regular bricks and keep the bricks at almost any angle.

building cleverly

When working on details, the crucial rule is to *match the pieces to the details, not the details to the pieces*. In other words, you should focus on how a detail looks and how to reproduce that look with LEGO pieces. Some builders make the mistake of focusing on some piece they want to use and then looking for a detail that looks vaguely similar.

Many objects have little details that are so distinctive that it's best to include them. For example, when building a Land Rover S2 model, I tried to re-create its distinctive tilted fuel cap. As Figure 25-23 shows, I eventually succeeded using a variant of the 1×1 brick held at an angle between two regular 1×2 Technic bricks.

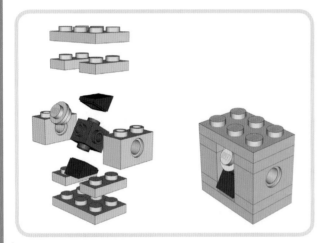

Figure 25-23: An exploded view and a complete assembly of my Land Rover S2 model's tilted fuel cap. The key was using a variant of a 1×1 brick and setting it at an angle.

A number of tiny pieces, especially LEGO minifigures' utensils, can be combined to great effect. For example, many tanks come with a commander's gun on top of the turret. In large-scale models, these guns have plenty of details, and their look is often unique for a given type of tank. When building a model of the Leopard 2A4 tank, I had the choice of using some simple piece that looked like a gun to me or using one of the few ready-made LEGO guns. Neither of these options produced an accurate-looking result, so I eventually combined a few minifigures' utensils, creating the gun shown in Figure 25-24. The gun was built around the body of a minifigure chainsaw, with a hatchet attached in back and a telescope and a fire hose's nozzle in front. The gun's distinctive, large box magazine was made from a few plates with a tile on top, and it was attached to the gun with a 1×1 plate with a clip. The gun was a total of nine simple pieces, and the result prompted some viewers to ask for instructions to build it or for the address to buy the gun.

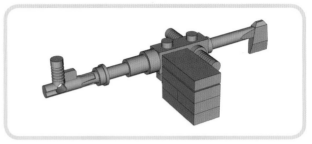

Figure 25-24: The commander's gun from my Leopard 2A4 tank model was built with nine pieces total, including minifigures' utensils, a few plates, and a tile.

the next step: controlling your models

Finally, remember that the fun doesn't have to end with building your model. Building a controller for complex models can be a challenge of its own, as exemplified by a model of the Demag H135 excavator built by Emil "Emilus" Okliński (see Figure 25-25). The model uses two NXT bricks in conjunction with another two bricks in the remote to enable realistic remote control. The remote includes complex joysticks built around NXT motors with internal rotation counters, and it takes advantage of the Bluetooth link to connect with the model. Some functions of the model, such as its internal pneumatic compressor, are controlled automatically, and some of its working parameters can be read from the remote. An extensive description of Emil's model is available at *http://www.eurobricks.com/forum/index.php?showtopic= 64131*.

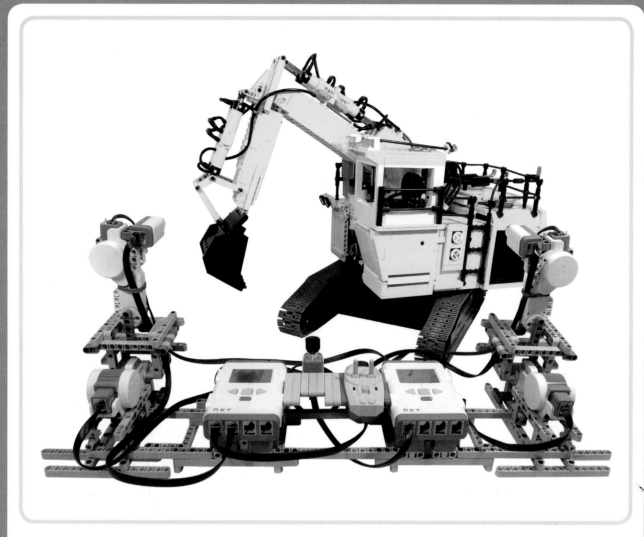

Figure 25-25: The Demag H135 model built by Emil "Emilus" Okliński employed four Mindstorms NXT bricks—two in the remote and another two in the model—to achieve realistic remote control. The complex joysticks based on NXT motors and the use of a Bluetooth link between the remote and the model provided the "driver" with an unparalleled experience.

afterword

I hope that by now you've gained a good understanding of the LEGO Technic system and how to build your own models. If you're looking for more avenues to explore, you'll find many among older LEGO sets. Some of the more unusual inventions include the barcode reader in the 8479 Barcode Multi-Set or the 9688 Renewable Energy Add-On set, which introduced a solar panel into the Power Functions system.

Even if you're a fan of old-school sets and digging up the past, it pays off to keep track of new LEGO products, too. LEGO is constantly introducing new elements and solutions, pushing the envelope even further, as exemplified by the MINDSTORMS EV3 robotics kit (set 31313), which includes programmable control units, motors, sensors, and more. If pure Technic is not enough and you feel like trying your hand at MINDSTORMS, there are a number of books published by No Starch Press that will help you along your way.

Having built well over 200 MOCs in the last few years, I can say that the trial and error of building your own constructions is the best part of building. Getting to play with your finished, working construction is a nice touch, but the real pleasure comes from successfully tackling problems, big and small, which crop up when you choose to design your own models rather than to build from instructions. With enough trial and error, the only real limit to what you can build is your own imagination.

It is my wish that this book helps you to experience that pleasure as you play with LEGO pieces.

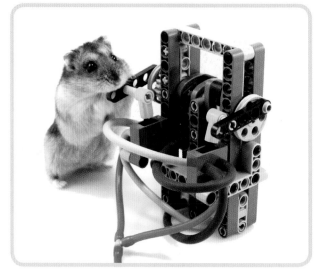

index

updates and additional resources

For updates, errata, and other information about the book, visit *https://nostarch.com/technicbuilder2/*.

While you're there, check out the online resources for this book, including gearing tools, a tire reference sheet, parts datasheets, a list of LEGO fan communities, and much more. To follow Sariel's work, visit him at *http://sariel.pl.*

More no-nonsense books from **no starch press**

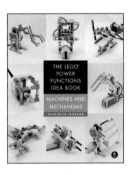

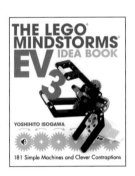

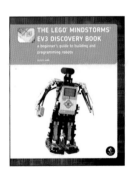

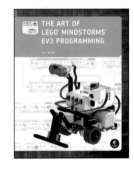

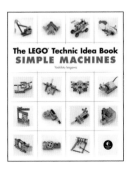

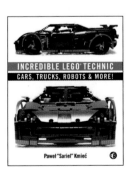

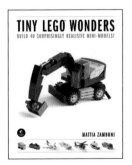

Visit *nostarch.com/ catalog/lego* for a full list of titles.

phone 1.800.420.7240 or 1.415.863.9900 | sales@nostarch.com | www.nostarch.com

COMMUNICATION AND COMMUNICATION DISORDERS

A Clinical Introduction

ELENA PLANTE

The University of Arizona

PÉLAGIE M. BEESON

The University of Arizona

Boston   New York   San Francisco
Mexico City   Montreal   Toronto   London   Madrid   Munich   Paris
Hong Kong   Singapore   Tokyo   Cape Town   Sydney

To our patients,
who continue to teach us.

Executive Editor and Publisher: *Stephen D. Dragin*
Series Editorial Assistant: *Barbara Strickland*
Marketing Manager: *Tara Whorf*
Production Administrator: *Annette Pagliaro*
Editorial Production Service: *Walsh & Associates, Inc.*
Composition Buyer: *Linda Cox*
Manufacturing Buyer: *Andrew Turso*
Cover Administrator: *Joel Gendron*
Text Design and Composition: *Publishers' Design and Production Services, Inc.*

For related titles and support materials, visit our online catalog at www.ablongman.com

Cataloging-in-Publication Data
Plante, Elena, 1961–
    Communication and communication disorders : a clinical introduction / Elena Plante, Pélagie M. Beeson. — 2nd ed.
        p. ; cm.
    Includes bibliographical references and index.
    ISBN 0-205-38922-8
    1. Communicative disorders. 2. Communicative disorders in children. I. Beeson, Pélagie. II. Title.
        [DNLM: 1. Communication Disorders. 2. Communication. 3. Speech-Language Pathology. WL 340.2 P713c 2003]
    RC423.P59 2003
    616.85'5—dc21

                                                                    2003041816

Printed in the United States of America

10 9 8 7 6 5 4 3 2 1   08 07 06 04 03

Photo credits on page x.

CONTENTS

iii

PREFACE

When we wrote the first edition of this textbook, our intention was to speak to the undergraduate student encountering speech, language, and hearing sciences for the first time. We strove to present concepts in a simplified, yet interesting manner. As we taught from the textbook and received feedback from others who used the book, we found that we hit the mark in many respects. But we also realized that some concepts were in need of further distillation and that the level of detail and complexity was too advanced in portions of the book. For that reason, as we updated the textbook for this edition, we directed considerable effort toward simplifying difficult concepts and removing excess detail. We also added more clinical cases within the various chapters because they proved to be effective in bringing the reality of the communication disorders and the professions to life. Another added feature is the inclusion of book lists from the popular literature at the end of the disorders chapters. These books include personal accounts of individuals with communication disorders written from various points of view. We feel that such readings offer a wonderful complement to the view of communication disorders and professions provided in the text.

For this edition, we decided to reorder the chapters so that normal aspects and disordered function are covered in sequence for each of the areas of speech, language, and hearing. This better approximated our preferred course sequence; however, the chapters remain sufficiently independent to allow other sequences. We also felt there was one content area that warranted expansion—the biological basis for hearing. We are pleased to include the addition of a new chapter on that topic written by our colleague, Theodore Glattke, Ph.D. The chapter serves to describe the amazingly elegant mechanism of hearing in a manner suitable for our readership and lays the foundation for the following chapters on hearing disorders in children and adults.

As we worked to revise this text, we were again impressed by the fact that we enjoy the breadth of our field and continue to be fascinated by the science within and outside our respective specialties. We also feel fortunate to have the privilege to work with such impressive and delightful colleagues in the process. We thank Drs. Julie Barkmeier, Anne Marie Tharpe, Linda Norrix, Fran Harris, and Ted Glattke for their excellent chapters and gracious responses to our editorial efforts to unify the tone of the book. We also thank Dr. Alice Smith for her guidance in the area of cleft palate. Thanks also go to Mike Beeson for his cheerful support and tolerance for piles of paper on the dining room table. We appreciate the time and input of reviewer Gayle H. Daly of Longwood College as well. Finally, we express our appreciation to Steve Dragin and Barbara Strickland at Allyn and Bacon for their superb guidance and support. We are pleased with the outcome of the combined efforts in this editorial process, and look forward to teaching from this new edition. We hope that others will find it useful as well.

ABOUT THE AUTHORS

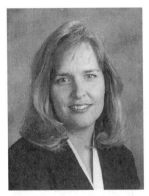

Elena Plante, Ph.D., CCC-SLP

Elena Plante completed bachelor's and master's degrees in speech-language pathology at Loyola College in Maryland. Before returning for a doctorate at the University of Arizona, she worked as a speech-language pathologist in the public schools. Since completing her doctorate and postdoctoral studies, she has been on the faculty at the University of Arizona. She also holds a research appointment with the National Center for Neurogenic Communication Disorders. Her research has focused on the behavioral and biological correlates of developmental language disorders using magnetic resonance imaging (MRI). Subsequent investigations have used electrophysiology and functional magnetic resonance imaging to examine the brain correlates of language processing. In addition, she has produced a series of studies that focus on identification of developmental language disorders in both children and adults through diagnostic testing. She has received support for her research from grants from the National Institutes of Health, National Institute on Deafness and Other Communication Disorders. Dr. Plante is a member of the American Speech-Language-Hearing Association. She is on the editorial board of the *Journal of Communication Disorders* and has reviewed for several of ASHA's professional journals. She speaks regularly at national and international conferences on the topic of developmental language disorders.

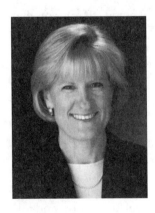

Pélagie M. Beeson, Ph.D., CCC-SLP

Pélagie (Pagie) Maritz Beeson received her bachelor's and master's degrees in speech-language pathology from the University of Kansas. She began her clinical career at a community speech and language center in Fairbanks, Alaska, where she provided service to a diverse clinical population. She later completed her doctoral work at the University of Arizona where she also served as the coordinator of the American Indian Professional Training Program in Speech-Language Pathology and Audiology. Currently, Dr. Beeson is Associate Professor in the Department of Speech and Hearing Sciences at the University of Arizona. Her research and clinical work has been devoted to neurogenic communication disorders in adults with a particular emphasis on the nature and treatment of aphasia, alexia, and agraphia. In Tucson, Dr. Beeson oversees the University of Arizona Aphasia Clinic where she remains active in clinical research and service delivery. She is board certified in Adult Neurogenic Communication Disorders by the Academy of Neurologic Communication Disorders and Sciences. Dr. Beeson is a Fellow of the American Speech-Language-Hearing Association and previously served as Coordinator of

the ASHA Special Interest Division 2: Neurophysiology and Neurogenic Speech and Language Disorders. She is also an active member of the Academy for Neurologic Communication Disorders and Sciences and the International Neuropsychological Society. She has contributed numerous publications to refereed journals, written several book chapters, and regularly speaks at professional meetings.

Julie Barkmeier, Ph.D.

Julie Barkmeier has extensive experience with assessment and treatment of voice and swallowing problems. She worked in the Department of Otolaryngology-Head and Neck Surgery at the University of Iowa Hospitals and Clinics for seven years where she initiated assessment and treatment services for patients with dysphagia. In addition, she coordinated and participated in the assessment and treatment of individuals with voice problems in the University of Iowa Voice Clinic. After completing her doctoral studies in speech pathology at the University of Iowa in 1994, Dr. Barkmeier worked as a Research Scientist in the Voice and Speech Section of the National Institute on Deafness and Other Communication Disorders (NIDCD). Her research at the NIDCD focused on modulation of laryngeal reflexes during swallowing as well as studying long-term effects of botulinum toxin treatment on adductor-type spasmodic dysphonia. Her clinical work while at the NIDCD focused on assessment and treatment of neurogenic voice disorders. Dr. Barkmeier is presently a member of the faculty in the Department of Speech and Hearing Sciences at the University of Arizona.

Theodore J. Glattke, Ph.D.

Theodore Glattke is a Professor in the Department of Speech and Hearing Sciences and the Department of Surgery at the University of Arizona. He is the former editor of the *Journal of Speech and Hearing Research* and currently edits the *Journal of Communication Disorders*. He provides clinical services in the areas of diagnostic audiology and electronystagmography and conducts research in noninvasive physiological measures of the auditory system. Dr. Glattke is a recipient of the Honors of the American Speech-Language-Hearing Association.

Frances P. Harris, Ph.D.

Fran Harris is an Associate Professor of Audiology and Hearing Science in the Department of Speech and Hearing Sciences at the University of Arizona. Among her specialty areas is rehabilitation of hearing loss in adults. She has also conducted research on the characteristics of otoacoustic emissions in adults with and without impaired hearing. She has over twenty years of experience as a clinical audiologist, primarily in an outpatient medical facility and in a state institution for individuals with developmental disabilities. She has published numerous scientific articles, primarily on otoacoustic emissions, and has presented her work nationally and internationally.

Linda Norrix, Ph.D.

Linda Norrix is a clinically certified audiologist who has experience assessing and treating individuals with hearing disorders. She worked at McFarland Clinic in Ames, Iowa, for two and one-half years where she performed audiologic testing and provided rehabilitation services that included counseling and the fitting of hearing aids. After completing her doctoral studies at the University of Arizona in 1995, she worked as a research scientist in the Center for Neurogenic Communication Disorders at the University of Arizona. Her research involved examining the perception and integration of auditory and visual speech. During her doctoral and post-doctoral studies she has continued to assess and treat individuals with hearing disorders at several medical facilities in Tucson. Dr. Norrix currently is an Assistant Research Scientist in the Cognitive Sciences program at the University of Arizona.

Anne Marie Tharpe, Ph.D.

Anne Marie Tharpe is Professor of Audiology in the Department of Hearing and Speech Sciences of the Vanderbilt Wickerson Center for Otolaryngology and Communication Sciences. Dr. Tharpe has been involved in the provision of clinical audiology services to the pediatric population for almost twenty years. In addition to clinical service, her activities include research, writing, and teaching. Her clinical and research work has focused on assessment and management of children with hearing loss, normal auditory development in infants, and practitioner education. She has published numerous scientific articles and pediatric audiology chapters and has co-authored a text on amplification in children.

Photo Credits: p. 1, Novastock/Photo Edit; pp. 19, 149, David Young-Wolff/Photo Edit; p. 39, Dwight Ellefsen/Omni-Photo Communications; p. 61, Will Faller; pp. 97, 253, Blair Seitz/Photo Researchers; p. 126, Michael Newman/Photo Edit; p. 173, Laura Dwight; p. 207, Spencer Grant/Photo Edit; p. 234, Elliott Smith/Silver Burdett Ginn; p. 287, Department of Speech and Hearing Sciences, The University of Arizona; p. 317, Stephen Simpson/Getty Images.

INTRODUCTION TO THE PROFESSIONS OF AUDIOLOGY AND SPEECH-LANGUAGE PATHOLOGY

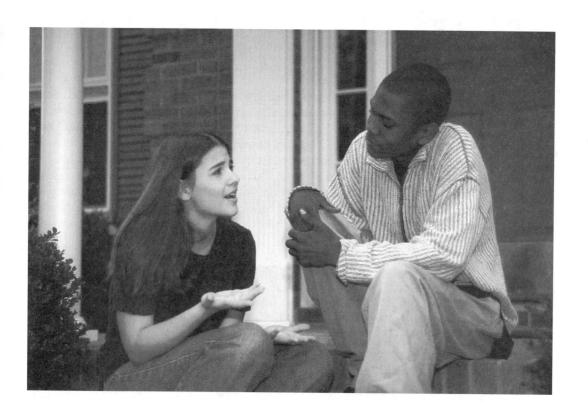

■ ■ ■ ■ ■ ▬▬▬▬▬▬▬▬▬▬▬▬▬▬▬▬▬▬▬▬▬▬▬▬▬▬▬▬▬

PREVIEW

Communication is so pervasive in daily life that we often take it for granted. In this chapter, we introduce the field of communication disorders. We begin by examining normal communication in its various modalities. Then six individuals with communication disorders are introduced who are among the estimated 10 percent of the population for whom communication is impaired. We can begin to understand the bases of these disorders by briefly examining the components of normal communication, which are discussed in detail in later chapters. For individuals with communication impairments, the services of a speech-language pathologist or audiologist may improve the quality of daily life. We will meet some professionals who work in the field of communication disorders and hear their perspectives regarding this dynamic field.

NORMAL COMMUNICATION

Human communication embodies a rich tapestry of information conveyed through elements of movement, emotional expression, and vocalizations. **Communication** includes all means by which information is transmitted between a sender and a receiver. By this definition, we know that animals communicate through posture, facial gestures, scent, and vocalizations. Humans are unique among animals because we have developed a system of symbolic communication we call language. Language may be written, spoken, or signed. Although all forms of language are used to communicate ideas, not all forms of communication involve language. A look at some real-life examples of normal communication illustrates that language and communication can take many forms.

> A father carried his 18-month-old son in his arms as he walked through a public park. His son leaned over and excitedly extended his arms into the air. "Da?" the toddler asked. The father looked to see what had caught his son's attention. A young girl from the neighborhood was walking her dog. "Oh, it's the dog," the father replied. "Da! Da!" the son exclaimed while bouncing with excitement.

With the use of a single "word," tone of voice, and gestures, this child begins to use language to ask a question, make a statement, and indicate interest. The father accepts the attempt at language as meaningful, even though it only approximates a word in its adult form. He uses the situational context, the child's gestures and emotional tone to support his interpretation of his son's meaning. Through context, it becomes obvious that the child is using "da" to mean "dog" and not "dad," "man," "teddy," "juice," or any of the other things that the child has referred to in the past with those sounds. The father's response to his son turns an attempt at a word into a conversation, to the enjoyment of both. As we will see, not all attempts at communication are equally successful.

Sixty-four students sat in a lecture room, one without any windows, listening to their professor. The professor, who had taught the course nine times before, was lecturing: "One might question, uh, the relational meanings that best describe, uh, the language of young children. Remember, that Bloom said (as well as Sinclair or, uh, and Bowerman) that it is possible to put in a logical order the kind of language experiences that occur in a typical order of, uh, let us say, emergence."

Some of the poorest communication may occur in the classroom. This lecturer's convoluted word order and interruptions due to word-retrieval pauses interfered with effective communication. The meaning of the subject matter may be difficult for the student to comprehend even without the teacher's poor sentence formulation. The students may not be listening for many reasons, such as the instructor's poor narrative, fatigue from a previous activity, worry about unrelated issues, or even the lack of ventilation in the closed room.

Effective use of language for communication is not restricted to spoken words. Humans have developed additional modalities for the expression of language. One alternative developed because some individuals are unable to perceive spoken language.

A 23-year-old student was hired as a classroom interpreter for a 19-year-old deaf engineering student. The interpreter had limited knowledge of the highly technical content of the engineering classes. To this was added the strain of translating the heavily accented and often broken English spoken by the foreign-born instructor into the completely different grammatical organization of American Sign Language. The engineering student, who had a pronounced playful streak in his personality, took advantage of these conditions for a little good-natured ribbing of the interpreter. At one point during the lecture, a fly was buzzing around the interpreter's nose and she swatted at it in mid-sentence. The student leaned forward, looked at her face, and repeated the gesture of swatting the fly, indicating he needed the gesture defined as if it were a word he did not know. When the interpreter ignored this obviously facetious request, the student only repeated it with increasing elaborations of the gesture and facial expressions. This act finally caught the attention of the instructor, who stopped the class to see if there was a problem. Thoroughly embarrassed, the student and interpreter finished out the lecture without further interruption.

American Sign Language (ASL) uses a system of manual gestures instead of spoken words to convey information. In ASL, hand and arm movements, facial expressions, and locations in space are used to express vocabulary and a grammatical structure that is different from that of other spoken, written, and manual languages. Rather than hearing the message, signed languages are perceived through the visual modality. Like other languages, ASL has a normal developmental sequence when learned as a first language. Fluent users are able to express the full range of human ideas and emotions. No matter the mode, all languages can be used for a variety of purposes, such as communicating, thinking, creating, learning, and even teasing and humor.

ASL, and other manual forms of language, provide an alternate modality for expression. Like signed language, written language also uses the visual modality for communication. Like spoken or signed language, written language may be used to inform and to regulate behavior.

> While traveling in the Southwest, we had occasion to visit the Ghost Ranch Living Museum in northern New Mexico. This center includes a small zoo of animals indigenous to the area. Signs in front of each animal habitat warned, "Do not feed your fingers to the animals. Their diet is carefully monitored."

This clever sign conveyed at least two important pieces of information: The animals should not be fed by visitors, and the animals will bite. In this case, the sign's creator used a humorous approach and indirect language to convey the message. The tone of the written message was particularly appropriate to the setting as it contributed to, rather than detracted from, the visitor's enjoyment of the sights. The use of indirect language is interesting here, in that much more is communicated than the words actually denote.

Normal communication encompasses verbal and nonverbal elements that, in combination, are used for a variety of purposes. Communication is successful when information is accurately transmitted from a sender to a receiver. Some aspects of communication, such as nonverbal elements, are not always intentional. Sometimes, our bodies "give us away." For example, posture, facial expression, and voice quality may combine to indicate fatigue, even when we may be very interested in the topic of a conversation. Other elements, such as proximity and gestures, are used to communicate the speaker's status, attitudes, and emotions.

Many of the nonverbal elements of communication are culturally regulated. For example, Anglo listeners tend to provide speakers with periodic feedback by nods and vocalized signals of affirmation. Navajo listeners provide less overt signs of attention; polite listeners attend unobtrusively. Some cultures maintain constant eye contact when listening; for others, "staring" at a speaker is rude. Even such aspects as the length of time one pauses between utterances is culturally determined. Although this may seem to be a minor component of communication, violations may have profound effects on the listener. A speaker who pauses too long may appear to be withholding and unsociable. One whose pauses are too short may appear to be impertinent and domineering. Most individuals are able to monitor and use an ongoing stream of nonverbal information for effective communication.

SIX INDIVIDUALS WITH COMMUNICATION IMPAIRMENT

Communciation is so pervasive in our lives that we sometimes take it for granted. However, those with a communication disorder feel the impact every day. There may be no better way for us to appreciate the diversity of these problems than to review a few cases of individuals with various forms of communication disorders.

As we will see from these cases, communication disorders affect both children and adults, and they do not discriminate by ethnic background or economic status.

Beth Feldman[1] is a 23-year-old student teacher who developed bilateral vocal nodules, or bumps on both vocal folds. By noon every day, she lost her voice completely, making it impossible to control the twenty-six children in her fourth-grade class. She was warned by her supervising teacher that she could not continue as a student teacher if she did not improve her voice. Seeking help in a voice clinic at a university hospital, she was told that she speaks at the bottom of her pitch range, clears her throat excessively, speaks in a loud voice, and exhibits other behaviors detrimental to her vocal health. She consulted two ear-nose-throat physicians (otorhinolaryngologists), each of whom told her that she had two small nodules, one on each vocal fold, that were not big enough to explain the severe voice symptoms she was experiencing. Both recommended voice therapy. Subsequent voice therapy attempts were thwarted by school and teaching activities that left her little time for either therapy or practice of voice techniques. Recent counseling efforts with Ms. Feldman were successful in making the point that her type of voice problem (hoarseness and loss of voice related to vocal nodules) could probably be resolved with voice therapy. However, she has not yet made her first therapy appointment.

Jim Fields is a 43-year-old promoter who arranges concerts for rock and pop musicians. His wife convinced him to have his hearing checked when she noticed that he was no longer hearing his wristwatch alarm and that he had difficulty understanding her over the telephone. His evaluation by an audiologist revealed a moderate to severe hearing loss of the type associated with noise exposure. The audiologist learned that his history of noise exposure dated back to his teens, when he sang in a band that in his words "substituted volume for talent." Since that time, there had been many occasions when he remembered leaving a performance with "ringing ears" or "fuzzy hearing." The audiologist explained the connection between exposure to loud sound and the hearing loss Mr. Fields was experiencing. He now uses hearing protection when exposed to loud music (and other loud sounds) to slow further hearing loss. He has enrolled in a lipreading course to help compensate for the loss he already has. In addition, he returns for regular hearing checkups to monitor his hearing acuity. He has elected to forgo a hearing aid at this time but understands that one may become a necessity in the future.

Rudolpho Torres, age 13 months, was evaluated by team members of a university orofacial-disorders clinic. He was born in Mexico with a bilateral cleft lip and palate. Although his cleft lip was surgically repaired within a few weeks of his birth, the roof of his mouth remained unrepaired. All of his attempts at speech (or when crying) appear to come out of his nose because there is open coupling of his oral and nasal cavities. He was examined by the plastic surgeon, who recom-

---

[1]We have changed the names of all individuals whose communication disorders are described in this book.

mended immediate surgery to finish the repair of his cleft. Both the audiologist and otolaryngologist found that the boy had a middle-ear infection, which was producing a moderate hearing loss. The speech-language pathologist felt that Rudolpho exhibited normal language comprehension for Spanish and urged early surgical intervention in an attempt to minimize his severe hypernasality. The boy and his mother were going to live temporarily with his uncle in Tucson, so the first stage of surgery could be started. The social worker on the team met with the speech-language pathologist, the plastic surgeon, and the boy's mother to arrange the temporary move from Mexico to Tucson.

Karen Burghart, a 33-year-old attorney, had stuttered all her life. She would repeat words over and over, and sometimes she would fix her mouth in a tight, twisted manner, unable to say anything. Although she received some speech therapy for her stuttering while in high school, she felt that it did not help her. While attending a university, she was the victim of a date rape. Her attacker was arrested and subsequently tried for his crime. Unfortunately, he was acquitted, which Karen blamed on her inability to speak during her attempts to testify against him during the trial. During counseling sessions with a psychologist, she was advised to receive speech therapy for her stuttering. She began receiving individual therapy twice weekly and participated in a young-adult stuttering group at the university speech clinic. She began to realize in therapy that most of her life had been spent trying not to stutter, and she found that she was beginning to do a lot of things to keep from speaking. In speech therapy she learned how to speak easily by prolonging the vowels in her speech. As the result of her courtroom experience and the injustice she experienced, she became fascinated with law and the criminal justice system. Upon graduation from the university, she went to law school and became an attorney. She continues in speech therapy to maintain her controlled fluency, but her speech now permits her to function as an assistant district attorney.

Bruce Murrich, age 69, was a retired executive who suffered a stroke while sleeping, awakening with a right-sided paralysis (hemiplegia) and aphasia (loss of language). His sudden symptoms transformed him from a golf-playing, fun-loving retiree in Arizona to a man unable to speak except for occasional profanity. He was also powerless to move his right arm and leg. He and his wife reacted initially to the severe disability with disbelief and denial, hoping that, with proper medical attention within the first few days of onset, his symptoms would go away. After several weeks of continued impairment, Mr. and Mrs. Murrich sought rehabilitation, which included speech-language pathology services. Mr. Murrich began receiving weekly group therapy and individual speech therapy (plus physical and occupational therapies). His wife attended a weekly spouse group and received individual counseling from a social worker in the rehabilitation center. As his language improved to the point where he could communicate many thoughts and needs in two-to-three word utterances with less profanity, his overall spirits improved dramatically. Now, about eighteen months after the stroke, both Mr. Murrich and his wife seem to accept the relative permanence of his disability.

Devon Douglas was 17 when we first met him. His younger brother had been diagnosed with a rare genetic condition that often affects development. The family lived

in a remote town and traveled two hours each way to reach our clinic where they participated in a research study to determine the communication aspects of the genetic disorder. When we first talked with Devon's mother, she had more concerns about him than her younger son, despite the fact that Devon did not have the genetic disorder. She reported that he had struggled his entire school history to maintain average grades. Over the years, she had asked the school system to evaluate Devon for a learning disability. The first time was when he was in second grade. Each time, the school staff indicated that they did not see Devon as having any educational handicaps, so he was never evaluated. Devon himself reported that teachers had told him that he was lazy and could do better if he tried. His mother was now worried that school was such a struggle that Devon might drop out. As part of our research program, we were able to evaluate his cognitive and linguistic skills. Testing revealed that his general cognitive abilities were in the high average range. However, he had great difficulty putting together grammatically correct sentences, following spoken directions, and understanding what he read. In fact, his overall language skills were quite weak. At age 17, we diagnosed a language-based learning disability for the first time in this young man's life.

These cases represent the challenges and diversity encountered by professionals in the field of communication disorders. Each of these people had been struggling to overcome a communication handicap. Ms. Feldman's vocal nodules had a direct impact on her effectiveness as a teacher. Mr. Murrich's stroke forever altered both his and his wife's plans for retired life. Devon's difficulty with language had a direct impact on his school success. Each case demonstrates how difficulty in just one aspect of communication can affect daily life.

CLASSIFICATION OF COMMUNICATION DISORDERS

Breakdowns in communication may be understood by looking at the components of normal communication. Communication requires the transmission of information from one person to another. Information can be conveyed through tone of voice, facial expressions, posture, and gestures. Language, however, is the medium of choice when we wish to communicate specific ideas. **Language** involves the coding of meaning into a system of arbitrary symbols that are recognized by members of the community. The way in which sounds are combined into words and words into sentences is arbitrarily determined across languages. For example, in English, words may begin with a "st" combination, as in "stairs," but not with a "ts" combination. However, Navajo includes words that start with the "ts" combination (e.g., tseí, meaning "rock"). These conventions within each language are completely arbitrary; English speakers are capable of producing the "ts" combination (e.g., "its"), but do not use it at the beginning of words. Other rules govern how words are combined into sentences (the grammar of a language). These are also arbitrary and vary among languages. For example, English requires the use of nouns or pronouns to specify the subject of a sentence. In Italian, however, the pronoun can be dropped from the sentence without any resulting confusion. We will explore the nature of language in more detail in Chapter 7.

For most individuals, language is communicated from speaker to listener through an oral-to-auditory pathway. The vocal mechanism and oral structures are used to form the individual sounds of language that we recognize as **speech**. A change in tongue placement is sufficient to differentiate a "t" from a "k." The addition of vocal fold vibrations changes the "k" to a hard "g." In other languages, further manipulations of sound contribute to speech. For example, Chinese is considered a tonal language because changes in the pitch of the voice are also used to differentiate between sound elements. Our vocal mechanism also allows us to vary the pitch and loudness of speech to convey emotion and emphasis. For the average person, these aspects come together seamlessly to produce a fluent flow of words. We introduce the physical structures that support speech in Chapter 2 and follow with a discussion of the sounds of speech in Chapter 3.

Because of their knowledge of the anatomy and physiology of the oral structures, speech-language pathologists have become involved with treatment of certain disorders that do not strictly involve communication. These include such conditions as tongue thrust and swallowing disorders. As we will see in Chapter 4, tongue thrust can be associated with a lisped "s" sound. It also has an impact on eating and on dental alignment, as the tongue pushes forward on the front teeth during swallowing. Other, more severe forms of swallowing disorders are covered in Chapter 6. Swallowing disorders often result from the same types of disease processes and acquired damage that can affect communication. Swallowing evaluation and treatment has become a prominent component of many speech-language pathologists' work in health-related settings.

Spoken language is received by the listener through the aural modality. This requires an intact auditory system. **Hearing** includes such aspects as the awareness of sound, the ability to distinguish among sounds, and the ability to process sound that occurs at a rapid rate. These abilities are central to being able to decode speech. When language is presented in the auditory-oral modality, normal hearing is also important. By hearing language spoken around us, we learn the rules of our native language, the sounds of speech, and even the accent and intonation patterns that characterize our regional dialect. When we speak, we monitor our own production and modify or correct our speech as we talk. The mechanisms of hearing, on which all these skills rely, are addressed in Chapter 10.

When impairments in communication occur, they typically involve a breakdown in one or more of the elements involved in speech, language, or hearing. In Figure 1.1, we see these three aspects of normal communication and how they relate to classes of communication disorders. Language disorders may include conditions that emerge as a child develops. These *developmental* language disorders may first appear during childhood, but may persist into adulthood. This was the case for Devon, whose difficulties were apparent in grade school. In contrast to developmental language disorders, acquired language disorders occur when an individual suffers an injury or disease that causes a loss of language skills. Mr. Murrich's case presents one type of *acquired* language disorder called aphasia. Although acquired language disorders can occur at any time during life, the major-

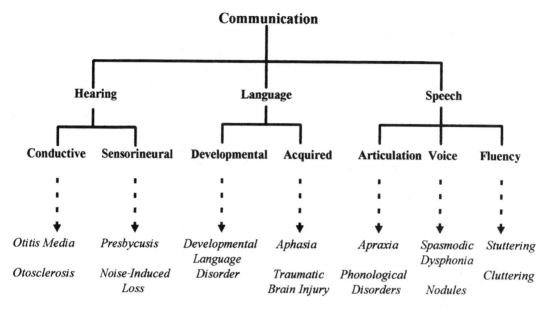

FIGURE 1.1   A conceptual representation of different types of communication impairments with examples of specific disorders (listed below the dashed arrows).

ity of individuals with acquired language disorders are adults. Disorders involving language skills in children and adults are discussed in Chapters 8 and 9.

Disorders of speech also may also occur in children and adults. These disorders may include aspects of **articulation**, or the way the sounds of words are produced. For Rudolpho, his cleft palate altered the oral structures needed for speech articulation. If left unrepaired, he would have little chance to develop normal speech. In other children, a developmental articulation disorder may appear without a known cause. As with language disorders, articulation disorders may be acquired following accident or disease. In other cases, difficulty with speech may involve the vocal mechanism. **Voice** disorders may alter the pitch, quality, or loudness of the voice. We saw in the case of Ms. Feldman that poor speaking practices may lead to physical changes of the vocal mechanism that interfere with speech over time. In her case, the voice disorder interfered with her professional life. In other cases, an overly breathy or harsh vocal quality or a loss of voicing may signal a health concern that requires immediate medical intervention.

Finally, a disorder of speech may involve **fluency**. Fluency disorders occur when the normally smooth flow of speech becomes interrupted. The individual may struggle to produce sentences that come effortlessly for others. Ms. Burghart had first-hand experience with the most prevalent of fluency disorders: stuttering. For most individuals, stuttering begins during childhood. Many of those who stutter will eventually overcome this difficulty. A few, like Ms. Burghart, will have to

monitor their fluency indefinitely. We will examine disorders of articulation, fluency, and voice in Chapters 4 through 6.

Disorders of hearing may arise from factors that prevent the conduction of sound into and through the hearing mechanism. These are referred to as a **conductive hearing loss**. Rodolpho had a conductive hearing loss due to fluid in the middle ear. Although children with cleft palate show high rates of this type of conductive loss, middle ear infection (otitis media) is also one of the most common afflictions of otherwise normal children. In contrast to conductive hearing loss, **sensorineural hearing loss** refers to a hearing loss caused by disease of the inner ear or the neural transmission of sound. In Mr. Field's case, exposure to loud sound over time produced a sensorineural hearing loss. In other cases, an individual may be born with a hearing loss or lose hearing after an illness. Although we classify hearing disorders as conductive or sensorineural, in some instances, hearing loss may involve a mix of both types. We will discuss disorders of hearing in Chapters 11 and 12.

CAREERS IN COMMUNICATION DISORDERS

As described in the cases at the beginning of this chapter, most individuals with speech, language, or hearing disorders can improve their communication. The professionals who provide front-line services for the remediation of communication disorders are **audiologists** and **speech-language pathologists**. The professional organization for audiologists and speech-language pathologists is the American Speech-Language-Hearing Association (ASHA). In 1989, ASHA passed a resolution that specified the fields of **Audiology** and **Speech-Language Pathology** as separate professions. Because of the common concern for human communication impairments and the historical association of these two professions, most individuals in either field have some knowledge and training in areas served primarily by the other. At the present time, for example, the undergraduate curriculum in most training institutes does not differ for the two fields. Instead, students specialize in one or the other profession as part of their graduate school training. Although there are some opportunities for individuals with less training (see Chapter 13 for a discussion of support personnel), a graduate degree is required to become certified as an audiologist or speech-language pathologist.

An aspiring speech-language pathologist must complete all graduate courses for a master's degree (or its equivalent) awarded from an accredited program. Upon completion of the degree, he or she will spend a clinical fellowship year working as a clinician under the supervision of a more experienced and certified speech-language pathologist. The path to clincal certification is currently in a period of transition for the aspiring audiologist. At the time this book went to press, audiologists were also required to complete a master's degree and a clinical fellowship year. As of 2007, certification requirements will increase the required education to 75 credit hours of post-baccalaureate study, and the clinical fellowship training will be enfolded into this training. In 2012, a doctoral degree (e.g., Ph.D., AuD., Sci.D.) will be the entry-level degree for audiologists. In addition to acade-

mic and clinical training, both audiologists and speech-language pathologists must pass a national certification examination before becoming certified to work independently in any of a wide variety of clinical settings.

The individuals who have careers in communication disorders are a diverse group. The membership survey of the American Speech-Language-Hearing Association (ASHA, 2001) reveals the variety inherent to the field. According to the survey, there are over 11,000 certified audiologists and over 82,000 certified speech-language pathologists. Like the U.S. population, they represent all major racial and ethnic groups, White, African American, Hispanic, Asian/Pacific Islander, and Native American. Most audiologists and speech-language pathologists (76 percent) are employed full time. For audiologists, the most common place of employment was in a healthcare facility (72 percent), which included hospitals, clinics, private practices, and as part of a physician's practice. Other employment settings included school systems (18 percent), industrial facilities, and colleges or universities. In contrast, 51 percent of the speech-language pathologists reported working in a school system. Other common employment settings for speech-language pathologists included healthcare facilities, colleges or universities, and private practice.

The results of the ASHA membership survey provide an overview of those who comprise the professions. To get a more personal view, we asked audiologists and speech-language pathologists from around the country to share their perceptions about their professions. Our informants included individuals who represent nearly all segments of the demographic groups that comprise the profession. We interviewed thirty-five individuals who had over 350 combined years of experience within the field.

Clinical Careers

We began by asking our colleagues why they chose to work in the field of Communication Disorders. As one might imagine, some were first introduced to the field because they knew someone with a communication disorder. That was the case for Nancy, who lives in Arizona and is a relative newcomer to the field with two years of experience. Nancy wrote, "I worked for a gentleman who had Parkinson's disease and he piqued my interest in the rehabilitation fields. He persuaded me to 'lose interest in the law' (a previous pursuit) and to become involved in a 'helping profession.' After doing some research, I found Speech-Language Pathology to be the most interesting." A few colleagues knew someone who was working in the field or had received clinical services themselves at some point. Kim, a speech-language pathologist from Colorado, reported that she received therapy for articulation as a young child. She "decided one day on my way to day care to be a 'Speech Therapist.' At the time, I only knew the 'r,' 'l,' 's,' part of the field." In her six years in the profession, Kim now has more extensive experience working in both school and hospital settings. Donna is an audiologist with thirty-five years experience who is employed as the director of a university clinic. She reported that a relative was a teacher of the deaf, and those experiences sparked her interest in

deafness. As an undergraduate, she was in the enviable position of having three fellowships, in theater, linguistics, and audiology, to choose among. She chose audiology and wrote "I have *never* regretted this decision."

Those with direct or indirect exposure to the field were in the minority. Others were attracted to the field because of a specific interest or desire that was encompassed by the field. Many of our colleagues noted a desire to enter a field where they could "make people's lives better." This sentiment was echoed by Jennifer, who wrote, "I knew I always wanted to work with children, but I wasn't sure how until I watched some Speech Pathologists work with some language-impaired preschoolers at a local hospital. Watching them, I realized how much impact a person could have in a child's life." Jennifer has had many opportunities to rediscover this impact in her own hospital-based position as a pediatric speech-language pathologist. Paula reported that she had an initial interest in languages and language development. "Then I took an Audiology course and became fascinated with the process of hearing and what can happen when people—especially children—are unable to hear." She has combined these interests for fifteen years as an educational audiologist in Colorado.

We are also seeing increasing numbers of individuals who come into the profession after having worked in another field. Zarina was a bilingual second grade teacher before deciding to go back to school. "I wanted to get out of teaching and I noticed that there were a lot of Spanish-speaking kids with language difficulties. I decided to go into Speech-Language Pathology to help bilingual children. I also wanted the option of working in other settings in addition to schools." Erin was a public relations account executive before returning to school for a master's in speech-language pathology. "What it all came down to was more meaningful work. I wanted a job helping people instead of just helping a company make money." She picked Speech-Language Pathology because it allowed her to combine her interests in languages (she speaks English and French) and allied health. Bret wrote, "I've had a long-standing interest in how we communicate (my B.A. is in Speech Communication). I was advised by a family friend to investigate Speech-Language Pathology . . . and learned just how diverse our field is and that it could provide a lifelong, stable career." He now works in a rehabilitation center in Colorado.

There is also what we like to think of as "the luck factor" that led people to discover the field. Consider Anne, who has been practicing for two years in Missouri. "I didn't really know what I wanted to do," wrote Anne. "I had several friends who talked me into taking a Speech-Language Pathology class, and (after enrolling) I decided then and there that I was in the right field." Carol, an audiologist of ten years in California, had a similar reaction to her initial academic exposure. "I found the coursework interesting and challenging. There didn't seem to be a single course in the program I wasn't interested in taking." For Ellen, who has now been practicing for eleven years in Tennessee, a problem with her own voice led to a career in Speech-Language Pathology. "I wanted to work with voice disorders as I was a voice major in music and experiencing problems. I took a class in phonetics and loved the content."

We were impressed with the variety of reasons that our colleagues entered the professions. This may be because the professions can accommodate the wide range of personality traits and backgrounds that these individuals bring to it. We saw this when we asked our colleagues to tell us about the personality traits that they saw as important to their job. Here are a few of the recurring themes that our colleagues expressed. Lane's experience in hospitals and skilled nursing facilities in Arizona has taught him that a "speech-language pathologist needs to be flexible, adaptable, a team player, a good communicator, and very clear about personal and professional integrity. These characteristics are crucial for survival in a rapidly changing healthcare system." Angie, a speech-language pathologist from Tennessee, commented, "I believe that you must be assertive in this field. People's quality of life is at stake and you must do whatever you can to help." The complementary position was expressed by Mike, a Colorado resident who wrote, "I think patience may be the key to some of my success as an audiologist [of twenty-three years], especially when working with families with young hearing impaired infants who need the gift of *time* to accept their child's impairments and to implement the many recommendations we make." In fact, patience was mentioned as a personality trait by almost all our respondents. Another common characteristic of our colleagues was an orientation toward solving problems. Ellen commented that "task analysis is at the center of what we do; identify problems then determine the best method of improving function." Not surprisingly, she feels traits like analytical skills and a questioning nature, mixed with enthusiasm and an action-oriented nature, apply to her. Rebecca, a speech-language pathologist of twenty-one years and the director of a hospital-based center for communication disorders in New York, adds qualities such as persistence, self-confidence, maturity, and a generous nature to the list.

Among the most frequently identified traits was independence. This trait characterized clinicians in private practice, university clinics, schools, hospitals, rehabilitation centers, and skilled nursing facilities. This is not surprising in that clinicians in most settings have a great deal of autonomy as to how they manage their caseload, develop programs, and provide quality service. Regardless of clinical setting or clientele, the field demands individuals with the motivation to identify areas of need and seek out information in this ever advancing field.

We were also curious about what keeps these professionals in the field year after year. Some cited specific aspects of their jobs, such as the experience of developing a new program for service delivery or working with cutting edge technology. Donna works with such new advances as programmable hearing aids and cochlear implants. She wrote, "Patients who are realizing dramatic functional gains do keep me going!" "I love the diagnostic process," writes Shara, a speech-language pathologist of eleven years. "To be able to identify strengths and weaknesses and explanations for behavior is very challenging. Also, to be able to change those behaviors, to see them 'get it' is exciting." Shannon, a Michigan-based speech-language pathologist echoed several common themes: "It's the versatility of being able to work with children or adults. I also like having a solid base of

knowledge in a variety of disorders. And there's always the advantage of always being able to find a job!" Angie expressed the sentiments of many of our colleagues. She wrote, "It's a fast-paced field. I am always encountering new situations that allow me to learn continuously." Lou, a speech-language pathologist of three years wrote, "The most exciting thing for me to experience is children's first words—the look in their eyes when they realize they are able to impact their environment using words." When asked what keeps her going, Jennifer put it succinctly, "Two words—the kids. Two more words—their smiles."

All clinicians have stories about particular clients that stand out, punctuating their careers like exclamation points along the way. This was the case for Angie who wrote about a difficult case involving a man who had had a stroke. "He once told me 'you remember those old movies where there are slaves rowing the boat and there is a man standing on deck cracking his whip. That is what you were for me. I never could have done it without you.' I never gave up on him, nor he on me." Ellen writes that one of her staff was able to identify an important medical issue for a patient that had been previously missed by several other professionals. "This speech-language pathologist referred the patient back to the ear, nose, and throat physician and highlighted her findings. The ENT diagnosed the actual cause of the swallowing disorder and was able to surgically repair it. The patient resumed a regular diet." Sometimes the smallest gains are the most important to the clinician. Susan, a speech-language pathologist in Minnesota, wrote of a severely autistic child who for the first time communicated a specific desire by selecting a picture of an activity. "We were so excited for him and what this skill will do for him in the future." She is now working to expand this child's first step into skills that will allow him to communicate with others through the use of pictures. The impact of these cases is captured by Lane, who commented that "the emotional rewards and the opportunity to powerfully impact and connect with people during a difficult time in their lives" are primary advantages to a career in this field.

Research Careers

Audiologists and speech-language pathologists impact lives through direct clinical services. But this is not the only avenue to effect change within the professions. The desire to advance the field beyond its current boundaries attracts professionals to incorporate research as a component of their career. Whereas direct clinical intervention improves the lives of one client at a time, research has the potential to improve the lives of many as new discoveries improve the profession's understanding, diagnosis, and treatment of communication disorders. Although opportunities for research exist in almost all job settings, less than 1 percent of the professionals see themselves primarily as researchers. Another 3 percent are college or university professors, for whom research is a typical component of their careers (ASHA, 2001). For most of these individuals, their education included doctoral studies, which provide core training in research methods. The majority of these researchers work in university settings. We asked some of these individuals

to tell us why they elected this career path and what it is like to be a researcher in the field of communication disorders.

Amy Skinder had just begun her doctoral studies at the University of Washington when we first talked with her. Prior to her enrollment, she had worked as a speech-language pathologist for four years, part of which was spent as a traveling clinician in a variety of settings around the country. "I am the last person out of my graduating class . . . that I expected to be going back for a Ph.D.," she reported. "My goal when I finished my master's was to be able to work with a broad range of disorders. After a while, I decided that instead of knowing a little about a lot, it would be nice to focus on one area. At the same time, I was working with a client in the public school system who had severe developmental apraxia of speech as well as attention deficit disorder and other learning disabilities. I went to a seminar . . . and asked lots of questions. I found out there weren't a lot of answers. After talking with the speaker [a noted researcher], I felt encouraged to go on for my doctorate. Doctoral studies are an opportunity to indulge in trying to answer all your burning questions."

When we next caught up with Amy Skinder she had obtained her doctorate, married, and has a faculty position at the University of Minnesota-Duluth. Dr. Skinder-Meredith filled us in on what it is like to start an academic and research career. "I enjoy my faculty position very much. It's good to be teaching! I work with wonderful people who value my work as a colleague, a teacher, and a researcher." She emphasized how important her own clinical background continues to be to her teaching and research endeavors. Besides conducting research in childhood apraxia, a communication disorder she saw as a clinician, she can draw on clinical issues to provide experiential learning in the classroom. In addition to continuing her own line of research, she has been forging contacts with others who work in her area of interest in order to foster collaborative research in the future.

This motivation has been echoed by many researchers we have talked with over the years. Anne Cordes Bothe, Ph.D., is on the faculty at the University of Georgia, where she conducts research in the area of stuttering. She realized during her master's degree that she wanted to go on for a doctorate. "The things that were catching my interest during my coursework and with my practicum clients were the things that we as a field didn't know or didn't yet understand—it wasn't the answers that I thought were interesting, it was the QUESTIONS! And the Ph.D. is a research degree, which is about questions, so it became pretty obvious that this is where I belonged."

Nancy Helm-Estabrooks, Sci.D., wrote, "In many ways I think I was always an informal researcher—trying new approaches, developing new materials, regarding every case as a case study—even before my doctoral studies, which I pursued in my thirties. I decided to get a doctorate to further my knowledge and to write grant proposals as a Principal Investigator so I could explore and test some ideas I had for new treatment approaches."

Steven Camarata, Ph.D., has been on the faculty at Vanderbilt University for over ten years. He wrote, "I wanted to teach at a university and was interested in

clinical research. Being able to follow my curiosity for research [is an exciting component of the job]. This freedom is a very precious gift. I knew that research would involve a lot of mundane work, but the discovery is worth it. Plus, I want to help children with speech and language problems and realized early on that I could best do this, not only by seeing patients (which I still do), but also by developing better treatments."

The efforts of getting a doctorate were definitely worth the time and effort for our colleagues. Barbara Lewis, Ph.D., of Rainbow Babies and Children's Hospital and Case Western Reserve University, has been conducting research for over ten years. Her work on the genetic basis of phonological disorders has drawn her into collaborations with psychologists, pediatricians, epidemiologists, and geneticists. She wrote to us, "I like the challenge of asking difficult research questions and finding results that do not always correspond to my prediction."

This was also apparent to Dr. Skinder-Meredith, when she was just beginning her research career. "It's not so easy to answer those big, burning questions. It's surprising how small you have to start out with your research. It's a lot more complicated than you anticipate." Those results, however unanticipated they may be, advance the state of professional knowledge.

Dr. Cordes Bothe wrote, "I love to pick up a new journal and read the report of a new study that flowed from a creative idea or from a creative way of approaching an old problem. If the method is good and sound so the results are believable, then it is such fun to enjoy the new findings and enjoy that sense of 'Well, of COURSE! Why hadn't anybody ever thought of that?' For the same reason, I love seeing a reference to my own published work in something that's almost unrelated, because somebody else saw some connection that I never even thought of." But the final impact of research is on clinical practice. We are one of the few therapeutic professions for which research advances are provided by its own membership, a situation that adds to the strength and autonomy of the professions as a whole.

Audiologist Theodore Glattke, Ph.D., expressed the importance of researchers within the profession, "If we fail to develop new knowledge, we will face extinction as service providers." Leslie Gonzalez Rothi, Ph.D., added, "We are the professionals best suited to perform this applied research—a bridge between basic research and clinical application."

Many of the most active researchers in our field are in academic positions. This brings with it the opportunity to interact with students. Dr. Cordes Bothe relates some of her favorite aspects of an academic position. "I like being able to sit with one student and figure out where she is and what the student's needs are and being able to point her in the right direction. I get a kick out of phrasing something just right in class so that I can see twenty light bulbs come on over the students' heads. And every so often, I get a kick out of the sudden realization that I DO know how to solve some problem after all." Dr. Glattke is on the faculty of the University of Arizona and has been in a faculty position for twenty-seven years. He has extensive experience mentoring students in research experiences. "It is a pleasure to witness the genuine excitement that the students express when they share their work. . . . Sometimes they discover something about themselves as a result of the

effort they put into writing about their research or synthesizing the literature base." He also had this to say about teaching in a university setting: "Contributing to the development of new knowledge, integrating the new knowledge into the curriculum, and adapting mentoring styles to respond to the needs of the students are invigorating activities. It is a privilege to be allowed to teach in a university setting."

Others conduct research within healthcare settings. Among the leading non-university research sites are some of the Veteran's Administration (VA) Medical Centers. Dr. Gonzalez Rothi is employed at the Gainesville Veteran's Administration Medical Center where she combines clinical practice with cutting edge research. She wrote that "my research background offers me a willingness to open doors that are not yet available to most. Second, no day is ever the same. Each time I come into the hospital, I find that new challenges are facing me, testing the limits of my abilities and always inspiring me to know more." Dr. Helm-Estabrooks has also worked in the VA system and has extensive experience conducting research in clinical settings. "Research appeals to my detective instincts, developing new assessment and treatment methods appeals to my creative instincts, and clinical research allows me to work directly with patients. Also, there are many aspects to my work—patient evaluations and therapy sessions, writing, teaching, mentoring, etc.—so that I'm always challenged and never bored."

Research careers present their own unique challenges. "One of the main challenges has been to remain focused on my primary interest—genetics of speech and language disorders," Dr. Lewis expressed. "There are many temptations to digress into related but very interesting areas. You have to realize that you can't do it all." Dr. Cordes Bothe agrees. "Balance and organization [are challenges]. My job gives me at least twice as many options as any one human being could reasonably keep track of. . . . An academic position is described as 'teaching, research, and service,' but what that really means is that the challenge is to find time for good teaching, good research, and a reasonable amount of service when it often seems that each day has about two days' worth of little stuff that has to get done. The challenge is to keep track of what's really important for the long term."

What advice do these individuals have to new generations of potential researchers? Dr. Lewis advises that "a student interested in research should learn as much as possible about research methodology and statistics while keeping a strong tie to the clinic. Most important is to identify an area of interest and explore related disciplines." Our research colleagues do not recommend so narrow a focus that outside studies and collaborations are ignored, however. Dr. Gonzalez Rothi urges students to "look for a program where you have an opportunity to look at a wide variety of perspectives. Set up an advisory committee that reflects this diversity. Take courses outside of your [major area of focus] that might be able to contribute to your knowledge base." Finally, Dr. Camarata provides this perspective: "Look in your heart and mind to determine whether satisfying your curiosity will sustain you. The key requirement for research is not 'intelligence' per se, but an interest in problem solving (with a large dose of persistence thrown in). If you like asking questions, a research career might be the most satisfying option."

CLINICAL PROBLEM SOLVING

We have introduced some of the types of communication disorders that concern the professions of audiology and speech-language pathology and have allowed some practicing professionals to share their insights about the field. The ensuing chapters will lay the groundwork necessary to understand normal and disordered communication processes in children and adults. We will consistently introduce the reader to clinical cases who bring to life the realities of the communication disorders. These individuals will help the reader appreciate the diagnostic and treatment processes that are at the heart of the professions.

Audiology and speech-language pathology are, by nature, fields in which memorization of facts is not enough for success. It requires the application of knowledge to real-life problems. For this reason, we will end each chapter with a section on clinical problem solving. This is an opportunity to take the information covered in a chapter and apply it to a case. We saw in this chapter how individual components of communication can break down in cases of disorder. Many communication disorders involve a combination of difficulties within the areas of speech, language, and hearing. Consider the following case:

Bonnie, age 8, was born with a severe hearing loss. Her loss was first diagnosed at age 18 months. She has some usable hearing for low-frequency sound and was fitted with hearing aids to help her capitalize on the little hearing she does have. Bonnie was placed in a preschool program that combined the use of hearing aid amplification with sign language and speech. Despite this early help, her spoken language skills were two years behind other children her age and her speech was grossly unintelligible when she entered first grade. Since then, she has made gains, but still struggles with grammar in both spoken and written language. Her speech is still difficult to understand, as she makes many articulation errors involving sounds that are out of her hearing range. Her voice has an effortful quality and sounds as if she is speaking from the back of her throat. Bonnie continues to receive academic tutoring and speech training. Her ability to communicate with spoken and written language lags far behind her ability to communicate through sign language.

1. Using Figure 1.1, identify which areas of communication (i.e., speech, language, hearing) are involved in Bonnie's case.
2. Identify the components of speech, language, or hearing that appear to be involved in this case.
3. Would Bonnie's communication disorder be classified as developmental or acquired?
4. Which professionals are likely to be involved with Bonnie to maximize her communication potential?

REFERENCES

American Speech-Language-Hearing Association (2001). *Semiannual counts of the ASHA membership and affiliation*. Rockville, MD: Author.

THE BIOLOGICAL FOUNDATIONS OF SPEECH AND LANGUAGE

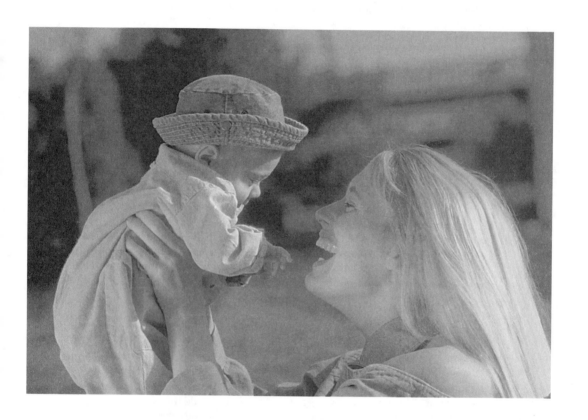

PREVIEW

Knowledge of the biological underpinnings of normal hearing, speech, and language is central to understanding the many ways in which communication can be disrupted. We will examine the vocal mechanism, which is responsible for sound production. The articulatory mechanism shapes the sound into the individual consonants and vowels that form words. Those words are perceived by the listener through the auditory system. Finally, they are comprehended by the brain, which then may store that information or formulate a response. The physical mechanisms normally do not function independently, but work together to support communication. When communication is disrupted by developmental disorder or acquired pathology, the disruption can often can be traced to one or more of these basic biological systems.

Speech-language pathologists and audiologists are confronted daily with clinical cases that require an understanding of the physical and neurological underpinnings of communication and how breakdowns in these systems lead to communication disorders. Consider the following scenarios:

Mr. Blades, age 71. In an acute-care hospital, a speech-language pathologist is asked to evaluate the speech and language of a 71-year-old man named Mr. Blades. He had been admitted to the hospital the day before, following a car accident in which he was a passenger. In addition to other injuries to his body, he had hit his head and lost consciousness for almost an hour. Although alert, he seemed to have difficulty understanding what was said to him. The clinician was concerned that the blow to the head may have damaged the parts of his brain that support language. Could the accident have caused difficulties in understanding language? Or could there be another cause for Mr. Blades' poor comprehension?

Alicia, age 3. Alicia was born with Down syndrome. This developmental disorder can be traced to a genetic abnormality that results in an extra copy of chromosome 21. For this engaging 3-year-old girl, the occurrence of this genetic abnormality could impact her communication skills in various ways. Low muscle tone associated with the disorder might interfere with her ability to move and explore her world. The changes to her oral-facial structure could interfere with speech articulation to some extent. Changes in the structure of the ear make children with Down syndrome prone to hearing loss. Her brain development has also been altered by the genetic abnormality, which has resulted in some degree of mental retardation. It might also have affected her capabilities for normal language development. An assessment team, consisting of a speech-language pathologist, an audiologist, a special educator, a psychologist, a physical therapist, and an occupational therapist, must determine how the effects of Down syndrome manifest in this child. The team will then determine how she can be assisted to maximize her overall development, including development of communication skills.

In both of these cases, the clinicians must have a thorough understanding of the physical mechanisms that support communication in order to determine the most likely sources of the communication problems these two individuals face. In the following sections, we will explore the biological systems that support normal communication and consider how they might be affected in clinical cases.

THE VOCAL MECHANISM

It is said that communication is an "overlaid function" that makes use of structures that have other primary functions. The same muscles and organs that allow us to breathe also provide the driving force behind sound production for speech. The larynx, which keeps us from choking on food or liquid that might otherwise be misdirected into the airway, also contributes to sound production. The structures of the mouth and throat that allow us to eat and drink also permit us to change the vocal tract in ways that result in the sounds that make up words and sentences.

The Respiratory System

The main function of the respiratory system is to sustain life through the continuous exchange of gases, primarily the exchange of carbon dioxide for oxygen. Because the body cannot store oxygen, it requires a continuous renewal of its oxygen supply, usually from twelve to eighteen inspirations-expirations (breath cycles) per minute. For the majority of persons without some kind of respiratory disease, the breath cycle continues almost unnoticed and without conscious effort.

Breathing is accomplished by movements of the rib cage and the **diaphragm**, a large muscle that separates the chest from the abdomen. The rib cage can be raised slightly by contraction of skeletal muscles. The diaphragm is shaped like an inverted bowl. When it contracts, it descends toward the abdomen, as shown in Figure 2.1. Because the lungs adhere to the inside of the rib cage and diaphragm, the lungs are stretched when the muscles of inspiration contract causing the rib cage to elevate and the diaphragm to descend. This increases the size of the lungs and results in a decrease in pulmonary pressure relative to air pressure outside the body. With the airways open, air flows into the lungs through the mouth or nose (or both) in order to balance the air pressure, and we inhale. Exhalation simply results from relaxation of the muscles of inhalation. The rib cage falls back to its resting state and the diaphragm ascends as it returns to its inverted bowl-shape. The lungs then decrease in size, causing an increase in pulmonary pressure relative to the atmosphere, and air rushes out. This cycle, shown in Figure 2.1 (p. 22), repeats itself continuously as we breathe in and out.

The inherent forces and active muscular contraction work, for example, during sleep in a natural, synergistic way. Our "in" breath is about as long as our "out" breath. When we sing or talk however, volitional forces are able to change the normal in-and-out pattern enabling us to take a quick inspiration and follow it

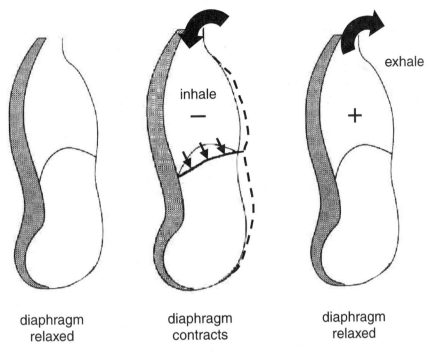

diaphragm   diaphragm   diaphragm
relaxed   contracts   relaxed

FIGURE 2.1   Schematic drawing of the torso during quiet breathing. Note that the diaphragm moves downward during inhalation and relaxes to a dome shape during exhalation. Adapted from Hixon (1973).

with a prolonged expiration, which we use for phonation. For a detailed understanding of aerodynamics of speech and voice, see Hixon and Abbs (1980), Kent, (1997), or Zemlin (1998).

The muscles of the torso that support respiration serve another function important to the support of speech breathing—that of postural control. These muscles support the body so that the lungs have room to expand. A person who lacks control of these muscles may have difficulty maintaining a stable posture for efficient speech breathing.

Many disorders can disrupt the musculoskeletal system that underlies control of speech breathing. Let us refer back to Alicia's case from the perspective of the respiratory system. When the evaluation team works with Alicia, several professionals will look at her musculoskeletal system. The physical therapist will examine postural support and gross motor movements. The occupational therapist will examine fine motor control, particularly in relation to age-appropriate play activities. The speech-language pathologist's primary concern will be whether Alicia has sufficient control over the muscles that support posture and respiration to permit connected speech. Alicia's muscle tone, although lower than normal, is adequate to support spoken communication. However, there are concerns about her ability to support her body and her motor skills.

The Phonatory System

Voice (or phonation) is produced by the vibration of the two vocal folds within the larynx. Although phonation is a vital part of communication, the primary function of the larynx is to guard the airway against **aspiration**, the inhalation of fluids or other matter into the airway. The larynx sits at the top of the trachea, where it plays this primary "watchdog" role, guarding the airway. When we swallow, the larynx elevates and muscles contract to protect the airway. In some individuals with structural damage to the vocal folds (a result of cancer, for example) or with muscular impairment of laryngeal function (perhaps part of a degenerative neuro-muscular disease), the valving mechanism can be compromised and the patient may experience life-threatening choking spells.

The human voice represents perhaps the highest function of the larynx in the mammal. To appreciate the perspective that the human voice may well not be an evolutionary accident, one has only to listen to the sheer beauty and control of the voice as heard in an operatic aria or popular ballad or the vocal interpretations of an accomplished actor. The communicative and artistic functions of the larynx take it well beyond its basic valving responsibilities. The average person, for example, is unaware of the valving role of the larynx, and when asked what the larynx (or "voice box") does, may answer, "We make sound with it."

The front and back view of the larynx can be seen in Figure 2.2. The **cricoid cartilage** forms the base of this structure and the **thyroid cartilage** sits above the cricoid. The thyroid cartilage is shield-shaped and forms the prominent anterior wall of the larynx. In many young men, we can see the prominent thyroid cartilage

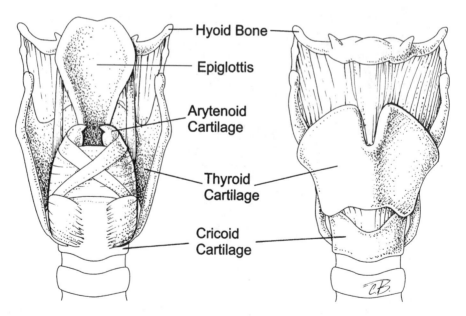

FIGURE 2.2   Structures of the larynx.

(Adam's apple). The vocal folds originate just below the thyroid notch that you can feel when you place your fingertips on your Adam's apple. From the thyroid cartilage, the vocal folds extend posteriorly to the base of two pyramid-shaped cartilages called the arytenoids. The vocal folds can be seen by looking down on the larynx from above, as seen in Figure 2.3. In this figure, we can see the open vocal folds and the arytenoid cartilages. The view of the thyroid cartilage is blocked by the **epiglottis**.

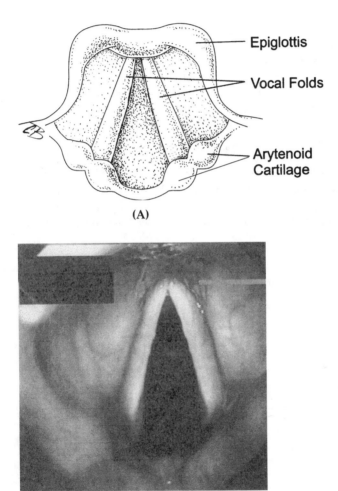

(A)

(B)

FIGURE 2.3   **The vocal folds can be viewed by looking down on the larynx from above. (A) Diagram of the vocal folds, arytenoid cartilages, and epiglottis. (B) Normal vocal folds.**

In Figure 2.2, the **arytenoid cartilages** sit on top of the posterior cricoid carti-lage. The arytenoid cartilages move and rotate on their mounts atop the cricoid cartilage by the action of several intrinsic muscles in the larynx. For example, when certain muscles contract, they move the arytenoid cartilages in such a way that they pull the vocal folds apart. The muscles that accomplish this movement are known as laryngeal *ab*ductors (they separate the folds). Laryngeal *ad*ductor mus-cles rotate the arytenoids in such a way that the folds come together. This muscle action is extremely quick, permitting the speaker to produce the rapid changes in voicing needed for continuous speech.

Another intrinsic muscle function is to lengthen (by stretching and tensing) or to shorten (by relaxing and thickening) the folds. Either action has an effect on pitch level. Thinner folds vibrate more quickly, producing higher frequencies (pitches); thicker folds vibrate more slowly, producing lower frequencies. The area between the vocal folds is known as the **glottis**. When the vocal folds are brought together (adduction), they are in the phonating position. The outgoing air builds up below the vocal folds, causing increased **subglottal air pressure**. When this pressure is greater than the pressure holding the folds together at the midline, it blows the vocal folds apart. A puff of air is released between the open folds, which then return to the midline. The closure results from the elastic recoil of the vocal fold tissues and is assisted by the movement of air across the surface of the folds. This opening and closing produce what is known as one cycle of phonation. Re-peated cycles produce sound, or phonation.

Because outgoing airflow causes the vocal folds to vibrate, changes in inten-sity or loudness of the voice are produced by changes in pressure below the level of the vocal folds. This pressure can be raised by increasing the muscular force that holds the vocal folds together or by increasing the respiratory drive. When the air-flow finally breaks through the vocal folds, they are blown apart with greater force. This, in turn, produces a greater lateral excursion of the vocal folds resulting in greater air displacement. In this way, a speaker can increase the loudness of the voice.

Along with loudness, changes in the pitch of the voice also occur as a result of changes in the action of the vocal folds. What we hear as pitch relates directly to the frequency at which the vocal folds open and close. The normal pitch of the speaking voice is primarily determined by the size and mass of the vocal folds. The tiny vocal folds in babies produce high voices because their vocal folds vibrate quickly. Nine-year-old children, for whom puberty has not begun, produce speak-ing voices just above middle C on the musical scale. We can describe this in terms of the number of vibrations per second, or cycles per second (**Hertz**). The speaking voice of an adult male, whose vocal folds have increased in size since puberty, is about an octave lower than it was when he was 9 years old. The adult female, whose larynx is usually half again as big as it was when she was 9, typically speaks at a pitch that falls between that of a male adult and a child.

The speed of the vibratory cycle is dependent on the mass, elasticity, and length of the vocal folds. These properties of the vocal folds can be changed by the action of the muscles of the larynx. When laryngeal muscles stretch the folds, they

become thinner, producing a faster vibratory rate (higher frequency). This translates to a higher vocal pitch. Likewise, when muscle action causes the folds to become shorter and thicker, the vibratory frequency decreases, and a lower pitch is heard. For a more detailed account of laryngeal functions and their relation to frequency and intensity, see Weismer (1988), Kent, (1997), and Zemlin (1998).

The Resonance System

Although the source of the voice is the larynx, sound waves are modified by the other structures within the throat, mouth, and nasal cavities. This is analogous to the way in which the body of a guitar modifies the sound produced by plucking the string. The sound waves that we recognize as the human voice result from both the sound produced by the larynx and the filtering of that sound by the resonance system.

The first area of the vocal tract through which the sound waves travel is immediately above the larynx. This cavity is called the **pharynx** (see Figure 2.4). The height of the pharynx changes as the larynx rises (shortens the pharynx) or lowers (lengthens the pharynx). The overall shape and width of the pharynx changes as the tongue moves forward or back and the pharyngeal walls move inward.

The pharynx can be studied using **videoendoscopy**, which involves placement of an illuminated lens to look down the back of the throat toward the larynx. The images of this structure can then be viewed on a video monitor. By doing this, we can see that the pharynx is constantly changing shape during speech. In a fascinating videoendoscopic tape distributed by the Voice Foundation (1985) of two famous impersonators, Rich Little and Mel Blanc, we can see that much of the muscle action used to produce many different voice impersonations takes place in the pharyngeal cavities. Although the pharynx plays an important role in shaping vocal resonance, it obviously plays another vital role as a conduit for the passage of air and food.

In addition to the pharynx, the oral cavity also shapes the resonance characteristics of the voice. The opening within the mouth is constantly changing size and shape during speech. The overall size of the oral opening is primarily determined by the position of the **mandible**, or lower jaw, which is continually lowering and elevating during speech. As the jaw drops for saying a low vowel, such as "ah," the tongue drops with it. However, the tongue has the greatest flexibility of any muscle group in the body, constantly changing its shape and position. When the tongue rides high, as in producing the "i" vowel, it occupies much of the anterior oral cavity. Vocal resonance is heavily influenced by the posture of the mouth, which is determined by the position of the mandible *and* the position of the tongue within the oral cavity (Boone & McFarlane, 2000).

The roof of the oral cavity is formed anteriorly by the bony hard palate and posteriorly by the muscular soft palate (also known as **velum**). The velum is a muscular structure, noticible for its dangling appendage, the *uvula*. The velum hangs down during normal breathing so that air can flow between the nasal cavity and the oral cavity. When eating or drinking, the opening between these two

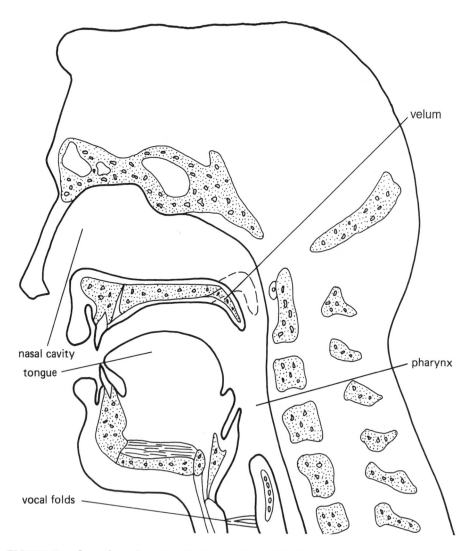

FIGURE 2.4 Sound produced at the larynx is modified by the resonance characteristics of the vocal tract, which consists of the pharynx and the oral and nasal cavities. At rest, the velum allows air to flow into the nasal cavity. When contracted (note dashed lines), it elevates to touch the pharyngeal wall.

cavities is closed as the velum raises and the pharyngeal wall constricts around it. During the production of most speech sounds, the velum is raised to close off the nasal cavity from the oral cavity. This allows for oral resonance of all the vowels and consonants in the English language except for the nasal sounds. When nasal sounds are produced, sound waves enter the nasal cavity through an open

velopharyngeal port. This nasal-oral coupling is the position required for the resonance of the three nasal consonants in English, "m," "n," and "ng." If we were to say *banana*, for example, the initial "ba" would require a raised velum. The "n" would require a rapid drop of the velum, with the next vowel, "a," requiring closure again, only to be followed by another rapid drop for the next "n," ending with an elevated velum again for the vowel "a."

Failure to move the velum rapidly enough to match the demands of the particular utterance can result in excessively nasal speech, called **hypernasality**. Many problems that involve hypernasality are related to faulty velopharyngeal closure, which could be related to a number of factors, such as cleft palate, short velum, injured palate, or paralysis or weakness of the velopharyngeal muscles (such disorders are discussed in several subsequent chapters). A less common resonance disorder is **denasality**, which is insufficient nasal resonance often related to excessive velopharyngeal closure. The *nasal cavity* may become blocked with swollen tissues (perhaps due to allergies and colds) that dampen sound waves and block the airflow through the nasal cavities. Excessive tonsil and adenoid tissue in the nasal cavity will sometimes create enough obstruction to give the voice a denasal vocal quality.

The resonance system gives each voice its distinctive quality. Changes in the quality of the voice can signal vocal pathology, as we will see in Chapter 6. Let us now look at the resonance system in the case of Alicia, the child with Down syndrome.

> Down syndrome can involve congenital malformations of the naso- and oropharynx. These can result in altered voice quality. For Alicia, the speech-language pathologist noted some instances of hypernasality. This can result from poor control of the velopharyngeal mechanism or from a defect in the articulatory mechanism, explained below. To differentiate between these two possible causes, the speech-language pathologist evaluated both the oral structures and velopharyngeal functioning.

THE ARTICULATORY MECHANISM

The Tongue

Looking at Figure 2.4 on page 27, we can see that the tongue occupies most of the space of the oral cavity. The tongue body is a composite of intrinsic muscles that run both the length and width of the structure and enable us to change its shape easily (curled, pointed, and so on). Other muscles of the tongue originate outside the tongue from various sites, such as the hyoid bone. These extrinsic muscles allow the tongue to be elevated, lowered, protruded, and retracted. How our tongue is postured influences the overall sound and resonance of the voice and is critical for the production of individual speech sounds. The vowels and diphthongs of our speech are produced primarily through changes in the shape and movement of the tongue (and elevation of the jaw). Most consonants are produced by vocal tract constriction, which results in some airflow restriction, more often than not caused by some precise movement of the tongue. Without the precision of tongue movements, there could be no articulate speech.

The Lips

The lips are made up primarily of facial muscles, which make it possible for them to pucker, spread, or make a circle. The lips are the most visible structures of the mouth and are easily shaped and altered to produce various facial expressions. They also play a vital role in such oral behaviors as sucking, kissing, chewing, and smiling. The lips represent the end of the oral vocal tract and also contribute to the resonance of the voice. For example, if one were to say an extended *"eee"* for five seconds and alternately pucker and then relax the lips while prolonging the sound, one would hear distinct changes in the vocal resonance with each pucker. This is because the lips extend or shorten the length of the oral cavity with each movement. The lips also play a primary function in the production of many consonants. Sounds such as "m," "p," "b," and "w" are produced by movements of the lip; "f" and "v" are produced with the upper teeth on or against the lower lip.

The Mandible

The movement of the mandible, or lower jaw, allows for the quick opening or closing of the mouth. Some mandibular movement contributes to change in the shape and size of the oral cavity needed for the production of different vowels. The normal speaker moves the mandible in quick synergistic movements with the lips and tongue during normal speech. If, however, a speaker were to talk with a pen in his mouth, the mandible would stay closed to trap the pen, which would require an immediate compensatory adjustment of the tongue and lips to maintain speech articulation. Optimal speech production and vocal resonance require continuous mandibular movement. Occasionally, we see patients with voice problems who speak with a clenched jaw most of the time, requiring the tongue to make all the muscle movements needed for vowel differentiation. Speaking this way is inefficient and often results in a muffled voice and sloppy articulation.

The Palate

The bony hard palate and the muscular soft palate make up the structures of the roof of the mouth, or **palate**. The hard palate extends from the alveolar ridge and tooth sockets of the maxillary dentition. It is an arched structure with a vaulted ceiling that contributes greatly to oral resonance. The tongue moves freely, making various articulatory contacts with the palate. Attached posteriorly to the hard palate just beyond the last molar tooth is the muscular soft palate. We discussed earlier the importance of the velum in its contact with the pharynx in separating the oral cavity from the nasal cavity for oral vocal resonance.

The Teeth

The teeth play a primary role in the chewing of food. Their contribution to speech articulation is somewhat secondary. However, a few English sounds, such as "f" and "v," are made by labial-dental contact, the lower lip being tucked under the

upper central incisors. The alveolar ridge behind the base of the maxillary teeth is an important contact point for the tongue for the production of such sounds as "n," "s," "z," "t," and "d." The tongue also extends out between the upper and lower central incisors for the production of "th" sounds.

When speech is slow to develop or the quality of spoken words is poor, it is important to rule out possible contributions by the oral and facial structures. In Alicia's case, the speech-language pathologist performed what is known as an **oral-peripheral examination**. This is an evaluation of the structure and function of the articulatory mechanisms.

> Alicia's oral-peripheral exam revealed several factors that could be important for communication. Some of her front teeth are quite crooked, which may interfere with sounds made against the teeth, such as "th" or "s." Her hard palate is highly arched, but does not contain any clefts or holes that would allow air to flow into the nasal cavity to produce hypernasality. Although her tongue appears large for her mouth and tends to protrude a bit, it is not actually too large, rather, it lacks the muscle tone to rest within the mouth. Alicia's face has a soft, rounded appearance, which also suggests low muscle tone of the facial muscles. Low tone in the oral and facial muscles can interfere with the movements needed to produce the sounds of speech. All these factors may account for the perception that Alicia's words sound "thick" and imprecise.

THE NERVOUS SYSTEM

The remarkable ability of human beings to communicate so efficiently is related primarily to a most complex nervous system that permits communication between a person and the environment, other creatures, and other people. The nervous systems of other animals may have features that permit them to perform a particular behavior "better" than human beings. For example, predator birds have more acute eyesight than humans, and the porpoise has a more advanced auditory system. However, it is the complex human brain that allows human beings to master the complexities and subtleties of human language. The brain is part of the **central nervous system** (CNS). It works in concert with the **peripheral nervous system** (PNS), which allows information to travel to and from the body. We will consider each separately.

Central Nervous System

The brain and the spinal cord, seen in Figure 2.5, are considered the two primary CNS structures. The brain enables humans to engage in high-level functions, such as learning from the environment and synthesizing information. Because of its critical role in such functions, factors that alter brain development or damage the brain underlie many types of communication disorders. Between the brain and spinal cord is the brainstem. The brainstem and spinal cord comprise the primary pathway for much of the sensory information that comes from the body. Con-

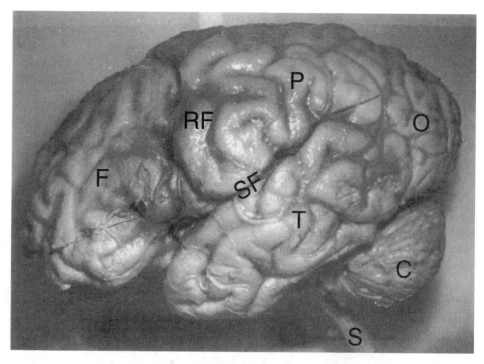

FIGURE 2.5 Structures of the human nervous system include the cerebrum, which can be divided into the frontal (F), parietal (P), occiptial (O), and temporal (T) lobes. Dividing the frontal from the parietal lobe is the Rolandic fissure (RF); dividing the parietal and temporal lobes is the Sylvian fissure (SF). Also seen are the cerebellum (C) and spinal cord (S).

versely, the brain sends motor commands through the brainstem to the spinal cord that result in our ability to support and move our bodies. Therefore, damage to the brainstem or spinal cord, with the resulting loss of muscular control, can disrupt the biological support necessary for speech.

The brain consists of the **cerebrum** and the **cerebellum** (see Figure 2.5). The cerebrum occupies the majority of the brain cavity within the head. The cerebellum sits below the cerebrum and behind the brainstem. Both the cerebrum and the cerebellum can be further divided into right and left **hemispheres**. The hemispheres of the cerebrum are joined at the midline by the **corpus callosum**, which is a large band of fibers that carries information between the cerebral hemispheres (see Figure 2.6, p. 32). The surface of the brain appears as a series of ridges, called *gyri*, and grooves, called *sulci*. Large sulci are referred to as fissures. The gyri and sulci can be individually identified by name, so that the location of both normal and pathological features of the cortex can be described in specific terms.

The cerebral hemispheres can be further divided into four lobes (see Figure 2.5), each of which contains regions that are associated with particular functions.

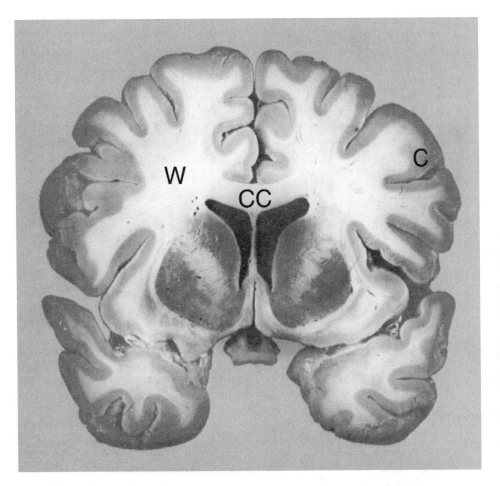

**FIGURE 2.6   A cross section of the brain. The corpus callosum (CC) can be seen
bridging the right and left hemispheres. The gray matter of the cortex (C) and white
matter (W)** *can be clearly distinguished.*

The **frontal lobes** contain the primary motor cortex that sends neural commands
to specific parts of the body. It also contains regions that are involved with attention, impulse control, and judgment. The **parietal lobes** contain the primary sensory cortex, which receives sensory information from the body, as well as other
regions that support a number of cognitive functions. The **occipital lobes**, at the
back of the brain, receive and process visual information. The **temporal lobes** contain the primary auditory cortex as well as regions important for language comprehension and memory.

   The specialized functions of each of the hemisphere's lobes are attributed to
differences in cells found within these regions. If we examine a cross section of the
cerebrum (see Figure 2.6), we can see the surface layer, or **cortex**. The cortex con-

tains layers of **neurons**, which are cells that support different types of brain activity. Because the bodies of these neurons appear gray, the cortex is also called *gray matter*. The layers of the cortex within the primary motor area of the frontal lobe, for example, contain many neurons that send signals to the body for the control of movement, whereas the primary sensory cortex contains many cells that receive incoming signals from the body. If we look at the cross section of the cerebrum (Figure 2.6), the lighter gray tissue beneath the cortex consists of cell fibers that originate in the gray matter. These fibers connect regions of the brain, receive sensory information from the body, and send impulses to move the muscles of the body. Such fibers are collectively referred to as *white matter*.

In the front half of the brain is a collection of subcortical bodies known as the **basal ganglia** (see Figure 2.6). These neural bodies are highly connected to the cerebellum and to cortical regions involved in movement. Disorders of the basal ganglia often result in impaired movements. In the posterior half of the brain, behind the basal ganglia, is another collection of subcortical neurons known as the **thalamus**. This highly complex region receives all types of information that is relayed between areas of the brain.

Several regions of the brain are particularly important for communication and are frequently involved when communication disorders occur. Neural impulses that occur in response to sound first reach the level of the cortex at the *primary auditory cortex* within the temporal lobes of both the right and left hemispheres. This region is on the superior surface of the temporal lobe inside the Sylvian fissure and is sometimes called *Heschl's gyrus* (see Figure 2.7). Within the left hemisphere, the primary auditory cortex is surrounded by cortical tissue that supports higher level auditory functions, including the comprehension of spoken language. Areas particularly important to this skill occupy the posterior regions of

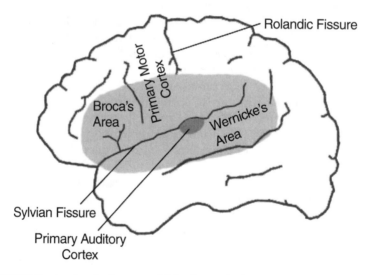

FIGURE 2.7   Anatomical areas within the perisylvian region (shaded in light gray).

the superior temporal lobe and parts of the parietal lobe. Sections of the left infe-rior frontal lobe, on the other hand, appear particularly important to aspects of lan-guage expression. Finally, the motor movements of speech are supported by the *primary motor area*, which is located in the frontal lobe of each hemisphere. This area works in conjunction with subcortical structures and the cerebellum to pro-duce the movements needed for speech.

In a normal, healthy brain, these various regions work in concert to support normal communication in all its complexity. However, when a brain is compro-mised during development or due to disease or injury, communication break-downs can occur.

> For Alicia, the effects that brought her to the developmental center began long be-fore the day of her birth. The genetic anomaly that leads to Down syndrome affects the development of the brain. Research with this population has revealed certain brain characteristics that co-occur with this disorder. In Down syndrome, changes in fetal brain development can be detected by ultrasound between 16 and 21 weeks gestation (Bahado-Singh, Wyse, Dorr, Copel, O'Connor, & Hobbins, 1992). These changes reflect neurobiologic features such as reduced brain size (particularly in the frontal lobes), fewer cells within specific layers of the cortex, and smaller cere-bellar size (see Schmidt-Sidor, Wisniewski, Shepard, & Seren, 1990 for a review of the brain correlates of Down syndrome). After birth, these neuroanatomic differ-ences can have functional correlates of concern for communication. For example, neuroimaging research has demonstrated reduced metabolic activity in the lan-guage areas of the brain associated with Down syndrome (Azari, Horowitz, Petti-grew, Grady, Haxby, Giacometti, & Schapiro, 1994).

Normal brain development is characterized by overproduction of neurons and of connections between cells. After birth, the brain normally begins a lifetime of refining itself by pruning back excess cells and connections and strengthening those connections that are most functional. What determines which cells and connections are most functional? A large determinant of functionality is the experience the young child receives. In other words, all babies' brains are shaped by the things they see, hear, and explore. Even for a baby like Alicia, brain development is not complete at birth. Experience continues to shape the brain throughout life. A child's early experiences are critical for realizing that child's full potential throughout life. This is one reason that professionals advocate for early intervention for children with communication disorders and those at risk for problems.

In other instances of communication disorders, the brain may have devel-oped normally, only to be damaged later by illness or injury. In fact, much of what we know about the brain's organization was learned by observing the behavior of individuals who suffered damage to localized regions of the brain. This work began in the 1800s with two landmark cases. Paul Broca described a case of a man who lost his ability to express himself through spoken language, but retained much of his ability to understand language and his general cognitive functioning. When this man died, Broca described the area of damage within the left frontal lobe, which has come to be known as Broca's area. Since that time, this area has

been closely associated with processes important for expressive language. Conversely, Carl Wernicke described a case of a man who lost the ability to comprehend spoken language whose brain lesion was in the posterior part of the left temporal lobe. This general area, associated with language comprehension, has come to be called Wernicke's area.

The work begun by Broca and Wernicke gave rise to the **cerebral localization** perspective on brain functioning. The premise of a localizationist approach is that certain regions within the brain appear necessary for a particular skill or function. For most people, the left hemisphere is specialized for language. In particular, the regions of the left hemisphere that surround the **Sylvian fissure** are critical language areas. This so-called **perisylvian region** includes the primary auditory cortex and the primary sensory and motor regions for the face that are located on either bank of the **Rolandic fissure**, which is roughly at right angles to the Sylvian fissure (see Figure 2.7). It also includes both Broca's and Wernicke's areas and additional areas of association cortex in the region. Damage within this broadly defined perisylvian region can lead to various types of language disorders, as we will see in Chapters 8 and 9.

The localization perspective focuses on regions that contribute to particular functions. However, we have become increasingly aware that brain areas do not act in isolation. Rather, systems composed of various brain structures and the connections between them act together to support behavior. This insight has given rise to a *connectionist* perspective, which emphasizes the interconnectedness of functionally related brain regions. For example, Geschwind described a connectionist model of language functioning that involved the sequential transfer of information through various left hemisphere regions in support of activities like reading aloud or repeating words (Geschwind, 1977). These types of models of brain functioning provide a basis for understanding the behavioral deficits that occur after brain damage.

For most individuals, language is a left hemisphere function; however, effective communication relies on many regions within both hemispheres of the brain. For example, listening to a lecture can involve all lobes simultaneously. As each person concentrates on the speaker, he or she tries to ignore other distractions (frontal and parietal lobes), take in the auditory and visual speech signal (temporal and occipital lobes), interpret its content (left temporal lobe), and visually monitor the facial expressions and affect of the speaker (occipital and right parietal lobes). It is the integrated function of all these brain regions that allows the listener to receive the verbal and nonverbal information and comprehend its meaning.

Peripheral Nervous System

To be functional, the brain must be connected to the outside world. This connection is made through the peripheral nervous system. The upper section of the peripheral nervous system includes twelve pairs of nerves that enter or exit the CNS within the cranial space occupied by the brain and brainstem. These are known as the **cranial nerves** (see Table 2.1).

TABLE 2.1. The Cranial Nerves

CRANIAL NERVE	NAME	PRIMARY FUNCTION	ROLE IN COMMUNICATION
I	Olfactory	Sense of smell	—
II	Optic	Vision	Face-to-face communication Reading Writing Sign Language
III	Occulomotor	Eye movement	Reading Writing Sign language
IV	Trochlear	Eye movement	Reading Writing Sign language
V	Trigeminal	Movement of jaw Sensation from face	Speaking
VI	Abducens	Eye movement	Reading Writing
VII	Facial	Movement of facial muscles Sensation from tongue, velum	Speaking
VIII	Auditory	Hearing and balance	Listening
IX	Glossopharyngeal	Movement of pharynx Sensation from posterior tongue, pharynx	Speaking
X	Vagus	Movement of larynx, pharynx, velum, diaphragm, heart, abdominal viscera Sensation from larynx, pharynx, internal ear, other body organs	Speaking
XI	Accessory motor	Movement of large muscles of the head, neck, shoulders	Speaking
XII	Hypoglossal	Movement of tongue, supralaryngeal muscles	Speaking

As one can see from Table 2.1, most of the cranial nerves play some role in communication. Therefore, injury or disease that affects individual nerves may also impair specific aspects of communication. It is not surprising, then, that speech-language pathologists and audiologists include assessment of functions related to cranial nerves when evaluating individuals with communication disorders.

Below the level of the cranial nerves are thirty-one pairs of nerves that enter or exit the spinal cord, known as the **spinal nerves**. The **spinal cord** is made up of ascending and descending nerve tracts. There are anterior and posterior nuclei at thirty-one levels of the spinal cord. From the anterior nuclei exit the thirty-one paired motor nerves (right and left) that innervate (depending on their level and site) the muscles of the chest, the abdomen, and the limbs. The posterior nuclei in the spinal cord have sensory functions. Sensory nerves come into the posterior spinal nuclei from various peripheral sites, such as glands, tissues, joints, and muscles. Some of the peripheral sensory information is "handled" at the spinal level, where various sensorimotor reflexes may occur. In other cases, the sensory information may be passed up into the central nervous system through the **brainstem** and cerebellum, where sensorimotor adjustments may be made. The sensory information may also travel to the thalamus, where it may be processed further. Some sensory impulses from the spinal nerves probably project directly (with little filtering or adjustment along the way) to the sensory cortex.

CLINICAL PROBLEM SOLVING

We opened this chapter with a case description of Mr. Blades, the man who had been in a serious car accident. The speech-language pathologist was asked to help determine why his comprehension may be poor.

1. Why would the clinician suspect that the car accident may have produced the language comprehension problem?
2. What other biological system(s) could also be the source of poor comprehension? Why?
3. If Mr. Blades also had difficulty speaking, what other biological system(s) could be involved? Why?

REFERENCES

Azari, N. P., Horowitz, B., Pettigrew, K. D., Grady, C. L., Haxby, J. V., Giacometti, K. R., & Schapiro, M. B. (1994). Abnormal pattern of cerebral glucose metabolic rates involving language areas in young adults with Down syndrome. *Brain and Language, 46,* 1–20.

Bahado-Singh, R. O., Wyse, L., Dorr, M. A., Copel, J. A., O'Connor, T., & Hobbins, J. C. (1992). Fetuses with Down syndrome have disproportionately shortened frontal lobe dimensions on ultrasonographic examination. *American Journal of Obstetrics and Gynecology, 167,* 1009–1014.

Boone, D. R., & McFarlane, S. C. (2000). *The voice and voice therapy* (6th ed.). Englewood Cliffs, NJ: Prentice Hall.

Geschwind, N. (1977). Specialization of the human brain. *Scientific American, 241,* 180–201.

Hixon, T. J. (1973). Respiratory function in speech. In F. D. Minifie, T. J. Hixon, & F. Williams (Eds.), *Normal aspects of speech, hearing, and language* (pp. 73–126). Englewood Cliffs, NJ: Prentice Hall.

Hixon, T. J., & Abbs, J. H. (1980). Normal speech production. In T. J. Hixon, L. D. Shriberg, & J. H. Saxman (Eds.), *Introduction to communi-*

cation disorders. Englewood Cliffs, NJ: Prentice Hall.

Kent, R. D. (1997). *The speech sciences*. San Diego, CA: Singular Publishing Group, Inc.

Schmidt-Sidor, B., Wisniewski, K. E., Shepard, T. H., & Seren, E. A. (1990). Brain growth in Down syndrome subjects 15-22 weeks gestational age and birth to 60 months. *Clinical Neuropathology, 9,* 181–190.

Voice Foundation. (1985). *The voice of the impersonator*. (Videocassette developed by R. Feder.) New York: Author.

Weismer, C. (1988). Speech production. In N. J. Lass, L. V. McReynolds, J. L. Northern, & D. E. Yoder (Eds.), *Handbook of speech-language pathology and audiology*. Philadelphia: B. C. Decker.

Zemlin, W. R. (1998). *Speech and hearing science: Anatomy and physiology* (4th ed.). Boston: Allyn and Bacon.

SOUNDS IN COMMUNICATION

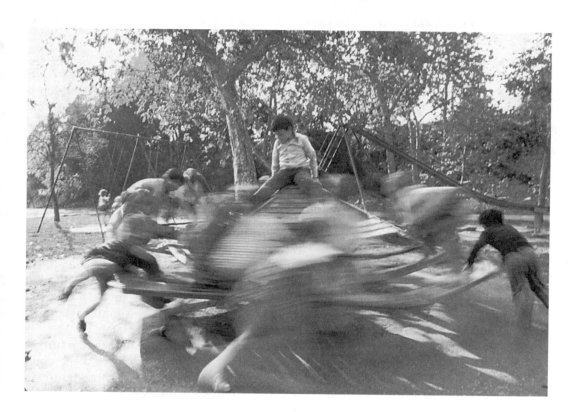

With contributions by Theodore J. Glattke, Ph.D.

■ ■ ■ ■ ■ ▬▬

PREVIEW

Sounds are the currency of auditory-oral communication. Both speech-language pathologists and audiologists are concerned with acoustic elements of sound as they are heard or produced. Because of this, they need a firm grasp of the basic physical nature of sound, how it is produced by humans, and how it can be described. Furthermore, the sounds of language must be acquired as an individual learns language. We will examine this process in a young child who is in the process of acquiring English as his native language.

Auditory functioning supports communication at many levels. A short bark at the back door lets us know that the dog wants to come inside. The phone's ring tells us someone is trying to reach us. With speech, humans are able to use sound to express an infinite variety of ideas, moods, and attitudes. We will examine sound first at its most basic level as an acoustic signal, and then as the signal is modified to form human speech.

ACOUSTIC ASPECTS OF SOUND

The essence of sound is motion. When someone talks to you from across the room, the vibrations created by his or her voice and articulation are carried through the air to your ears. Sound energy "travels" because air molecules that are adjacent to a source of vibration bump up against neighboring molecules and push them a bit. The individual molecules do not move far before they rebound back in place, but they set off a chain reaction of motion that radiates from the source. Those molecules likewise displace their neighbors, and so on, so that the vibration is propagated. As depicted in Figure 3.1, the disturbed molecules alternately bunch close together (causing areas of *compression*) and then spread apart as they return to their original locations (causing regions of *rarefaction*). This vibratory motion produces a sound wave that travels through the air, but can also be carried through other media like water or solid structures, such as dormitory walls.

Frequency

The rate of vibration is referred to as the **frequency** of the sound. It is the number of complete cycles of to and fro motion that occur in one second. The units of measurement for frequency are named Hertz to honor a scientist who made important contributions to the development of the radio. Young persons are able to hear sounds that range in frequency from about 20 to 20,000 Hertz (Hz). Sounds at different frequencies are each perceived as having a different **pitch**. In other words, frequency refers to that actual number of vibrations per second, whereas pitch reflects how those frequencies sound to us.

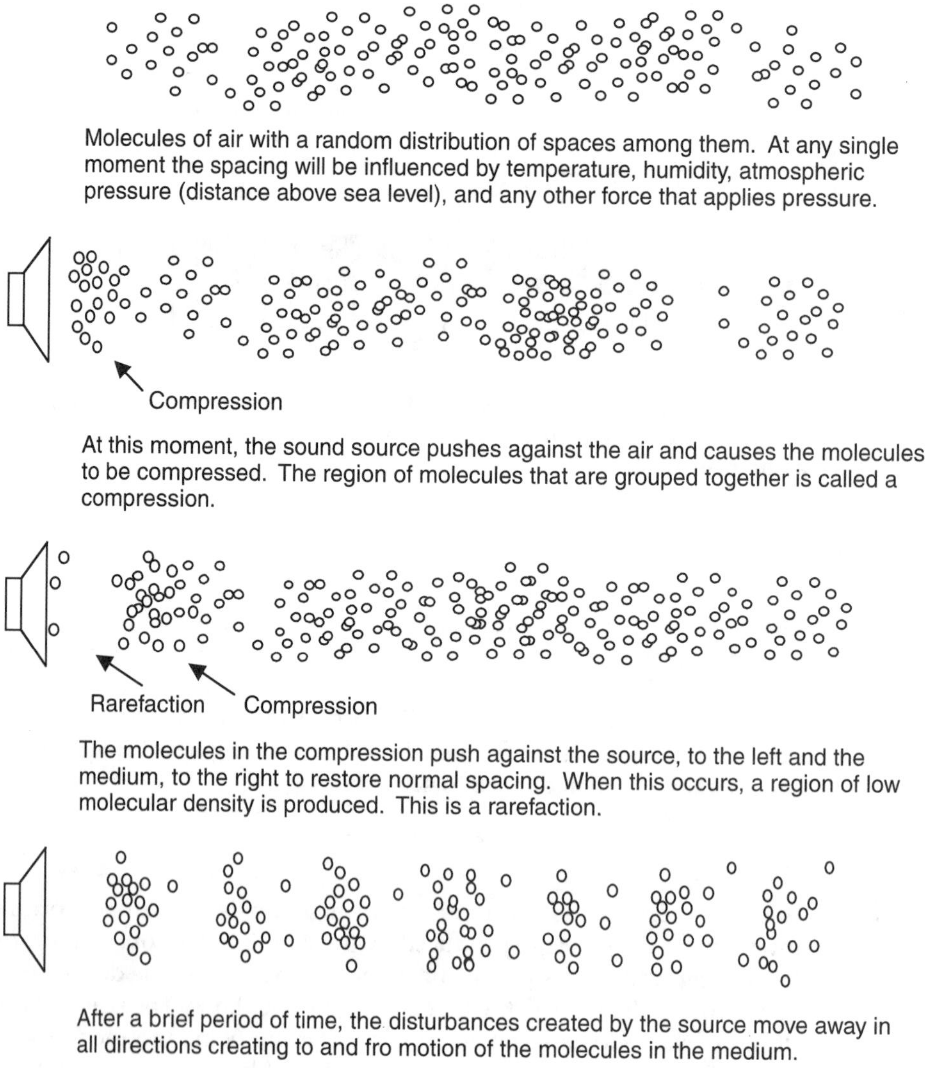

Molecules of air with a random distribution of spaces among them. At any single moment the spacing will be influenced by temperature, humidity, atmospheric pressure (distance above sea level), and any other force that applies pressure.

Compression

At this moment, the sound source pushes against the air and causes the molecules to be compressed. The region of molecules that are grouped together is called a compression.

Rarefaction   Compression

The molecules in the compression push against the source, to the left and the medium, to the right to restore normal spacing. When this occurs, a region of low molecular density is produced. This is a rarefaction.

After a brief period of time, the disturbances created by the source move away in all directions creating to and fro motion of the molecules in the medium.

FIGURE 3.1   Illustrations of compressions and rarefactions in air, which serve to propagate sound.

The notes on a piano keyboard span the frequency range from about 20 to 4000 Hz. The voices of people, the sounds of speech, and most of the music that we enjoy are within that frequency range. Figure 3.2 (p. 42) illustrates a standard piano keyboard. Middle C (C4) on the piano corresponds to a frequency of 256 Hz, which means that when the piano string is struck, it vibrates 256 times in one second. This frequency is typical of the fundamental frequency of the voice of an adult woman.

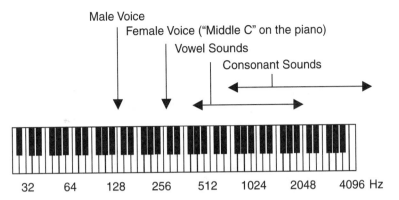

FIGURE 3.2 **Frequency of sound in Hertz. Note that the frequencies that allow us to distinguish between vowels and consonants are higher than those that distinguish among voices.**

The voice of a man has a fundamental frequency that is about 128 Hz, or half the typical frequency of a woman's voice. When the frequency of sound is increased by a ratio of 2:1, it is increased by one octave, so a typical woman's voice is about one octave higher than a typical man's voice. Additional information in a speaker's voice is carried at higher frequencies. The most important frequencies for speech sounds range from about 500 to 4000 Hz.

Intensity

What we perceive as the loudness of a sound is determined primarily by its **intensity**, or the pressure produced by the vibrating motion. Sound pressure level (SPL) is typically measured using a **decibel** (dB) scale. The decibel was named to honor Alexander G. Bell, the inventor of the telephone. The scale is based on logarithms of the ratio between an arbitrary starting point and the pressure, or intensity, to be measured. The starting point, 0 dB SPL, is approximately the smallest pressure that can be detected by a person with no hearing loss. The logarithmic scale is such that the loudness of sounds increases faster than the decibel values assigned to them. To illustrate, the range of pressure from the threshold of hearing to the threshold of discomfort is about a million to one (Kelly, 1985), but on the logarithmic scale the difference between these two sounds is only about 120 dB. The sound pressure levels for some common sounds are shown in Table 3.1. Of interest to us at this point is the relative loudness of the human voice compared to various environmental sounds. You can see that conversational speech falls in the middle of this range of intensities. It is obvious that hearing speech is easier when we are not also confronted with louder sounds.

TABLE 3.1. **Possible Sound Pressure Levels of Common Sounds**

10–20 dB	Whispering heard from over five feet away
40 dB	A quiet room
50 dB	A dog burping
57 dB	The dial tone of a phone
60–70 dB	Conversational speech
74 dB	A door closing
79 dB	A dog barking
89 dB	A door slamming
100 dB	A household fire alarm

Complex Sounds

The motion patterns that produce sound take many forms. One way to study sounds is to produce a graph of the moment-to-moment position of the sound source (or a molecule that is moving in response to the force applied by the source). Such a graph is called a **waveform**. Three examples of waveforms are provided in Figure 3.3 (p. 44). The horizontal axis provides a time scale that is marked in intervals of hundredths of a second (or milliseconds). The unit of measurement along the vertical axis reflects displacement from a starting or resting point.

The waveform in Figure 3.3A shows a uniform pattern of vibration, with three complete cycles over the 3 millisecond time span. This waveform represents a single frequency at 100 Hz, so that over the course of a full second the cycle would repeat 100 times. This type of waveform is called a *sine wave*, or a **pure tone**, because it reflects energy at only one frequency. Such pure tones do not occur naturally but can be produced in the laboratory and are used to test hearing at specific frequencies. All other sounds are produced by energy located at more than one frequency.

The waveform in Figure 3.3B was produced by an adult male producing the vowel "ah." It is an example of a *complex waveform*, which means that more than one frequency is produced by the source. The motion pattern is complicated, with several peaks and troughs. Nonetheless, it is possible to see that the pattern is repeated three times within the time frame illustrated in Figure 3.3. In other words, the repetition rate of the complex pattern is the same as that of the 100 Hz pure tone shown in the figure. The lowest frequency of those that make up this complex tone is 100 Hz. This is called the *fundamental frequency*.

The waveform illustrated in Figure 3.3C is also complex, but it does not reveal any regular or repeated pattern of motion. This type of motion pattern produces *noise*, such as that produced by a waterfall or jet engine, or simply the sound made by producing /s/ or /sh/. When noise is produced by motion that is completely random, it is called *white noise* because it contains all frequencies. This is analogous to white light, which contains all colors. We hear white noise on the

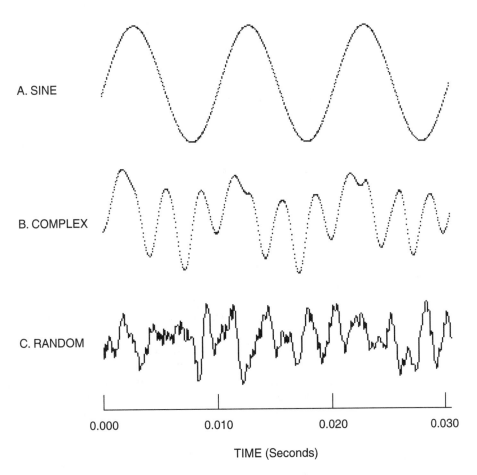

A. SINE

B. COMPLEX

C. RANDOM

| 0.000 | 0.010 | 0.020 | 0.030 |

TIME (Seconds)

FIGURE 3.3   **Examples of simple and complex waveforms.**

television when we try to tune in a station that is not broadcasting, or that is not available through our particular cable company. Noise also can be produced by abrupt or brief sounds, such as consonants produced without voice (e.g., /p/, /t/, /k/).

Speech can also be displayed in terms of their intensity over the period of time that the sounds are spoken. This display is known as a **spectrogram** (see Figure 3.4). Using the spectrogram, we can see the difference among the words *bit, bat,* and *bait,* which is readily apparent to the listener. These words differ along the two parameters of sound that we have already discussed: frequency and intensity. For each of these words, we can see the distribution of sound energy at different frequencies. The energy appears as bands on the spectrogram with higher intensities shown as darker bands at particular frequencies.

For each of the words in Figure 3.4, we see differences in the relative intensity and duration of each sound that makes up the word. The portion of speech corre-

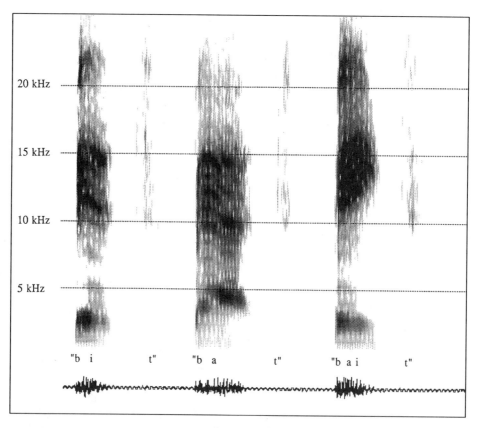

FIGURE 3.4   Complex speech sounds can be analyzed to show the component frequencies that we hear as different speech sounds. The words shown here are *bit*, *bat*, and *bait*.

sponding to vowel sounds contains regions of strong acoustic energy, which appear as dark bands on the spectrogram. When we listen to words, we pick up information about the speaker's voice primarily from vowels, because of the relatively long duration of voiced sound production. In contrast to the vowels, the unvoiced consonant "t" produces a short and relatively weak burst of energy, which is represented by a much lighter shade of gray on the spectrogram. These differences in the frequency and intensity of speech sounds may seem subtle when examined visually. However, they are adequate to distinguish between words, for those with normal hearing.

The spectrogram also reveals a third parameter that differentiates the sounds of speech: time. It is the combination of the distribution of sound energy over certain frequencies and the particular timing patterns that lead to the perception of three different vowels, and thus, three different words. Changes in the spectral energy and timing differentiate consonants as well as vowel production.

THE SPOKEN SOUNDS OF COMMUNICATION

Vocalization

As we learned in Chapter 2, the production of speech sounds relies on the coordinated action of many physical elements, including muscles of the larynx, throat, face, and oral structures. **Vocalization** requires a sound generator—the larynx—and a force to drive this generator—air. During normal breathing, the vocal folds of the larynx are open, allowing air to flow in and out unobstructed. For speech, the vocal folds are open during the production of voiceless sounds and are closed to produce voiced sounds. When exhaled air hits the closed (or closing) vocal folds with sufficient force, the folds blow apart and the exhaled air hits the stationary air above the folds, setting off a sound wave.

The frequency of the sound created by the vibrating vocal folds depends on the size and elasticity of the folds. Larger vocal folds tend to vibrate fewer times per second and therefore produce sounds at a lower frequency. Thus, men's voices tend to be lower than women's, and women's voices are lower than children's. Table 3.2 shows some frequencies of different voices for comparison. The fundamental frequency of the voice is carried by the vowel sounds in speech. The frequency of air rushing through narrowed oral cavities to produce consonant sounds is much higher than the fundamental frequency of the voice.

Speech Sounds

As clinicians, we need a precise system for differentiating among the sounds that people produce. The written word, as produced with the English alphabet, is inadequate for this task because one letter can correspond to more than one sound. Consider the "o" in *off* versus in *over*, or the "c" in *cat* versus in *certain*. For other consonants, more than one letter represents the sound (e.g., "th," "sh," "ng"), and the same sound can be represented in more than one way (e.g., "f" and "ph"). Further complicating matters is the occurrence of "silent letters" (e.g., "p" in *ptomaine*,

TABLE 3.2.   The Fundamental Frequency of the Human Voice

SOURCE	FREQUENCY LEVEL OF THE VOICE
FUNDAMENTAL FREQUENCIES	
An infant cooing	380 Hz
Boys and girls, age 9, talking	260 Hz
An adult woman saying "hat"	256 Hz
An adult man saying "hat"	128 Hz
CONSONANT SOUNDS	
s or z	4000–8000 Hz
t or v	6000–7000 Hz
th	7000–8000 Hz

"gh" in *weight*) in English orthography. For these reasons, clinicians use the *International Phonetic Alphabet* (IPA). The IPA symbols for consonants appear in Table 3.3 (see page 49), along with their corresponding sounds in words. In all, forty-one different symbols are needed to specify the sounds of English, compared with the twenty-six letters of the English alphabet. These forty-one symbols allow us to specify the different sounds, or **phonemes**, of the English language. The actual production of a sound by a speaker is referred to as a **phone**. The term **allophone** refers to the variations in phones that are still categorized as the same phoneme. For example, we say the "t" in *tap* slightly differently than in *setting*, although both are considered versions of /t/.

Vowels

The vowel system (vowels and **diphthongs**) requires twenty-six symbols and combinations of symbols in the IPA alphabet. Diphthongs are distinguished from vowels in that they are a combination of two vowel sounds. Vowels and diphthongs are produced with vocal fold vibration, or voicing. The sound generated by the vocal fold vibration is then modified in the vocal tract through movements of the pharynx, soft palate, tongue, jaw, and lips. These modifications of the initial voicing allow for production of the vowels that characterize any given language. For each vowel, there is a distinctive configuration of the vocal tract. For example, in the production of the /i/ ("ee" as in *beet*) vowel, the vocal tract is shaped by the tongue positioned as high and forward as possible, with the jaws relatively close together and the lips slightly withdrawn. The differences in the acoustic characteristics of vowels are dependent upon the position and height of the tongue in the oral cavity as well as the configuration of the lips. As shown in Figure 3.5, for

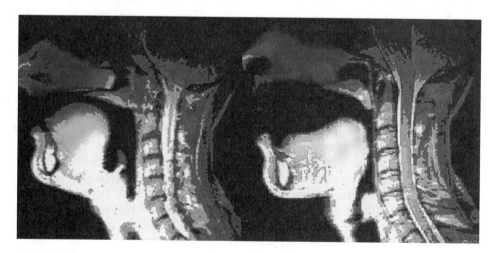

FIGURE 3.5   **A side view of the articulators showing the differences in tongue and jaw position during the production of the vowels /i/ (on the left) and /ɑ/ (on the right). Note that the tongue and jaw are elevated for /i/, wheraeas they are lowered for /ɑ/. Used by permission of B. Story, Ph.D., The University of Arizona.**

example, we can see that the /i/ vowel is produced with the tongue high and anterior in the mouth. Conversely, we see that the /ɑ/ ("o" as in *bop*) vowel is produced, with the jaw dropped and the back of the tongue held low in the oral cavity. None of the vowels require vocal-tract constriction as is necessary for consonant production. Diphthongs, such as /aɪ/ or /ɔɪ/ in b*uy* and b*oy*, are assimilated blends of two separate vowels, producing a two-vowel glide. Production of a diphthong requires a quick sequence of vocal-tract adjustments, usually requiring rapid movements of the tongue from low to high (or vice versa) and back to front (or vice versa).

As mentioned earlier in this chapter, it is the vowels that allow us to hear the voice of the speaker. The sound of one's voice, for example, whether it is hoarse or hypernasal, is determined by listening to vowel production. Although consonants play a primary role in how well speech is understood, or its *intelligibility*, the vowels we utter also contribute to how well someone can understand us. Each vowel found in a particular language has its own distinctive production characteristics. For example, listening to an Australian speaker and an American speaker, one will perceive the same English language with the same consonants embedded in markedly different vowels and diphthongs. These differences may cause difficulties for the listeners as they try to understand one another.

Consonants

As discussed above, vowels are distinguished primarily by their place of production. Consonants, in contrast, can be characterized by three general parameters: their *place* of articulation, the *manner* in which the sound is produced, and whether the consonant is voiced. The place-manner-voicing system can be used for describing the production of specific sounds. It can also be used to highlight differences in the consonant systems of different languages. For example, English contains only one glottal sound (a place distinction), the glottal continuant /h/, whereas other languages, like Navajo, include glottal stops. On the other hand, English contains certain consonants (e.g., /l/ and /r/) not found in some other languages, like Chinese. Sometimes, what we perceive as the "accent" of a nonnative speaker of English relates to a subtle alteration in either the place, manner, or voicing aspects of the consonants. Likewise, as we will see in Chapter 4, the ability to characterize sounds by place, manner, and voicing can help reveal common patterns when articulation disorders occur.

In Table 3.3, the consonants in English are listed to show how each phoneme is distinguished by its place, manner, and voicing characteristics. The anatomical sites of production, or the *place of production*, are listed from front (bilabial) to back (glottal), indicating the various structures of articulation: lips, teeth, tongue, hard palate, velum, and glottis. If the consonant is voiced, an asterisk is placed above it. We see the manner of production in the left-hand margin. There are six consonants (/p/, /b/, /t/, /d/, /k/, /g/) that are classified as stops or **plosives**, produced by a brief cessation of airflow, followed by a sudden release of the sound. The consonants that are paired in Table 3.3 (e.g., /p/ and /b/; /t/ and /d/) are called

TABLE 3.3.   The Consonants in English

MANNER OF ARTICULATION	PLACE OF PRODUCTION						
	Bilabial	*Labiodental*	*Interdental*	*Alveolar*	*Palatal*	*Velar*	*Glottal*
Stop or Plosive	p (*p*at)			t (*t*oe)		k (*k*ick)	
	b̊ (*b*at)			d̊ (*d*oe)		g̊ (*g*ap)	
Fricative		f (*f*at)	θ (*th*in)	s (*s*ip)	(*sh*oe)		
							h (*h*ip)
		v̊ (*v*at)	ð̊ (*th*at)	z̊ (*z*ip)	ʒ̊ (mea*s*ure)		
Affricate				tʃ (*ch*op)			
				d̊ʒ (*j*ob)			
Nasal	m̊ (*m*om)			n̊ (*n*un)		ŋ̊ (si*ng*)	
Lateral				l̊ (*l*ap)			
				r̊ (*r*are)			
Glide	ẘ (*w*all)				j̊ (*y*es)		

*Consonant is voiced.

cognates. These sounds have the same manner and place of production, differing only on the dimension of voicing. The **fricative** consonants (/f/, /v/, /θ/, /ð/, /s/, /z/, /ʃ/, /ʒ/, and /h/) are created by articulators forming a tight constriction that produces some audible noise from the airflow (voiced or unvoiced). All of the nine fricatives are also **continuants**, as they can be continued as long as the airflow is present. The **affricate** consonants (/tʃ/, /dʒ/) are combinations of a stop and a fricative. Only three consonants in the English language (/m/, /n/, and /ŋ/) are produced with the velopharyngeal port open, allowing their production to be nasalized. There are two commonly recognized liquids, or lateral, consonants: first, the lateral (/l/), produced by the tongue tip raised to contact the central alveolar ridge with openings along the sides of the tongue where the air stream passes during sound production; second, the consonant /r/, produced by two points of lingual constriction on the anterior hard palate (just posterior to the alveolar ridge) and on the anterior velum. The last consonant grouping in Table 3.3 is the glide sounds (/w/, /j/), which are often classified as semivowels that become consonants because of added constriction.

The flow of articulatory movements used for the series of phones produced in running speech is continuous and constantly changing. Any one sound in isolation has a specific series of requirements or "targets, ideal places of contact, forces

of contact, particular shapes, particular airflows, and particular patterns of movement necessary for a given speech sound" (Daniloff, 1973, p. 198). Speech articulation is a motor behavior that requires muscular specificity (one has to be on target or listeners will hear another phone) with a continuously variable rate and rhythm. The sounds that precede or follow a particular sound influence the production of that sound, a process often called sound assimilation. For example, if we said, "Tea, too," the production of the /t/ phone in each word will be slightly different; the high vowel in *tea* will bring the tongue tip slightly more forward than for the production of /t/ in *too*. Assimilation provides some evidence that speech production is organized by the nervous system in larger units than the single phone. Production of a phone in running speech is often simultaneous with the production of an adjacent phone preceding or following the target phone, a process known as **coarticulation**.

Prosody
So far, we have discussed those constituents of speech that make up the individual sounds within words (i.e., the consonants and vowels). However, additional aspects of sound are critical in conveying meaning in conversation. These aspects include the tempo, rhythm, and intonation with which the sounds and words are spoken. These elements make up the **prosody** of speech.

In conversational speech, there are two distinct types of prosodic information. One differentiates between classes of sentences. For example, the words "You liked rhubarb pie" can be expressed as a statement (as in, "You had it before and you liked it.") or as a question (as in, "You really liked it?"). What conveys the difference between a statement and a question in English is the steady or falling intonation in the statement form and the rising intonation in the question form. In other sentences, prosodic cues include short pauses that set off the phrase embedded within the sentence (separated by commas in written text) as in "The report, which appeared to be composed by monkeys typing at random, received a failing grade." These types of prosodic cues are referred to as *linguistic prosody* and they provide information concerning the grammatical structure of the spoken sentence.

Emotional prosody is different from linguistic prosody. Whereas linguistic prosody is used purposefully to differentiate sentences of different grammatical forms, emotional prosody is often unintentional. This is why those who know us well can detect, from the tone of our voice, whether we are upset or secretly pleased, even when the words we use are relatively neutral. In other cases, we purposefully mismatch the content of our words with the emotional tone of our speech to express sarcasm or irony. Most individuals are exquisitely sensitive to the myriad of overtones that can be added to speech via emotional prosody. In fact, when there is a mismatch between what we say (i.e., the words used) and how we say it (i.e., the emotional prosody), our listener is likely to feel that the prosodic information conveyed our true meaning. For this reason, we hear comments like "She said it was OK, but she didn't seem too happy about it."

SPEECH SOUND DEVELOPMENT

When a child is born with a normally functioning hearing mechanism and is raised by people who speak to him or her, the child will systematically acquire the perceptual capabilities needed to understand the language he or she hears. As the baby develops, we see a corresponding development of the sound system (see Table 3.4). In order to understand the development of the child's auditory and early sound production capabilities, let us look at the experiences of a single child.

Birth

Abraham was born in the early morning of May 15. He was the first child in his family. Within days of Abraham's birth, his hearing was screened for the first time in his life. Neonatal hearing screenings have become widely used as part of a well-baby checkup. The relative cost of widespread screenings is minor compared with the advantages gained by early intervention with children who have hearing loss at birth. In Abraham's case, the results confirm a normally functioning hearing mechanism.

The development of Abraham's sound system actually began while he was still in the womb. A developing fetus responds to sound by the third trimester of gestation (Birnholz & Benacerraf, 1983). The fetus will change positions and

TABLE 3.4   Approximate Ages for Milestones in the Comprehension and Production of Sound

AGE	MILESTONE
0 weeks	Startles at loud sound Prefers mother's voice to strangers' Produces reflexive, vegetative sounds
4 months	Responds to household sounds Can discriminate among many speech sounds Produces differentiated cries Produces vowel-like sounds
7 months	Produces canonical babbling Uses sound with communicative intent
10 months	Produces "protowords" Repeats sounds made by others Produces jargon Understands some words
12 months	Produces words with simplified forms

increase heart rate in response to sound. If the sound persists, these behavioral signs of hearing will wane, only to return if the characteristics of the sounds change (Leader, Baillie, Martin, & Vermeulen, 1982). However, the sounds that reached Abraham in utero were probably more limited in scope than what he can now hear. First of all, his mother's body tissues attenuated, or dampened, more common sounds, particularly at the higher frequencies (Walker, Grimwade, & Wood, 1971). Because the voice of Abraham's father had to travel from the air through his wife's body to reach his developing child, Abraham probably heard only a muffled version of his father's voice in the womb. The lower frequencies carried by vowel sounds, and the pitch, rhythms, and intonation of the father's voice were probably more clearly heard than the higher frequency sounds that distinguished the consonants of his speech. In contrast, his mother's voice had a direct route to her fetus, via internal sound vibrations that traveled through her body to the womb. This advantage makes maternal speech more intelligible when recorded within the womb than the speech of others (Armitage, Baldwin, & Vince, 1980; Bench, 1968).

The influence of prenatal auditory experience can be measured in babies soon after birth. Researchers use techniques such as "high amplitude sucking" in which infants suck on a pacifier that is wired to data-recording instruments. Infant abilities are explored by conditioning babies to change their rate of sucking in response to what they hear. DeCasper and colleagues conducted a series of studies that show infant preference for sounds available in the prenatal environment; infants show preferences for hearing recordings of the sound of an intrauterine heartbeat (DeCasper & Sigafoos, 1983) and the voice of their own mother (DeCasper & Fifer, 1980). Therefore, it is no surprise that Abraham is comforted by being held against his mother's body as she speaks gently to him. The warmth of her body and the sounds of her heartbeat and voice are already familiar to him.

At home, Abraham is already a beginning communicator. However, much of this is unintentional on his part. As his uncle holds him, Abraham makes a series of lip smacks. In response, his uncle responds playfully as if the baby had just related a shocking secret about his parents. Later, as his mother gives him a sponge bath, Abraham is fussy and emits a series of cries. His mother "explains" to him that she is bathing him and that she is trying to do this as fast as she can. She then picks him up in a towel to rock him, telling him he is okay. While dressing him, she "trades" sounds with him by repeating his short cries and other vocalizations. Soon, his parents begin to recognize the different types of cries he is now making. For example, Abraham's father recognizes a cry of protest as he removes a bottle of formula from Abraham's mouth in order to reposition him. These early interactions provide the infant with important information about communication. The infant learns that his or her vocalizations have the positive effect of parental attention and response. The close proximity of the parent's face allows the infant to see his or her parent's facial expressions. The give-and-take interchanges lay the ground work for conversational turn-taking.

Six Weeks

Abraham awakens from his nap. His legs and arms stretch and move about as he makes a series of sounds. His mouth is open and he emits a series of short vowel-like sounds as well as lip and tongue smacks. Sometimes these sound like exclamations, comments, or complaints. Early on, infants' cries and other vocalizations often occur with the velopharyngeal port open, giving sounds a nasal quality (Oller, 1980). Infants may produce sounds on both expirations and inspirations. Each infant is quite variable in how he or she produces sounds from one time to the next. It may be that the infant is "trying out" the many combinations of positions and movements that can be used to produce grunts, cries, and other vocalizations (Boliek, Hixon, Watson, & Morgan, 1996).

Abraham's father enters the nursery and gets down on eye level with his son. When he calls his son's name, Abraham turns his head and looks at his father's face. His father asks, "Are you waking up? Are you waking up now?" Abraham gives his father a big smile. These types of interactions demonstrate the infant's early interest in and preference for familiar faces and voices. In return, Abraham's interest in his father's voice is rewarded by more verbal attention from his father. In fact, Abraham's parents speak to him quite a lot. They name his body parts as they wash him. They tell him about his fashion options while dressing him for the day. They recite nursery rhymes while changing his diaper. Although all this language stimulation may seem beyond his level of comprehension, it provides him with an ongoing stream of information from which he is already beginning to gain knowledge about his native language.

Like parents around the world, Abraham's parents talk to him with exaggerated stress and pitch variations, slower rate, and liberal use of repetitions. This type of speech is often called *child-directed speech*, or sometimes *motherese*. Adults and older children often use child-directed speech when speaking to infants and toddlers, and babies seem to prefer this type of speech. Researchers feel that the exaggerations of child directed-speech may also play an important role in assisting the young child in cracking the code of communication by helping to segment the ongoing sound stream into units of phrases, words, and individual sounds (Jusczyk, 1997; Kuhl & Iverson, 1995).

Four to Six Months

At four months, Abraham's major activity for the day is putting things in his mouth, with a secondary emphasis on drooling. He tries putting his hand, his feet, his toys, and leaves on the ground into his mouth, then makes a grab for his grandmother's earrings. This is the typical infant's favored mode for exploring the world at this age. Whether or not his mouth is full, he makes a variety of vowel sounds. Sometimes, these vowels are prolonged while pitch is varied (e.g., "aaaaaah"), and other times they are staccato-like exclamations (e.g., "eh!"). These sounds are not necessarily directed toward anyone, although they stop when his mother approaches. His mother gets down on the ground with him and exclaims "How's

my big boy?! How's my big boy?!" He looks at her intently and then squeals in response. Although Abraham does not yet understand just what was said to him, he has already begun the job of recognizing the sounds and patterns that comprise his native language.

We know that very early on infants have perceptual capabilities that allow them to begin to segment the ongoing sounds within running speech. As we saw in our discussion of consonant production, the production of individual sounds varies from one word to the next due to coarticulation effects. Nonetheless, we perceive all the variations of sounds like "b" as the phoneme /b/, and all the variations of "p" as the phoneme /p/. The auditory systems of mammals, including humans, appear equipped to handle such variation among sounds by accomplishing what is known as *categorical perception*. This trait of the auditory system allows us to perceive a range of acoustic signals whose voicing characteristics actually lie midway between a [b] or [p] as one or the other of these sounds. For the infant, this provides the advantage of delimiting the infinite variation in acoustic speech signals into a relatively small set of consonants (and vowels) that repeat over and over again in their own native language. An early study by Eimas, Siqueland, Jusczyk, and Vigorito (1971) showed that infants could distinguish between such acoustic contrasts at four weeks after birth. Subsequent work (e.g., Burnham, Earnshaw, & Clark, 1991; Streeter, 1976; Werker & Lalonde, 1988) has shown that infants initially perceive contrasts that include sounds not found in their native language. Over time, however, these nonnative contrasts appear to lose salience for the developing child. Thus, children's experience with the language (or languages) of their community shapes their perception of the sounds of speech.

A parallel situation occurs for the processing of vowel sounds. Like consonants, a specific vowel can be pronounced with a range of acoustic variation, depending on the speaker, the word, and the context. However, by 6 months of age, infants show that they consider variants of the same vowel as perceptually similar, whereas variants of different vowels are considered distinct. This phenomenon has been called the *perceptual magnet effect* (Kuhl, 1994; Kuhl & Iverson, 1995) because the perceived difference between vowel variants appears to be less than the actual acoustic difference would otherwise suggest. In other words, when we hear variants of a particular vowel, our perception of those variants is drawn, like a magnet, toward the prototypical vowel of that type. In contrast, variants that correspond to different vowels seem more perceptually distinct than the acoustic differences between vowels would suggest. Cross-linguistic work indicates that infants show a perceptual magnet effect for prototypical vowels that occur only in their native language (Kuhl, Williams, Lacerda, Stevens, & Lindblom, 1992). This work suggests that the perceptual change reflects a developmental effect that requires exposure to spoken language.

Seven to Nine Months

At 7 months of age, Abraham celebrated his first Christmas. Wearing his pajamas and a red Santa's hat, he sat on the couch and reached for the small gifts that fell

out of his Christmas stocking. His parents began to rip the wrapping paper for him, but once started, he was able tear the remaining paper off his gifts. He mouthed each individual piece of wrapping paper, before tossing it aside. In all, handling wrapping paper appeared to be the most interesting part of the process to him. He patted the box with his open hand. Each gift held his interest and he looked at each while his parents named and commented about it. This "joint reference" between parent and child provided Abraham with the opportunity to observe objects and actions at the same time that he heard the words that related to them. His breathing was rapid and heavy, and he waved his arms with excitement.

During this period, Abraham reached a new milestone in the development of the speech sound system. His production of sounds no longer consisted solely of vowels. The first consonants were added to his repertoire. Abraham exclaimed "Da!" as he reached for an as-of-yet untasted piece of wrapping paper. These first consonant-vowel (CV) and consonant-vowel-consonant-vowel (CVCV) utterances are referred to as **canonical babbling**. This type of babbling is nonspecific, in that babies Abraham's age do not use these CV or CVCV combinations to refer to specific objects or intentions. However, Abraham, like other babies, produced these sound combinations with the prosody of speech, so that it seemed as though he was speaking, even though no true words were produced.

Abraham's initial production of canonical babbling at 7 months was about average for developing infants. Eilers and Oller reported that normally hearing infants may enter the stage of canonical babbling as early as 3 months or as late as 10 months (1994). Auditory experience seems critical for the development of this milestone. Hearing impaired infants are delayed in developing this milestone, with the onset of canonical babbling occurring after 11 months of age. In contrast, infants with other developmental problems that do not involve hearing loss may show little or no delay in reaching this milestone (Eilers & Oller, 1994).

The vocalizations of babies at 6 and 7 months of age include elements seen at earlier ages. They continue to make vowel-like sounds in addition to CV combinations. They make sounds regardless of whether another person is interacting with them. However, there are qualitative changes in sound production at this stage as well. For example, Abraham often seemed fascinated with his own babbling. He seemed to play with variations of his own babbling. He tried out one string of sounds and repeated them with a slight change in the overall pattern. For example, while playing, he produced "di da...di..da...daaaaaah..da." As at earlier ages, these sounds appeared to be a form of vocal play, without reference to any one thing in particular.

Another change is the emergence of communicative intent behind Abraham's use of sound. This preverbal use of sound is typical among babies at this age. Parents recognize their baby's use of sounds to direct their attention to an object, to request actions ("give me"), or just as a social interaction. At this age, Abraham used sounds to signal refusal, for example. His mother offered him a spoon full of strained peas, which appeared to be out of favor at the time. He exclaimed his disgust and turned his cheek away from the offending food. These first intentional vocalizations are quite probably true precursors of linguistic behaviors yet to come.

In fact, babies at this stage begin to comprehend a few spoken words, signaling the onset of the first true linguistic stage of development.

Ten to Fourteen Months

Abraham learned to walk before his first birthday. Initially, he used a coffee table or the couch to lift himself up and then "cruised" around the room holding onto the edges of the furniture. Then he walked without support. But often, he was only able to take a few steps before landing on his seat. His most efficient mode of locomotion was still crawling at that point.

Abraham also expanded his sound repertoire. In addition to the single syllables that were heard at 7 to 9 months, he learned to produce consonants in combination. As he stood ready to walk to his mother's outstretched arms, we heard "yee yeah adee di hee." Then Abraham's father, holding a video camera, caught his attention. His mother asked, "Do you want to walk to Daddy?" Abraham piped in with an enthusiastic "da! dee!" Although this approximated the word "daddy," it was not yet a true word for Abraham. In fact, a few minutes later, we heard Abraham utter a chorus of "da dees" when attempting to walk toward his mother but also when attending to neither his mother nor father. In this particular case, "da dee" reflected a different milestone in the development of speech sounds: the ability to repeat sound strings produced by others. We saw this new ability to repeat more explicitly when Abraham's mother was encouraging him to show off for the camera. She told him "Wave to the camera. Wave! Wave!" He echoed back "ey . . . ey" as a shortened form of "wave." Then he waved his hands, first with one hand and then with both hands. Next, his mother told him "Say 'Hey!' You know how to say 'Hey!' Say hey!" And he repeated "Hey!"

At this age, we often heard a chain of syllables with sentence-like inflectional patterns, such as "ba to aa aa na ?" We refer to these speech-like sound strings as *jargon*. Such an utterance is directed toward a listener, with the baby often searching to make eye contact, causing the listener to feel almost obligated to answer the jargon question with "yes" or "no." Abraham appeared to demand an object from the listener, give it back, and then demand it again. He changed his role within the communicative exchange, first becoming the asker, then the giver, and then the asker again. The sound of his voice carried as much of the message as the reaching gestures or looking at the object.

Jargon includes many combinations of consonants and vowels, and there does not appear to be a one-to-one representation for a particular object or desire. That is, the baby is not using the same combination of sounds to represent particular words. Although many of the consonant-vowel combinations are repeated, many are unique. The intention of the utterance is carried more in the inflection and prosody than in the consonant-vowel combination. At earlier ages, vocalizations flowed easily and there was no demand that babies produce any specific sounds. When they use vocalized jargons as intentional communication, however, babies begin to use the inflectional patterns that have been heard in their native language that represent particular needs and wants. At this stage, we hear front,

middle, and back vowels sandwiched between many different consonant-like sounds. Many of the consonant attempts will drop out of babies' repertoire as they get older and attempt to say words.

Like other babies at this stage, Abraham was fun to play with. He enjoyed playing sound games, often reacting to his parents' model with exact or altered vocalization patterns of his own. Babies at this age may amaze their parents with novel, innovative jargon not previously heard. How well babies this age interact with others and the quality of their vocalizations may have clinical implications for future communicative competence. Normal babies 9 to 10 months of age enjoy vocal play with others and seem to enjoy the human interaction both in play and during various caregiving tasks (feeding, bathing, diapering). Early parent-child interactions provide the baby with experiences that reinforce the positive aspects of communication. Such comfort and success in communication may go a long way toward giving the baby the confidence needed for future attempts at communication. The absence of such enjoyment in babies this age may be symptomatic of future communicative interaction problems. As Van Riper and Emerick (1984) wrote, ". . . in this socialized babbling or vocal play of the baby we find the basic pattern of communication, of sending and receiving, although it is only sounds, not meaningful messages, that are batted back and forth" (p. 93). Perhaps the baby whose play attempts and reaching out toward others go unheeded does not experience the give-and-take of **dyadic** (two-people) **communication** required for successful communication skills development. Some future language problems may have their genesis in the first year if babies receive little satisfaction or reinforcement from their early attempts to communicate. Other babies seem to lack the interest in others that would lead to vocal play with another person. Such children are at risk for continued social and communicative problems as they grow.

Around the age of 11 months, Abraham entered a stage characterized by "nonreduplicated or variegated babbling" (Schwartz, 1984), meaning the jargon sounds were individualized and not often repeated. The infant begins to show real control over the stress and intonation of vocalization with the jargon pattern closely resembling the language the baby has been hearing. Ingram (1976) presented a number of diary studies that described particular babies at 11 to 12 months who were beginning to repeat the same vocalization pattern in a give situational context. There was still enough phonetic variability to prevent the utterance from being classified as true words. Most of the vocalization utterances at this age often sound more like phrases in that they are longer than that which would be perceived as single words.

The baby this age produces the immediate precursor to true words, in what Schwartz (1984) describes as vocalizations that are characterized by phonetically consistent forms known as **protowords** (primitive, early forms of an actual word). Whereas jargon vocalization appears to be more related to the affective, emotional state of the infant and is therefore rather free-flowing and without tight structure, the protowords have much greater specificity and appear to be more object- or action-specific. Sometimes, babies this age embed a protoword in the prosodic jargon. At other times, we observe a combination of prosodic jargon, then a slight

pause, followed by the production of a protoword. It would seem that the first true words that often appear at 12 to 13 months do not come suddenly but have developed gradually, from babble to jargon to protowords and then finally to a true word with relative phonetic stability.

Despite the arrival of the first few words, typical 1-year-olds seem to attempt most of their communication by continuing differentiated jargon. The first words are not said very often. The jargon pattern becomes longer, sounding more like real language and occasionally containing a real word. Much of the intended message, when understood by the listener, is communicated not by the occasional word but by the general intonational pattern of the utterance and by the situational context.

Leonard and colleagues pointed out that children this age may comprehend the meaning of words that are beyond their phonologic capability to produce (Leonard, Schwartz, Folger, & Wilcox, 1978). It would appear that the selectivity process for production is basically related to the child's ability to produce the sounds of a particular word. However, before the first word is spoken, toddlers at this age produce many of the speech sounds that are used in their language community in the form of jargon. From about 10 months onward, their sound repertoire expands to include at least approximations of all the phonemes of their language. Although a wide variety of sounds may be heard in the babbling of children, relatively few are heard in their first words.

When imitating the sounds of others, there is some selectivity regarding the kinds of sounds chosen for play. We also see this pattern as babies begin to produce their first words (Ferguson, 1978). Babies imitate the sounds they can physiologically produce; if the sounds are too complex to make, the babies will usually simplify the utterance, perhaps changing the consonant to one they can produce and preserving the vowel that was in the model. Abraham was heard doing just this when he produced "tita" when looking at a tiger in a picture book. As the first words are produced, there is some phonologic selectivity; the first words are those that are less motorically complex. Many of the first words may involve similar sounds, often voiced, front consonants. Sounds such as /m/ and /b/ appear in early speech in most languages. Babies often use the same consonant-vowel combination for several different words. For example, /ba/ may be used for words as different as *ball* or *car*. Over time, as children add to their repertoire of speech sounds, the pronunciation of these two words becomes distinct.

Fifteen Months and Older

At this age, Abraham entered the true verbal stage of communication development. We will look in some detail at his development from single words to sentences in Chapter 7. However, Abraham will continue to add to his sound system as well during this time. As he grows, he will add sounds in a fairly predictable way. Irwin and Wong (1983) described the sequence with which typically developing children like Abraham add sounds to their repertoire between 1½ and 3 years of age. Their work shows most children at 18 months have one or two distinct vowels and a few consonants that they use to produce approximations of

their first words. By 24 months, many of the vowels are produced distinctly, and a few new consonants are added. By 3, children have expanded their consonant repertoire, which greatly aids the overall intelligibility of their speech. Over time, children learn to use the sounds that they have acquired in different positions within words (Dyson, 1988). The job of learning the sounds of speech, and using them correctly in connected speech, takes years to complete. Some normal 5-year-olds, for example, may still be mastering some of the latest acquired sounds like /r/ and /l/ (Kenney & Prather, 1986), although these sounds begin to emerge much earlier. Likewise, normally developing children may make sound errors in some words and not in others. This is because the production of a particular sound is influenced by all the other sounds contained in the word. As children mature, their speech is less affected by these coarticulatory effects (Nittrouer, Studdert-Kennedy, & McGowan, 1989). By age 4, most children can be readily understood, even by those who do not know them well.

CLINICAL PROBLEM SOLVING

Kim was born with a severe hearing loss affecting both of his ears. He responded reliably to sounds of 500 Hz to 1000 Hz at 40 dB HL; sounds at 2000 to 4000 Hz were heard at 50 to 60 dB HL; and sounds above 4000 Hz required even greater intensities (up to 80 dB HL).

1. What does this mean for Kim in terms of everyday hearing experiences? What types of environmental sounds will he hear and what will he miss?
2. Give examples of how his experience with the sounds of speech might affect development of this aspect of communication.
3. Which components of speech (i.e., vowels, consonants, prosody) will be most difficult for him to hear?
4. Some children (and adults) who experience a hearing loss become proficient lipreaders. Which aspects of speech sound production can be best discriminated by this method and why? What aspects of conversational speech make lipreading difficult?

REFERENCES

Armitage, S. E., Baldwin, B. A., & Vince, M. A. (1980). The fetal sound environment of sheep. *Science, 206,* 1173–1174.

Bench, J. (1968). Sound transmission to the human fetus through the maternal abdominal wall. *Journal of Genetic Psychology, 113,* 85–87.

Birnholz, J. C., & Benacerraf, B. R. (1983). The development of human fetal hearing. *Science, 222,* 516–518.

Boliek, C. A., Hixon, T. J., Watson, P. J., & Morgan, W. J. (1996). Vocalization and breathing during the first year of life. *Journal of Voice, 10,* 1–22.

Burnham, D. K., Earnshaw, L. J., & Clark, J. E. (1991). Development of categorical identification of native and non-native bilabial stops: Infants, children, and adults. *Journal of Child Language, 18,* 321–260.

Daniloff, R. G. (1973). Normal articulation processes. In F. D. Minifie, T. J. Hixon, & F. Williams (Eds.), *Normal aspects of speech, hearing, and language.* Englewood Cliffs, NJ: Prentice Hall.

DeCasper, A. J., & Fifer, W. P. (1980). Of human bonding: Newborns prefer their mother's voices. *Science, 208*(1), 1741–1776.

DeCasper A. J., & Sigafoos, D. (1983). The intrauterine heartbeat: A potential reinforcer for newborns. *Infant Behavior and Development, 6,* 19–25.

Dyson, A. T. (1988). Phonetic inventories of 2- and 3-year old children. *Journal of Speech and Hearing Disorders, 53,* 89–93

Eilers, R. E., & Oller, D. K. (1994). Infant vocalizations and the early diagnosis of severe hearing impairment. *Journal of Pediatrics, 124,* 199–203.

Eimas, P. D., Siqueland, E. R., Jusczyk, P. W., & Vigorito, J. (1971). Speech perception in infants. *Science, 171,* 303–306.

Ferguson, C. (1978). Learning to pronounce: The earliest stages of phonological development in the child. In F. Minifie & L. Lloyd (Eds.), *Communicative and cognitive abilities: Early behavioral assessment.* Baltimore: University Park Press.

Ingram, D. (1976). *Phonological disability in children.* New York: Elsevier North Holland.

Irwin, J. V., & Wong, S. P. (1983). *Phonological development in children 18 to 72 months.* Carbondale: Southern Illinois University Press.

Jusczyk, P. W. (1997). *The discovery of spoken language.* Cambridge, MA: MIT Press/Bradford Books.

Kelly, J. P. (1985). Auditory system. In E. R. Kandel & J. H. Schwartz (Eds.), *Principles of neural science.* New York: Elsevier

Kenney, K. W., & Prather, E. M. (1986). Articulation development in preschool children: Consistency of production. *Journal of Speech and Hearing Research, 29,* 29–36.

Kuhl, P. K. (1994). Learning and representation in speech and language. *Current Opinion in Neurobiology, 4,* 812–822.

Kuhl, P. K., & Iverson, P. (1995). Linguistic experience and the perceptual magnet effect. In W.

Strange (Ed.), *Speech perception and linguistic experience.* Baltimore, MD: York Press.

Kuhl, P. K., Williams, K. A., Lacerda, F., Stevens, K. N., & Lindblom, B. (1992). Linguistic experience alters phonetic perception in infants by 6 months of age. *Science, 255,* 606–608.

Leader, L. R., Baillie, P., Martin, B., & Vermeulen, E. (1982). The assessment and significance of habituation to a repeated stimulus by the human fetus. *Early Human Development, 7,* 211–219.

Leonard, L., Schwartz, R., Folger, M., & Wilcox, M. (1978). Some aspects of children's imitative and spontaneous speech. *Journal of Child Language, 5,* 403–416.

Nittrouer, S., Studdert-Kennedy, Y. M., & McGowan, R. S. (1989). The emergence of phonetic segments: Evidence from the spectral structure fricative-vowel syllables spoken by children and adults. *Journal of Speech and Hearing Research, 32,* 120–132.

Oller, D. (1980). The emergence of speech sounds in infancy. In G. Yeni-Kamshian, J. Kavanaugh, & C. Ferguson (Eds.), *Child phonology. Vol. 1: Production.* New York: Academic Press.

Schwartz, R. (1984). The phonologic system: Normal acquisition. In J. Costello (Ed.), *Speech disorders in children.* San Diego: College-Hill Press.

Streeter, L. A. (1976). Language perception of two-month-old infants shows effects of both innate mechanisms and experience. *Nature, 259,* 39–40.

Van Riper, C., & Emerick, L. (1984). *Speech correction: An introduction to speech pathology and audiology* (7th ed.). Englewood Cliffs, NJ: Prentice Hall.

Walker, D., Grimwade, J, & Wood, C. (1971). Intrauterine noise: A component of the fetal environment. *American Journal of Obstetrics and Gynecology, 109,* 91–95.

Werker, J. F., & Lelond, C. E. (1988). Cross-language speech perception: Initial capabilities and developmental change. *Developmental Psychology, 24,* 672–683.

DISORDERS OF ARTICULATION

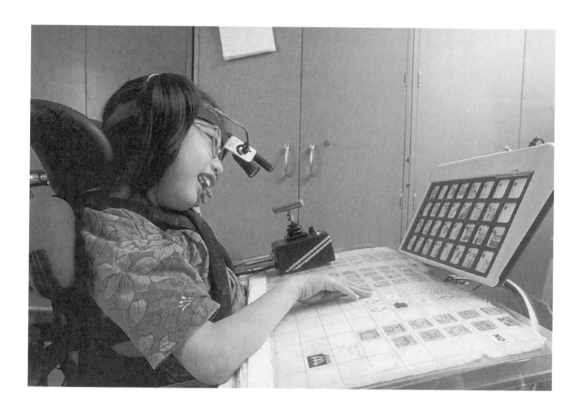

■ ■ ■ ■ ■

PREVIEW

Disorders of articulation affect both children and adults. Sound errors may range from a mild lisp to nearly unintelligible speech that results from many sound substitutions, omissions, and distortions. Childhood articulation problems may be caused by structural abnormalities such as a cleft palate, but are more frequently related to faulty or incomplete learning of the sound system. Some adults show the residual signs of a childhood articulation disorder. In others, articulation disorders result from damage to the central nervous system. Brain damage may produce the slurred or labored speech of dysarthria, the unpredictable articulation errors of apraxia, or even the complete loss of speech in cases of mutism. In evaluating the wide range of articulation disorders, the speech-language pathologist must recognize the factors that cause and maintain the disorder. Intervention typically includes behavioral therapy, alone or in combination with medical management.

The emergence of spoken words is one of the most important milestones in a toddler's life. We commonly hear from excited parents who report hearing the word "papa" or "mama" in the babblings of their child well before the child is using these sounds as true words. As long as the baby's word attempt contains sufficient phonemes to be recognized, the listener accepts it as the target word. In the first three years of life, parental concern focuses on the emergence of new words, new combinations of words, and communication, rather than on the precision of articulation. If the young child's speech can be understood, there is usually little concern about articulation. During the preschool years, children's articulation improves and approximates adult sound production. However, some children persist in using immature patterns of speech, often interfering with their ability to make themselves understood. In the case of acquired articulation disorders, an adult may begin to make speech errors following an illness or injury. Persistent articulation errors in either adults or children may warrant concern.

TYPES OF ARTICULATION ERRORS

In Chapter 2, we studied the speech mechanisms required for the production of normal speech; and in Chapter 3, we considered the consonants, vowels, and diphthongs of English speech patterns. We also learned that sounds are strung together to form words in connected speech. We say these sounds very rapidly. It is often in the rapid production of sounds required for normal speech that articulatory errors become most noticeable. Whether heard in a single syllable, a single word, a phrase, or sentences, such errors are known as **misarticulations**. There are four forms of misarticulation: **substitution errors** (*fith* for *fish*), **omission errors** (*fi'* for

fish), **distortion errors** (a lisped sh in *fish*), and **addition errors** (*fisha* for)
error types can be easily remembered by the acronym SODA (substitutio
sion, distortion, addition).

Substitutions

Substitutions are a common articulation error in young children. Preschool children often substitute one phoneme for the target phoneme, with a certain logic or
predictability. In many cases, the incorrect sound is similar to the target sound in
terms of the place and manner of articulation and voicing characteristics of the
sound (see also Chapter 3). For example, the child who says, *I tee the wabbit* has
used two common substitutions heard in the speech of young children with articulatory errors of substitution. Like the /s/ in *see*, the substituted /t/ is a voiceless
sound that is made near the same spot in the front of the mouth; the /w/ has many
production similarities to the target sound /r/ that it replaces. In other cases, the
incorrect sound shares similarities with other sounds within the word. For example, when a child says *bate* for *bake*, the /t/ replaces /k/ because /t/ is produced
forward in the mouth, closer to where /b/ is produced. This is a case of progressive, or forward, assimilation, because a sound at the beginning of the word (the
/b/ in *bake*) influenced the production of a later sound, the /t/ for /k/ in this case.
Regressive, or backward, assimilation occurs when sounds following the target
phoneme influence its pronunciation as when a child says *guck* for *duck*.

Until children acquire a particular sound of the adult phonemic system, they
often replace it with a sound they have some success in making. Many of the
substituted sounds are ones that are acquired by children at earlier ages than the
target sound. For example, if 4-year-olds cannot say an /s/, they might well substitute a sound that they can say, such as /t/. Substitution is perhaps the most
common articulatory error in the child who is learning to talk. However, these errors may persist or may be far more frequent in a child with a speech disorder.

Omissions

When speakers omit sounds from words, their speech is difficult to understand.
Consider the following exchange between a 28-month-old boy and his father:

Dad:	Look at all that stuff!	
Child:	I bri a boo. A bir boo.	(I bring a book. A bird book)
Dad:	(Looks at book.) Is it a bird book?	
Child:	I ge thi un, you ge tha un.	(I get this one, you get that one.)
Dad:	Oh. Ok, I get this book about shells.	
Child:	I a pi un.	(It's a pink one.)
Dad:	It's a pretty pink shell.	

it is difficult to tell what this child is saying from his words alone. ther, who provides a running translation, we might not know what ctually saying.

omissions may occur anywhere within a word, they are more often final position. A particular sound or a whole class of sounds may asionally, a young child will leave all endings off words. Shriberg t the omission of consonants, known as a syllable-simplification process, is a natural part of phonological development. In some children, simplification processes can lead to the omission of an entire syllable, which is what occurs when the young child says *nana* for *banana* or *amblance* for *ambulance*. In each case an unstressed syllable has been omitted from the word. These omissions of either sounds or syllables occur frequently in the speech of toddlers and become less common as the child grows. However, when a 4-year-old child persists in making sound omissions, or an adult begins to produce them after years of normal speech, these omissions signal an articulation disorder.

Distortions

As we saw in Chapter 3, the production of a sound must be relatively close to the target to be perceived by listeners as correct. Slight variations of a sound that still sound like the target sound are acceptable *allophones*, but marked variation in sound production is classified as a distortion. In a distortion error, the target sound is produced with some change of the sound, although not enough to be classified as a substitution or an addition. One of the most common distortions and among the easiest to identify is the lateral lisp, in which the target /s/ or /z/ phonemes sound slushy (the /s/ or /z/ sounds as if it has an unvoiced /l/ as part of its production).

Additions

A fourth type of articulatory error involves an addition of a sound. We might hear an individual with an addition error saying *boata*. In other cases, an extra vowel may be inserted between the two consonants of a consonant blend (e.g., *galass* for *glass*). As in these examples, the addition error is often an unstressed vowel. Unlike other types of articulation errors, addition errors are not typically seen as a part of normal development. They can occur when an individual adds a voicing dimension to a word or is unable to stop the flow of air (voiced or voiceless) at the end of it. Occasionally, an individual with a disorder such as cerebral palsy or other physical disability affecting motor control will make voicing additions.

ARTICULATION DISORDERS IN CHILDREN

It is often difficult to isolate a specific cause of articulation problems in children. The great majority of young children who have difficulties pronouncing words basically do not differ emotionally, mentally, or physically from their age-peers. In most cases of developmental articulation disorders, children's success in commu-

nicating is limited by their ability to make themselves understood. Their pattern of articulation errors may make them sound younger than they are. This type of articulation disorder would be classified as a developmental phonological disorder, probably related to central nervous system factors that are yet unknown. Disorders of speech articulation affect approximately 3.8 percent of 6-year-old children (Shriberg, Tomblin, & McSweeny, 1999). Boys are identified as having articulation difficulties slightly more frequently than girls. Although a small percent of these children also have language difficulties, most of the children identified with speech delay have no other obvious problems.

Phonological Disorders

Some children's poor articulation skills are not readily attributable to structural abnormalities. Parents become concerned when their child's speech seems to lag behind their playmates. For some children, speech articulation errors are limited to just a few sounds. In other cases, articulation errors are so numerous that the young child's speech is nearly impossible to understand.

When a child is referred for an articulation disorder, a speech-language pathologist will attempt to characterize the child's sound errors. Some children will mispronounce only a few sounds, such as /r/, /l/, or /s/. Since children tend to master these sounds relatively late (4 years old or older), the speech-language pathologist may recommend a "wait and watch" approach. Intervention may be limited or deferred while the child is given a chance to self-correct articulation through normal maturation. For school-age children, even a few sounds produced in error is unusual. A 10-year-old boy's lisped /s/ rarely interferes with his ability to communicate his ideas. It can, however, negatively affect the way other children view him (Hall, 1990). Such children are typically candidates for therapy and are often quite motivated to correct their speech.

The phonological approach to articulation disorders recognizes that the child has some difficulty in mastering the adult phonology of the language. In his or her attempts to use language, the child in effect makes systematic simplifications of the phonology. From this point of view, children with a phonological disorder continue to use a simplification process beyond the time when others their age use them.

As Dunn (1982) wrote, "The term phonological process, however, is frequently used as a way to describe the systematic simplifications observed in child speech" (p. 147). The articulatory productions of young children who make articulation errors are systematic and seem to be the result of the same processes that normal children use (Ingram, 1981). Some common phonological processes are found in Table 4.1 (p. 66). It would appear, however, that children with articulatory errors persist in using simplification processes beyond the time when their age-peers use them (Grunwell, 1980). To test a child's use of phonologic processes, it is important to have a method of identifying the different processes that are used, control for the number of times a process is sampled, and identify the actual number of times that it has occurred. Several such tests are commercially available, particularly for young children who show developmental articulation disorders.

TABLE 4.1   **Phonological Processes**

EXAMPLES

Natural Phonological Processes	*Adult Word*	*Child Word*
SYLLABLE-SIMPLIFICATION PROCESSES		
Deletion of the final consonant	ball	"ba__"
Deletion of the unstressed syllable	away	"__way"
Cluster reduction	stop	"__top"
ASSIMILATION PROCESSES		
Regressive (backward) assimilation	doggie	"goggie"
Progressive (forward) assimilation	television	"televivion"
SUBSTITUTION PROCESSES		
Stopping—fricatives are replaced by stop-plosives	shoes	"tood"
Fronting—palatal and velar sounds are replaced by alveolar sounds	bake	"bate"

Used with permission of Prentice Hall. From L. D. Shriberg. Developmental phonological disorders, in *Introduction to Communication Disorders*, ed. T. Hixon, L. Shriberg, and J. Saxman (Englewood Cliffs, NJ: Prentice Hall, 1980).

Because children's errors are systematically related to these phonological processes, articulation therapy concentrates more on correcting the processes than on treating individual sound errors. Robbie is one such child.

At age 4, Robbie was brought to a university speech-language clinic by his concerned parents. The parents, most other family members (including three older siblings), and neighbors had difficulty understanding him. He had normal hearing, normal cognitive ability, and normal speech mechanisms at the time of the speech evaluation. His articulation errors were abundant. In the initial position of a word, he could correctly say m, p, b, t, d, n, and he correctly said m, p, b in the medial position. He produced no final consonants correctly. Most of his consonant errors were actually omissions (he left the sounds out completely), although he made a few consonant substitutions (substituting another sound for a target sound): t/k, d/g, t/f, b/v, t/θ. Of the twenty-five English consonants, he said only six of them correctly; most of his vowel sounds were produced correctly. His overall attempts at conversation were restricted to two- or three-word utterances, many of which were not intelligible. He appeared to limit his mean length of response to two or three words as a conscious gesture to accommodate his listeners; he apparently had learned that if he said more than that, no one would understand him.

Because Robbie could say six consonants correctly in the initial position, a phonological approach to his problem focused on making him aware that many words had consonant endings that he could say. At the start of therapy, the stop consonants that he could produce correctly (/p/, /b/, /t/, /d/) were presented at

the beginning and the end of a word. The phonological approach was to teach him the place in a word to say the sound. In therapy, he was soon able to produce most of the six target sounds (the ones he could say at the evaluation) at both the beginning and the end of a word, such as *pop, top, mop, Bob, tub, mom, Pam* (his sister), and so forth. Saying two words in a rapid series, in which the last consonant of the first word and the first consonant of the second word were the same, such as *mom-mop,* seemed to facilitate the production of the omitted consonant in the medial position. Later therapy sessions included working on phonetic sounds that Robbie should have been making correctly; not only was production practiced in therapy, but also some phonological instruction was included, providing him with the rules for applying his newly acquired sounds.

A phonological profile of children who are brought to the attention of a speech-language pathologist can be obtained by examining the features that co-occur with phonological disorders (Ruscello, St. Louis, & Mason, 1991; Shriberg, Kwiatkowski, Best, Hengst, & Terselic-Weber, 1986). About two-thirds of the children referred for services for phonological disorders are boys, the majority of whom have a history of ear infections that may have affected their hearing at some time. Frequently, there are signs of general neuromotor problems. These children may be described as "clumsy," with many of them showing mild signs of muscle weakness and incoordination. Frequently, a developmental language disorder co-occurs with the phonological disorder. Difficulty with language production is more common than problems with language comprehension. Half of the children with phonological problems also have difficulty learning to read. Problems with academics may persist long into the school years, even after speech is no longer an obvious impairment (Shriberg & Kwiatkowski, 1988). Sometimes, a family history of phonological as well as other speech-language disorders can be documented for these children (Lewis, 1990).

Probably the majority of young children with developmental articulation problems can profit from a phonological-process approach in therapy. Some children show isolated, residual errors, even after the more general processes have been corrected. These children seem to know the phonological rules of production but may have learned a faulty muscular pattern for producing a particular sound. They may require additional therapy with a focus on the individual sound in error.

Tongue Thrust

Several generations of Americans have been evaluated and treated for **tongue thrust** as part of an orthodontic management program. Children with tongue thrust use an unusual sequence of oral movements when swallowing. The tongue pushes forward against the anterior teeth (particularly the upper incisors). This forward tongue movement while swallowing has led some to refer to tongue thrust as reverse swallowing. The forward tongue movement is accompanied by high tension in the muscles controlling lip movement, which is needed to prevent the tongue from protruding as it pushes forward during swallowing. This abnormal and inefficient pattern of swallowing tends to make children with tongue thrust

messy eaters. In addition, the frequent forward pressure of the tongue forces the teeth out of alignment. For this reason, many orthodontists are reluctant to fit a child with braces until the tongue thrust habit has been overcome. This problem frequently requires direct intervention with special procedures know as **myofunctional therapy** to develop optimal intraoral tongue postures for swallowing (Barrett & Hanson, 1978).

Some children with identified tongue thrust also have an associated articulation disorder, most commonly heard by others as a lisp because the anterior sibilants (particularly /s/ and /z/) are mispronounced. Speech-language pathologists who have been trained in myofunctional therapy techniques may choose to treat the articulation disorder and tongue thrust simultaneously. When there is tongue thrust but no articulation disorder, the speech-language pathologist may elect to administer myofunctional therapy to correct abnormal tongue and lip postures and movements (ASHA, 1991).

Anomalies of the Oral and Facial Structures

Various acquired or genetic abnormalities of the facial skeleton can cause severe articulation problems. Many of these facial abnormalities are part of a broader pattern of anomalies that are known collectively as a **syndrome**; that is, a certain number of predictable features (e.g., skeletal anomalies, distinctive facial features, motor involvement, cognitive difference) co-occur. For example, a child may be classified as having the Berry-Treacher Collins syndrome, characterized by a lack of mandible-facial growth, a downward slanting of the eyes, a notching of the lower eyelid, and microtia (a lack of external ear development). This syndrome is genetic in origin and may often be observed in several members of the same family. A syndrome is usually named after the physician(s) or other professional who first described the group of signs that co-occurred in their patients. Other syndromes, such as fetal alcohol syndrome, are named for the factors that cause the condition. Besides oral-facial abnormalities, problems in communication may be part of the symptom complex that includes hearing loss, language delay, mental retardation, or problems in speech articulation.

Sometimes we see children in speech-language clinics who were born with facial or tongue muscles that lack neural innervation. One girl, age 8, was unable to smile because the necessary facial muscles had no innervation; by extensive neuro- and plastic surgery, some of the nerve fibers used to move the jaw were transplanted to innervate the muscle fibers used in smiling. The operation was successful, giving her a smile and enough functional control of her lips to improve her faulty articulation.

Occasionally, tongue problems may contribute to articulation difficulty. Another structural problem of the tongue is that it may appear to be too large (macroglossia) or too small (microglossia). Macroglossia, seen with certain developmental syndromes, has been thought to contribute to poor articulation. At one time, tongue reduction surgery was recommended for these children, but follow-up studies have failed to document improved articulation (Lynch, 1990). Some-

times the tongue appears to be too large because it is riding forward in the mouth and protruding, possibly because of abnormalities in the back of the oral cavity, such as enlarged tonsils. In other cases, a forward tongue carriage may be the result of muscle weakness and inadequate neural innervation of the tongue muscles. These types of problems will be discussed as part of the physiological problems observed in dysarthria later in this chapter.

A tight lingual frenulum is another feature of the tongue that has been blamed for articulation problems. The lingual frenulum is the small band of tissue on the base of the tongue's underside. When it is too tight, forward and upward movement of the tongue tip is restricted. In rare cases, this could interfere with the production of sounds, like /l/, for which the tongue tip must be elevated. This condition is sometimes called tongue tied. When protruded, the tongue will often appear to be heart-shaped, indented at the tip. Most "tongue-tied" children, however, experience no difficulty with articulation. In the rare case when this condition interferes with speech articulation, some parents may elect to have the lingual frenulum clipped by a surgeon. However, this practice is declining because the necessity of surgical intervention in these cases is open to question.

Dental abnormalities have also been blamed for articulation problems. Shelton and colleagues (Shelton, Furr, Johnson, & Arndt, 1975) looked closely at the influence of various dental abnormalities on improvement in articulation therapy, concluding that even children with severe malocclusion could learn to articulate normally. Severe malocclusions, as seen in underbite or overbite, may or may not have an effect on articulation. Sometimes the orthodontic correction of malocclusion, the wearing of braces or bands, will interfere with tongue precision, creating a possible articulation problem. Such problems are temporary, and the child usually learns to adjust speech movements to accommodate the orthodontia.

Cleft Lip and Palate

In Chapter 2, we saw the importance of the oral structures to the production of speech. When children are born with anomalies that disturb the structure or growth of these structures, speech development may be impeded. Among the more common structural anomalies are cleft lip and palate. Clefting occurs in early pregnancy, when different sections of the embryo first form, between the fifth and twelfth weeks. Clefts may occur to either side of the midline of the upper lip, to the right or left of the bone that holds the upper front teeth (the **alveolar ridge**), and along the midline of the velum or hard palate. These predictable locations for clefts relate directly to the fact that these structures grow as segments that must fuse together during embryonic development.

Estimates of the incidence of cleft lip or palate range between one in 500 to one in 750 babies (Peterson-Falzone, Hardin-Jones, & Karnell, 2001). Clefts range widely in severity. A small defect may involve a partial division in the uvula and a gap within the soft tissues of the velum. Severe clefts may involve both sides of the lip and alveolar ridge (in which the top front teeth are rooted) and a cleft that extends from the velum forward into the hard palate so that the nasopharynx is

open to the mouth. For many children, the cleft is part of a syndrome that affects additional aspects of development (Shprintzen, Siegal-Sadewitz, Amato, & Goldberg, 1985). For example, a child born with velocardiofacial syndrome may have other facial anomalies and heart defects in addition to cleft palate. These children frequently have problems with language development as well. For other children, the cleft lip or palate is the only problem.

Perhaps we can best appreciate the impact of a cleft on the life of a child by considering the case of Andres.

> Andres is an engaging 3-year-old who was born with a left unilateral complete cleft lip and palate. In the country of his birth, his mother lacked the resources to feed and care for her child, and Andres was brought to an orphanage. When he was adopted at 14 months, he was small for his age, weighing only 14 pounds. In addition, his language skills lagged well behind age expectations. Whereas children of 14 months are typically producing some words, Andres was not yet producing anything that even sounded like the speech sounds of his native language. His adoptive parents were an American couple who brought him to the United States. Andres' adoptive mother was a speech-language pathologist who had special expertise in cleft palate.
>
> Because Andres' parents adopted him knowing he had a cleft palate, they did not experience the initial emotional shock that most parents who discover their baby has this condition must contend with. Moreover, Andres' parents had a much better understanding of the implications of raising a child with a cleft palate from a medical and communication standpoint. For example, they were aware that some of the corrective surgery that Andres should have would need to be scheduled quickly. In fact, many babies born with cleft lips and palates have already had a repair of the lip well before Andres' age. Therefore, Andres' parents arranged for an initial evaluation with an ear, nose, and throat doctor and with a plastic surgeon soon after arriving home with him. By 16 months, Andres had his first surgery, during which his lip cleft was closed and preliminary work was begun to close the palate. In addition, tubes were inserted through Andres' eardrums so that the fluid that frequently accumulated inside the middle ear could drain.
>
> Much to his parents' delight, the day after his first surgery, Andres produced his first speech sound, an /m/. As his mother related, "His eyes just lit up." He seemed to recognize that this sound was an important development, and he produced several more in succession. His first words approximations, *more, mom,* and *milk* built on this early appearing sound. Subsequently, he added /h/, /n/, and /p/ and nasalized /b/ to his repertoire of sounds along with several different vowels. These additional sounds allowed him to expand his repertoire of words to include social routines like *hi* and an approximation of *please.* He also produced some sound approximations that were unidentifiable as English sounds.
>
> Andres made a return trip to the hospital for a second round of surgery at 18 months. This time, surgery targeted repairs of the soft and hard palate. Andres and his parents stayed overnight, which was required by the hospital staff to assure that he was alert and able to drink independently before he was released. After an episode the next day in which he ran down the hall with his mother gamely attempting to keep up with his IV pole and tubing, the staff decided he was fit to be

released. Another postsurgery challenge was that Andres was fitted with arm splints to prevent him from reaching his stitches. However, these did not always remain on this active boy. On several occasions, Andres handed the splints to his mother to indicate she should put them back on.

It is safe to say that Andres' cleft lip initially had an impact on every aspect of his life. However, we also see how quickly intervention with these children can improve both their communication skills and the quality of their lives. As we see with Andres, a good home environment and medical and behavioral treatment transform a child who had delayed development along with a cleft lip and palate into a active little boy whose cleft was just one more fact of his life.

Andres' case illustrates that treatment of the child with cleft palate typically involves both medical and behavioral interventions. Indeed, Andres' treatment to date has involved his parents, a plastic surgeon, an ear, nose, and throat physician (an ENT), and a speech-language pathologist. The cleft palate team may also include additional members like an pediatrician or orthodontist for other children. An audiologist is also frequently involved because of hearing loss due to structural anomalies affecting the auditory system. In Andres' case, tubes that allow middle ear fluid to drain will help him maintain normal hearing. This source of hearing loss is common in children with cleft lip and palate (Handzic-Cuk, Cuk, Gluhinic, Risavi, & Stajner-Katusic, 2001). In Chapter 13, we will see how these various professionals function together as a team.

By 23 months, Andres was putting two words together, but his spoken vocabulary was still quite limited. In addition, the words he did use were difficult to understand because they only approximated the adult form. For example, he rarely used sounds that required contact of the tongue to the alveolar ridge. He also did not use "back" consonants (i.e., /k/, /g/). His sound preferences probably reflected a combination of factors, some related to his cleft and some that were perhaps compensatory. Children with complete clefts often have difficulty producing the tongue-to-palate contact and movement of the soft palate for back consonants, and thus they may avoid them. His mother also wonders whether his tendency to hold his security blanket in his mouth limited his opportunity to produce alveolar sounds like /t/ and /s/. If so, this would be another example of a physical impediment that affected speech sound development. In contrast, he seemed to understand very well for his age. At 28 months, his parents made the decision at this time to enroll him in language therapy with the goal of expanding his vocabulary and increasing his utterance length. This focus was intended to help him achieve parity with his preschool classmates, whose skills were somewhat more advanced.

The configuration of the oral and nasal structures of children with cleft lip and palate often lead to altered resonance (see Chapter 2 for an explanation of Resonance). These altered oral structures also may affect the child's ability to produce certain sounds normally. For example, a cleft palate would preclude a normal-sounding /k/ or /g/ as the child attempts to contact the clefted velum with the

back of the tongue. Often, these children may adopt compensatory articulatory contacts that we do not see in the English language (Peterson-Falzone et al., 2001). For example, a child with a cleft palate may use a pharyngeal stop in which the back of the tongue touches the pharynx. This tongue placement allows the child to stop the airflow at the level of the pharynx, whereas attempts to stop the airflow at the velum would be unsuccessful if the velum is cleft. As in Andres' case, we also see a preference for the types of sounds that are most easily produced (i.e., nasal sounds) in the first fifty words learned by children with clefts (Estrem & Broen, 1989).

> Today, Andres is continuing with both preschool and speech-language therapy. Therapy now directly targets his articulation, as well as his language. The goal is to encourage use of the full range of speech sounds by training the place of articulation for sounds he does not use or uses inconsistently. Andres often is able to produce a new sound when told how to do it, and he seems to recognize words that contain sounds he is working on. This awareness of the sounds of words is a good predictor of later ability to master reading and is an encouraging sign for his parents. His parents intend to continue with therapy and will have an evaluation of his velopharyngeal function for speech when he is a little older. This will help determine whether there is an organic contribution to his poor articulation, which may need to be addressed in addition to the behavioral therapy.

Speech outcome for children with cleft palate is generally good (e.g., Grunwell, Brondsted, Henningsson, et al., 2000). However, Andres' speech and language development may be monitored for quite some time into the future. This is because some children with cleft palate may exhibit additional problems as they mature. For example, a number of children with surgically repaired clefts will nonetheless have difficulty moving the velum and pharyngeal muscles to completely close off the oral cavity from the nasal cavity during speech (see Chapter 2). This condition is known as *velopharyngeal insufficiency*. In some cases, this failure results in nasal-sounding speech and even audible airflow through the nose during speech. In addition to these types of physical problems, Andres will be monitored for problems with oral language and reading, as these problems can co-occur with cleft lip and palate. Fortunately for Andres, he is showing early indicators that his ability to develop language and literacy skills is good.

> Andres has made enormous strides in other areas of development. His motor skills and self-help skills are on par with the other children in his preschool class and his ability to understand language continues to be a strength. He also now has a new baby sister, also born with a cleft lip and palate, whom he dotes on.

Developmental Dysarthria and Apraxia

Although structurally based and phonological articulation disorders account for the majority of cases in children, a few children exhibit signs of speech disorders

typically associated with brain damage in adults. These are children with signs of developmental dysarthria or apraxia of speech. Children identified as having developmental dysarthria typically have abnormal muscle tone in facial muscles, which may be worse on one side than the other. Low muscle tone may result in a soft, somewhat drooping facial expression. Muscle tone that is abnormally high may produce a taut appearance or contribute to facial distortions and grimaces. Some children may have trouble with drooling or eating. Children with dysarthria have difficulty producing rapid speech or nonspeech movements. Affected children typically are late in acquiring their first words. As they grow older, their speech often remains very difficult to understand. Dysarthria may be associated with conditions such as cerebral palsy (see below), but may also occur in the absence of a more pervasive disability.

Children with developmental apraxia of speech are somewhat more difficult to identify. Often, they lack the more apparent motor signs that characterize developmental dysarthria. Apraxia has been defined as an impairment in the ability "to program, combine, and sequence the elements of speech" (Jaffee, 1984, p. 166). A child with a pure apraxia of speech would demonstrate relatively normal comprehension of language but be unable to imitate a simple spoken word, despite having no muscular weakness or paralysis. A case presentation of a 6-year-old girl with apraxia of speech illustrates the problem:

> Esme was a friendly and enthusiastic 6-year-old who was enrolled in a public school kindergarten. From her first day, it was apparent that her speech skills were well below average. Esme was nearly impossible to understand. Her kindergarten teacher was also concerned about Esme's language skills. The kindergarten program was largely built around language arts, and Esme had difficulty participating in many of the classroom activities. The kindergarten teacher asked the school's speech-language pathologist to observe Esme in the classroom. The speech-language pathologist noted that Esme was rarely understood by her teacher or classmates and often showed signs of frustration and distress while trying to communicate. Immediate intervention was needed.
>
> The speech-language pathologist contacted Esme's mother to obtain permission to see Esme for a formal evaluation and for therapy. Esme's mother confided that her child had been evaluated once before. At the age of 2, Esme had been seen at the county's developmental disabilities center because she had not yet started to speak. At that time, based on her poor motor and speech development, she was diagnosed as mentally retarded. Her mother was so distressed at this diagnosis that she refused all preschool services and refused to release the records of that diagnosis to anyone. She was sure her child was bright and was afraid Esme would be stigmatized and held back by a diagnosis of retardation. Instead, the mother kept Esme at home and spent a great deal of time taking her on field trips and engaging in other creative activities with her. The mother waited until Esme was 6 to enroll her in kindergarten, hoping that the extra year would give her a developmental advantage to compensate for her poor communication. Although her mother remained wary of therapists and special education professionals, she agreed after some discussion to allow the speech-language pathologist to see the child again.

Esme's formal evaluation revealed that she rarely pronounced any words correctly, even when speaking only single words. She often made sound errors on the initial sounds in words and omitted the ending altogether. Her sentences tended to be short, with an average of three words per sentence. A battery of language tests indicated that her receptive language skills were slightly above average and her expressive language skills were poor.

During subsequent therapy sessions, Esme made slow and inconsistent progress. The speech-language pathologist began noticing signs suggesting that Esme may have had more than the typical phonological disorder. She sometimes showed facial tension while speaking. Once, when trying to imitate the speech-language pathologist, she used her fingers to move her tongue in position to say a [d] sound. Sometimes she would reach for a card and grab the wrong one while telling herself "no!" These behaviors suggested problems with sequencing and executing movement. The speech-language pathologist made a diagnosis of developmental apraxia of speech. Esme's mother was convinced, after much counseling, to take her child back to the developmental disabilities center so that she could be evaluated by a physical therapist. The physical therapist confirmed that Esme had a mild limb apraxia in addition to apraxia of speech. With this information, the mother, school staff, and therapists met to discuss how classroom materials and procedures could be modified to minimize the effects of Esme's apraxia. The speech-language pathologist provided a teacher inservice on the expected impact that Esme's apraxia would have on her academic progress, including writing, test taking, and oral skills.

Apraxia of speech is more of a phonetic problem than an overall language problem; however, apraxia creates a marked discrepancy between receptive language and the ability to express language through speech. Often the affected children are forced to struggle at the single-word level. Even when they can produce multiword sentences, their speech lacks the normal prosody. Preschool children with apraxia require intensive individual therapy as well as language-based intervention in which efforts are made to encourage the development of a variety of communication skills.

Cerebral Palsy

Some children who display motor impairment early in their lives, often from the time of birth, have **cerebral palsy**. This is not a disease per se but rather a term used to label a number of motor-sensory conditions that result from damage to or imperfect development of the central nervous system. According to McDonald and Chance (1964), about three in every 1,000 newborns could be classified as having cerebral palsy. This neurological impairment may occur before birth, during birth, or during the first three years of life. Therefore, there is often motor delay in many aspects of the child's life: crawling, sitting, standing, walking, chewing-swallowing, self-feeding, and talking. The finer the required motor skill, such as

talking, the more likely the child will have a problem. In cerebral palsy, the motor deficits may be grossly divided into four types:

Spasticity. **Spasticity** is characterized by severe tightness of the muscles. Speech prosody is often interrupted by respiratory and voice breaks. Articulation is often severely defective.

Athetosis. **Athetosis** is characterized by a series of involuntary muscle contractions, with flailing of extremities and much facial grimacing. Lack of respiratory control causes a monotonic voice, often lacking sufficient loudness. There are many phonemic distortions.

Mixed. This type of cerebral palsy represents a mixture of both tight spasticity and flailing athetosis, sometimes called tension athetoid.

Ataxia. **Ataxia** is characterized by a lack of balance, with severe problems in coordination of movements. Ataxic speech sounds like the slurred, arhythmical speech of someone inebriated.

The motor speech problems of the child with cerebral palsy can be classified as a type of dysarthric speech. Dysarthria also occurs in adults who suffer brain damage and is discussed in greater detail below. Cerebral palsy implies a motor disorder of speech that is developmental in nature. If the condition is severe, the affected child enjoys few normal developmental experiences and a marked delay in speech. The treatment of the dysarthria for the child with cerebral palsy, therefore, may be quite different from that of one who acquires dysarthria after normal speech patterns have been established.

Often the child with cerebral palsy is so physically active with muscle contractions or unstable head and trunk posture that speaking appears almost impossible. Therefore, the child must first develop some postural control and some control of extraneous movements before work can begin on the fine motor control required for speech (Mysak, 1980). For example, learning to sit erect (with or without support) and keeping the mouth in a controlled, closed position are often prerequisite behaviors for attempting speech (Boone, 1972). The speech-language pathologist working with the child coordinates the speech-language program closely with other treatment specialists, such as the orthopedic surgeon, the physiatrist (a physician specializing in physical or restorative medicine), the physical therapist, the occupational therapist, and the special educator.

For some severely involved children with cerebral palsy, articulate speech is not a realistic goal; for these children, some form of nonvocal communication system must be introduced. A manually or electronically operated communication board has been found to be an effective alternate communication system. The child has several items (e.g., pictures, objects, symbols) mounted on a board and selects the appropriate one by indicating with a hand, a foot, or perhaps a headstick or headlight mounted on a helmet or by eye gaze. With the improvement of electronic

assistive devices, it is possible to activate stimulus selection by electronic switches attached to the chest, arm, or leg. Eye movements have been used to activate stimulus panels on some electronic boards (Broen, 1981; Coleman, Look, & Myers, 1980). Thanks to modern technology, there are assistive communication devices available to meet the basic communication needs of the most severely handicapped child with cerebral palsy.

Hearing Loss

In Chapters 10 and 11 we will see the importance of the hearing mechanism in the development of normal communication. Human communication is primarily an oral-aural interaction. A conductive or sensorineural hearing loss can seriously impair the aural reception of language. Some young children with articulation delay have had a series of middle-ear infections, each of which caused a temporary hearing loss. As discussed in Chapter 11, hearing loss is a frequent cause of a developmental communication problem (articulation and language). Some children simply cannot hear certain phonemes. When children lack the ability to hear spoken sounds, it is difficult for them to learn to produce them. Common causes of hearing loss and its effect on speech sound development are described at length in Chapter 11.

EVALUATION OF CHILDHOOD ARTICULATION DISORDERS

Articulation Screening

Most articulation screening programs are used in the public schools, particularly in kindergarten and the first few elementary grades. Such programs are typically set up in the fall, and all new children in the particular school district (kindergarten and other grades) meet with the speech-language pathologist or a speech-language assistant (see Chapter 13) for a brief screening. The screening might focus on naturalistic dialogues with the children to observe their articulation and their overall language function, voice quality, and speech fluency. However, many young children are reticent about talking to a "stranger," making a natural conversation impossible. Therefore, it is usually necessary to structure the screening so that a maximum amount of information can be obtained from a relatively brief speech sample.

It should be noted that certain speech sounds are stressed in the screening program—usually those that young children typically mispronounce throughout the early years. Perhaps the most common articulation errors identified during screening programs are distortions and substitutions for /s/ and /z/ and the common w/l and w/r substitutions. The focus of the screening program is to identify the children who misarticulate, not to identify the reason for the problem or study the possible processes involved. Ideally, the screening test should identify

those children who will outgrow their problem with maturation and those with articulation problems who need remediation. Unfortunately, speech-language pathologists in the schools sometimes find that identifying children who "need" therapy does not necessarily satisfy the parents who want their 5-year-olds who make an /r/ substitution to begin therapy, whether the screening test indicates a need or not. More and more often, screening programs are heavily supplemented by teacher and parent referrals to the speech-language pathologist for a full speech evaluation.

Articulation Evaluation

Articulatory precision in the production of the phonemes of a language naturally facilitates communication. Formal articulation evaluation may begin by engaging the child (or adult) in a real conversation. The conversation may be between the client and other children, between parent and child, or between clinician and child. This may involve discreet observation of a school-aged child at home, on the playground, or in the classroom. Other children may be seen in a clinic testing suite (which often looks like a playroom for young children) that have observation mirrors permitting the clinician to observe the child in as natural a communication setting as possible. A conversation during spontaneous play will often reveal how the child actually talks outside of the testing situation. With an older child, an actual conversation about topics of interest will reveal the communicative ability, offering information about articulation proficiency as well as about voice, language, and fluency.

The experienced and well-trained speech-language pathologist is able to observe the child's productions systematically and make a useful summary statement based on the observations relevant to the articulatory adequacy, specifying type and number of errors, place of error, and so forth. It is possible, however, that observation of play and conversation will not reveal all of the client's articulatory errors, nor will conversation alone provide the diagnostic information that a more structured evaluation will include. Therefore, the evaluation is likely to include conversational speech and more formal testing.

Audiometric Testing. Audiometric testing, at least as a screening measure, should be part of every articulation evaluation. As we will see in Chapters 11 and 12, various levels of hearing loss can have devastating effects on phonology. The child's ability to perceive the sounds of words is an important part of the evaluation. Therefore, audiometric testing may include evaluation of speech sound reception and discrimination levels.

Oral Peripheral Evaluation. A oral peripheral evaluation provides the speech-language pathologist with information relative to the adequacy of oral structure and function. As discussed earlier in this chapter, sensory losses, structural defects, and incorrect movements of the articulators can all contribute to faulty articulatory

production. An oral peripheral examination form (see Figure 4.1) lists the clinician's judgments about various structural areas of the vocal tract and how well they may function. The particular form pictured has been completed for an adult man with normal articulation who has a voice problem. The slight departures from normal described for this man apparently do not contribute in any way to faulty articulation. His ability to produce rapid alternating movements for speech (oral **diadochokinesis**), like other parts of the peripheral oral examination, was within normal limits.

The advantage to the speech-language pathologist of using a form to summarize the data from the oral examination probably lies in the need to be complete and systematic. The form, in effect, provides a checklist for each part of the oral mechanism in terms of its structural and performance adequacy. For the patient with dysarthria or a major structural defect (such as a cleft palate), a more detailed and supplementary examination would be required.

ORAL PERIPHERAL EVALUATION

	Structure	Function
Lips	Symmetry *normal* Scarring *none*	Pursing *normal* Smiling *normal* Close lips, puff out cheeks *normal*
Teeth	Alignment *slight overjet* Gap or Missing Teeth *none*	
Tongue	Scarring *none*	Moves side to side *normal* up and down *normal* in and out *normal*
Hard Palate	Vault Height *normal* Vault Width *normal* Scarring *none*	
Soft Palate	Symmetry *normal* Scarring *none*	Lifts on "ah" *normal* Symmetry of movement *normal*

Diadochokinesis:	Pa (20 repetitions)	*4* seconds
	Ta (20 repetitions)	*5* seconds
	Ka (20 repetitions)	*5* seconds
	PaTaKa (20 repetitions)	*4* seconds

FIGURE 4.1   An oral peripheral evaluation form.

Articulation Inventory.   Many commercially available articulation tests provide the clinician with a ready inventory of speech sounds. Most tests can identify not only the actual sounds produced incorrectly but also the place in the word where the error occurs (initial, medial, or final position) and the type of error (omission, substitution, distortion, or addition). A typical articulation inventory will provide the type of information found in Figure 4.2. This form shows the results of a

ARTICULATION TEST				
Name: Katie		**Age:** 5.0 years		
SOUND	**ITEM**	**I**	**M**	**F**	**PHONOLOGICAL PROCESS**
p	pencils, zipper, cup	✓	✓	-/p	Final consonant deletion
m	matches, Christmas, drum	✓	✓	-/m	F.C.D.
n	knife, Santa, gun	✓	✓	-/n	F.C.D.
w	window	✓			
h	house	✓			
b	rabbit, bathtub	✓	✓	-/b	F.C.D.
g	gun, wagon, flag	✓	✓	-/g	F.C.D.
k	cup, chicken, duck	✓	✓	-/k	F.C.D.
f	fishing, telephone, knife	p/f	p/f	-/f	F.C.D., Stopping
d	duck, window, bed	✓	✓	-/d	F.C.D.
ŋ	finger, ring		g/ŋ	-/ŋ	F.C.D., Stopping
j	yellow	✓			
t	telephone, bathtub, carrot	✓	✓	-/t	F.C.D.
ʃ	shovel, fishing, brush	t/ʃ	t/ʃ	-/ʃ	F.C.D., Stopping
tʃ	church, matches	t/tʃ	t/tʃ	-/tʃ	F.C.D., Stopping
l	lamp, yellow, squirrel	w/l	w/l	-/l	F.C.D., Liquid Simplification
r	rabbit, carrot, car	w/r	w/r	-/r	F.C.D., Liquid Simplification
dʒ	jumping, pajamas, orange	d/dʒ	g/dʒ	-/dʒ	F.C.D., Stopping
θ	thumb, bathtub, bath	t/θ	-/θ	-/θ	F.C.D., Stopping
v	vacuum, shovel, stove	b/v	b/v	-/v	F.C.D., Stopping
s	scissors, pencils, house	d/s	t/s	-/s	F.C.D., Stopping
z	zipper, scissors	d/z	d/z	-/z	F.C.D., Stopping
ð	this, feather	d/ð	d/ð		Stopping

FIGURE 4.2   Articulation test results for Katie, age 5 years. Note F.C.D. = final consonant deletion. Items adapted from the *Goldman-Fristoe Test of Articulation* (Goldman & Fristoe, 1986) and the *Khan-Lewis Phonological Analysis* (Khan & Lewis, 1986).

single-word articulation test given to 5-year-old Katie, who demonstrated a number of speech-sound errors. This form shows how the errors may be described individually as substitutions (e.g., p/f) or omissions (e.g., f) in the initial (I), medial (M), or final (F) position in the word. In the column labeled Phonological Process, errors are ascribed to one of three phonological processes used. *Stimulability* testing and deep testing would follow the formal articulation test to see whether, under the special conditions of those tests, the incorrect sounds could be produced correctly. Both types of testing will be discussed shortly. A phonological-process evaluation (considered later in the chapter) might follow, particularly if stimulability and deep testing were unsuccessful in eliciting correct phonemic productions.

Phonological Process Analysis.   For many children, the problem is not limited to a few consistently misarticulated sounds. More often, the speech-language pathologist finds errors on many of the consonant sounds. These errors may at first glance seem inconsistent. Certain consonants may be correctly produced in a few words, whereas in others they are omitted, distorted, or replaced with another consonant. A careful examination of these speech-sound errors almost always reveals a pattern. For example, when a child says *Tuta too my tir* for *Susan took my shirt*, the errors might be classified in the two ways shown in Table 4.2. Substitution errors are shown by writing the error sound followed by a slash (/) and the target sound. Omitted sounds are noted by a minus (-) sign.

When the sound errors are listed individually in Table 4.2, we notice that the child is inconsistent in the use of the /t/ sound. The child uses it correctly when attempting the word *took* but substitutes it for each /s/ in *Susan* and /ʃ/ in *shirt* and omits it altogether at the end of *shirt*. This use would be puzzling if we concentrated only on the individual sound errors. However, all these errors, plus those not involving /t/, can be accounted for by two general patterns, or **phonological processes**. The substitutions of /t/ for /s/ and /ʃ/ are all examples of a process

TABLE 4.2   Examples of Sound Errors in Children's Speech

	INDIVIDUAL ERRORS	PHONOLOGICAL PROCESSES
ATTEMPTED STATEMENT: Susan took my shirt.		
CHILD'S STATEMENT: Tuta too my tir.	Initial t/s t/ʃ	Stopping
	Medial t/s	Stopping
	Final -n -k -t	Final consonant deletion

called *stopping*, in which a stop consonant (e.g., /t/, /d/, or /g/) is substituted for a continuant (/s/, /f/, or /v/). All the errors of omission occur on the final consonant, indicating a process of final consonant deletion. Many phonological processes are seen in normally developing children, but persist in children with phonological disorders.

Distinctive Feature Analysis.   Each phoneme (consonant and vowel) has one or more **distinctive features,** or production characteristics, that distinguish it from other phonemes. When analyzing articulation errors, the features of the incorrect sound are compared with those of the adult-model sound in the hope that a particular feature error may be identified and corrected.

Two examples of a feature error are substituting a voiceless production for a voiced production, such as /t/ for /d/ (the voicing feature) and using a /t/ for a /k/ (a placement feature). If one were to make a feature-contrast analysis between two phonemes, it might resemble the one in Table 4.3. A distinctive-feature list has been included and is applied to the consonants /s/ and /t/, which are two sounds often confused by young children (who usually substitute the /t/ for /s/). We see that all phonemes share seven common features (no wonder the simpler /t/ is often used instead of the more complex /s/). The two consonants differ from each other in only three ways. For some clients, distinctive feature analysis identifies commonalities among sound errors that can be targeted for therapy. It may be the case that a child does not produce a single distinctive feature, which accounts for a range of sound errors. For example, if a child does not produce continuant sounds (those that involve prolonged production of sounds as in /s/, /v/, /r/), concentrating on this feature may help the child to bring in a whole class of sounds to his or her speech repertoire.

Severity Estimation.   Sound inventories and the analysis of speech sound errors are important prerequisites to selecting therapy goals. However, these forms of

TABLE 4.3   A Distinctive-Feature Analysis for /s/ versus /t/

DIFFERING FEATURES	/s/	/t/	
PLACE			
Alveolar	+	+	
MANNER			
Continuant	+	−	(differs)
Stop	−	+	(differs)
Strident	+	−	(differs)
VOICING			
Voiceless	+	+	

analysis do not always reflect the overall severity of a client's problem. For example, consider the speech of the following two children:

> **Maria:**   He go bi tee (he's got big teeth). Bu i no a he (But it's not a he). I a she! (It's a she!)
>
> **Joseph:**   I see a amblance (I see a ambulance). Let me see. I see an elphant (I see an elephant).

Both of these children have one phonological process that describes their speech errors. Maria tends to delete final consonants, and Joseph shows a pattern of weak syllable deletion. Although both children's errors can be described with a single process, Maria is much more difficult to understand than Joseph. This illustrates that knowledge of specific error types does not always provide accurate insight concerning overall severity. Kent, Miolo, and Bloedel (1994) reviewed the wide variety of available methods for estimating the overall intelligibility of speech. They noted that these measures tend to emphasize different aspects of speech analysis. A clinician may select among measures that emphasize phonetic contrasts, phonological error patterns, whole word identification in isolation or in connected speech, or measures that require listeners to rate how well speech can be understood. Some of these measures were developed with the characteristics of a particular type of articulation problem in mind (e.g., speech associated with hearing impairment, dysarthria, phonological disorders). Therefore, the clinician's decision concerning which measure to select may reflect the type of client he or she needs to evaluate and even the types of speech sound errors the client shows (Kent et al., 1994; Shriberg, Austin, Lewis, McSweeny, & Wilson, 1997).

Stimulability.   An important part of the articulation evaluation is to see how well the client can produce incorrect sounds when they are presented by the clinician as repeated auditory, visual, and tactile models. This is known as *stimulability*. For those children who can correct their sound errors when given visual, auditory, or tactile cues, the prognosis for correction is much better than for those who cannot. After the formal articulation test is completed, the speech-language pathologist selects several incorrect sounds to determine if the client is stimulable for that sound.

Stimulability testing can occur at several levels. The higher the level at which the child is able to produce the sound correctly, the easier it is to correct the production of the sound. At the highest level, the clinician may ask the child to say a mispronounced word over again by prompting, "Can you say that better?" If the child does not self-correct the articulation, the clinician might ask the child to repeat the word after a model is given. If the child's attempt is incorrect, the clinician might draw attention to visual cues to aid articulation by instructing the child to "watch how I say it." If the addition of visual cues is not effective, the clinician might ask the child to produce a misarticulated sound in a consonant-vowel combination, like *la-la-la*. If necessary, visual and tactile cues may be added to help the child. These steps are taken to determine what capacity the child has for producing the sound and how much support and cueing the child needs to do so.

Language Testing.   A phonological problem may be a sign of an overall language difficulty. At the time of the articulation evaluation, the speech-language pathologist should certainly determine the overall adequacy of the child's language skills.

Certain phonological processes may interfere with the clinician's ability to assess specific aspects of language. For example, processes such as final-consonant deletion will eliminate parts of speech like -ed. Other processes, such as stridency deletion, will eliminate the plural and possessive /s/. Often, comparing phonological and language testing can help distinguish between the effects of the phonological disorder and a spoken language disorder. Because phonological disorders frequently co-occur with other language difficulties, many clinicians routinely include one or more language measures in their assessment.

Older children with isolated articulation defects, such as the persistence of a lateral lisp, are less likely to have an associated language problem. Rather, the child exhibits a phonetic problem related to executing speech movements with the precision required for production of the adult model. Similarly, the adult patient who acquires an articulation problem (perhaps due to dysarthria or even from a loose denture) is unlikely to exhibit an associated language problem.

ARTICULATION THERAPY FOR CHILDREN

Let us now consider several approaches to articulation therapy. Speech-language pathologists work with children (and adults) with articulation disorders in many ways. Earlier in the chapter, many possible causes of faulty articulation were reviewed. We could probably find as many advocates of particular approaches to therapy as there are causes of a problem. Causation, which is difficult to identify, can rarely be treated directly as a first step in the management of an articulation problem. That is, if a hearing loss were identified as a possible cause of a developmental articulation problem in a child, correction of that loss (sometimes possible in a conductive loss) will not magically cure the faulty articulation. It may still be necessary to make the child aware of the desired target behavior, work directly to modify the articulation, and develop strategies for generalization of the newly acquired pattern into everyday speech.

The most effective speech-language pathologists working with articulation disorders may be those who are familiar with different approaches and employ the one most appropriate for the individual with the defect. The least effective clinicians, in our opinion, use the same remediation steps for all their clients. The diagnostic evaluation data should provide the information needed to plan individualized treatment. Let us consider briefly what is done in articulation therapy, dividing the topic in two: acquisition training and generalization training.

Acquisition Training

Helping the child or adult acquire target sounds is a common goal of all forms of articulation therapy. Many informal approaches and published programs attempt

to accomplish this goal. Therapy programs are typically tailored to meet the individual needs of each client and may incorporate a variety of different techniques. We will examine a few of these techniques here.

A *semantic* approach to articulation therapy emphasizes the changes in meaning that sometimes accompany phonological errors. Let us look at an example of a semantic approach to therapy.

> Brian is a school-based speech-language pathologist who has formed a group of three first-grade children with phonological disorders. All of these children make systematic substitutions of one class of sounds for another. For example, Amon, one of his students, reduces clusters like /st/ or /bl/ to one sound (/t/ or /b/). Another student, Marta, uses stop consonants in the place of fricatives (see Table 4.1 for example of phonological processes). Brian is able to address each of these children's different patterns of sound errors through a semantic approach. He has selected pairs of picture cards that contrast the error sound with the sound pattern each child needs to master. For example, one card shows a stop sign and its pair shows a toy top. The words *stop* and *top* contrast the cluster /st/ with the word that would be produced if the child reduced the cluster from /st/ to /t/. Other pairs of cards contrast the error patterns of the other children. Brian and the children play a modified game of *go fish*. There are two sets of each picture, so that a child holding one picture can ask another child for that picture in an attempt to obtain matching pairs. Each child has to show the picture he or she requests so that Brian can tell whether each child produces the target sound. Amon is holding the stop sign card, but asks "Do you have any top signs?" Brian replies, "No, I don't have any tops, but I do have a stop." This highlights for Amon the difference between what he asked for and what he meant to ask for. Likewise, when Marta asks Amon for a "tail" when she meant to say "sail," Amon has the opportunity to model the correct word. This approach works for these children because they are able to produce the sounds they are working on, but don't necessarily do so when they need to. It doesn't take long before the children realize that to get what they want, they have to produce the sound patterns that correspond to the correct word.

Many children need only a few examples of these minimal pairs before they are able to produce the target sounds in additional words (Elbert, Powell, & Swartzlander, 1991). The semantic method serves to alert the children to the fact that there is a difference between what they are saying and what they should be saying and that this difference is important. This method does not require children to think about the sounds themselves, an advantage for young children, who have little awareness of sounds as units smaller than words.

Some clients will not benefit from a semantic approach. They may see the differences in meaning between their sound errors and the correct production but be unable to produce the sound correctly without additional assistance. A *cross-modality* approach may provide that assistance. Cross-modality approaches utilize sensory information to facilitate correct articulation. For example, a client and clinician may face a mirror while the clinician demonstrates the target sound. The client may then attempt to repeat the sound while monitoring his or her movements visually in the mirror. In another case, a clinician may rub a child's alveolar

ridge with a mint so that the child can "taste" where the tongue belongs for /t/ and /d/. Or clients are instructed to put their hand over their larynx to feel the difference between /s/ and /z/. This additional sensory input can be an effective way for adults or children to monitor their performance.

For some sounds there are few available cues that the client can see or feel. Sometimes it is possible to take advantage of the *coarticulatory context* to promote correct sound production. Coarticulatory context refers to the fact that the sounds preceding and following a phoneme will influence the way that phoneme is produced. For a phoneme like /r/, for which there are few visual cues, coarticulatory context can help in learning correct production. For example, the /g/ and /k/ in /gr/ or /kr/ blends require a high, back tongue carriage, which carries over to facilitate a correct production of /r/. Once this correct tongue placement is established in blends, it can be used in words with other sound combinations. Let's take a look at an approach that capitalizes on co-articulatory context.

> Makayla has teamed up with her school's art teacher to integrate her articulation therapy into her students' classes. The art teacher's lesson plan involved constructing hand puppets in the shape of dragons. Makayla sat at the table with one of her students, Emily, who was working on the production of /r/. A number of other students were seated at the table as well. As Makayla assisted these students with the construction of their puppets, she asked them what sounds dragons might make. Several children offered that they may have made a sound like /grrrrr/. Makayla readily agreed that /grrr/ was a strong candidate for dragon speech. She encouraged each of the children to make their puppets imitate sentences that contained extended /gr/ blends. Soon, the children were pronouncing sentences like "Grrrr, I will grrrrab the grrrreasy grrrrrapes!" or "Grrrr, grrrasshoppers are grrrross!" By saying /grrrr/ at the start of each sentence, Emily had an opportunity to position her tongue for a correct /r/ before it came up in a full word. The use of /gr/ in words blends facilitated tongue position during running speech. Finally, by extending the /gr/ to /grrr/, Emily could slow down production of the blend to increase her chances of correct productions. Though this activity, Emily got an opportunity to work on her speech without missing out on art class. In addition, because many children were engaged in "dragon talk," she didn't feel singled out.

These different techniques can be used in conjunction with behavioral techniques. Many behavior-modification programs are commercially available for children with articulation disorders. They offer a number of attractive therapy materials designed to make the learning task interesting and fun for the young child. As a first step, the speech-language pathologist establishes a baseline of what the child is able to produce. For example, a particular target sound is selected, and the number of productions the child is able to say correctly, either spontaneously or by prompting, is established as the child's general proficiency for that sound. The treatment program for that sound then begins, following the systematic presentation of a particular program. The child is given an occasional prompt (a helping suggestion) to aid in production tasks, and as the typical program progresses, the clinician fades out support (doing less and less). A particular sound is usually

taught to a particular success level (percentage correct); for example, the child who makes an /r/ error must produce that sound correctly 80 percent of the time before going on to the next (usually more difficult) task in the program.

Operant conditioning techniques can be integrated with articulation therapy. The goal of correct articulation for certain sounds (or classes of sounds) may be broken down into stages. An initial goal may be an approximation of the sound as it occurs at the beginning of words. When the client has mastered this step, closer approximations may be required until correct productions are made. Clients are rewarded for these closer and closer approximations. Rewards may be tangible or intangible. Very young children or mentally retarded individuals might receive a treat or tokens for meeting their goals. Other children may be rewarded by taking their turn in an articulation "game." For many older children and adults, articulatory and communicative success is frequently its own reward.

Generalization

If clients have learned the correct pronunciation of the /r/ sound, it does them little good if they can produce it only in /gr/ blends or only in the therapy setting. The goal of articulation therapy is for clients to be able to use the newly corrected sounds in all words and in all situations. When clients are able to transfer their newly learned articulation skills to untrained words and new settings, we say that they are demonstrating generalization of articulation skills. Generalization does not always occur automatically. The therapist should incorporate activities that promote generalization into the therapy program.

Generalization goals may be broken down into categories, such as generalizations to other sound contexts, to different speaking tasks, and with different speaking partners. Research has shown, for example, that training children on developmentally late-appearing sounds facilitates more generalization to other untrained sounds than when children are trained on earlier-appearing sounds (Gierut, Morrisette, Hughes, & Rowland, 1996). Therefore, through careful consideration of which sounds to train, a clinician can see gains on other sounds "for free." In some cases, the therapist may be able to find a few words in which the client is able to correctly produce the target sound. Generalization then involves transferring this limited skill to greater numbers of words (Prather & Whaley, 1984). For example, the client may lateralize the /s/ (air escapes over the sides of the tongue) in /sl/ blends but produce /st/ blends accurately. In this case, the therapist may present /sl/ blends in conjunction with /st/ blends to facilitate generalization. If the target sound is never produced correctly, the therapist may select a small set of words that begin with the target sounds for initial training. When these are mastered, the therapist may incorporate new words containing the target sounds into the therapy sessions. This set of words is expanded to include words with the target sounds in the medial and final position. The therapist may also include combinations of sounds within words that are more difficult for the client. Different words will be included in each session to promote generalization to new words.

Single-word responses can be expanded into short phrases and sentences. Sometimes a standard carrier phrase can be used initially to facilitate articulation

in longer utterances. For example, a group of children might play a game of twenty questions in which each child asks, "Is it a . . . ?" to find out what card the therapist holds. Older children and adults can practice articulation while reading sentences and short passages. The use of carrier phrases or reading tasks allow clients to practice their articulation skills without having to concentrate on the content of the message. As articulation skills become increasingly automatic, the clinician will incorporate conversational tasks into the therapy session.

As therapy progresses, children and adults become increasingly adept at monitoring their articulation during the therapy session. This self-monitoring process appears to relate to the client's ability to generalize articulation skills (Shriberg & Kwiatkowski, 1990). Outside of the therapy session, clients are typically more concerned with the content of their speech than their articulation. To promote generalization to other settings, the therapist may enlist the cooperation of others. For a child, the therapist may provide parents with tips for facilitating correct articulation at home. Teachers may monitor articulation in the classroom. A peer may be enlisted for activities outside the therapy setting. McReynolds (1982) writes that bringing other people into generalization sessions as critical listeners will sometimes accelerate generalization; however, she notes that we must caution others "not to overdo their help, so that the person does not become overly self-conscious about the problem" (p. 136). Generalization occurs primarily in a practice atmosphere. Individuals should be treated gently when they make mistakes and given realistic positive reinforcement when they produce sounds well.

ACQUIRED ARTICULATION DISORDERS IN ADULTS

Adults who have developed normal speech and language abilities give little attention to their articulation processes when they speak. The motor patterns for speech are well established and relatively automatic under most circumstances; however, adults may acquire structural or neurological impairments that disrupt their articulation abilities. Treatment of such impairments differs from treating developmental articulation disorders because adults may need to change their articulation patterns, and formerly automatic processes may need to become more intentional.

Articulation Impairments Due to Structural Impairments

Structural changes of the articulators can result from traumatic damage or surgical removal of all or portions of the larynx, tongue, jaw, teeth, or lips. Removal of the larynx results in the dramatic loss of the laryngeal voice and is discussed in Chapter 6. In some cases, portions of the tongue must be surgically removed because of cancer. The procedure is called a **glossectomy**, and it may be either partial or total, depending on the extent of the disease. Articulation is a challenge without the tongue; recall from Chapter 2 that many of the sounds of English are differentiated by movements of the tongue. The speech therapy goal following glossectomy is to adjust the placement of the remaining articulators to produce the most intelligible

speech possible. There are many subtle adjustments that can be made to approximate speech produced without the tongue. For example, the sound /t/ normally requires the tongue to touch the alveolar ridge, just behind the teeth, but in the absence of the tongue, the patient might touch the lower lip behind the front teeth in a manner that stops and then releases the airflow. Because the manner of production is still a plosive and it is produced at the alveolar ridge, listeners may be tricked into thinking they heard a /t/. In fact, it is typically easier to understand the speech of a glossectomy patient if you do not look at the mouth, where some surprising articulatory placements are being made.

In some cases, structural changes of the articulators can be compensated for by specially designed artificial replacements, such as a prosthetic tongue and jaw (Arcuri, Perlman, Philippbar, & Barkmeier, 1991; Leonard & Gillis, 1982, 1983). The artificial tongue does not move, but fills in the gap resulting from tongue removal. This improves the speaker's ability to use the remaining articulators to overcome the changes in the oral structures. Some speakers adapt to their new anatomy by making appropriate articulatory adjustments. When therapy is needed, the speech-language pathologist works with the patient to come up with the most satisfactory approximation of sounds that are in error due to structural changes. In some cases the rate of speech must be slowed to allow the necessary time to articulate in a manner that is different from lifelong speech patterns.

Motor Speech Disorders

The most commonly acquired articulation disorders in adults are due to neurological impairments that affect the motor control for speech. They are collectively referred to as motor speech disorders and include the disorders of dysarthria and apraxia of speech. As we saw earlier in this chapter, these disorders can occur in children as well. When they occur in adults, they are typically caused by damage or dysfunction of the motor control centers in the central or peripheral nervous systems, or both. The disturbances may affect any or all aspects of speech production, including respiration, phonation, resonance, and articulation.

Dysarthria.   The dysarthrias are a group of motor speech disorders caused by weakness, paralysis, slowness, incoordination, or sensory loss in the muscle groups responsible for speech. The muscle weakness and poor control typically result in imprecise articulation, so that speech is difficult to understand. The sounds may be distorted or involve the substitution of an incorrect sound. The specific characteristics of dysarthria tend to reflect the location of the damage to the nervous system, so that certain clusters of symptoms have been associated with certain diseases (Duffy, 1995). Some of the causes of dysarthria are stroke, Parkinson's disease, Huntington's disease, amyotrophic lateral sclerosis (Lou Gehrig's disease), and cerebellar diseases. In addition to imprecise articulation, other symptoms include hypernasality because of poor motor control of the soft palate; disturbed voice quality including harsh or breathy voice because of poor control of the lar-

ynx; and abnormal prosody because of poor control of the variations of pitch, loudness, and timing. If motor control is so severely impaired that no understandable speech can be produced, it is called **anarthria**.

Apraxia. **Apraxia of speech** differs from dysarthria in that there is no muscle weakness, paralysis, or incoordination but there is impaired ability to plan the movements for speech production. Thus, apraxia of speech has been referred to as an impairment of the motor planning for articulation. Speech is difficult to understand because of substitution errors, sound repetitions, and some inappropriate sound additions. The errors are often inconsistent, so that repeated attempts at the same word come out differently on each attempt. Apraxia of speech often co-occurs with the language impairment of aphasia, and in those cases it is difficult to separate the speech and language disorders. However, apraxia of speech can exist independently of aphasia, so that language formulation, reading, and writing are unimpaired, but speech production is disturbed (Duffy, 1995).

Treatment of Motor Speech Disorders

The goal for the management of motor speech disorders is to improve communication. This can be accomplished through therapy designed to improve the intelligibility, naturalness, and efficiency of speech production, but may also be achieved by the use of assistive devices. There are excellent resources that provide treatment approaches specific to particular syndromes (Duffy, 1995; Moore, Yorkston, & Beukelman, 1991; Square-Storer, 1989; Yorkston, Beukelman, & Bell, 1988). Treatment may be directed toward the restoration of normal speech production processes or the compensation for impaired motor control. In some cases, adjustments need to be made to overcome the impairment. For example, Parkinson's disease often results in a dysarthria that is characterized by imprecise articulation, decreased loudness, and flat prosody. A treatment approach called the Lee Silverman Voice Treatment trains patients to increase the effort that they exert while speaking by adjusting their loudness. With increased loudness, the Parkinson patients also increase their articulatory precision and thus remarkably improve their speech intelligibility (Ramig, Countryman, Thompson, & Horii, 1995).

Although the symptomatology of apraxia and dysarthria differs, there are similarities in some of the behavioral treatment approaches appropriate to these speech disorders. For both types of disorders, treatment is designed so that there is an orderly progression of treatment tasks and extensive drill to reestablish and stabilize the motor movements. For example, a treatment continuum for apraxia of speech begins with the clinician saying the target word, followed by the patient and clinician producing the target together. If the patient correctly produces the response simultaneously with the clinician, then the clinician reduces support by mouthing the word along with the patient, and ultimately the patient produces the response to a question, without support from the clinician (Wertz, LaPointe, & Rosenbek, 1984). In cases where speech production is not adequate for everyday communication, augmentative communication devices may be appropriate.

AUGMENTATIVE COMMUNICATION SYSTEMS

Some adults and children have physical limitations so severe that oral speech may not be an attainable goal. For these individuals, alternate methods must be found for communication. These range from a simple signaling device, like the call bell on a bedside nightstand, to sophisticated electronic devices that are tailored to the client's individual needs. The speech-language pathologist's challenge is to find the combination of features in a communication device that best matches the client's needs and abilities. A child who can identify pictures, but cannot yet read, may start with a picture board that includes objects and actions common to his or her daily life (see Figure 4.3). An adult who can read may do well with an electronic device that can produce both synthetic speech and written output (see Figure 4.4).

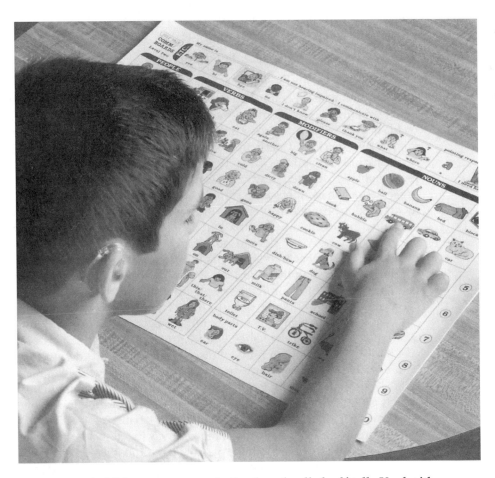

FIGURE 4.3   A child uses a communication board, called self-talk. Used with permission of Communication Skill Builders, San Antonio, TX.

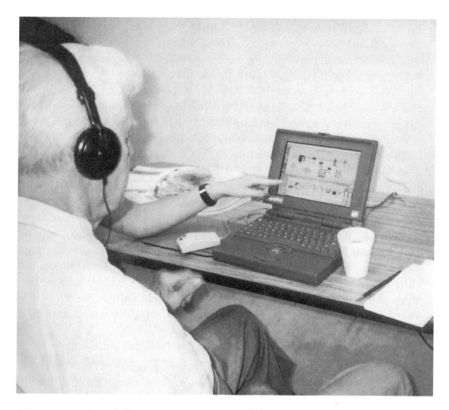

FIGURE 4.4   **An adult uses the Lingraphica® (Tolfa) system to communicate recent events in his life. (Courtesy of The University of Arizona, Department of Speech & Hearing Sciences)**

Before a device can be selected, an initial assessment of the client's abilities must be obtained, often through the coordinated efforts of a variety of professionals such as audiologists, vision specialists, psychologists, speech-language pathologists, and physical and occupational therapists. These individuals contribute information concerning the client's sensory, motor, cognitive, and language abilities. This evaluation is designed to determine the client's limitations as well as strengths that might be used for communication. For example, an individual with limited visual acuity may do better with simple line drawings than with glossy photos. An individual with severe cerebral palsy may have sufficient control of eye movement, head movement, or even foot movement to allow the use of certain switches with an electronic device. Perhaps different devices are needed to allow the child or adult to communicate from different positions, such as sitting in a wheelchair or lying on the floor or in bed. The devices selected must be able to accompany the client and be usable whenever the client needs to communicate.

The decision about how the child or adult will communicate is closely related to what information will be communicated. Communication involves a code that

is passed from sender to receiver. For normal speakers, this code is oral language. For a patient who is recovering from surgery that removed the larynx, the code might be written language. For a child who cannot write, the code might be a symbol system. For a child of more limited language or cognitive abilities, pictures might be used. In selecting the code, both the client's abilities and the people they need to communicate with must be considered. It makes no sense to train clients to expert levels with a new symbol system, for instance, if their families, teachers, and classmates prefer not to learn this new symbol system to communicate with them.

After one or more communication systems are selected, training is vital for developing successful communication. Training is geared toward the client's developmental level and daily needs. For a toddler, it may mean starting with toys and activities that develop turn-taking skills and communicative intent. For a school-aged child, it might include the use of language for academic purposes as well as for interpersonal communication. For the adult, the goal may be to reestablish communication that has been affected by illness or injury. Training often involves trial and error on the part of both the client and the clinician. Imagine the dilemma of the clinician who must try to adapt a communication system to meet the particular needs of the client before the client has the means of communicating those needs. Imagine the frustration of the client who must wait until the clinician figures it out!

A client with the desire and means to transmit a message is still only half of a successful communication. Communication requires other people. Family members often receive direct training on how to use and maintain augmentative devices, but the client is also likely to encounter others who have never seen an augmentative device. Unfortunately, some people may not want to take the considerable time and effort involved in communicating through an alternative system. Communication is inevitably slower and is often less accurate. It can be tiring for both the sender and receiver. However, for many nonverbal individuals, the basic need to interact with other people provides the motivation and reward for the effort involved. This can clearly be seen in the case of Mr. Moser.

Mr. Moser had been a high-school science teacher until he suffered brain damage at the age of 43. An artery at the base of his brain was thin-walled and weak. Eventually, this section of the artery ballooned out, forming an aneurysm, which ultimately burst. Immediate surgery was able to halt the bleeding but not before sections of his brainstem and cerebellum were damaged. When he recovered from surgery, he was left with a variety of permanent deficits.

Damage to the auditory tracts in the brainstem cause a rare form of an acquired auditory disorder. Although he could hear sounds and tell when two sounds were different, Mr. Moser could not attach meaning to what he heard. Consequently, he could not understand spoken language, although he understood written language quite well. Damage to the motor tracts running through the brainstem and cerebellum left him confined to a wheelchair. He suffered from ataxia of movement. When he would reach for objects, his hands and arms would waver back and forth. He would frequently over- or undershoot his reach for the object he

wanted. His speech was similarly affected. His voice was a monotone and low in pitch. He spoke with great effort, and his face often contorted as he struggled to get out the words. He spoke only when asked specifically to do so.

Because of his difficulty in producing the movements needed for speech and his inability to monitor his speech through audition, he became mute. In place of speech, he relied on an electronic communication system that allowed him to type in a message that was displayed on a small screen. Messages were typed with an ever-wavering index finger, one letter at a time. When he wished to convey a longer message, which he frequently did, the device printed the message on paper. His laboriously produced messages revealed his intelligent, inquisitive, and outgoing personality. Armed with his communication system and a large amount of persistence and charm, Mr. Moser was able to interact with others through written language.

CLINICAL PROBLEM SOLVING

Kiesha, age 6, was brought into our research lab to participate in a language study. While she was there we taped the following conversation:

Kiesha: Hey, Piget (Piglet)!

Dad: There he is. You found him. There's Piglet.

Kiesha: Shhhhh.

Dad: Oh, is it because he's sleeping?

Kiesha: Kaiet (quiet)!

Dad: Ok, I'll be quiet. Are they all asleep?

Kiesha: We da he seep (Where does he sleep?)

Dad: What are they doing?

Kiesha: Let's make 'em seep (sleep). He's at home.

Dad: Who's this guy.

Kiesha: Gover (Grover). And Ernie. Cookie Monser (Cookie Monster).

1. Does this speech sample indicate an articulation disorder? Would you feel the same if the child had just turned 3? (To review normal development, consult Chapter 3).
2. Using Table 4.1 can you identify any phonological processes among the sound errors? Remember that identification of a phonological process requires evidence of a pattern that affects more than one individual sound.
3. What factors would you need to rule out as causes of these speech errors before considering therapy?
4. Which therapy approaches might you consider for remediation in this case? Which would not be appropriate? Why?

REFERENCES

Arcuri, M. R., Perlman, A. L., Philippbar, S. A., & Barkmeier, J. M. (1991). The effects of a maxillary speech-aid prosthesis for the combined tongue and mandibular resection patient. *Journal of Prosthetic Dentistry, 65*(6), 816–22.

ASHA. (1991). The role of the speech-language pathologist in management of oral myofunctional disorders. *Asha, 33*, (Suppl. 5), 7.

Barrett, R. H., & Hanson, M. L. (1978). *Oral myofunctional disorders* (2nd ed.). St. Louis: Mosby.

Boone, D. R. (1972). *Cerebral palsy.* New York: Bobbs-Merrill.

Broen, P. (Ed.). (1981). *Language, speech and hearing services in the schools* (Special issue on nonvocal communication), 4:12.

Coleman, C., Look, A., & Myers, L. (1980). Assessing no-oral clients for assistive communication devices. *Journal of Speech and Hearing Disorders, 45*, 515–526.

Duffy, J. R. (1995). *Motor speech disorders: substrates, differential diagnosis, and management.* St. Louis, MO: Mosby-Year Book.

Dunn, C. (1982). Phonological process analysis: Contributions to assessing phonological disorders. *Communicative Disorders, 7*, 147–163.

Elbert, M., Powell, T. W., & Swartzlander, P. (1991). Toward a technology of generalization: How many exemplars are sufficient? *Journal of Speech and Hearing Research, 34*, 84–87.

Estrem, T., & Broen, P. A. (1989). Early speech production of children with cleft palate. *Journal of Speech and Hearing Research, 32*, 122–119.

Gierut, J. A., Morrisette, M. L., Hughes, M. T., & Rowland, S. (1996). Phonological treatment efficacy and developmental norms. *Language, Speech, and Hearing Services in Schools, 27*, 215–230.

Goldman, R., & Fristoe, M. (1986). *Goldman-Fristoe Test of Articulation.* Circle Pines, MN: American Guidance Service.

Grunwell, P. (1980). Developmental language disorders at the phonological level. In F. M. Jones (Ed.), *Language disability in children.* Lancaster, PA: MTP Press.

Grunwell, P. (1981). *The nature of phonological disability in children,* New York: Academic Press.

Grunwell, P., Brondsted, K., Henningsson, G., Jansonius, K., Karling, J., Meijer, M., Ording, U., Wyatt, R., Vermeij-Zieverink, E., & Sell, D. (2000). A six-center international study of the outcome of treatment in patients with clefts of the lip and palate: The results of a cross-linguistic investigation of cleft palate speech. *Scandinavian Journal of Plastic and Reconstructive Surgery and Hand Surgery, 34*, 219–229.

Hall, B. J. C. (1990). Attitudes of fourth and sixth graders towards peers with mild articulation disorders. *Language, Speech, and Hearing Services in Schools, 22*, 344–340.

Handzic-Cuk, J., Cuk, V., Gluhinic, M., Risavi, R., & Stajner-Katusic, S. (2001). Tympanometric findings in cleft palate patients: Influence of age and cleft type. *Journal of Laryngology & Otology, 115*, 91–96.

Ingram, D. (1981). *Procedures for the phonological analysis of children's language.* Baltimore: University Park Press.

Jaffee, M. B. (1984). Neurological impairment of speech production: Assessment and treatment. In J. Costello (Ed.), *Speech disorders in children.* San Diego: College-Hill Press.

Kent, R. D., Miolo, G., & Bloedel, S. (1994). The intelligibility of children's speech: A review of evaluation procedures. *American Journal of Speech-Language Pathology, 3*, 81–95.

Khan, L., & Lewis, N. (1986). *Khan-Lewis Phonological Analysis.* Circle Pines, MN: American Guidance Service.

Leonard, R. J., & Gillis, R. (1983). Effects of a prosthetic tongue on vowel formants and isovowel lines in a patient with total glossectomy (an addendum to Leonard and Gillis, 1982). *Journal of Speech & Hearing Disorders, 48*(4), 423–6.

Leonard, R. J., & Gillis, R. (1982). Effects of a prosthetic tongue on vowel intelligibility and food management in a patient with total glossectomy. *Journal of Speech & Hearing Disorders, 47*(1), 25–30.

Lewis, B. A. (1990). Familial phonological disorders: Four pedigrees. *Journal of Speech and Hearing Disorders, 55*, 160–170.

Love, R., Hagerman, E., & Taimi, E. (1980). Speech performance, dysphagia and oral reflexes in cerebral palsy. *Journal of Speech and Hearing Disorders, 45*, 59–75.

Lynch, J. I. (1990). Tongue reduction surgery: Efficacy and relevance to the profession. *Asha, 32*, 59–61.

McDonald, E. T., & Chance, B. (1964). *Cerebral palsy.* Englewood Cliffs, NJ: Prentice Hall.

McReynolds, L. V. (1982). Functional articulation problems. In G. H. Shames & E. H. Wiig (Eds.), *Human communication disorders: An introduction.* Columbus, OH: Charles E. Merrill.

Moore, C. A., Yorkston, K. M., & Beukelman, D. R. (Eds.). (1991). *Dysarthria and apraxia of speech.* Baltimore, MD: Paul H. Brookes.

Mysak, E. (1980). *Neurospeech therapy for the cerebral palsied* (3rd ed.). Totowa, NJ: Teachers College Press.

Peterson-Falzone, S. J., Hardin-Jones, M. A., & Karnell, M. P. (2001). *Cleft palate speech* (3rd ed.). St. Louis: Mosby.

Prather, E., & Whaley, P. (1984). Articulation training based on coarticulation. In H. Winitz (Ed.), *Treating articulation disorders: For clinicians by clinicians.* Baltimore: University Park Press.

Ramig, L. O., Countyman, S., Thompson, L., & Horii, L. (1995). A comparison of two intensive speech treatments for Parkinson disease. *Journal of Speech and Hearing Research, 39,* 1232–1251.

Ruscello, D. M., St. Louis, K. O., & Mason, N. (1991). School-age children with phonologic disorders: Coexistence with other speech/language disorders. *Journal of Speech and Hearing Disorders, 34,* 236–242.

Shelton, R. L., Furr, M. L., Johnson, A., & Arndt, W. B. (1975). Cephalometric and intraoral variables as they relate to articulation improvement with training. *American Journal of Orthodontics, 67,* 423–431.

Shprintzen, R. J., Siegal-Sadewitz, V. L., Amato, J., & Goldberg, R. B. (1985). Retrospective diagnosis of previously missed syndromic disorders among 1000 patients with cleft lip, cleft palate, or both. *Birth Defects, 21,* 85–92.

Shriberg, L. (1980). Developmental phonological disorders. In T. J. Hixon, L. Shriberg, & J. Saxon (Eds.), *Introduction to communication disorders.* Englewood Cliffs, NJ: Prentice Hall.

Shriberg, L., Austin, D., Lewis, B. A., McSweeny, J. L., & Wilson, D. L. (1997). The percentage of consonants correct (PCC) metric: Extensions and reliability data. *Journal of Speech Language and Hearing Research, 40,* 708–722.

Shriberg, L. D., & Kwiatkowski, J. (1988). A follow-up study of children with phonologic disorders of unknown origin. *Journal of Speech and Hearing Disorders, 53,* 144–155.

Shriberg, L. D., & Kwiatkowski, J. (1990). Self-monitoring and generalization in preschool speech-delayed children. *Language, Speech, and Hearing Services in Schools, 21,* 157–170.

Shriberg, L. D., Kwiatkowski, J., Best, S., Hengst, J., & Terselic-Weber, B. (1986). Characteristics of children with phonological disorders of unknown origin. *Journal of Speech and Hearing Disorders, 51,* 140–161.

Shriberg, L. D., Tomblin, J. B., McSweeny, J. L. (1999). Prevalence of speech delay in 6-year-old children and comorbidity with language impairment. *Journal of Speech, Language, and Hearing Research, 42,* 1461–1481.

Square-Storer, P. (Ed.). (1989). *Acquired apraxia of speech in aphasic adults.* Salisbury, UK: Lawrence Erlbaum Associates.

Wertz, R. T., LaPointe, L. L., & Rosenbek, J. C. (1984). *Apraxia of speech in adults: The disorder and its management.* Orlando, FL: Grune & Stratton.

Yorkston, K. M., Beukelman, D. R., & Bell, K. R. (1988). *Clinical management of dysarthric speakers.* Boston: College-Hill Press.

READINGS FROM THE POPULAR LITERATURE

Albom, M. (1998). *Tuesdays with Morrie.* New York: Doubleday. (amyotrophic lateral sclerosis, ALS, or Lou Gehrig's disease)

Gordon, S., & Tempel, L. (1992). *Parkinson's: A personal story of acceptance.* Boston: Branden. (Parkinson disease).

Grady-Fitchett, J. (1998). *Flying lessons: On the wings of Parkinson's disease.* New York: Forge. (Parkinson disease)

Grealy, L. (1994). *Autobiography of a face.* New York: Harper Perennial. (facial cancer)

Handler, L. (1998). *Twitch and shout: A Touretter's tale.* New York: Dutton. (Tourette syndrome)

Hasse, J. (1996). *Break out: Finding freedom when you don't quite fit the mold.* Berea, OH: Quixote Publications. (cerebral palsy)

Kondracke, M. (2000). *Saving Milly: Love, politics and Parkinson's disease.* New York: Ballantine Books. (Parkinson disease)

McDermott, J. (2000). *Babyface: A story of heart and bones.* Bethesda, MD: Woodbine House. (Apert syndrome)

Montague, A. (1999). *Elephant man* (3rd ed.). New York: E. P. Dutton. (Facial disfigurement)

Rabin, R. (1985). *Six parts love: One family's battle with Lou Gehrig's disease*. New York: Scribner. (ALS)

Reeve, C. (1997). *Still me*. New York: Random House. (spinal cord injury, ventilator dependency)

Robillard, A. B. (1999). *Meaning of a disability: The lived experience of paralysis*. Philadelphia: Temple University Press. (motor neuron disease).

Sacks, O. (1973). *Awakenings*. New York: E. P. Dutton. (cases of diminished movement and communication related to Parkinsonism)

Sienkiewicz-Mercer, R., & Kaplan, S. (1989). *I Raise my eyes to say yes*. West Hartford, CT: Whole Health Books. (cerebral palsy)

Stehli, A. (1995). *Dancing in the rain*. Westport, CT: The Georgiana Organization. (stories by parents of children with special needs)

Webster, B. D. (1989). *All of a piece*. Baltimore: Johns Hopkins University Press. (multiple sclerosis)

Wexler, A. (1995). *Mapping fate*. New York: Times Books: Random House. (Huntington disease)

DISORDERS OF FLUENCY

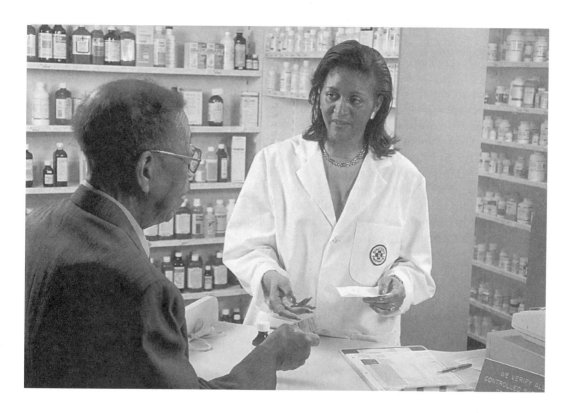

■ ■ ■ ■ ■ ▬▬▬▬▬▬▬▬▬▬▬▬▬▬▬▬▬▬▬▬▬▬▬▬▬▬▬▬▬▬▬

PREVIEW

The area of fluency and fluency disorders has been one of the most dynamic areas within the profession of speech-language pathology. Principal among disorders of fluency is the phenomenon of stuttering. The various definitions of stuttering reflect a wide range of perspectives that experts have brought to bear in trying to understand this disorder of communication. Indeed, developmental, familial, psychological, neurological, and motoric factors all appear to interact in cases of stuttering. Although stuttering is the most common fluency disorder, there are other disorders characterized by changes in fluency. We will briefly consider disruptions of fluency associated with cluttering and cases of acquired stuttering in adults.

When Abraham[1] was about 3 years of age, his mother noticed that his sentences did not always flow smoothly. Sometimes he would repeat the same word several times before he was able to get the rest of the sentence out. There were pauses midsentence. In fact, at times Abraham sounded quite disfluent. This concerned both of his parents because they each had a family history of **stuttering**. The mother's brother had stuttered during most of his childhood, although he was described as completely fluent as an adult. The father's sister began stuttering as a child and continued to stutter into adulthood. The parents did not want Abraham to struggle to communicate the way their siblings had, and they were naturally concerned when Abraham seemed to go through periods when he was particularly disfluent. At age 3 years, 3 months, we had the following conversation with him:

Author: What's Wishbone?

Abraham: Um, he's one of the shows that I watch. He's a dog. The story of Wishbone is really . . . um, really a show.

Author: He's a dog. And he has his own show?

Abraham: No, there's a . . . there's a boy in it.

Author: What do they get to do?

Abraham: They do everything. But only in the shows, they get to do . . . I don't know.

[*Abraham notices the barnyard toys and goes to them.*]

Author: Let me see what's in this barn. There's a lot of animals in here.

Abraham: Yeah, I . . . [silence]

Author: All right. Well, there's a cow. And there's a baby cow. That's a . . . that's a brown cow.

---

[1]We followed the speech and language development of Abraham in Chapters 3 and 7.

Abraham: No, that's a white cow. That's called . . . that's called . . . These two are cows.

Author: Oh yeah? What kind of cows?

Abraham: Black ones and white ones.

Author: Black ones and white ones. And this is a dog.

Abraham: This is . . . This is a dog.

Author: Do you think he's a sheep dog?

Abraham: Nooo.

Author: Do you think he's a cow dog? Does he have to watch out over the cows?

Abraham: [*Nods in agreement.*]

Author: Well, I've got some hay. [*Picks up a cow.*] Do you think he's a hay eater?

Abraham: Yes he is. I'll put hay on his . . . in his . . . in his . . . .in there so he can't eat anything.

[*Abraham puts animals in the hay loft.*]

Author: Now we have two cows in the hay.

Abraham: Is this one the . . . .the . . . the . . . the baby one?

Author: I don't know. It's kind of small. Maybe he is a baby one.

During this brief conversation, we were able to observe a number of interruptions in the flow of communication. These included whole word repetitions ("the . . . the . . . the . . . the baby one"), phrase repetitions ("This is . . . this is a dog."), and interjections ("um"). However, Abraham seemed completely unfazed by his disfluencies. His focus was on the toys and our play, and he was probably unaware of his own speech patterns. Notice, too, that Abraham was not the only one to show speech repetition. The author repeated part of a sentence ("That's a . . . that's a brown cow.") during the conversation as well. In fact, everyone experiences a minor interruption in the flow of speech at some time or another. Differentiating between "normal" disfluencies and stuttering is an ongoing challenge to those working in the area of fluency disorders.

It is not always easy to identify an episode of disfluency that characterizes stuttering unequivocally from an episode that is a momentary lapse of fluency. This is particularly true in the case of young children. As young children are learning to put together sentences, it is very common to hear them make false starts (I . . . he did it!), revise mid-sentence ("He's in . . . he's on T.V."), hesitate over the next word to come ("I want . . . juice."). We often get the sense that these interruptions in fluency have more to do with the child's partial grasp of the language than any struggle making the words come out. Likewise, we frequently hear a child who is so excited that word or phrase repetitions come pouring forth ("Mommy! Mommy! Mommy! Mommy! Mommy! Can I, can I, can I have one?!"). For most

ren, these episodes reflect normal development, rather than the onset of stut-
g. In fact, for Abraham, this proved to be the case. As he continued to develop
ch and language skills, the episodes of disfluency decreased. By $4\frac{1}{2}$, no one,
uding his parents, had any concerns about his speech fluency.

NORMAL DISFLUENCIES VERSUS STUTTERING

Conture (1990) noted that deciding who is and who is not stuttering is a relative, rather than an absolute decision, in that there is no behavior that children who stutter display that normal children *never* exhibit. Although normally developing children (and adults on occasion) sometimes experience breakdowns in these speech parameters, there is a much more normal flow of speech than is observed in a child who stutters. For example, normal children, such as Abraham, may repeat words or phrases at the age of three. However, by the age of $4\frac{1}{2}$, children usually repeat utterances only when they wish to emphasize something (Curlee, 1980).

Early Signs of Stuttering

Although no method is foolproof for identifying the young child who will persist in stuttering, a number of behavioral signs are considered to be "red flags" for stuttering (see Table 5.1). In the case of stuttering, speech is frequently characterized by changes in duration, rate, and rhythm, with frequent interruptions of smooth fluency from sound to sound and from word to word. One distinction that has been suggested involves the unit of speech on which the disfluency occurs (Andrews, Craig, Feyer, Haddinott, Neilson, & Howie, 1983; Wall, 1988). The type of speech unit in which the individual is most likely to produce normal disfluency is the word, phrase, or sentence; those who stutter are most likely to do so on single sounds and syllables. A child showing normal disfluency may say "I want . . . I want it," whereas a child who stutters may say "I wwwwwant it." The frequency of disfluent episodes is also different for children with normal disfluencies and for those who stutter. Wingate (1962) found that nonstuttering children seldom make repetitions for more than 3 percent of their total speech utterances; children who stutter were found to have a frequency of syllable disfluencies ranging from 7 to 14 percent.

The signs of stuttering are not restricted to interruptions of speech. Children who stutter are also likely to differ from their peers in facial movements accompanying episodes of disfluency. Conture and Kelly (1991) reported that young children who stutter could be differentiated from nonstuttering children by the types of facial behaviors they exhibit. For example, children who stutter were likely to look away, blink their eyes, raise their upper lip, or press their lips together during periods of disfluency, whereas their fluent peers showed these behaviors less frequently. Stuttering children may show signs of struggle or tension while attempting to speak, whereas children with normal disfluencies typically seem unaffected by the disfluent episode.

TABLE 5.1 Signs Often Associated with Normal and Stuttered Speech

NORMAL DISFLUENCIES

Word repetitions	I like that . . . that book.
Phrase repetitions	I want a . . . want a big one!
Sentence repetitions	Watch me! Watch me! Watch me!
Hesitations	He took . . . my juice.
Interjections	We, um, got to go too.

STUTTERING

Syllable repetitions	We saw a vi-vi-vi-video.
Sound repetition	I g-g-g-got it from school.
Sound prolongations	Wwwwwwait for mmmme.
Sound blocks	[starts word but no sound comes out]
Nonspeech behaviors	[e.g., blinks, facial tension, limb movement]

Several investigators (Schwartz, Zebrowski, & Conture, 1990; Yairi & Ambrose, 1992) have examined the earliest signs of stuttering by studying the behaviors of young children whose parents reported that stuttering had begun recently (within the previous twelve months). Yairi and Ambrose interviewed parents concerning the age of their children and the characteristics of their disfluent speech when stuttering began. Parents reported that their children were sometimes quite young, between the ages of 20 months to 5 years of age, when stuttering was first recognized. Just under half of the parents reported that their children began to stutter suddenly, whereas other parents remembered the onset of stuttering as evolving gradually over the course of several weeks. Schwartz and colleagues recorded the speech of such children on videotape to assess the behaviors associated with the earliest stages of stuttering. The investigators reported that the disfluencies of these children frequently included sound prolongations (33 to 60% of all disfluent episodes). They also frequently exhibited nonspeech behaviors, such as eye movements or eye closings during disfluent episodes. Somewhat surprisingly, the stuttering behaviors of children who were at the younger end of the age range did not differ remarkably from those at the older end. Although prolongations were somewhat more frequent for children who had been stuttering longer, the authors emphasized that there were more similarities among the behaviors of children at different ages than differences.

The signs that suggest the onset of stuttering, as opposed to developmental disfluencies, can vary between children and even within a single child. However, we have seen that there are some signs that signal that a child is struggling with more than just the normal disruptions of fluency that all children sometimes experience. These signs can be seen in the case of a young boy who was brought to the clinic for a fluency evaluation.

Jackson was 6 years old when he was first seen in the clinic. His mother brought him in because "he stutters." She reported that he started stuttering two years

before, but she had always assumed that he would grow out of it. Now that Jackson was in school, however, she was concerned that other children were teasing him. She had already noticed that Jackson seemed aware that his speech was different from other children. She reported that he sometimes got frustrated when trying to talk. As far as she knew, no one in her family had ever stuttered, and she couldn't recall anyone having had any kind of developmental problems at all.

When we talked with Jackson, it was apparent that his speech showed more than the typical amount of disfluency. In fact, sometimes it seemed as if he could hardly get his thoughts out. His speech was frequently disrupted by sound prolongations and blocks, when no sound came out at all. During these episodes, his mouth seemed to lock into a tense position from which he was unable to break free. His brows knit together; sometimes he would blink or contort his face until the disfluent period passed and speech resumed its normal flow. When asked why his mother brought him to the clinic, he replied "I-i-i-t's . . . because I t-t-t-t-t . . . alk . . . I can't talk."

In contrast to his fluency, a formal assessment of his language showed average to above average skills. Likewise, when he was not stuttering, he did not show problems with speech articulation. An examination of his oral mechanism (see Chapter 4) revealed normal structure, muscle tone, and nonspeech movement. Likewise, he could repeat nonsense words and say entire sentences in a sing-song cadence, which indicated he possessed the physical mechanisms to support normal speech.

Persistent Stuttering

A majority of the children who show early disfluencies will eventually develop fluent speech. However, some children will not. Yairi and colleagues reported that children destined to recover from early stuttering-like behaviors may initially show more disfluencies than children who continue to be disfluent. However, the children who recover begin to show reductions in their number of disfluencies within the first year after stuttering-like disfluencies began. In contrast, children who failed to recover were relatively stable in their rate of disfluency (Yairi, Ambrose, Paden, & Throneburg, 1996). Although there is a chance that some of these children will recover still later in childhood, they are at risk for struggling with fluency throughout their lives. Let us look at the case of one such man:

> Mr. Andrews, age 32, has stuttered since childhood. Although he had received therapy several times, he continued to show a variety of stuttering signs. His stuttering consisted primarily of silent blocks, during which his mouth and face contorted as he struggled to break free. Occasionally, he would also experience part-word repetitions, where the first sound of a word was repeated over and over. He had recently contacted the clinic because he thought that his stuttering was preventing him from advancing in his career as fast as he thought he could. He expressed, "T————eam work is very important in my c-c-c-c-company, and I knnnnnnnnnow that the others would rather not have me on the team b————cause of my stuttering. When I present m——y ideas, they d————on't take them as ssssseriously." He reported that he was able to speak fluently "most of the time" after his last experience with therapy in high school. However, to maintain fluency,

he felt he had to concentrate harder on how he was speaking than on what he was actually trying to say. Over time, his disfluency slipped back to pre-therapy levels. He was willing to try again to reduce his stuttering severity.

Adults who stutter may continue to show some of the same characteristics of childhood stuttering. They may continue to produce sound repetitions and prolongations, along with silent interruptions, called blocks, in the flow of speech. "Secondary" characteristics of stuttering, which may have been present during childhood, may be more pronounced. These characteristics include facial tension, facial contortions, and extraneous movements during the stuttering episode. In addition, these adults typically have had years of frustration with their difficulty in communicating ideas with the ease that comes naturally to others. This frustration can become as problematic as the actual episodes of fluency breakdown.

It is not uncommon for nonstuttering individuals to stereotype those who stutter with a variety of negative traits, including being anxious, tense, insecure, or nervous (Kalinowski, Lerman, & Watt, 1987). Indeed, several studies have examined physiological correlates of stress and found evidence of increased levels of stress and anxiety among those who stutter (Blood, Blood, Bennet, Simpson, & Susman, 1994; Weber & Smith, 1990). The question remains whether stuttering results from internal stress and anxiety, or if those traits are a consequence of repeated negative experiences with communication. Several studies suggest that the latter is the case. For example, Miller and Watson (1992) reported that their subjects who stuttered were no more anxious overall than nonstuttering subjects. However, the two groups differed in terms of their attitudes toward communication, with attitudes worsening with increased stuttering severity. Craig (1990) showed that adults who stutter were significantly more anxious during a communication task than control subjects prior to treatment for stuttering. After reducing their level of disfluency through treatment of stuttering behaviors, anxiety was reduced to a level characteristic of nonstuttering adults. Such findings may be leading to a shift in clinician perceptions of stuttering as involving characteristic personality traits such as anxiety or other negative affective states (Cooper & Cooper, 1996).

One of the more puzzling features of persistent stuttering is that speech can become completely fluent under certain circumstances. Let us consider the following case:

Mr. Tirai, age 27, was a graduate student who had come to this country to study three years earlier. Although he spoke two other languages with native proficiency, he had only rudimentary English at that time. He spent his first academic year in the United States studying primarily for his English language proficiency exam. He needed to pass this exam to continue his studies in engineering. An outgoing man, he also spent his time going to campus and community cultural events, through which he developed a number of U.S. friends. Through his determined study, his circle of English-speaking friends, and a measure of talent for learning languages, he steadily gained proficiency in English over the next three years. Other than his accent, his English seemed largely unremarkable. He had long since acquired the common grammatical forms of English. His vocabulary had grown to a point where

he rarely needed to search for words in conversation. However, in his final year of study, he was beginning to show occasional episodes of stuttering-like disfluencies. Although "stuttering" was not a word he had acquired in English, he managed to convey that he did indeed stutter in his two native languages. He had initially thought that he had escaped from stuttering through English, but that it appeared to have caught up with him just as he was feeling comfortable with this new language.

Mr. Tirai was fluent for an extended period of time during which he was learning English. Others have discovered that short-term fluency can be induced under a number of speaking conditions. Fluency may be achieved under conditions of delayed auditory feedback. This involves use of instrumentation that presents the speaker's own voice, through headphones, at a slight time delay. So, as the speaker is talking, what he or she hears lags behind what is currently being said. Choral reading or speaking, during which people speak in concert, also tends to promote fluency. Likewise, intentional changes in the rhythm of speech, as in chanting or singing, will produce fluency. All of these speaking conditions, from learning a foreign language to chanting, involve either an increase in effort or a change in the timing of speech production. It appears that such changes may "override" whatever mechanisms may lead to disfluent episodes in regular speech. Unfortunately, as Mr. Tirai found, as speakers grow proficient with these "unusual" speaking conditions, stuttering may reappear.

STUTTERING IN THE POPULATION

The **prevalence** of a disorder is the number of people in the population who have a particular problem at any given time. There have been several prevalence studies of stuttering over the years. The National Institute of Deafness and Other Communication Disorders (NIDCD) of the National Institutes of Health (NIH) estimated that approximately 2 million Americans stutter (1992). This corresponds to a prevalence of approximately 0.8 percent. This figure is comparable to estimates of 0.8 percent derived by Hull, Mielke, Willeford, and Timmons (1976), 0.7 percent by Young (1975), and 0.8 percent by Morley (1952).

Although less than 1 percent of the population may be identified as stutterers at any given time, the percent of people who stutter varies across the life span. Morley (1972) followed approximately 1,000 children in Newcastle-upon-Tyne for fifteen years to examine various aspects of development. The **incidence** of stuttering, or the number of new cases identified during a period of time, in this particular study was about 4 percent, or one in 25 children. NIDCD estimates that one in 30 children will go through a period of disfluency that lasts a minimum of six months.

Stuttering is typically first identified before the age of 5 and many resolve to normal fluency before puberty (Morley, 1972; Wingate, 1976). Wingate (1976) sum-

marized fourteen studies and concluded that approximately 80 percent of children recover from stuttering. Although there has been some dispute about the exact number, it appears that for the majority of children who stutter at an early age, stuttering will disappear before they graduate from high school. Curlee (1980) came to the following conclusion: ". . . if the incidence of stuttering among the general population does approximate 4 percent, a recovery rate of 80 percent would account for a 0.7 percent prevalence of stuttering" (p. 281).

In some respects, stuttering is an "equal opportunity" disorder. It affects people of all racial and socioeconomic backgrounds. However, it does appear that some individuals are at higher risk for developing the disorder than others. Stuttering affects more boys than girls. NIDCD (1992) estimated that four times as many boys stutter as girls. Others have placed the male:female ratio at the somewhat lower figures of 3:1 (Hull et al., 1976) or 2:1 (Morley, 1972; Yairi & Ambrose, 1992). These differences may reflect, in part, the different age groups examined in these studies. The male:female ratio tends to increase with older ages, which has led some to suggest that girls may show higher rates of recovery with age than boys (Yairi, Ambrose, & Cox, 1996).

In addition to the surplus of males among individuals identified as stutterers, a family history of stuttering increases an individual's risk for the disorder. Although the population prevalence for stuttering is thought to hover around 0.7 to 0.8 percent, the prevalence among the relatives of an individual who stutters is much higher (Andrews & Harris, 1964; Howie, 1981; Kidd, 1980; Yairi & Ambrose, 1992, Yairi, Ambrose, & Cox, 1993). Yari and Ambrose reported that almost half (46.6%) of their sample of young children who stutter had parents or siblings who also stuttered at some time. If blood relatives in the extended family were considered, two-thirds (66.3%) of the children had a positive family history for stuttering. The pattern of family aggregation for stuttering may signal the presence of a single major gene that contributes to expression of the disorder (Yairi et al., 1993). However, the actual components that contribute to the development of stuttering may be more complex. Some have suggested that genetic factors may confer a risk for stuttering, but that certain environmental factors are needed to trigger the disorder (Andrews et al., 1983; Howie, 1981).

Family history for stuttering may account for some of the variability seen among individuals who stutter. Janssen, Kraaimaat, and Brutten (1990) examined a variety of traits in subjects who stuttered with reference to family history for stuttering. Compared with those who lacked any relatives who stuttered, those with a positive family history for stuttering had more sound prolongations and silent blocks in their speech. They also showed differences on measures of duration and variability in the acoustic stream than those without a positive family history. In contrast, the two stuttering groups did not differ on measures of reading, autonomic nervous system response, or responsiveness to therapy. Janssen and colleagues suggest that these results indicate that familial or genetic contribution to stuttering may impact the motoric aspects of stuttering more than other associated features of the disorder.

DEFINITIONS

Definitions of stuttering are many and varied. Let us consider a few of the definitions that have appeared in the literature over the years.

> *1955, Johnson:* "Stuttering is an anticipatory, apprehensive, hypertonic avoidance reaction" (p. 23). According to Johnson, stuttering is what speakers do when they expect stuttering to occur: dread it, tense in anticipation of it, and attempt to avoid doing it.
>
> *1977, World Health Organization:* Stuttering includes "disorders in the rhythm of speech, in which the individual knows precisely what he wishes to say, but at the time is unable to say it because of an involuntary, repetitive prolongation or cessation of sound" (p. 227).
>
> *1978, Wingate:* "Stuttering is characterized by audible or silent elemental repetitions and prolongations. These features reflect a temporary inability to move forward to the following sound" (p. 249).
>
> *1980, Perkins:* "Stuttering is the abnormal timing of speech sound initiation."
>
> *1987, Speech Foundation of America:* Stuttering is defined as "a communication disorder characterized by excessive involuntary disruptions or blockings in the flow of speech, particularly when such disruptions consist of repetitions or prolongations of a sound or syllable, and when they are accompanied by avoidance struggle behavior" (p. 183).
>
> *1991, Perkins, Kent, and Curlee:* "Stuttering is a disruption of speech experienced by the speaker as a loss of control" (p. 734). They differentiate stuttering from nonstuttered forms of disfluencies by identifying the latter as "abnormal as well as normal sounding disfluency not experienced as loss of control" (p. 734).
>
> *1995, Cooper and Cooper:* "Stuttering . . . is a clinical syndrome characterized by abnormal and persistent disfluencies in speech accompanied by characteristic affective, behavioral, and cognitive patterns" (p. 126).

There is no one definition of stuttering that is uniformly accepted by experts in the field. The differences among these and other definitions available in the literature reflect the fact that stuttering is a complex disorder that is not simply characterized. These definitions highlight the differences in perspective among stuttering experts. Several of the definitions are limited to the description of stuttering behaviors (e.g., prolongations, repetitions), from a listener-based perspective. Three include the perspective of the individual who stutters by including their perception of it (i.e., loss of control) or their reaction to it (e.g., apprehension, avoidance). The interpretation that disfluent episodes are involuntary in nature further reflects the perceptions of the person who stutters. A few definitions make inferences concerning the underlying cause of the disorder (e.g., psychological reaction to disfluency, timing disruptions). In all, the definitions reflect the changing

trends within the field that have emphasized different aspects of the disorder at different times.

Consider how the components of these various definitions might apply to a particular case.

> Laura's parents report that she has stuttered since she was 3 years old. At the time of her speech evaluation at age 7, she was found to repeat the first sounds and syllables of many words at the beginning of a phrase or sentence. At times, she seemed to posture her mouth and blink, and no sound could be heard. She made no attempt to avoid talking and had moments of normal fluency; suddenly the fluency would end, seemingly without warning. During her stuttering, she would often purse her lips, close her eyes, and appear as if she were trying to push out the word she was attempting to say. Laura's parents reported that she has expressed frustration at times over her inability to speak fluently.

In this brief case description, we recognize some of the common components of many definitions of stuttering:

1. Repetition and prolongation of sounds and syllables
2. Sudden or involuntary fluency interruptions
3. Often accompanied by physical signs of struggle
4. Often perceived negatively by the speaker

Therefore, despite the differences in definitions of stuttering, it is possible to observe the various components that these definitions present within a single case.

THEORIES OF STUTTERING

There is probably no clinical area in speech-language pathology that has generated more controversy than our understanding of the cause and nature of stuttering. The number of causative theories is astonishing and reflects an evolution in thought over the last century. At any given time, one theoretical position becomes more popular as research advances and changing social mores shift the clinical perspective on this disorder. As Van Riper indicated in 1971, the pendulum of popular and clinical opinion tends to swing between physical and psychological causes. Despite these shifts in theoretical perspective over time, we will clearly see the impact of these various theories reflected in approaches to intervention later in this chapter. Let us consider a few of the more prominent theoretical positions that have appeared over time.

Diagnosogenic Theory of Stuttering

Wendell Johnson is considered one of the founding fathers of the field of speech-language pathology. He spent his professional life studying the onset of stuttering.

He concluded that the normal disfluencies experienced by many children were often labeled by their parents and other listeners as stuttering (Johnson, 1959). His **diagnosogenic theory of stuttering** was built on the belief that stuttering begins when normal disfluencies are labeled as stuttering. This theory recognized that normal children often pass through a period of nonfluent speech as they are in the process of language acquisition. Parents may hear their young children's normal episodes of disfluent speech and react negatively to them. They may call attention to their children's speech by telling them to "slow down" or to "take a deep breath and start over." Johnson suggested that these children are sensitive to their parents' reactions and become nervous or self-conscious about their speech. This leads them to become more disfluent in response, until stuttering becomes a learned behavior.

During his years of research at the University of Iowa, Johnson was never able to document any biological or psychological differences between those who do and do not stutter. However, his research occurred during a period that predated many more recent techniques for investigating potential biological correlates of the disorder. For many years, the lack of evidence to the contrary shaped the belief that people learned to stutter and that those who stutter were not otherwise different, as a group, from anyone else. For Johnson, the genesis of stuttering lay in the interactions between the listener and speaker. He believed that stuttering existed "in the ear of the listener." This causative idea is known as the *interaction theory of stuttering*.

As we saw earlier, Johnson (1955) defined stuttering as an "anticipatory, apprehensive, hypertonic avoidance reaction." In his view, the fear of stuttering is conditioned over time, and this fear becomes at least as great a problem as the actual stuttering. Sheehan (1970) considered the anticipatory fear of those who stutter and developed his *approach-avoidance theory*, so called because those who stutter were thought to be in a struggle over whether to speak. Feeling that they are going to stutter, they begin to use all kinds of avoidance behaviors (grimacing, eye blinking, and noise making) that they have learned instead of making an easy, open sound or syllable repetition. Sheehan suggested that without these distracting behaviors, "little stuttering would remain."

Psychological Aspects of Stuttering

As we saw earlier in the chapter, those who stutter can show physiological signs of stress and anxiety (Blood et al., 1994; Weber & Smith, 1990). These signs of anxiety associated with speaking led to the idea that stuttering might be a manifestation of an underlying emotional conflict (Blanton, 1965; Bryngelson, 1971; Glauber, 1958; Travis, 1971). Lee Travis (1971) was one of the strongest proponents of a psychological cause of stuttering. He developed the *repressed-need theory*. In his view, stuttering is the surface symptom of repressed needs, often disguised hostility. Children's primitive likes and wants, which may be socially unacceptable, are thwarted by those around them. "The parents not only induced in the child the drives of fear, guilt, and shame as checks on the child's primary drives, but they

and their helpers in society perpetuated these checks" (p. 1020). Stuttering becomes a way to get around these societal checks.

In his classic chapter, "The Unspeakable Feelings of People with Special Reference to Stuttering" (Travis, 1971), Travis detailed what he considered to be the repressed needs and feelings of adults who stutter. Rather than working directly on stuttering, Travis and others (Barisara, 1962; Glauber, 1958) recommended psychotherapy with the intent of uncovering the hidden prohibitions that were at the root of an individual's stuttering. Travis concluded that "those stutterers who recovered and expressed what we have termed unspeakable feelings and thoughts did enjoy increased speech fluency and less anxiety over speech blocks" (p. 1032).

Psychotherapists commonly believe that most patients come for help when their personal misery is intense. The same is true for those who stutter. If they seek treatment because they are miserable about their stuttering, they may require counseling to develop some degree of perspective about their stuttering. In recognition of this, Bryngelson (1971) urged speech-language pathologists not to become so concerned with stuttering symptomatology that they neglect the "patient's need to be an acceptable human being." A counseling approach may reduce anxiety and negative self-image sufficiently to permit subsequent work on controlling fluency through behavioral techniques.

Neurological Theories of Stuttering

The idea that a physical, rather than psychological cause for stuttering existed was popular early in this century. One early organistic theory was the *cerebral dominance theory* of stuttering. The idea that a disturbance in the normal hemispheric specialization for and control of behaviors might underlie developmental disorders was made popular by Orton in the 1920s. Although Orton is best known for his work in dyslexia, the basic ideas of cerebral dominance were applied to stuttering as well. Likewise, Travis pursued the cerebral dominance theory before he embraced the repressed need theory of stuttering (see Van Riper, 1971, for a discussion).

The cerebral dominance theory recognized that one cerebral hemisphere (usually the left) plays a dominant role in speech and language. Although one hemisphere may lead in the sequencing of sounds and words, the actual execution of these sounds requires well-coordinated bilateral innervation. The paired muscles of speech production must receive their impulses at exactly the same time. The cerebral dominance theory hypothesized that the arrival of impulses at the peripheral muscles is poorly timed. This lack of precise timing is known as *dysphemia*. In the case of stuttering, the flow of nervous impulses to the paired speech musculature might break down with the slightest provocation. The bilateral coordination that is essential for normal speech would be compromised when one side received innervation before the other. As Van Riper (1971) put it, it is very difficult to lift "a wheelbarrow with one handle."

A number of early investigations seemed to support the cerebral dominance theory. Researchers used such techniques as dichotic listening, which involves simultaneous presentation of different auditory stimuli to each ear as a measure of

brain lateralization. Others looked at the pattern of ongoing electrical activity measured from electrodes placed on the scalp. However, this early research failed to reveal robust differences between those who stutter and those who do not. In summarizing years of research on the topic, Andrews and colleagues (1983) concluded that there was no clear evidence that those who stutter have poorly lateralized speech or gross neurological abnormalities. Despite this history, biological investigations may yet enjoy rebirth with the advent of new biomedical technologies. For example, Ingham and colleagues used positron emission tomography (PET) to reexamine the issue of baseline physiological differences. They reported slight differences in bloodflow within the resting brain, which were localized to areas associated with speech and hearing functioning. However, the directionality (left vs. right hemisphere) of the effect was inconsistent (Ingham, Fox, Ingham, Zamarripa, Martin, Jerabek, & Cotton, 1996).

Perkins and colleagues (1991) provided a paradigmatic shift away from the cerebral dominance theory with their *neuropsycholinguistic theory* of stuttering. This theory posits that disfluencies in general result from dyssynchronies in the timing and coordination of any one of the neural systems that support communication. This theory differentiates between disfluencies that are attributable to an identifiable interruption (e.g., a momentary distraction) and those unknown sources that interrupt or delay the neural systems that support communication. Stuttering only occurs when the speaker encounters a breakdown in fluency without apparent reason and tries to press through. The unknown nature of the breakdown accounts for the perception of a loss of control central to their definition of stuttering. The causes of these breakdowns may include biological factors (e.g., developmental, genetic, acquired factors) that predispose the nervous system to dyssynchronies, as well as environmental factors that may exacerbate processing problems. The complexity embraced by this theory gives it a great deal of flexibility in accounting for the range of symptoms that has made stuttering so difficult to characterize in any unified way.

Perkins and colleagues based their theory on a few fundamental premises. The first is that oral communication is a complex behavior that requires the coordination of multiple brain systems. For example, the linguistic and emotional components of communication appear to be served by different brain systems. Furthermore, there is evidence that different systems support different components of the linguistic aspects of communication (see Chapter 2). We can imagine that if the timing of just one of these components was delayed (e.g., retrieval of the specific sounds that make up the words), then the synchronization needed to bring sounds, grammar, and emotional content together into an utterance would be interrupted. Furthermore, the speaker would be unaware that phonemic retrieval was at heart of the processing breakdown, as this process happens without conscious awareness. From the perspective of this theory, it is easy to account for developmental disfluencies, which occur during that period when children are in the process of acquiring and coordinating the various components of oral language, and why they disappear as these systems mature. It would also account for why persistent stuttering sometimes seems to involve different linguistic components

(e.g., sound repetitions, blocks at the beginning of syntactic clauses) during different stuttering episodes. This variation in the surface manifestation may relate to variation in the coordination of underlying neural systems involved in oral communication.

Motor Theories of Stuttering

The neurological theories of stuttering focused on the central nervous system as the source of fluency breakdown. With motor theories, we see a shift in focus to the peripheral nervous system control of speech. Schwartz (1976) was one of the leading supporters of the view that stuttering was caused by a disorder of the vocal mechanism. In 1976, he published a book with the relatively immodest title *Stuttering Solved*, in which stuttering was attributed to an abnormal airway dilation reflex. Normally, the airway dilation reflex is a rapid opening of the glottis during inspiration that occurs due to rising subglottal air pressure. It will occur reflexively if there is a subglottal obstruction and a need for a greater air supply. According to Schwartz, as the individual who stutters speaks, the vocal folds may reflexively open, creating a stuttering block. Phonation is suddenly out of synchrony for the speaker, whose mouth is already postured for the intended sound.

Work by others supported the idea of a laryngeal role in stuttering. Adams and Reis (1974) found less stuttering when individuals read a passage designed to have no voiceless sounds, thus maximizing time spent with the vocal folds together. Conture (1984) reported that the vocal folds, viewed fiberoptically, seemed to open and close inappropriately during stuttering. Furthermore, stutterers seem to need more neural response time for various verbal acts that require a quick reaction (Netsell & Daniel, 1974; Reich, Till, & Goldsmith, 1981; Till, Reich, Dickey, & Seiber, 1983). Although many investigations of motor functioning have focused on the speech mechanism, some have attempted to find evidence of a more generalized problem in motor functioning. However, these studies have not resulted in a clear consensus concerning peripheral motor movements.

Other investigators have suggested that the motor component of stuttering may involve both central and peripheral mechanisms. Neilson and Neilson (1991) proposed that the phenomenon of stuttering is the manifestation of inadequate or poorly functioning neural resources for speech production. In their *Adaptive Model Theory*, they posited that speech production involves both systems involved in motor movements and feedback mechanisms that allow online, moment-to-moment monitoring of speech. However, the neural resources needed to accomplish these complex interactions may be limited or inefficient in those who stutter. They used an auditory tracking task during which subjects hear a tone and adjust the pitch of a second tone, by either hand or jaw movements, to match the first. This is parallel to hearing one's own speech and making motor adjustment to the vocal tract, based on the auditory feedback. Adults who stuttered were deficient at this task, even though they did well with a visual tracking task. Neilson and colleagues suggested that the source of this limitation may be in the cortical and subcortical components of the motor system (Neilson, Neilson, & O'Dwyer, 1992).

EVALUATION OF DEVELOPMENTAL STUTTERING

The broad goals of a fluency evaluation are to determine whether clinically significant disfluencies are present, to understand (to the extent possible) the nature and potential cause of these disfluencies, and to understand the impact of these disfluencies within the context of the client's life. As we have discussed throughout the chapter, everyone experiences disfluent speech from time to time, and many young children typically pass through a period of normal disfluency as they acquire language skills. One of the first jobs of the clinician is to assess the likelihood that the client's disfluencies fall outside the range of normal. Typically, the clinician will consider the types of disfluencies observed, their frequency and duration, associated nonspeech behaviors (e.g., struggle, avoidance), and the client's (or parents') attitudes toward the periods of disfluencies. The clinician may need to assess fluency in more than one context, because stuttering severity can change remarkably depending on the situation. School-based clinicians, for example, may observe a child in the classroom, out on the playground, or even request a taped speech sample from home. Different task demands, such as making a phone call or providing an explanation, often alters the frequency of disfluent speech as well.

As we will see later in this chapter, there are other forms of disfluent speech besides stuttering. Disorders such as cluttering can produce disruptions in fluency that are qualitatively different from stuttering. The clinician must also differentiate between the breakdowns in fluency that result from an expressive language disorder or that occur in conjunction with it. A sudden disruption of fluency, particularly in later childhood, may be the first sign of a neurological disorder, which would prompt referral to a neurologist. Formal and informal measures of speech and language, as well as a detailed case history, are invaluable in distinguishing among disorders that affect fluency. Failure to do so can lead to inappropriate attempts to manage these conditions.

Finally, the perceptions and attitudes of clients who stutter can have an enormous impact on the degree to which their lives are altered by stuttering and their readiness and motivation for change. Gaining this information is an ongoing process that starts with an initial interview and continues over the course of intervention. Clients may have very specific intervention goals ("I need to be able to conduct interviews for my job") or completely unrealistic ones ("I want my child to stop repeating himself all the time when he's excited"). A client's internal anxiety or lack of confidence about speaking may interfere with his or her ability to benefit from speech modifications. Unless we know what these attitudes and perceptions are, subsequent intervention may be fruitless or even offensive to the client.

STUTTERING THERAPY

Stuttering can be successfully treated. There are now numerous reports in the literature that show that clients can develop and maintain fluency over time (e.g.,

Blood, 1995; Hasbrouck, 1992; Onslow, Costa, Andrews, Harrison, & Packman, 1996; Packman, Onslow, & van Doorn, 1994). The primary questions in intervention are who should receive treatment, when it should begin, and what form it should take. For adults, the decision to seek treatment is a personal one. For children, a number of factors may influence parents' decisions to initiate treatment. Because many children who show early signs of stuttering will overcome this difficulty, some professionals have advocated vigilant waiting, with parent counseling, and regular monitoring of the child's speech (Zebrowski, 1995). In contrast, Starkweather (1990) noted a growing emphasis on early intervention for stuttering. He noted that a wait-and-see attitude is more risky than the cost of treatment for a child who would have recovered later on his or her own. In addition, he reported that recovery rates with treatment routinely exceed the rate of spontaneous recovery. Finally, there is some evidence to suggest that waiting to initiate treatment with the child who stutters is associated with more time spent in treatment. All these factors support the trend toward early intervention for children who show early signs of stuttering.

Parental Involvement

There are a number of components of fluency therapy. For children, one critical component may be the assessment of parent and family attitudes. Subsequent family involvement in the therapy process may be key to its success (e.g., Healey, Scott, & Ellis, 1995; Rustin & Cook, 1995). Kelly (1995) noted that mothers and fathers often differ in how they interact with their children and may require different advice and guidance in order to best improve their child's fluency. We can see the need to understand the parent's perspectives in the following case:

> Gerry and Anna had very different reactions to their 4-year-old son's periods of disfluency. Anna told of her anxiety whenever Gerry Jr. would stutter: "It hurts me to see him struggle. I don't want other kids teasing him, either." She went out of her way to "not call his attention to it." As a result, she would allow her son to interrupt her conversations with others, and often intervened when she thought his brothers and sisters might upset him and cause him to stutter. Gerry Sr. interpreted his wife's actions as "spoiling the boy." He didn't see his son's disfluencies as a problem. If anything, he thought that stuttering was one way that Gerry Jr. could get more attention in a household that included four other children. Needless to say, these differences in how each parent reacted to their son's disfluencies were a source of friction between them. It was apparent that intervention would have to include the parents' reactions to their child's disfluencies. This began with discussions to help the parents differentiate between the actual disfluent episodes and their reactions to it. The parents were provided with weekly "homework assignments" that were designed to help them develop workable and appropriate means of responding to specific situations that had been problematic from either a fluency or a social-interaction perspective (e.g., Should Gerry Jr. be allowed to interrupt at will?). For these parents, this approach allowed them to develop new perspectives on their son's disfluencies.

Parents may have many roles in the intervention process. They are often the ones to first seek help on behalf of their children and should be involved in setting long and short term goals for their child. As we saw in Gerry's case, parents may hold a range of attitudes and beliefs about stuttering. They may need information about what changes they can reasonably expect from therapy (Healey et al., 1995). They can also become invaluable assets in the intervention process. For example, Stephenson-Opsal and Bernstein Ratner (1988) reported that slower parental speaking rates have been associated with positive outcome in therapy. Parents may be asked to reinforce the goals established for their children outside of the therapy session. Some intervention programs have used parents as the primary service provider with success (e.g. Craig, Hancock, Chang, et al., 1996).

Treatment Approaches

Speech therapy for stuttering in both children and adults may take different forms, depending primarily on the treatment philosophy of the speech-language pathologist. To simplify our discussion of the treatment of stuttering, let us identify three main approaches:

Psychological approach: Counseling and psychotherapy are given to improve the individual's attitude toward the problem, decrease avoidance, and create a better self-image.

Modifying speech: Therapy is given to facilitate speech that is free of stuttering by modifying rhythm, rate, and voicing.

Modifying the stuttering: Therapy is given to modify the stuttering behaviors, helping the individual to stutter more fluently.

Although these approaches can be thought of as philosophically and practically distinct, in practice, speech-language pathologists tend to combine and adapt these approaches to fit the needs of individual clients. Gregory (1995), for example, stated that therapy may emphasize a certain approach or component more than others at any given time. However, change for the client may involve behavioral and psychological components simultaneously. In order to understand the potential contributions of the individual approaches, we will consider them each separately.

Psychological Approach. You would not have to stutter for very long before you might develop negative feelings about speaking. Some go to great lengths to avoid speaking and begin to employ avoidance behaviors of various kinds (being silent, not using words they "know" will come out stuttered, and so on). Counseling or psychotherapy may help clients who stutter to see themselves as a whole, having a complete life that includes many different kinds of experiences, including stuttering. Such therapy is often helpful in giving clients who stutter a perspective on the problem, so that the stuttering does not loom larger than it should.

As mentioned earlier in this chapter, psychotherapy has been used as a treatment for stuttering, particularly as described by Travis (1971). From the psychotherapy view, stuttering is only a symptom of an underlying psychological conflict. To treat the symptom (stuttering) per se would not diminish the *need* for the stuttering. Thus, counseling and psychological therapy are needed to provide the client who stutters with a healthier mental perspective.

There is little documentation that a psychotherapeutic approach alone will give patients permanent fluency. However, clinicians frequently find that counseling can be a valuable support to programs that focus on the behavioral aspects of stuttering. Cooper and Cooper (1995) stated that stuttering can be thought of as having three components (the ABCs): *A*ffective (feelings), *B*ehaviors (moments of stuttering), and *C*ognitive (thoughts and attitudes). They expressed that "While the Bs (disfluencies) may be the most attention-getting aspect of the problem, the As and Cs are far more significant in assessing and treating stuttering syndromes" (p. 127). Their intervention program includes specific goals to reinforce feelings, attitudes, and behaviors that enhance fluency. In some cases, a poor self-concept, which may result from constant struggles with fluency, may begin to taint reality, imposing itself on every dimension of the patient's life. For example, some who stutter blame stuttering for all their misfortunes. A woman who stuttered told us, "If I didn't stutter, I would have gone on to law school, but no one wants to go see a lawyer who can't even say, 'Your Honor,' don't you agree?" A poor self-image begins to taint reality, imposing itself on every dimension of the patient's life. Counseling and psychotherapy have been found to be most important in giving the stuttering client a better (more realistic) self-concept (Wingate, 1976).

Modifying Speech.   In the treatment of stuttering during the mid-1970s, there was a shift away from its modification and toward the shaping of fluent speech. It remains an important component of many current intervention methods today (e.g., Cooper & Cooper, 1991; Healey & Scott, 1995; Ramig & Bennet, 1995). The fluency-shaping approach came directly out of learning theory, in which a baseline behavior (such as a baseline of fluency) is followed by shaping approaches designed to extend or refine that behavior. One of the early practitioners of fluency shaping was Webster (1974), who established fluency by primarily mastering five target behaviors: the stretched syllable, syllable transition, slow change, full breath, and gentle voicing onsets. Webster's patients were required to spend three weeks of intensive, daily training mastering the five target behaviors in sequence. Schwartz (1976) required massive therapy practice (as much as three months of three-times-weekly therapy, two hours per day) to overcome the laryngeal airway problem (airway dilation reflex), which he felt precipitates the stuttering. Schwartz emphasized the preparation for speech, attempting to establish a passive flow of air to initiate easy-onset voicing. In fluency shaping, effort is made to find an easy, fluent way of speaking (easy onset, reduced rate, and prolonged speech). Massive practice is then used to establish this fluent speech as a method of talking. There is less need for a change of attitude through counseling because this change is

"thought to occur secondary to improved speech control" (Guyette & Baumgartner, 1988, p. 646).

Wingate (1976) offered a fluency-shaping program that focused on the rate and prosodic flow of speech. In stuttering, these aspects are seriously interrupted. To establish more normal fluency, Wingate recommended the rate of speech be slowed down, primarily by prolonging the length of vowels. As he explained in his monograph, *Stuttering and Laryngeal Behavior: A Review*, Starkweather (1982) stated that although Wingate's vowel lengthening is effective in reducing stuttering, it is effective also because of the reduced rate of speaking and the regularity of rhythm that are induced. Adams (1974) shaped fluency by focusing on the timing and smoothness of voicing onsets, with some attention given to extending the duration and ease of expiratory airflow. Starkweather concluded that although some stuttering may be precipitated by laryngeal-system dysfunction, some is also the result of an oral-system breakdown (poor coordination of lips, tongue, and jaw).

Techniques that facilitate fluency are highly individualized for each person who stutters. What works for one person may not be helpful for another. Among the battery of techniques used by the speech-language pathologist are prolonging speech (usually achieved by prolonging vowels), reducing speaking rate and maintaining fluency, increasing breathiness at the onset of speech, and otherwise reducing tension during speech (Perkins, 1984; Schwartz, 1976; Shames & Florence, 1980). Such symptomatic therapy for stuttering as fluency shaping is often aided by some counseling, designed to give the client who stutters a more positive perspective toward communication (Cheasman, 1983).

Modifying the Stuttering.   At the turn of the century in the United States, the primary treatment for stuttering was to work on easy voicing onsets, developing a rhythm of some kind, and maintaining speech fluency. Modifying the stuttering (instead of the fluent speech) developed as an opposite form of therapy and is still widely used as a treatment for stuttering. In modifying stuttering, the belief is "that the root of stuttering is in the struggle to be fluent," as described by Perkins (1980). Consequently, most such therapy is of a dual nature: improving the attitude toward speaking and learning to stutter with less effort and reduced tension.

After a lifetime's experience, both first hand and clinical, with the problem of stuttering, Van Riper (1990) concluded, "The stutterer already knows how to be fluent. What he doesn't know is how to stutter. He can be taught to stutter so easily and briefly that he can have very adequate communication skills. Moreover, when he discovers he can stutter without struggle or avoidance most of his frustration and other negative emotions will subside" (p. 318). Many clinicians agree with this position. In modifying the stuttering, the belief is "that the root of stuttering is in the struggle to be fluent," as described by Perkins (1980). Others (e.g., Healey & Scott, 1995) turned to stuttering modification techniques for clients whose stuttering included marked avoidance behaviors or who were unsuccessful with fluency enhancement techniques alone.

Clients can be taught to stutter with less tension, avoidance, and interruption to the flow of communication with specific techniques (Peters & Guitar, 1991).

Treatment may include intentional stuttering that is relaxed in order to reduce the fear and embarrassment associated with involuntary stuttering episodes. A client's awareness of the difference between typical stuttering and the new, modified stuttering may be enhanced by practice that contrasts tense, struggle-prone stuttering with intentional, easy stuttering, and nonstuttered speech. Clients may learn to monitor their ongoing speech for instances of problematic disfluencies. These can be "cancelled" by pausing after the onset of a stuttered word and a fresh attempt at the word with easy, slower, struggle-free stuttering.

OTHER DISORDERS OF FLUENCY

Cluttering

Clinical Signs.   Another clinical disorder associated with altered fluency is **cluttering**. Like those who stutter, children who are described as clutterers have abnormally high frequencies of word and phrase repetitions. In contrast to stuttering, cluttering involves fewer sound or syllable-level disfluencies (e.g., prolongations, sound repetitions). In addition, cluttering usually occurs without signs of struggle, tension, or avoidance that occur in stuttering (St. Louis, Hinzman, & Hull, 1985). Although the prevalence of cluttering is unknown, speech-language pathologists in the United States tend to report familiarity with a few cases of cluttering in their practices. Children are more likely than adults to be seen by a speech-language pathologist for cluttering, and the prevalence in caseloads declines from grades 1 to 12.

Wood (1971) defined cluttering as "rapid, nervous speech marked by omissions of sounds and syllables" (p. 10). This definition gives equal prominence to the symptoms of rapid rate and articulatory errors and is similar to that of Wingate (1978), who defined cluttering as "a fluency disorder of unknown origin characterized by sporadically excessive rate and incomplete and distorted articulation" (p. 268). In one of the few monographs written on the topic, Arnold (1966) reviewed detailed European literature, which described cluttering as a disorder that included symptoms of rapid rate, faulty articulation, and related reading and writing problems. All three speech-language problems were often associated with "disorders of lateral dominance." Wall (1988) said that cluttering is characterized by rapid speed and disordered articulation but added this important part to the definition: "a lack of awareness of the problem on the part of the speaker" (p. 637). It would appear that most clutterers, unlike stutterers, are not upset by their continuing disfluency.

Clutterers speak much faster than stutterers; in fact, the word *tachyphemia*, which is sometimes used as a synonym for cluttering (although it is not), literally means "rapid speech." Clutterers may be differentiated from stutterers by the former's slurred and omitted phonemes, periods of unusually rapid rate of speech, lack of awareness of their poor speech, and the fact that they neither avoid nor feel tense about the act of speaking. In addition, clutterers are often observed to exhibit

faulty thought processes, some problems in auditory language comprehension, and some problems in reading and writing (St. Louis et al., 1985). Such problems may lead services for language and learning disabilities during the school years (St. Louis & Hinzman, 1986). By combining the views of several writers, let us define cluttering:

> Cluttering is rapid speech characterized by fluency and articulation errors, sometimes accompanied by language difficulties, usually without the speaker's awareness or concern.

Treatment of Cluttering.   Although both stuttering and cluttering involve disfluencies, the differences between the two disorders dictate very different treatment approaches. St. Louis and Meyers (1995) offered a series of working principles to guide treatment of cluttering. St. Louis and Meyers begin with a recognition that stuttering and cluttering are, in fact, independent disorders. For the child who clutters, disfluencies are a direct combination of fast speaking rate combined with a weak ability to handle the phonologic, syntactic, or semantic aspects of spoken language.

Children who clutter can increase their fluency by slowing their rate. However, as anyone who has tried to change their speaking rate knows (e.g., slowing down speech for a class presentation), maintaining a different speaking rate at the same time one is thinking about what to say is difficult. We can use direct methods to address rate. The speaker might pace his or her speaking rate to different rates of a metronome to raise awareness about rate of speech. Later, a clinician might provide visual feedback, such as an arrow indicator of whether speech is too fast, just fine, or too slow. The following case provides an example of an indirect method of addressing rate, by having the speaker alter loudness (which later can be reduced to normal levels when rate has been reduced). This 17-year-old was asked to listen to a recording of himself followed by one of a normal male speaker near the client's age:

Clinician: You must talk twice as fast as that other kid. Did you hear that?

Client: He donna wanna go fatter than me.

Clinician: Maybe if we just had you talk a little louder, like this: "I'm going to speak loudly for a bit." That sure makes me sound better, doesn't it?

Client: Talin' loud is easy for me. I tal' loud at home and they all hear me.

Clinician: Well, let's make a recording of you talking louder, and we'll see how that sounds.

Rather than working on the components of rate and articulation, both of which were far from normal in this case, the clinician elected to work holistically on making the patient aware that he could speak better by changing his speaking habits. Given a tangible method of changing his speech, the patient could better monitor

his speech when he spoke more loudly, which served to slow the rate of speech and improve his articulation.

Sometimes, indirect methods can be used to decrease rate, by concentrating on another element of speech or language. For example, if a child's poor articulation contributes to cluttering, exercises designed to remediate articulation may have the side effect of reducing speaking rate. Likewise, if fluency breakdowns are occurring because of linguistic deficits such as word-finding problems or difficulty with syntactic constructions, then it makes sense to remediate these linguistic problems directly. In many cases, improved fluency is a side effect of a linguistic approach.

St. Louis and Meyers (1995) pointed out that a synergistic approach that focuses on improved communication may be best. Linguistic formulation problems may be aided when rate is slowed because the individual has more time to organize his ideas and give them linguistic structure. Improved self-monitoring may help the individual concentrate on correct articulation, which in turn will tend to slow speaking rate. Word-finding strategies may help prevent semantic breakdowns that reduce fluency. This dynamic approach may also include coordinated services with others (e.g., family members, teachers, psychologists) who can help to manage social and educational aspects associated with this disorder.

Acquired Disfluency

Most adults who stutter have a history of childhood stuttering. There are, however, numerous cases of previously fluent adults who have an abrupt onset of stuttering (Market, Montague, Buffalo, & Drummond, 1990). In most instances, acquired stuttering is associated with neurological damage from a stroke, head injury, progressive neurological disease, or exposure to toxins (Helm-Estabrooks, 1998; Ringo & Dietrich, 1995). Less frequently, acquired stuttering may have a psychological origin related to anxiety, depression, or other psychological disturbance (Baumgartner & Duffy, 1997). Although the symptoms of neurogenic and psychogenic stuttering may be difficult to distinguish from one another, a review of the patient's history is usually helpful in distinguishing its probable cause. We were asked recently to help interpret the disfluencies of 69-year-old man.

> Mr. Nelson was referred by his neurologist following a series of transient ischemic attacks or possibly small strokes. The most recent episode was followed by what appeared to be stuttering. The disruption of speech was a concern to Mr. Nelson, who was a highly educated, articulate man and a frequent public speaker as president of a volunteer organization. Despite his neurological history, the referral letter from the neurologist described Mr. Nelson's disfluency as "a functional acquired stuttering, possibly secondary to some sort of depression or anxiety."
>
> Prior to his visit, Mr. Nelson was asked to write a narrative of his recent medical history to describe any changes in his speech or language. His description clarified that he had experienced two episodes that involved neurological signs that occurred two years apart. The first episode included persistent numbness and

tingling on the left side of his body that lasted for about a week. The second included a more dramatic onset of right-sided weakness and some problems speaking. Mr. Nelson was hospitalized following the second episode and put on blood thinning medication because of his risk for stroke. He wrote that he was recovering fully from the second episode but he began to have increasing difficulty talking within a month. He had some trouble coming up with the names of things, but his most vexing problem was stuttering, which he described as having "a lot of hesitation" in his speech.

An evaluation of Mr. Nelson's speech revealed many disfluencies. For example, as he read a 100-word passage aloud, he was disfluent on 10 words: 5 were tense pauses, 3 were sound prolongations, and 2 were sound repetitions. His conversational speech was similarly disrupted by pauses—although his articulators were postured correctly to produce a word, he seemed unable to proceed. No secondary stuttering characteristics such as facial grimacing, hand clenching, or head movements were observed. In fact, Mr. Nelson appeared to be annoyed by his disfluencies, but not overly upset by them.

Mr. Nelson's disfluencies and his medical history suggested that he had acquired neurogenic stuttering. Although an MRI brain scan revealed some small areas of white matter changes, and it was not clear that Mr. Nelson had suffered a stroke, his medical history clearly indicated some compromise of his neurological functions. Neurogenic stuttering is not limited to damage to a particular region of the brain, but has been related to left and right hemisphere damage, cortical and subcortical damage, as well as damage to the cerebellum and brainstem. It co-occurs with aphasia about a third of the time (Baumgartner & Duffy, 1997). In Mr. Nelson's case, he evidenced some mild word finding problems (anomia), but his overall performance was excellent for spoken and written language.

Neurogenic versus Developmental Stuttering.   Neurogenic stuttering refers to an acquired disruption of fluency that can be linked with an identifiable neurological event, such as a stroke or head injury. This is in contrast to developmental stuttering, which may also have an underlying neurological component as described earlier. The disruptions in normal speech production that are observed in neurogenic disfluency are similar in some ways to developmental stuttering, but there are some differences. Whereas instances of disfluency in developmental stuttering occur most often on words that start with consonants than with vowels, neurogenic stuttering occurs similarly often on words beginning with consonants and vowels (Ringo & Dietrich, 1995). Likewise neurogenic stuttering occurs equally often on substantive and function words, whereas content words are more likely to be disfluent by adults who have stuttered since childhood. As was true with Mr. Nelson, most individuals with neurogenic stuttering are notably free of anxiety about their speech and characteristics such as accessory behaviors and facial tension that are common in stuttering having a developmental origin.

Neurogenic versus Psychogenic Stuttering.   Mr. Nelson's disfluencies differed from psychogenic stuttering in several ways. Although psychogenic stuttering can

be similar to neurogenic stuttering, Baumgartner and Duffy (1997) found several distinguishing features. Unlike neurogenic stuttering, psychogenic stuttering may be intermittent and associated with specific speaking situations, struggle behaviors and other signs of anxiety are not uncommon, and unusual or bizarre speech patterns that are not observed in other speech or language disorders, such as using "me" for the pronoun "I," are often present. Moreover psychogenic stuttering usually responds quickly to behavioral treatment.

Intervention.   After we determined that Mr. Nelson's disfluencies were consistent with those of a neurogenic origin, we needed to decide whether treatment was warranted. Cases reviewed in the literature indicated that neurogenic stuttering often resolves on its own without treatment within a month or two of onset. Therefore, we assured Mr. Nelson that his stuttering appeared to be related to the neurological episodes he had experienced and told him that we suspected his fluency would improve on its own. He was scheduled for a follow-up visit six weeks later, at which time he showed considerable improvement in fluency. Some brief pauses were still observed as he spoke, but they were relatively subtle, and he reported that they were not as bothersome to him. In fact, he said that he was most annoyed by his occasional word-finding difficulty at that time, a problem he minimized during his initial visit.

Had Mr. Nelson's stuttering persisted and had he wanted treatment, we might have treated it behaviorally in much the same way as developmental stuttering. Approaches that enhance fluency such as slowed speaking rate and easy onset of voicing have been used with success in neurogenic stuttering (Market et al., 1990). Fluency can also be facilitated by pacing speech production so that it is not disrupted by hesitations, prolongations, or repetitions (Helm-Estabrooks, 1998). In some cases, medications have been shown to improve neurogenic disfluency, although some cases of acquired dysfluency appear to have been caused by medication (reviewed in Helm-Estabrooks, 1998). Thus, a careful a review of a patient's history and medications are essential in instances of adult-onset disfluency.

CLINICAL PROBLEM SOLVING

Annette first came to the attention of the school speech-language pathologist through a phone call from the district director of Special Education. Annette's parents had been phoning both his office and home requesting that their daughter be treated for her stuttering. Annette's father was an adult stutterer, and both parents wanted Annette's speech to be "corrected before her stuttering became permanent." They also reported that Annette began speaking somewhat late, but they had no concerns about her speech or language other than the stuttering. Annette was enrolling in kindergarten that fall. After school began, the clinician was able to observe Annette on several occasions in the classroom, during which her speech was consistently fluent. The clinician reported her observations to the parents, advising them to allow Annette time to settle into the school routine. The parents

were adamant that Annette stuttered frequently at home and were insistent that she be treated through the school. At the parents urging, the clinician set up a classroom monitoring program to permit the classroom teacher to systematically document Annette's speech. From September to December, only two disfluent episodes were noted. After receiving this news, the parents sent the clinician a taped sample of Annette's speech at home. The tape revealed frequent episodes of disfluent speech, including part word repetitions, sound prolongations, and silent episodes, which may well have reflected blocks.

1. Do you think that Annette does stutter? What makes you think so/not?
2. What risk factors for stuttering appear in Annette's history?
3. Select two theories and discuss how this case profile might relate to each theory.
4. Speculate on the reasons why Annette may stutter at home, but not in her new kindergarten.
5. Do you think that Annette should receive therapy for stuttering? If so, what factors would you consider in developing a plan of intervention for Annette?

REFERENCES

Adams, M. R. (1974). A physiologic and aerodynamic interpretation of fluent and stuttered speech. *Journal of Fluency Disorders, 1,* 35–67.

Adams, M. R., & Reis, R. (1974). Influence of the onset of phonation on the frequency stuttering, a replication and re-evaluation. *Journal of Speech and Hearing Research, 17,* 752–754.

Andrews, C., Craig, A., Feyer, A., Haddinott, S., Neilson, M., & Howle, P. (1983). Stuttering: A review of research findings and theories circa 1982. *Journal of Speech and Hearing Disorders, 48,* 226–245.

Andrews, C., & Harris, M. (1964). *The syndrome of stuttering.* London: Heinemann Dynamic Medical Books.

Arnold, C. (1966). *Studies in tachyphemia: An investigation of cluttering and general language disability.* New York: Speech Rehabilitation Institute.

Baumgartner, J., & Duffy, J. R. (1997). Psychogenic stuttering in adults with and without neurologic disease. *Journal of Medical Speech-Language Pathology, 5,* 75–95.

Barisara, D. (1962). *The psychotherapy of stuttering.* Springfield, IL: Charles C. Thomas.

Blanton, S. (1965). Stuttering. In D. Barbara (Ed.), *New directions in stuttering.* Springfield, IL: Charles C. Thomas.

Blood, G. W. (1995). A behavioral-cognitive therapy program for adults who stutter: Computers and counseling. *Journal of Communication Disorders, 28,* 165–180.

Blood, G. W., Blood, I. M., Bennett, S., Simpson, K. C., & Susman, E. J. (1994). Subjective anxiety measurements and cortisol responses in adults who stutter. *Journal of Speech and Hearing Research, 37,* 760–768.

Bryngelson, B. (1971). Speech and personality. In L. Travis (Ed.), *Handbook of speech pathology and audiology.* Englewood Cliffs, NJ: Prentice Hall.

Cheasman, C. (1983). Therapy for adults: An evaluation of current techniques for establishing fluency. In P. Dalton (Ed.), *Approaches to the treatment of stuttering.* London: Croom Helm.

Conture, E. C. (1984). Observing laryngeal movements of stuttering. In R. F. Curlee & W. H. Perkins (Eds.), *Nature and treatment of stuttering: New directions.* San Diego: College-Hill Press.

Conture, E. G. (1990). Childhood stuttering: What is it and who does it? *ASHA Report Series, 18,* 2–14.

Conture, E. G., & Kelly, E. M. (1991). Young stutterers' nonspeech behaviors during stuttering. *Journal of Speech and Hearing Research, 34,* 1041–1056.

Cooper, E. B., & Cooper, C. S. (1991). *Personalized fluency control therapy—Revised.* New York: DLM-Teaching Resources.

Cooper, E. B., & Cooper, C. S. (1995). Treating fluency disordered adolescents. *Journal of Communication Disorders, 28,* 125–142.

Cooper, E. B., & Cooper, C. S. (1996). Clinicians' attitudes toward stuttering: Two decades of change. *Journal of Fluency Disorders, 21,* 119–135.

Craig, A. (1990). An investigation between anxiety and stuttering. *Journal of Speech and Hearing Disorders, 55,* 290-294.

Craig, A., Hancock, K., Chang, E., Mccreay, C., Shepley, A., Mccaul, A., Costello, D., Harding, S., Kehren, R., Masel, C., & Reilly, K. (1996). A controlled clinical trial for stuttering in persons age 9–14 years. *Journal of Speech and Hearing Research, 39,* 808–826.

Curlee, R. F. (1980). A case selection strategy for young disfluent children. *Seminars in Speech, Language, Hearing, 1,* 277-287.

Glauber, I. P. (1958). The psychoanalysis of stuttering. In J. Eisenson (Ed.), *Stuttering. A symposium.* New York: Harper and Row.

Gregory, H. (1995). Analysis and commentary. *Language, Speech, and Hearing Services in Schools, 26,* 196-200.

Guyette, T. W., & Baumgartner, J. M. (1988). Stuttering in the adult. In N. J. Lass, L. V. McReynolds, J. L. Northern, & D. E. Yoder (Eds.), *Handbook of speech-language pathology and audiology.* Philadelphia: B. C. Decker.

Hasbrouck, J. M. (1992). FAMC intensive stuttering treatment program: Ten years of implementation. *Military Medicine, 157,* 244-247.

Healey, E. C., & Scott, L. A. (1995). Strategies for treating elementary school-age children who stutter: An integrative approach. *Language, Speech, and Hearing Services in Schools, 26,* 151–161.

Healey, E. C., Scott, L. A., & Ellis, G. (1995). Decision making in the treatment of school-age children who stutter. *Journal of Communication Disorders, 28,* 107–124.

Helm-Estabrooks, N. (1998). Stuttering associated with acquired neurological disorders. In R. F. Curlee (Ed.), *Stuttering and related disorders of fluency* (pp. 255–268). New York: Thieme Medical Publishers.

Howie, P. M. (1981). Concordance for stuttering in monozygotic and dizygotic twin pairs. *Journal of Speech and Hearing Research, 24,* 317–321.

Hull, F. M., Mielke, P. W., Willeford, J. A., & Timmons, R. J. (1976). *National speech and hearing survey.* Final Report, Project 50978. Washington, DC: Office of Education, Bureau of Education for the Handicapped, Department of Health, Education, and Welfare.

Ingham, R. J., Fox, P. T., Ingham, J. C., Zamarripa, F., Martin, C., Jerabek, P., & Cotton, J. (1996). Functional lesion investigation of developmental stuttering with positron emission tomography. *Journal of Speech and Hearing Research, 39,* 1208–1227.

Janssen, P., Kraaimaat, F., & Brutten, G. (1990). Relationship between stutterers' genetic history and speech-associated variables. *Journal of Fluency Disorders, 15,* 39–48.

Johnson, W. (1955). A study of the onset and development of stuttering. In W. Johnson & R. R. Leutenegger (Eds.), *Stuttering in children and adults.* Minneapolis: University of Minnesota Press.

Johnson, W. (1959). *The onset of stuttering.* Minneapolis: University of Minnesota Press.

Kalinowski, J., Lerman, J., & Watt, J. (1987). A preliminary examination of the perceptions of self and others in stutterers and nonstutterers. *Journal of Fluency Disorders, 12,* 317–331.

Kelly, E. M. (1995). Parents as partners: Including mothers and fathers in the treatment of children who stutter. *Journal of Communication Disorders, 28,* 93–106.

Kidd, K. K. (1980). Genetic models of stuttering. *Journal of Fluency Disorders, 5,* 187-202.

Market, K. W., Montague, J. C., Buffalo, M. D. & Drummond, S. S. (1990). Acquired stuttering: Descriptive data and treatment outcome. *Journal of Fluency Disorders, 15,* 221-233.

Miller, S., & Watson, B. C. (1992). The relationship between communication attitude, anxiety and depression in stutterers and nonstutterers. *Journal of Speech and Hearing Research, 34,* 789–798.

Morley, M. E. (1952). A ten year survey of speech disorders among university students. *Journal of Speech and Hearing Disorders, 17,* 25–31.

Morley M. F. (1972). *The development and disorders of speech in childhood.* Edinburgh: Churchill Livingstone.

National Institutes of Deafness & Other Communication Disorders (NIDCD). (1992). *Research in human communication.* (NIH Publication No. 93–3562.) Washington, DC: U.S. Government Printing Office.

Neilson, M. D., & Neilson, P. D. (1991). Adaptive model theory of speech motor control and stuttering. In H. F. M. Peters, W. Hulstijn, & C. W. Starkweather (Eds.), *Speech motor control and stuttering.* New York: Excerpta Medica.

Neilson, P. D., Neilson, M. D., & O'Dwyer, N. J. (1992). Adaptive model theory: Application to disorders of motor control. In J. J. Summers (Ed.), *Approaches to the study of motor control and learning*. Amsterdam: Elsevier Science Publishers.

Netsell, R., & Daniel, B. (1974). Neural and mechanical response time for speech production. *Journal of Speech and Hearing Research, 17,* 608–618.

Onslow, M., Costa, L., Andrews, C., Harrison, E., & Packman, A. (1996). Speech outcomes of a prolonged-speech treatment of stuttering. *Journal of Speech and Hearing Research, 39,* 734–749.

Packman, A., Onslow, M., & van Doorn, J. (1994). Prolonged speech and modification of stuttering: Perceptual, acoustic, and electroglottographic data. *Journal of Speech and Hearing Research, 39,* 724–737.

Perkins, W. H. (1980). Disorders of speech. In T. Hixon, L. Shriberg, & J. Saxman (Eds.), *Introduction to communication disorders*. Englewood Cliffs, NJ: Prentice Hall.

Perkins, W. H. (1984). Techniques for establishing fluency. In W. H. Perkins (Ed.), *Stuttering disorders*. New York: Thieme Stratton.

Perkins, W. H., Kent, R. D., & Curlee, R. F. (1991). A theory of neuropsycholinguistic function in stuttering. *Journal of Speech and Hearing Research, 34,* 734–752.

Peters, T. J., & Guitar, B. (1991). *Stuttering: An integrated approach to its nature and treatment*. Baltimore, MD: Williams & Wilkins.

Ramig, P. R., & Bennett, E. M. (1995). Working with 7- to 12-year-old children who stutter: Ideas for intervention in the public schools. *Language, Speech, and Hearing Services in Schools, 26,* 138–150.

Reich, A., Till, J., & Goldsmith, H. (1981). Laryngeal and manual reaction times of stuttering and nonstuttering adults. *Journal of Speech and Hearing Research, 24,* 192–196.

Ringo, C. C., & Dietrich, S. (1995). Neurogenic stuttering: An analysis and critique. *Journal of Medical Speech-Language Pathology, 3*(2), 111–122.

Rustin, L., & Cook, F. (1995). Parental involvement in treatment of stuttering. *Language, Speech, and Hearing Services in Schools, 26,* 127–137.

Schwartz, M. F. (1976). *Stuttering solved*. Philadelphia: Lippincott.

Schwartz, H. D., Zebrowski, P. M., & Conture, E. G. (1991). Behaviors at the onset of stuttering. *Journal of Fluency Disorders, 15,* 77–86.

Shames, G. H., & Florence, C. L. (1980). *Stutter-free speech: A goal of therapy*. Columbus, OH: Charles E. Merrill.

Sheehan, J. G. (1970). *Stuttering: Research and therapy*. New York: Harper and Row.

Speech Foundation of America. (1987). *Self-therapy for the stutterer* (6th ed.). Publication 12. Memphis, TN: Author.

St. Louis, K. O., & Hinzman, A. R. (1986). Studies of cluttering: Perceptions of cluttering by speech-language pathologists and educators. *Journal of Fluency Disorders, 11,* 131–149.

St. Louis, K. O., Hinzman, A. R., & Hull, F. M. (1985). Studies of cluttering: Disfluency and language measures in young possible clutterers and stutterers. *Journal of Fluency Disorders, 10,* 151–172.

St. Louis, K. O., & Meyers, F. L. (1995). Clinical management of cluttering. *Language, Speech, and Hearing Services in Schools, 26,* 187–195.

Starkweather, C. W. (1982). *Stuttering and laryngeal behaviors: A review* (ASHA Monograph 21). Rockville, MD: American Speech-Language-Hearing Association.

Starkweather, C. W. (1990). Current trends in therapy for stuttering children and suggestions for future research. *ASHA Report Series, 18,* 82–90.

Stephenson-Opsal, D., & Bernstein-Ratner, N. (1988). Maternal speech rate modification and childhood stuttering. *Journal of Fluency Disorders, 13,* 49–56.

Till, J., Reich, A., Dickey, S., & Seiber, J. (1983). Phonatory and manual reaction times of stuttering and nonstuttering children. *Journal of Speech and Hearing Research, 26,* 171–180.

Travis, L. E. (1971). The unspeakable feelings of people with special reference to stuttering. In L. D. Travis (Ed.), *Handbook of speech pathology and audiology* (2nd ed.). Englewood Cliffs, NJ: Prentice Hall.

Van Riper, C. (1971). *The nature of stuttering*. Englewood Cliffs, NJ: Prentice Hall.

Van Riper, C. (1973). *The treatment of stuttering*. Englewood Cliffs, NJ: Prentice Hall.

Van Riper, C. (1990). Final thoughts about stuttering. *Journal of Fluency Disorders, 15,* 317–318.

Wall, M. J. (1988). Disfluency in the child. In N. J. Lass, L. V. McReynolds, J. L. Northern, & D. E. Yoder (Eds.), *Handbook of speech-language pathology and audiology*. Philadelphia: B. C. Decker.

Weber, C. M., & Smith, A. (1990). Autonomic correlates of stuttering and speech assessed in a

range of experimental tasks. *Journal of Speech and Hearing Research, 33,* 690–706.

Webster, R. (1974). A behavioral analysis of stuttering: Treatment and theory. In K. Calhoun, H. Adams, & K. Mitchell (Eds.), *Innovative treatment methods in psychopathology.* New York: Wiley.

Wingate, M. E. (1962). Personality needs of stutterers. *Logos, 5,* 35–37.

Wingate, M. E. (1976). *Stuttering theory and treatment.* New York: Irvington.

Wingate, M. E. (1978). Disorders of fluency. In P. Skinner & R. Shelton (Eds.), *Speech, language, hearing: Normal processes and disorders.* Reading, MA: Addison-Wesley.

Wood, K. S. (1971). Definitions and terms. In L. D. Travis (Ed.), *Handbook of speech pathology and audiology* (2nd ed.). Englewood Cliffs, NJ: Prentice Hall.

World Health Organization (WHO). (1977). *Manual of the international statistical classification of diseases, injuries, and causes of death,* Vol. I. Geneva: Author.

Yairi, E., & Ambrose, N. (1992). Onset of stuttering in preschool children: Selected factors. *Journal of Speech and Hearing Research, 35,* 782–788.

Yairi, E., Ambrose, N. G., & Cox, N. (1996). Genetics of stuttering: A critical review. *Journal of Speech and Hearing Research, 39,* 771–784.

Yairi, E., Ambrose, N. G., Paden, E. P., & Throneburg, R. N. (1996) Predictive factors of persistence and recovery: Pathways of childhood stuttering. *Journal of Communication Disorders, 29,* 51–77

Young, M. A. (1975). Onset, prevalence, and recovery from stuttering. *Journal of Speech and Hearing Disorders, 40,* 49–58.

Zebrowski, P. M. (1995). The topology of a beginning stutterer. *Journal of Communication Disorders, 28,* 75–92.

READINGS FROM THE POPULAR LITERATURE

Bobrick, B. (1996). *Knotted tongues.* New York: Kodansha International.

Jezer, Marty. (1997). *Stuttering: A life bound up in words.* New York: Nasic.

Shields, D. (1998). *Dead languages.* New York: Random House. (novel)

St. Louis, K. O. (2001). *Living with stuttering.* Morgantown, WV: Populore.

DISORDERS OF VOICE AND SWALLOWING

JULIE BARKMEIER

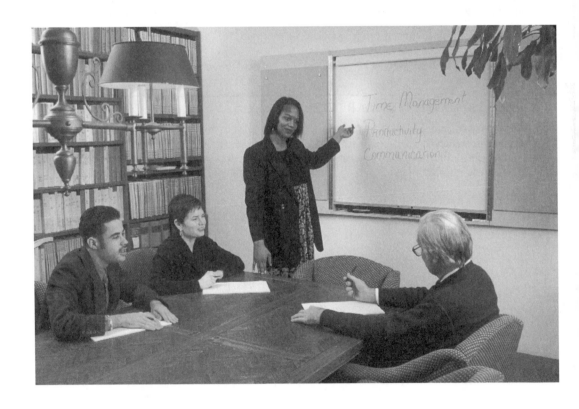

■ ■ ■ ■ ■

PREVIEW

The larynx serves to protect the airway during eating and is the source of our voice for speaking. Damage to the larynx or structures of the vocal tract may result in voice or swallowing problems. Most people experience problems with their voice due to improper voicing habits. Such voice disorders can usually be treated or improved by voice therapy that identifies and changes damaging voicing behaviors to healthy ways of voicing. Voice disorders related to physical damage to the laryngeal structure(s) may also be treated effectively with voice therapy; however, in some cases, medical intervention is needed. Using adapted postures or changing the consistency of food eaten frequently helps problems with swallowing. Sometimes, exercises are used to strengthen oral and pharyngeal structures for safe and effective eating.

VOICE DISORDERS

As described in Chapter 2, vocal fold vibrations produce sound, which is modified by the vocal tract. Individual differences in the vocal mechanism and its resonance characteristics contribute to the individual characteristics of each person's voice. Many temporary conditions, such as a stuffy nose or the effects of prolonged yelling, can change the voice. These types of problems tend to resolve on their own and typically do not require professional attention. However, permanent changes to the voice may occur with damage or disease. These conditions often require professional intervention.

The exact number of individuals who experience voice disorders in the population is not known. For children, the incidence of voice disorders has been estimated to range from 3 (Hull, Mielke, Willeford & Timmons, 1976) to 23.4 percent (Silverman & Zimmer, 1975). The prevalence in adults has been estimated at 7.2 percent for men and 5 percent for women, based on voice screenings (LaGuaite, 1972). Occupations carrying the highest risk for developing voice problems include sales-related work (13%), teaching (4.2%), and other jobs for which workers were considered professional voice users (Titze, Lemke & Montequin, 1996). Of these occupations, teaching is estimated to have the highest incidence of voice disorders (Fritzell, 1995; Smith, Gray, Dove, Kirchner, & Heras, 1997). A majority of voice patients report that their problem had a negative impact on their career options, social interactions, and other aspects of their daily lives (Smith, Verdolini, Gray, et al., 1996).

Voice disorders can be described as problems related to pitch, loudness, vocal quality, and resonance. Voice problems may stem from vocal misuse, disease, congenital defects, laryngeal trauma, aging affects on the voice, and neurological disorders. Emotional and psychological factors may also contribute to acquired voice disorders. Treatment of voice disorders usually requires the combined specialties

of the ear-nose-throat doctor (otolaryngologist) and a speech-language pathologist with expertise in assessing and treating voice disorders.

VOICE DISORDERS RELATED TO VOCAL FOLD TISSUE CHANGES

Most voice disorders arise from overuse or frequent improper use of the voice, which can result in tissue changes that disrupt normal fold vibration.

> Susan, age 17, was a cheerleader for her high school varsity football team for three years. During her first two years as a cheerleader, she experienced temporary bouts of hoarseness following each game. These usually subsided in a couple of days. During her third year as a cheerleader, however, she began to experience longer periods of hoarseness that did not fully resolve before the next game. By the end of the football season, her voice almost always sounded hoarse and she had difficulty being heard in the football stands. Eventually, she was no longer able to cheer.
>
> An otolaryngologist found bilateral nodules on her vocal folds (see Figure 6.1). The nodules prevented her vocal folds from coming together unless she increased her loudness. She was discouraged from participating in cheerleading until the vocal nodules diminished. She was also referred to a speech-language pathologist for voice therapy. The speech-language pathologist helped Susan identify ad-

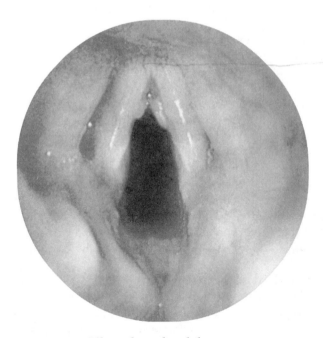

FIGURE 6.1   Bilateral vocal nodules.

ditional habits that were contributing to physical damage, such as coughing, clearing her throat frequently, and yelling at her younger brother when he teased her. Susan reduced the frequency of these behaviors and learned better ways to produce her voice. After one month, the size of the vocal nodules had reduced dramatically, and Susan's voice was significantly improved.

Traumatic Laryngitis

In the early stages of her voice disorder, Susan experienced repeated bouts of **traumatic laryngitis**. This condition is characterized by swollen and red vocal folds resulting from excessive yelling, screaming, or other traumatic uses of the voice (see Figure 6.2). Traumatic laryngitis is common and usually resolves within days of its onset. It often results from continuous vocal misuse such as yelling, or

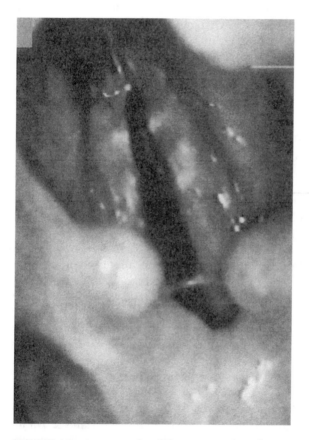

FIGURE 6.2   An example of the appearance of traumatic laryngitis obtained using videoendoscopy. (Courtesy of The University of Arizona, Department of Speech & Hearing Sciences)

cheering throughout an exciting athletic event. In such situations, people yell at high intensity over loud environmental noise so that the vocal folds are slammed together at high velocities. This causes trauma to the tissue at the site of impact. As a result, the vocal folds become swollen and irritated (Brodnitz, 1971). Tissue swelling along the length of the vocal folds disrupts normal vocal fold vibration, causing changes in voice quality. In severe cases, there may be a complete loss of voice (**aphonia**). The best treatment for traumatic laryngitis is to rest the voice, allowing the vocal folds to heal. After two to five days, depending on the extent of damage, vocal fold swelling and irritation typically resolve and the normal voice returns. In Susan's case, she experienced this cycle of trauma and recovery during her first two years of cheerleading.

If the vocal misuse continues, vocal fold irritation can become chronic. The mucosa that covers the vibrating portion of the vocal folds may thicken. Chronic irritation may result from attempts to talk over environmental noise (e.g., in a factory or during construction work) or talking for long periods of time. Once thickening of the mucosa occurs, changes need to be made in daily voice use to prevent further permanent damage and allow healing. Voice therapy may be necessary to identify poor vocal habits and to teach improved techniques for using the voice.

Vocal Nodules

Vocal nodules are small bumps that develop on the medial border of the vocal folds (see Figure 6.1). These bumps consist of fibrous tissue (Gray, Hammond, & Hanson, 1995), much like calluses that develop on the hands or feet. Nodules occur along the anterior one-third of the membranous vocal folds as a result of persistent improper voicing patterns. Prolonged periods of vocal fold inflammation are also common. Vocal nodules can occur on one vocal fold, but most frequently develop on both vocal folds at the site of impact. In early stages, nodules may appear as small swollen areas on the vocal folds. In later stages, the nodules become hard and impair normal vocal fold vibration. If the nodules become large enough, they can prevent the vocal folds from coming together completely, as occurred with Susan. She also demonstrated signs of traumatic laryngitis that preceded the development of nodules. She could have prevented the development of vocal nodules with modification of her voice use. Instead, Susan's vocal fold tissue adjusted to the continual irritation and traumatic impact by developing vocal nodules. Although vocal nodules certainly are not life-threatening, they can result in significant voice problems. The symptoms of vocal nodules arise gradually and manifest as increasing hoarseness and difficulty projecting the voice. This condition can be treated effectively with voice therapy that identifies voice misuse and teaches improved voicing habits (McCrory, 2001; McFarlane & Watterson, 1990; Yamaguchi, Yotsukura, Kondo, et al., 1986). Improved voicing habits are taught by reducing harmful voicing habits and teaching individuals better methods for producing and projecting their voices.

Vocal Polyps

Vocal polyps are small, fluid-filled sacks that develop on the vocal folds as a result of yelling, screaming, and other excessive uses of the voice (Kleinsasser, 1979, 1990). However, unlike the prolonged vocal misuse that leads to vocal nodules, it is believed that as little as a single event of vocal misuse can lead to development of a polyp (McFarlane & Von Berg, 1998). Compared to nodules, which are fibrous, polyps are soft and compliant. They may occur anywhere in the larynx such as on the vocal folds, or ventricular folds, or between the arytenoids. They usually occur on one side only. They are thought to be caused by a single intense event of harmful laryngeal behavior such as screaming or even intense coughing.

> Mrs. Delvechio, age 56, began to experience gradual onset of hoarseness after an upper respiratory infection with severe coughing episodes. She was seen by an otolaryngologist who identified a polyp located near the posterior segment of the vibrating portion of the left vocal fold. The physician suspected the polyp resulted from traumatic vocal fold impact during repeated episodes of severe coughing. The physician referred Mrs. Delvechio to a speech-language pathologist for counseling concerning excessive coughing and throat clearing. During counseling, Mrs. Delvechio mentioned that her husband was hard of hearing and she often tried to talk to him over the television or from another room in the house. She was encouraged to speak at comfortable loudness and not to speak over noise. In addition, she was instructed to talk to her husband only when they were in the same room. After six weeks, her polyp was reduced in size and her voice was almost completely normal.

A vocal polyp may result in significant voice problems that include breathiness or hoarseness. The polyp may also cause each vocal fold to vibrate at a different rate, causing a double voice or **diplophonia**. Frequently, treatment for a vocal polyp entails identification of the behaviors that led to the problem (e.g., yelling, throat clearing, coughing). In Mrs. Delvechio's case, once she became aware of the behaviors that were contributing to the voice problem, she could eliminate those habits. Subsequently, the polyp reduced in size as the laryngeal tissues healed. In other cases, the individual may need specific therapeutic instruction by a speech-language pathologist to improve use of the voice. In some cases, surgical removal of a polyp by an otolaryngologist is necessary (Kleinsasser, 1979, 1990).

Papilloma

Papillomas are wart-like growths found along the vocal tract and respiratory system. They are caused by a virus and are found predominantly in preschool children. Papilloma growths do not usually appear after puberty (Kleinsasser, 1979), so adults infrequently present with this disorder. The onset of this condition may be characterized by breathiness and hoarseness. If the papilloma grows large enough, a stridor or whistling sound may be heard during breathing. Papillomas may be treated with laser surgery, but unfortunately, they grow back quickly and

multiple surgeries may be necessary. Frequent laser surgeries may result in vocal fold scarring that cannot be repaired. Eventually, the vocal folds may become so scarred that the voice cannot be produced due to the stiffness of the scarred vocal folds. Voice therapy can sometimes help these individuals make the best of their voices after surgery.

Carcinoma

Cancer, or **carcinoma**, of the larynx can be a life-threatening disease if not identified during its early stages. Persistent vocal hoarseness is the most common symptom associated with laryngeal cancer. Other warning signs include swallowing problems, swelling in the throat and neck region, and pain.

> Mr. Mahr, age 45, smoked a pack of cigarettes per day for twenty-five years. He also enjoyed a cigarette along with several drinks during cocktail hour every night before dinner. Over a period of six months, his voice became increasingly hoarse. He did not experience any illness during this time, although he noticed that he felt more fatigued than usual and sometimes felt as though he could not breathe in enough air. Mr. Mahr loved his work as an attorney and usually had a lot of energy. He finally went to see an otolaryngologist, who discovered that his vocal folds were covered with a whitish mass that impaired their normal movement. The physician scheduled surgery to remove a piece of the mass and determine its pathology. The biopsy revealed that it was cancer. Mr. Mahr was told that the cancer had invaded much of the larynx and that the entire larynx would need to be removed. After surgery, Mr. Mahr also needed to undergo a series of radiation treatments to reduce the risk that the cancer would reoccur. Fortunately, Mr. Mahr's laryngeal cancer was caught early enough that survival was likely. However, the treatment would cost him his voice. Mr. Mahr was referred to a speech-language pathologist who offered alternatives for creating a new voice after the laryngectomy.

As in Mr. Mahr's case, those who develop laryngeal cancer usually smoke and drink alcohol (McKenna, Fornataro-Clerici, McMenamin, & Leonard, 1991; Rafferty, Fenton, & Jones, 2001). When caught in its early stages, laryngeal cancer frequently can be treated using conservative medical approaches. These include radiation, chemotherapy, and surgery to remove the cancer, leaving the larynx as intact as possible (Mendenhall, Parsons, Stringer, Cassisi, & Million, 1988). In its later stages, laryngeal cancer is typically treated by surgical removal of the entire larynx.

When the larynx is removed, the trachea is attached to a permanent opening in the neck called a **tracheostoma** (see Figure 6.3). After his **laryngectomy**, Mr. Mahr will be able to breathe normally except that the air will now enter and exit the body through an opening in his neck rather than the nose or mouth. Food and drink are still taken by mouth, although the sense of taste is diminished because airborne odors no longer are breathed through the nose.

After surgery, a speech-language pathologist will work with Mr. Mahr to develop alternative ways of generating a sound source for speech. One method

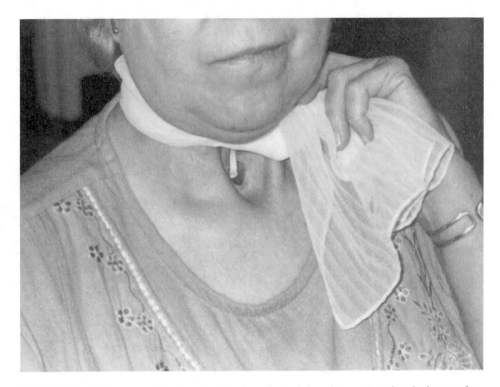

FIGURE 6.3   **This woman is showing the location of the airway opening in her neck called a tracheostoma. She now breathes through the tracheostoma since undergoing a laryngectomy. The white tab attached to the skin outside the tracheostoma secures a one-way valve. This valve shunts air into the esophagus to create a voice by causing tissue to vibrate in a similar, but less predictable way to the vocal folds.**

is esophageal speech. To use this method, Mr. Mahr must learn to trap air in his mouth and project it into the esophagus (McKenna et al., 1991). Once the air is trapped in the esophagus, it is belched back up, creating sound by vibration of esophageal tissues. This sound source is transformed into words by the articulatory movements of the teeth, tongue, and lips, as with normal speech.

A second method of speech production involves an electronic device called an **electrolarynx**, or artificial larynx (Casper & Colton, 1993). The electrolarynx is a hand-held device that makes a buzzing sound as a substitute for vocal fold vibration. The device is placed against the neck so that the sound travels through the skin into the vocal tract, providing a "voice" that is modified into speech by mouthing words (see Figure 6.4, p. 134). The speech-language pathologist provides therapy to help improve intelligibility using the electrolarynx.

A popular surgical method to provide voice is a tracheo-esophageal puncture. This surgical procedure involves creating a hole for the placement of a small tube into the tissue that divides the trachea from the esophagus (see Figure 6.3).

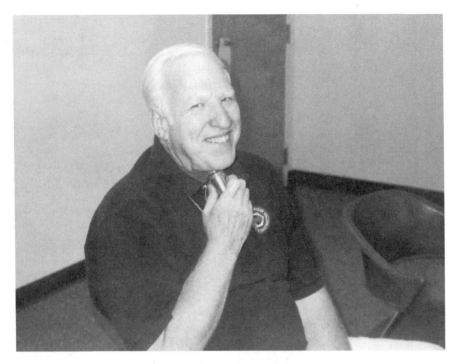

FIGURE 6.4   **This gentleman is holding an electrolarynx securely against the front side of his neck to provide his "voice" for speech.**

The tube has a one-way air valve that shunts air from the trachea into the esophagus when the tracheostoma is covered by the individual's thumb or finger. The shunted air vibrates the esophageal tissue in the same way as the belching does in esophageal speech, resulting in a voice.

Whichever method Mr. Mahr uses to communicate, training and practice will be necessary to maximize speech intelligibility. Many individuals such as Mr. Mahr are grateful that they have another chance at life and resume their activities with great enthusiasm. Others may fall into depression and need professional care to help them deal with the psychological and social issues that arise.

NEUROLOGICAL VOICE DISORDERS

Mrs. Finley, age 45, developed a voice problem after undergoing surgery to remove her thyroid gland. She awoke after the surgery with a breathy voice and choked whenever she drank liquids too quickly. She was evaluated by an otolaryngologist who diagnosed paralysis of the right vocal fold. The doctor suggested that the nerve innervating the vocal fold was probably injured during thyroid surgery. Because this nerve may recover from such damage, the physician decided to wait for six months before considering surgical intervention for the condition. In the

meantime, Mrs. Finley was referred to a speech-language pathologist to learn techniques to stimulate the functioning left vocal fold to vibrate against the paralyzed right vocal fold. In addition, the speech-language pathologist needed to address Mrs. Finley's swallowing problem. She was able to avoid choking by taking small sips of liquid while tilting her chin toward her chest. This position protected her airway during swallowing.

Through voice exercises, Mrs. Finley learned to produce a soft voice instead of a breathy one. By five months postsurgery, her voice had become stronger and closer to normal, indicating that nerve innervation was returning. By six months, her voice was clear and strong. The otolaryngologist reexamined her larynx at that time and determined that her right vocal fold had regained near normal function.

Vocal Fold Paralysis

The recurrent laryngeal nerve is a branch of cranial nerve X (the vagus nerve). It provides neural input to muscles that move the vocal folds during voicing and swallowing (see Chapter 2). Vocal fold paralysis may result from damage to one or both recurrent laryngeal nerves on either side of the larynx. Unilateral vocal fold paralysis is most common. As in Mrs. Finley's case, damage to the nerve can occur when it is cut or compressed during surgery. Nerve damage can also result from a tumor or viral infection. In some cases, there is no known cause for nerve damage. Once the nerve to the laryngeal muscles is damaged, the vocal fold on the same side as the nerve is immobilized. Because the vocal folds cannot close completely, the voice is breathy and patients often choke on liquids. In many cases, the impaired nerve recovers or regenerates within six months, resulting in recovery of the voice (Hockauf & Sailer, 1982; Mu & Yang, 1991).

To compensate for the paralyzed vocal fold, patients are taught to use greater effort to help increase the movement of the working vocal fold. With increased exertion, the healthy vocal fold may be able to vibrate against the paralyzed vocal fold to produce voicing. If the impaired nerve does not recover within six months, several surgical procedures are available to improve voice production. The surgical procedures move the immobile vocal fold medially so that the working vocal fold can vibrate against it. This was not necessary in Mrs. Finley's case because her vocal fold function recovered over time.

Paralysis of both vocal folds is a more serious problem than one-sided vocal fold paralysis. This disorder is typically caused by an impairment to the central nervous system such as a tumor or stroke that interferes with the generation of the neural signals that control movement of the vocal folds. Bilateral paralysis may result in difficulty breathing when the vocal folds are paralyzed in the closed (or nearly closed) position. Surgical intervention is usually necessary to create an open airway adequate for breathing.

Spasmodic Dysphonia

Spasmodic **dysphonia** is a rare voice disorder characterized by a strained-strangled voice quality. The cause of this disorder was once thought to be related

to psychological dysfunction (Arnold, 1959). It is currently thought to result from a dysfunction involving the neural signals that control the vocal folds during speaking (Ludlow, 1995b). There are two types of spasmodic dysphonia: *ABductor* and *ADductor* type. The ADductor type occurs when the vocal folds close together too tightly during voiced speech sounds resulting in a strained-strangled voice quality. The ABductor type occurs when the vocal folds spasm apart during production of unvoiced speech sounds resulting in excessive breathiness. Thus, the difference between the two types of spasmodic dysphonia can be remembered by these two rules:

1. The "AD" part of ADductor means that the vocal folds spasm together.
2. The "AB" part of ABductor means that the vocal folds spasm apart.

ADductor spasmodic dysphonia is characterized by intermittent onset of the strained-strangled voice quality, or voice stoppage. Additional muscular force is needed to move the folds and results in effortful voice production. The ABductor type of spasmodic dysphonia occurs less frequently than the ADductor type and is characterized by intermittent bursts of breathy voice quality. The breathiness results from vocal fold spasms that keep the vocal folds apart during speech. Thus, these individuals may complain that they cannot make their voice loud enough to be heard.

> Mr. Sparks, age 42, began to experience a catch in his voice while giving business reports to his employer. When this first began, he thought it was related to being nervous. However, he noticed the catches in his throat occurred more frequently over time. They also occurred at times when he was not nervous, such as after a church service or at home. Over the course of a year, the condition worsened. He put such effort into forcing his voice to function that he often became exhausted after a short period of talking. As the voice problem increased, his employer became displeased with Mr. Sparks's productivity and inability to provide regular business presentations. In desperation and frustration, Mr. Sparks went to see his doctor.
>
> Mr. Sparks's primary care physician thought the problem was related to stress, but agreed to refer him to a speech-language pathologist specializing in voice disorders. The speech-language pathologist recognized Mr. Sparks problem as spasmodic dysphonia. Voice therapy was initiated to modify some of the problematic voice patterns he had developed to compensate for his uncooperative larynx. The speech-language pathologist also recommended consultation with an otolaryngologist for further evaluation. The otolaryngologist diagnosed Mr. Sparks with ADductor-type spasmodic dysphonia and recommended medical treatment that consisted of injections of a toxin (Botox®) into the muscles of the vocal folds to reduce spasms during talking.

The injection of toxin into the vocal folds is the current treatment of choice for ADductor-type spasmodic dysphonia. The toxin is Botulinum Type A, most often referred to as Botox®. Botox impairs the ability of nerve endings to cause contraction of the vocal fold muscles. This results in weakened vocal fold muscles that cannot spasm closed during talking. However, the vocal folds may be so weak that

they cannot come together to create a strong voice or protect the airway during swallowing. After a few weeks, the Botox is absorbed by the body and new nerve endings grow. At this point, the vocal folds begin to move more normally, resulting in an improved voice quality. After three to six months, the Botox wears off and the symptoms of spasmodic dysphonia typically return, requiring reinjection of Botox to maintain an improved voice.

In some individuals, Botox does not effectively weaken the vocal fold muscles. In those cases, an alternative is surgery to cut one of the laryngeal nerves to create unilateral vocal fold paralysis (Dedo & Behlau, 1991; Dedo & Izdebski, 1983; Weed, Jewett, Rainey, et al., 1996). Although the resulting voice is slightly breathy, it allows the individual to function more normally in daily communication. In approximately 20 percent of individuals who undergo surgical cutting of the laryngeal nerve, the nerve regrows and the symptoms of ADductor spasmodic dysphonia return within one to three years after the surgery (Dedo & Behlau, 1991). Although it is a treatment of last resort, newer methods of cutting the nerve show promise for more successful long-term benefits for those who do not respond well to Botox treatment (Weed et al., 1996).

Despite its success in the treatment of ADductor-type spasmodic dysphonia, Botox injections are not as effective with ABductor spasmodic dysphonia. Botox treatment is typically attempted with ABductor spasmodic dysphonia to see if it will effectively weaken the laryngeal muscles that pull the vocal folds apart during a spasm. However, the improvement is typically minimal and lasts only two to four weeks. These individuals often experience an extremely breathy voice for several weeks after treatment before their voice improves (Ludlow, 1995a). Presently, there is no known effective way to treat ABductor spasmodic dysphonia.

VOICE ASSESSMENT AND MANAGEMENT

The goal of a voice evaluation is to determine the nature of a problem, its probable cause, and the options available to treat the problem. Some people go to their primary care physician first, who then refers them to an otolaryngologist or a speech-language pathologist. Others seek help on their own and go directly to the otolaryngologist. Otolaryngologists with specialized interest in voice disorders often work with a speech-language pathologist with similar interests. Thus, medical evaluation and treatment may be augmented by voice therapy from a speech-language pathologist. Depending on the setting and equipment available to those assessing the voice problem, various methods of evaluation may be undertaken.

Voice evaluations begin with gathering information about the history of the problem and the symptoms present at the time of the examination. This information influences the evaluation procedures as well as the treatment plan.

Ms. Norwood worked as a real estate agent for the past six years and was one of the top salespeople in her company. Her company relocated to a new building two years ago. Since the relocation, numerous renovation projects were necessary, such

as putting in new carpet and paint. She noticed that whenever she worked in her new office, her voice became increasingly hoarse over the course of the day. When her productivity dropped significantly and she felt increasingly anxious about her work, she sought medical help from an otolaryngologist.

The otolaryngologist looked at Ms. Norwood's larynx and noted that both vocal folds were swollen and red and did not vibrate normally during voicing. Thinking that she probably developed improper voicing patterns that led to changes in the vocal folds, the otolaryngologist referred her to a speech-language pathologist for voice therapy. The speech-language pathologist thoroughly documented events leading to Ms. Norwood's voice disorder and discovered her problems began after her office was relocated to the new building. More specifically, her voice problems coincided with the new carpet and paint in her office. The speech-language pathologist suspected that Ms. Norwood was sensitive to chemicals in the air from the renovations. Ms. Norwood also had begun to cough frequently and clear her throat to try to get her voice to improve. Furthermore, she reported drinking a lot of coffee and only small amounts of water each day. The caffeine from the coffee and the low amount of other fluids may have caused dehydration that exacerbated her voice disorder. The speech-language pathologist helped Ms. Norwood monitor and eliminate the daily habits that were irritating her voice and taught her techniques to improve the sound of her voice. In addition, she was instructed to avoid the office for two weeks to determine if the chemicals from the new carpet and paint were irritating her vocal folds.

Ms. Norwood's voice improved dramatically over the two weeks she was away from her office. Upon her return, the voice problem returned despite her efforts to speak using the techniques she was taught by the speech-language pathologist. Thus, it appeared that Ms. Norwood's voice problem was caused by her sensitivity to the chemicals in her office. She decided not to work in her office to avoid exposure to the chemical fumes until the renovation was completed.

In the example above, the true source of Ms. Norwood's voice problem was uncovered after all the information related to the onset of her voice disorder was obtained. The physical appearance of her larynx was similar to that associated with chronic improper and effortful use of the voice. However, use of the following case history guidelines helped to determine the probable causes of a voice problem and, consequently, influenced the course of treatment:

1. Obtain the client's description of the voice problem.
2. Determine whether the onset of the voice problem was associated with an illness, accident, or other significant circumstance.
3. Note the duration and consistency of the symptoms of the voice problem.
4. Note patterns or variability in the reported symptoms or severity of the voice problem on a daily, weekly, monthly, and seasonal basis.
5. Obtain a description of the client's daily voice use.
6. Obtain a description of the client's work, home, and social activities.
7. Note whether the client's voice changes across different environments, speaking situations, or times of the day.

The case history provides information concerning development and impact of the voice disorder on the client's life. It also provides an opportunity for the speech-language pathologist to get to know the client as an individual. As in Ms. Norwood's case, an examination of the circumstances leading to the voice problem helped reveal the true cause of the voice problem, resulting in an effective voice treatment plan.

In addition to the case history, a voice evaluation also includes examination of the vocal mechanism. In Ms. Norwood's case, the otolaryngologist examined the larynx to determine whether vocal pathology was present. To observe the pharynx and larynx, the physician may need to use a tongue depressor, a light to illuminate the structures, and a laryngeal mirror to reflect their image. Other ways of viewing the soft palate and throat utilize fiberoptic equipment to obtain a picture of the soft palate or throat. This procedure is called videoendoscopy. Videoendoscopy can be done using a scope placed through the mouth or nose. The scope that is placed through the nose (i.e., **nasoendoscope**) is a small tube with fiberoptic cables that illuminates and allows viewing of the nasal passages, soft palate, pharynx, and larynx (see Figure 6.5). Another type of scope that can be used to view the larynx is

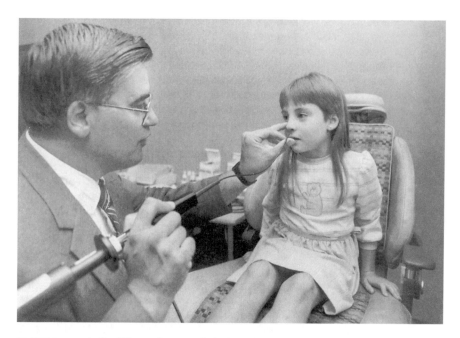

FIGURE 6.5   **A flexible endoscope is being placed into the left nasal passageway of this young girl. Once inserted, it can be advanced to obtain views of the soft palate, pharynx, and larynx. Used with permission of S. C. McFarlane, University of Nevada Medical School, Reno.**

a rigid scope. This scope looks like a steel rod with a lens on the end. It acts like a periscope in that it is placed over the tongue and provides a view of the larynx as it is placed just beyond the back of the tongue. The image obtained by either scope is displayed on a television monitor and can be recorded on a videotape. The rigid scope obtains a closer view of the vocal folds than the flexible scope. However, the client cannot talk with the rigid scope in his or her mouth. The flexible scope is a good way to obtain a recording of the structures in the throat while someone is talking. The lighting used for both scopes can be changed into a strobe light while the client sustains a vowel sound such as "ee." The strobe light illuminates only a fraction of the vocal fold vibrations so that they appear to occur in slow motion.

The voice evaluation may also assess the facial muscles, lips, teeth, soft and hard palate, tonsils, and pharynx because these structures may be affected when a voice disorder is present. Other components of a voice evaluation include respiration testing, acoustic measurements of the voice (e.g., frequency and intensity), and descriptions of the voice quality (e.g., breathy, hoarse) as perceived during different speaking tasks. The combined information from observation and measurements help the speech-language pathologist to determine the best approach for treating the client's voice problem and can be compared to findings after therapy.

Ms. Alvarez worked as a kindergarten teacher. During the first six months of her job, she began experiencing increased hoarseness that worsened from morning to night. By the end of each week, she could barely make herself heard in the classroom. Ms. Alvarez became frightened that she may have laryngeal cancer, so she went to see an otolaryngologist. The otolaryngologist looked at Ms. Alvarez's larynx and noted the development of two small bumps on her vocal folds, called vocal nodules. In addition, her vocal folds were red and swollen. Ms. Alvarez was referred to a speech-language pathologist for further evaluation of her voice and voice therapy.

The speech-language pathologist performed videoendoscopy on Ms. Alvarez using the rigid scope and a strobe light to assess vocal fold vibration. The speech-language pathologist also tape recorded Ms. Alvarez's voice during sustained phonation of *ah* and *ee* and while reading. The speech-language pathologist asked Ms. Alvarez about her work, family, and social life to obtain a better idea of how she uses her voice in different environments. From this information, the speech-language pathologist determined that Ms. Alvarez's problems were primarily related to how she used her voice at work. She often needed to shout above noise to get the children's attention. The speech-language pathologist suggested using a microphone system so that Ms. Alvarez could project her voice above the noise without using much effort. In addition, they developed instructional strategies such as using a whistle to get attention and using more visual aids that helped preserve her voice. Finally, the speech-language pathologist taught Ms. Alvarez how to project her voice without straining. After one month, Ms. Alvarez's voice had improved noticeably. On reexamination, the vocal nodules appeared smaller than they were initially.

In Ms. Alvarez's case, the strain on her voice at work led to the development of vocal nodules. The speech-language pathologist was able to determine the likely cause of the voice problem by getting information surrounding the onset of her voice problem. In addition, the speech-language pathologist knew that vocal nodules usually occurred with chronic misuse of the voice. The type of therapy done with Ms. Alvarez could be described in two ways:

1. Elimination of harmful daily vocal habits.
2. Learning new techniques to effectively use the voice without strain.

These are the two primary approaches used to treat voice disorders resulting from harmful vocal habits. In severe cases, surgical removal of a growth may be necessary; however, more frequently, voice therapy is successful in treating clients such as Ms. Alvarez and Ms. Norwood (discussed earlier). Medical intervention (e.g., surgery, medication) is provided by a physician such as an otolaryngologist. When medical interventions are used, the speech-language pathologist often provides voice therapy prior to and afterwards to help the client improve vocal techniques and to eliminate or prevent the use of harmful vocal habits.

DYSPHAGIA

Eating is vital to maintaining life and providing the energy for basic bodily functions. The process of ingestion begins with chewing and swallowing food, a complex process that we do not often give much thought. However, when swallowing is impaired, we become more aware of how large a role eating plays in our daily living. In addition to nutrition, eating is the focus of many social functions. Impaired eating, called **dysphagia** (pronounced dis-fay-ja), may create such difficulties during eating that social occasions are avoided and eating may become an unpleasant activity.

Most individuals diagnosed with dysphagia are over 55 years of age. In that age group, the prevalence is estimated to range between 16 to 22 percent (Bloem, Lagaay, van Beek, Haan, Roos, & Wintzen, 1990; Kjellen & Tibbling, 1981). This includes a wide range of problems with eating that are related to stroke, neuromuscular problems, traumatic brain injury, progressive neurological diseases, surgery to structures involved in ingestion and digestion, head and neck cancer, and cognitive problems such as dementia. Although older individuals more frequently experience symptoms of dysphagia, infants, children, and young adults may also have this condition. In young people, dysphagia may be due to illness, surgeries of the head and neck, or congenital malformations.

In order to understand dysphagia, one must appreciate the components of normal eating. There are four stages to consider, any of which may be impaired in someone with dysphagia. These can be seen in Figure 6.6.

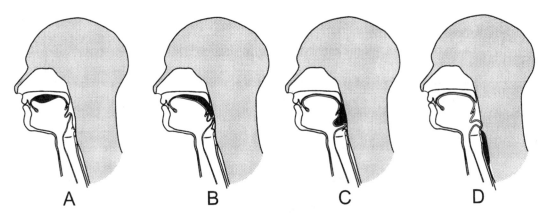

FIGURE 6.6   The four stages of eating are shown. (A) The oral preparatory stage. (B) The oral transport stage. (C) The pharyngeal stage. (D) The esophageal stage.

Stage One

The first stage when eating is referred to as the *oral preparatory stage* (see Figure 6.6A). This stage is important for preparing food placed in the mouth for transport to the stomach. During this stage, the lips, tongue, and soft palate play a major role in holding the food within the oral cavity. The tongue moves the food around so that it can be chewed and, finally, gathered into a central groove formed by the tongue prior to swallowing. The collection of food held together by the tongue is referred to as a food **bolus**. During this stage, saliva produced by glands in the mouth begins the digestion process. Saliva coats the food so that it is moist, and the digestive chemicals soften the food prior to swallowing. Problems with the oral preparatory stage may arise because of changes in the oral structures from congenital malformations, age-related changes, surgery, trauma, and neurological problems.

> Mrs. Baker, age 71, lost her teeth and could not afford dentures to replace them. As a consequence, she was unable to eat any food that required chewing such as meat, popcorn, salad, or fruit. Her self-imposed diet was restricted to soups, applesauce, oatmeal, and fluids. After six months, Mrs. Baker lost considerable weight and became malnourished. She sought help from her doctor who recognized the difficulties related to her diet and chewing problems. Mrs. Baker was admitted to the hospital where she was given intravenous fluids to rehydrate and rebalance her body chemistry. She was seen by a dietician who recommended the addition of a nutritional drink to supplement her meals. It was also recommended that Mrs. Baker obtain dentures to allow her to eat more normally. Once Mrs. Baker regained weight and was healthy, she was released from the hospital and instructed to check back with her doctor and dietician periodically to monitor her health and diet.

In this example, Mrs. Baker's lack of teeth resulted in difficulties chewing that limited her food options. She did not make wise food choices to ensure adequate nutritional and caloric intake. As a consequence, she lost weight and jeopardized

her health due to poor nourishment. Mrs. Baker's situation was easily remedied by obtaining dentures. However, if dentures were not an option for her, Mrs. Baker would need to continue using nutritional supplements to make sure her diet was well-balanced and to ensure adequate caloric intake.

Stage Two

Once food is chewed and ready to be swallowed, the tongue gathers it into a cohesive bolus held between the tongue and hard and soft palate. The tongue propels the bolus posteriorly into the pharynx by pressing up against the hard palate and pushing the bolus backwards. This stage of transporting the bolus from the oral cavity into the pharynx is called the *oral transport stage* of the swallow (see Figure 6.6B).

> Mr. Roswell, age 85 years, suffered a stroke that impaired his ability to control tongue and lip movements. As a consequence, it was difficult to control the food in his mouth while chewing. Food and fluids often spilled out of his mouth because his lips were too weak to keep them in his oral cavity. Mr. Roswell also had difficulty collecting the food in his mouth into a cohesive bolus for swallowing. After swallowing, food remained in his mouth.
>
> The speech-language pathologist assessed Mr. Roswell while he ate and determined that his primary difficulty was controlling food in the mouth. A *Flexible Endoscopic Examination of Swallowing* (FEES) was performed to visualize the pharynx while he swallowed measured amounts of milk and then applesauce. It was observed that after a teaspoon of milk was placed in his mouth, the milk ran back into the pharynx before he initiated a swallow. Milk also spilled through his lips. Mr. Roswell was able to control applesauce so that it did not spill into the pharynx or out through his lips. He was also able to swallow all of the applesauce so that none remained in his mouth.
>
> The speech-language pathologist recommended that Mr. Roswell's wife try thickening liquids and soups using cornstarch or a food-thickening product. This allowed Mr. Roswell to place a spoonful of food with a consistency similar to applesauce on his tongue and immediately swallow without having to chew first. Adding thickener to liquids also allowed Mr. Roswell improved oral control so that liquids did not spill out of his mouth or into his throat before initiating a swallow. Treatment included exercises to strengthen his tongue, lips, and jaw and to increase the range of their motion in order to control food in his mouth. The combination of strengthening exercises and the use of foods with preferred consistencies helped Mr. Roswell recover most of his oral control so that he could enjoy a wider variety of foods.

As seen in the example of Mr. Roswell, difficulty with the oral transport stage can prevent an individual from moving food out of the oral cavity to be swallowed. However, simple measures can be taken to help compensate for this problem by restricting foods to those the client can manage best. In addition, weakness of the oral musculature may be improved by strengthening and range-of-motion exercises with the tongue, lips, and jaw (Logemann, 1983).

Stage Three

The *pharyngeal stage* is characterized by movement of the bolus of food through the pharynx and into the esophagus (see Figure 6.6C). The bolus is propelled into the pharynx and, as it passes the back of the tongue, muscles of the pharynx contract to continue the propulsive action initiated by the tongue. As the superior portion of the pharynx contracts, the airway closes and the larynx elevates. This raised position during the swallow maximizes protection from *aspiration* of food into the airway. After the bolus enters the esophagus, the pharyngeal structures return to their resting positions. This stage is less than 1 second in duration.

> Mrs. Lasser, age 65 years, began having difficulty getting food to clear from her throat when she swallowed. She felt as though there was something caught in her throat and she needed to drink lots of fluids to clear the food that was stuck. In addition, she began choking on the fluids she drank to clear food stuck in her throat. Her swallowing difficulties required so much time and effort that she was embarrassed to eat in front of her friends and stopped enjoying meals. Thus, she reduced the amount of food eaten and declined invitations to join friends for meals. After losing weight and becoming malnourished, Mrs. Lasser went to see her doctor.
>
> Mrs. Lasser's doctor, in turn, referred her for a swallowing examination, which was performed jointly by a radiologist and speech-language pathologist. During the test, Mrs. Lasser experienced all of the swallowing difficulties described earlier. The examination revealed that Mrs. Lasser's pharyngeal muscles appeared weak and her larynx was not elevating completely during swallowing. Not all food swallowed was cleared completely from her throat. The speech-language pathologist showed Mrs. Lasser a way to swallow while tilting her chin downward. Mrs. Lasser used this posture while eating and found it less difficult to swallow. However, she still needed to follow each bite of food with water or juice to clear her throat completely.

As shown in this case, impairment of the pharyngeal stage of the swallow can often be compensated for by simple posturing changes while swallowing. When food does not clear the throat during this stage of the swallow, the individual risks aspiration of food into the airway. This can lead to inflammation of the lungs, which is a potentially serious illness called aspiration pneumonia. A team assessment by the radiologist and speech-language pathologist is the best way to assess the pharyngeal stage of swallowing. A procedure called a modified barium swallow is performed in which the patient is given food or liquid mixed with a radio-contrast material, barium, which is detected using an x-ray procedure called **videofluoroscopy**. This allows visualization of the pharyngeal structures and their movement during the pharyngeal stage of the swallow. Videofluoroscopy also allows identification and estimation of the amount of food aspirated into the airway before, during, and after the swallow. The videofluoroscopy also allows assessment of whether changes in posture improve the clearance of food from the mouth and throat. The effects of different food consistencies (e.g., fluid, paste, solids) can also be determined using videofluoroscopy.

Stage Four

The fourth, *esophageal stage* includes transportation of the bolus to the stomach by the esophagus (see Figure 6.6D). The esophagus pushes the bolus toward the stomach using muscle contractions that squeeze each portion of the esophagus from the top to the bottom, called **peristaltic contractions**. This contraction is similar to that which propels a worm as it moves along the ground. That is, each muscle segment surrounding the esophagus contracts in sequence from the upper esophageal sphincter to the stomach so that the bolus is squeezed through the esophagus into the stomach.

> Mr. Gilford, age 56, started experiencing problems with food that had been eaten during meals coming back up. This regurgitation, or **reflux**, became increasingly worse over a six-month period before he sought medical assistance. His physician examined his throat and noticed that the pharyngeal tissues appeared red and irritated. Given Mr. Gilford's symptoms, his physician suspected reflux. Mr. Gilford was referred to a gastroenterology specialist who determined that Mr. Gilford had an adequate swallow to clear food from the throat; however, undigested food appeared to come back up rather than continue through the esophagus toward the stomach. The gastroenterologist requested a barium swallow examination to assess Mr. Gilford's esophagus and digestive tract. The radiologic test entailed swallowing cupfuls of barium contrast while a videofluoroscopic image was monitored to follow the path of the barium. This test revealed that Mr. Gilford's esophagus was not contracting strongly enough to push the barium into the stomach. As a result, most of what Mr. Gilford drank during the test remained in the esophagus and some of it squeezed back into the pharynx as reflux. The gastroenterologist prescribed a medication that increased the contraction of the esophageal muscle to improve propulsion of food toward the stomach. The medication helped reduce Mr. Gilford's symptoms dramatically.

As all of the above examples demonstrate, dysphagia occurs when there is a problem with any or all of the four stages described previously. Common signs of dysphagia include:

- Difficulty initiating a swallow.
- Difficulty chewing food due to poor dentition (as in Mrs. Baker's case).
- Difficulty controlling food in the oral cavity so that it spills out of the mouth or spills into the airway before the larynx closes to protect the airway (as in Mr. Roswell's case).
- Choking when swallowing food, and food sticking in the throat (as Mrs. Lasser experienced).
- Reflux of food from the esophagus or stomach to the throat (as in Mr. Gilford's case).

Various methods exist for assessing the swallow, as demonstrated by the above examples. Imaging techniques are most frequently used to visualize the oral and pharyngeal structures such as the FEES method (Langmore, Schatz, & Olsen,

1988) and the modified barium swallow (Logemann, 1993). Although the speech-language pathologist can perform the FEES method if properly trained, an oto-laryngologist may also obtain FEES images while the speech-language pathologist administers the test food substances. During a modified barium swallow, the radiologist or radiology technician performs the videofluorographic imaging while the speech-language pathologist administers the barium contrast substances and determines which postures or consistencies appear to be successfully swallowed during testing. The gastroenterologist and radiologist are best trained to assess esophageal and other digestive organs during the barium swallow.

Many professionals may be involved in assessing and providing care to someone with dysphagia, including a speech-language pathologist, radiologist, gastroenterologist, otolaryngologist, neurologist, dentist, nurse, social worker, dietician, occupational therapist, and psychologist. The speech-language pathologist plays a major role in the assessment procedures, making recommendations to compensate for the dysphagia and referring the individual for further assessment by other dysphagia team members. Treatment of dysphagia most frequently entails simple measures such as changing the posture of the head and body during eating and swallowing, altering the consistency of the types of foods eaten, changing the temperature of foods eaten to improve initiation of the swallow, and performing exercises to improve strength and range of motion of oral structures. Other treatment methods provided by medical specialists entail use of drugs to improve smooth muscle contraction, non-oral feeding using a nasogastric or gastric tube, and surgical intervention.

CLINICAL PROBLEM SOLVING

Mrs. Hepple, age 65 years, underwent surgery to remove a portion of her esophagus that was cancerous. After surgery, her voice was breathy and she choked every time she drank water. In addition, the food she swallowed came back up. She was sent to an otolaryngologist who examined her vocal folds and noted that the left vocal fold was not moving during voicing. She was referred to a speech-language pathologist who further evaluated her voice. Rigid videoendoscopy using a strobe light was used to assess vocal fold vibration. However, Mrs. Hepple's vocal folds did not come together completely when vibrating. The speech-language pathologist was concerned about Mrs. Hepple's difficulties with swallowing and suggested a modified barium swallow. During this testing, the speech-language pathologist noted that liquids entered Mrs. Hepple's trachea during the pharyngeal stage of the swallow. Subsequently, she choked and coughed to clear the liquid from her airway.

1. Why does Mrs. Hepple have a breathy voice quality?
2. What do you think caused her left vocal fold to stop moving?

3. How might the speech-language pathologist try to help her improve her voice quality?
4. Might the voice problem go away with voice therapy?
5. What stage of the swallow is impaired?

REFERENCES

Arnold, G. E. (1959). Spastic dysphonia: I. Changing interpretations of a persistent affliction. *Logos, 2,* 3–14.

Bloem, B. R., Lagaay, A. M., van Beek, W., Haan, J., Roos, R. A. C., & Wintzen, A. R. (1990). Prevalence of subjective dysphagia in community residents aged over 87. *British Medical Journal, 300,* 721–722.

Brodnitz, F. S. (1971). *Vocal rehabilitation.* Rochester, MN: Whiting Press.

Casper, J. K., & Colton, R. H. (1993). *Clinical manual for laryngectomy and head and neck cancer rehabilitation.* San Diego, CA: Singular Publishing Group.

Dedo, H. H., & Behlau, M. S. (1991). Recurrent laryngeal nerve section for spastic dysphonia: 5- to 14-year preliminary results in the first 300 patients. *Annals of Otology, Rhinology, and Laryngology, 100*(4), 274–279.

Dedo, H. H., & Izdebski, K. (1983). Intermediate results of 306 recurrent laryngeal nerve sections for spastic dysphonia. *Laryngoscope, 93,* 9–16.

Fritzell, B. (1995). *Occupation and voice problems.* Paper presented at the Proceedings from XXIII World Congress of IALP [abstract].

Gray, S. D., Hammond, E., & Hanson, D. F. (1995). Benign pathologic responses of the larynx. *Annals of Otology, Rhinology, and Laryngology, 104*(1), 13–18.

Hockauf, H., & Sailer, R. (1982). Postoperative recurrent nerve palsy. *Head and Neck Surgery, 4,* 380–384.

Hull, F. M., Mielke, P. W., Willeford, J. A., & Timmons, R. J. (1976). *National speech and hearing survey* (Final Report Project 50978). Washington, DC: Bureau of Education for the Handicapped, Office of Education, Department of Health, Education, and Welfare.

Kjellen, G., & Tibbling, L. (1981). Manometric oesophageal function, acid perfusion test and symptomatology in a 55-year-old general population. *Clinical Physiology, 1,* 405–415.

Kleinsasser, O. (1979). *Microlaryngoscopy and endolaryngeal microsurgery: Technique and typical findings.* Baltimore: University Park Press.

Kleinsasser, O. (1990). Restoration of voice in benign lesions of the vocal fold by endolaryngeal microsurgery. In R. T. Sataloff (Ed.), *Voice perspectives.* San Diego: Singular Publishing Group.

LaGuaite, J. (1972). Adult voice screening. *Journal of Speech and Hearing Disorders, 37,* 147–151.

Langmore, S. E., Schatz, K., & Olsen, N. (1988). Fiberoptic endoscopic examination of swallowing safety: A new procedure. *Dysphagia, 2,* 216–219.

Logemann, J. A. (1983). *Evaluation and treatment of swallowing disorders.* Austin, TX: Pro Ed.

Logemann, J. A. (1993). *Manual for the videofluorographic study of swallowing* (2nd ed.). Austin, TX: Pro-Ed.

Ludlow, C. (1995a). Treating the spasmodic dysphonias with botulinum toxin: A comparison of results with adductor and abductor spasmodic dysphonia and vocal tremor. In J. Tsui, & D. Calne (Eds.), *The Dystonias.* New York: Dekker.

Ludlow, C. L. (1995b). Management of the spasmodic dysphonias. In J. S. Rubin, R. T. Sataloff, & G. S. Korovin (Eds.), *Diagnosis and treatment of voice disorders* (pp. 436–434). New York: Igaku-Shoin.

McCrory, E. (2001). Voice therapy outcomes in vocal fold nodules: A retrospective audit. *International Journal of Language and Communication Disorders, 36*(Suppl), 19–24.

McFarlane, S. C., & Von Berg, S. (1998). Facilitative techniques in intervention for dysphonia. *Current Opinion in Otolaryngology and Head and Neck Surgery, 6,* 161–165.

McFarlane, S. C., & Watterson, T. L. (1990). Vocal nodules: Endoscopic study of their variations and treatment. *Seminars in Speech and Language, 11,* 47–59.

McKenna, J. P., Fornataro-Clerici, L. M., McMenamin, P. G., & Leonard, R. J. (1991). Laryngeal cancer: Diagnosis, treatment and speech rehabilitation. *American Family Physician*, 44(1), 123–129.

Mendenhall, W. M., Parsons, J. T., Stringer, S. P., Cassisi, N. J., & Million, R. R. (1988). T1-T2 vocal cord carcinoma: A basis for comparing the results of radiotherapy and surgery. *Head and Neck Surgery*, 12, 204–209.

Mu, L., & Yang, S. (1991). An experimental study on the laryngeal electromyography and visual observations in varying types of surgical injuries to the unilateral recurrent laryngeal nerve in the neck. *Laryngoscope*, 101, 699–708.

Rafferty, M. A., Fenton, J. E., & Jones, A. S. (2001). The history, aetoiology and epidemiology of laryngeal carcinoma. *Clinical Otolaryngology*, 26(6), 442–446.

Silverman, E., & Zimmer, C. (1975). Incidence of chronic hoarseness among school-age children. *Journal of Speech and Hearing Disorders*, 40, 211–215.

Smith, E., Gray, S., Dove, H., Kirchner, L., & Heras, H. (1997). Frequency and effects of voice problems in teachers. *Journal of Voice*, 11, 81–87.

Smith, E., Verdolini, K., Gray, S., Nichols, S., Lemke, J., Barkmeier, J., Dove, H., & Hoffman, H. (1996). Effect of voice disorders on quality of life. *Journal of Medical Speech-Language Pathology*, 4(4), 223–244.

Titze, I. R., Lemke, J., & Montequin, D. (1996). Populations in the U.S. workforce who rely on voice as a primary tool of trade. *NCVS Status and Progress Report*, 10, 127–132.

Weed, D. T., Jewett, B. S., Rainey, C., Zealear, D. L., Stone, R. E., Ossoff, R. H., & Netterville, J. L. (1996). Long-term follow-up of recurrent laryngeal nerve avulsion for the treatment of spasmodic dysphonia. *Annals of Otology, Rhinology, Laryngology*, 105(8), 592–601

Yamaguchi, H., Yotsukura, Y., Kondo, R., Horiguchi, S., Imaizumi, S., & Hirose, H. (1986). Nonsurgical therapy for vocal nodules. *Folia Phoniatrica*, 38, 372–373.

LANGUAGE

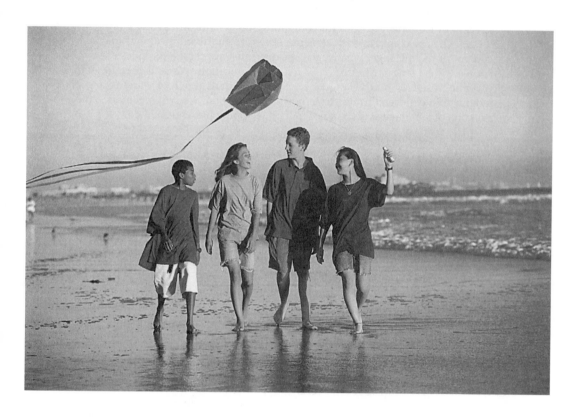

■ ■ ■ ■ ■

PREVIEW

Human communication includes a wide range of activities. Much of it is nonverbal: A pointed stare or a strategic clearing of the throat is often sufficient to convey an emotion or prompt the recipient to action. A speaker's body posture and hand gestures convey aspects of attitude, emphasis, and emotion. Often, these nonverbal forms of communication are unintentional and nonspecific. When a specific message must be conveyed, people typically employ language. Language, whether spoken, written, or signed, involves a system of symbols that conveys meaning. Language involves the interaction of many skills, which combine for effective communication. A speaker must know the rules for combining sounds into words and words into sentences. The speaker uses both sentence structure and word meanings to convey the content of the message. Finally, the speaker must appreciate the rules of social discourse to use language effectively for communication. We will present some approaches used to study language acquisition that highlight various aspects of language in children. To illustrate normal acquisition, we will summarize the progression of language skills in a normally developing preschool child.

Human communication provides an opportunity for the exchange of feelings, knowledge, and wants between two or more people. In the first year of life, the baby communicates primarily through changes in the voice with accompanying facial expressions and gestures. These nonverbal vocalizations in the early part of life, primarily expressions of internal biological states, are affective in nature, and are interpreted by those around the baby as communicating emotion. The vocalizations soon begin to take on the melody of speech. When we left our discussion of infant vocalization in Chapter 3, Abraham, a child whose development we have been following, was just beginning to say his first words. At this point, the child's knowledge of the language (language competence) begins to show by the actual use of the language (language performance).

THE COMPONENTS OF LANGUAGE

As effortless as language appears to be for most people, effective use involves the interaction of many skills. To understand language better, it is sometimes useful to examine the skills that contribute to overall language functioning. Bloom (1988) suggested that language skills can be described in terms of form, content, and use. **Form** includes phonology, syntax, and morphology. **Content** includes the meaning, or **semantics**, of words and utterances. **Use** includes pragmatic skills such as the rules of social discourse and the speaker's purpose for communication.

Form

Phonology.   **Phonology** is the study of the sounds of speech. Linguists have been studying the phonological development of children since the early 1900s (Ingram, 1981). Much of current phonological investigation focuses on uncovering the rules required for speech sounds (or phonemes) as used in combination in syllables and words. As we saw in Chapter 1, any given language contains only a subset of the possible sound combinations that can be produced. For example, the phonology of English permits the /st/ blend at either the beginning or end of words, but /str/ can only appear at word beginnings. Likewise, there are specific rules for voicing or unvoicing in pluralization. If we were to pluralize the words *hat* and *hit*, we would add the unvoiced consonant /s/. Pluralization of a noun ending in a voiced consonant requires the use of the voiced cognate of /s/, the phoneme /z/. So, if we were to pluralize the word *bed*, we would add the /z/ phoneme, writing the word in phonetics as [bɛdz]. Such rules for how sound is used are part of the phonology of the language.

Syntax.   **Syntax** refers to the structure of sentences. The structure can be described in terms of hierarchically ordered components, as illustrated in Figure 7.1. A syntactic theory describes the rules by which words may be combined into grammatically acceptable sentences. For example, in English, the subject of a declarative sentence (a noun or noun phrase) must precede the predicate of a sentence (a verb or verb phrase). Therefore, a sentence such as "He is swinging" is

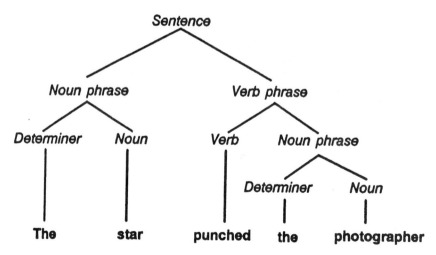

FIGURE 7.1   The syntactic structure of a sentence.

acceptable, whereas "Is swinging he" is not. Syntactic rules also describe the constraints in combining words and phrases of particular types. For example, for the predicate "is swinging," there are a limited number of phrases that might follow it in a sentence. We might say, "He is swinging wildly" or "He is swinging on the porch swing" or "He is swinging the baby." The predicate "is swinging" belongs to a class of verbs that can be followed by an adverbial phrase, prepositional phrase, or noun phrase. For most people, the rules for combining words into sentences are unconscious and automatic. Knowledge of these syntactic rules allows a speaker to produce grammatical utterances effortlessly. In any language there is a limited number of acceptable syntactic structures. Therefore, knowledge of these structures allows listeners to anticipate the words they will hear and draw conclusions about how the words relate to one another to convey meaning. For example, in "Jamie asked Adelida . . . " there is a high probability that the sentence will continue with either a prepositional phrase (e.g., "about . . . ") or a verb infinitive (for example, "to go . . . " or "to call . . . "). The listener, from the conversational context, may even be able to anticipate the precise phrase. Given the complete sentence "Jamie asked Adelida to go," the syntactic rules tell the listener that Jamie is doing the asking and that Adelida is being asked to go. In this way, the syntax has represented the general meaning of the utterance in a structured, rule-governed way. This phenomenon is referred to as mapping a deep structure (meaning) to a surface structure (syntax).

We will talk more about syntax in the next section of this chapter when we discuss language acquisition. Problems in syntactic comprehension and production in language-impaired children and adults will be presented in Chapters 8 and 9.

Morphology. **Morphology** refers to how meaning is represented by the use of words, affixes, various grammar tenses (such as past tense), and plurality. A **morpheme** is the smallest unit of a language that has meaning. It can be a whole word, one of several parts of a word, the beginning of a word (i.e., a prefix, such as *un-*), or a word ending (i.e., a suffix, such as *-ing*). The following words contain one morpheme; they cannot be divided into any smaller units and still carry meaning:

quick	(one morpheme)
build	(one morpheme)
structure	(one morpheme)

Words that can stand alone are called *free morphemes*. A second class of morphemes is called *bound morphemes* because they must be attached to other words. Bound morphemes include the suffixes in:

quickly	(two morphemes)
builder	(two morphemes)
structured	(two morphemes)

Each of these words contains two morphemes, one free and one bound. Notice that the bound morpheme changes the meaning of the word in each case. In some cases the addition of a morpheme actually changes the syntactic classification of the word. The addition of *-ly* changes *quick* from an adjective to an adverb. The addition of *-er* changes *build* from a verb to a noun. Conversely, the addition of *-ed* to *structure* changes it from a noun to an adjective. In other cases, morphemes add meaning without changing the class of the word (e.g., *dog* versus *dogs*).

Children's acquisition of morphology seems to follow predictable stages. After analyzing the utterances of children over time, Brown (1973) developed five stages of sentence construction that seem to parallel (or mirror) overall language development. The five stages were developed according to the number of morphemes a child said per utterance, known as the MLU, or mean length of utterance, in morphemes:

Stage I (1.75 morphemes). The child is using single words and is starting to put noun-verb sequences together, such as "Car go."

Stage II (2.25 morphemes). The child starts to change word endings to portray grammar, as in "Cars going."

Stage III (2.75 morphemes). The child begins to use questions and imperatives, for instance, "That a car?"

Stage IV (3.5 morphemes). The child begins to use complex sentences, for example, "Where's car going now?"

Stage V (4 morphemes). The child may use connectors and more functions, as in "Mom's in the car."

Although there is obvious overlap between successive stages, Brown and his colleagues conducted a number of studies over time that showed a progression from saying a single word to the two-word utterance, to the telegraphic sentence, with the gradual refinement of grammar leading to complete sentences compatible with the adult model.

Content

Content includes the meanings of individual words and words in combination. The study of word meanings is sometimes referred to as semantics. Our basic use of language as a tool for communication is to transmit meaning to someone else. Hubbell (1985) noted, "Meaning is the bridge between the thoughts and experiences of individuals and the sequences of sounds they produce to symbolize those thoughts and experiences. Words symbolize concepts, and concepts represent experiences or reality" (p. 33).

Of interest here is how young children attach meaning to a particular phonological sequence they have been hearing and how their meaning for a word develops into the adult-like meaning. As children hear words associated with particular actions and behaviors in social contexts, they begin to assign meaning to those

words. Eventually, a word stands for those actions and feelings, without the need for the original context. As the child develops cognitively through various experiences, there is greater coupling of words with meaning. The child begins to use "words to refer to or represent external objects and events" (Clark, 1979, p. 193).

Two kinds of meaning may develop for words, denotative and connotative. Denotative meaning is the literal meaning of the word. For example, for the word *milk*, we can use the dictionary definition of "a whitish fluid that is secreted by the mammary glands of female mammals for the nourishment of their young" as a literal, denotative meaning. (Few of us have thought of this meaning very often.)

Besides the literal, denotative meanings, words carry connotative meanings, which include the subtle overtones that distinguish words of very similar meanings. Thus, we would probably prefer to be called "unique" or even "unusual" rather than "atypical" or "abnormal." Connotative meanings often set the emotional tone of what is said. For example, "She requested it" has a more formal tone than "She asked for it." Connotative meanings also reflect concepts associated with particular words. For example, if we associate the concept of physical nourishment with milk, we can make the connection to spiritual nourishment to understand an alternate meaning of milk in the metaphorical "milk of human kindness." Speakers learn the rules of the semantic system by hearing and using words in ways appropriate to both their connotative and denotative meanings.

The sentence context influences the specific meanings that we attach to individual words. The meanings of nouns and verbs are modified by the use of adjectives and adverbs. The listener's expectations about the meaning of a sentence may change as later words cause its meaning to shift. For example, the noun *shoe* typically produces in the mind of the listener a picture of a leather covering of the foot mounted on a thicker sole. We can see how the sentence context is used to produce many different meanings for this word:

If the shoe fits, wear it.	(a nonliteral, proverbial meaning)
It fits like an old shoe.	(from experience, old shoes feel good on the foot)
Make a ringer with a horseshoe.	(*horse* morpheme changes meaning, and *ringer* requires specialized knowledge of horseshoe game)
You can't stop with worn shoes.	(a brake shoe is ineffective when worn)

In the preceding examples, we see that the noun *shoe* (which we may first think of as the object we wear on a foot) can have many other meanings. We understand the particular meaning in the context in which the utterance was made. Disagreements in interpreting what someone intended to say may sometimes be related to different interpretations of word meaning. Someone speaks to a gathering of people in the hope that everyone assembled will make the same interpretation of the words; however, the literal meanings of the words may compete with

their connotative meanings, often resulting in many different interpretations than that intended by the speaker.

Use

How we use words, and in what situations, is the focus of language use, or pragmatics. This is the study of the use of language in context. After the first six months of life, spontaneous vocalization begins to be replaced with intentional vocalization accompanied by expression and gesture (Oller, 1980). Bates (1976) and Bruner (1975) pointed out that the human interaction the baby experiences in the first year of life establishes various pragmatic roles long before the baby is using actual language. The preverbal behaviors described in Chapter 3 are basically employed to control and manipulate the environment. From about the age of 9 months, the baby enjoys interaction with the caregiver, using vocalization appropriately for such games as pat-a-cake and peek-a-boo. In these early games, the child is using vocalization to interact with others, which Bates (1976, p. 426) calls "preverbal performatives." Even between 12 and 18 months, the baby uses single-word responses like "bye-bye" more as part of a physical interaction with the caregiver than as true words that represent concepts. These utterances are called "performative acts" by Bates. The performative act serves a communicative purpose for the child, such as declaring, promising, asking questions, and so forth (Bates, Benigni, Bretherton, Camaioni, & Volterra, 1977).

The speech acts theory, developed by Searle (1969), focuses on the speaker's intention rather than on the words one uses. Searle described three types of intents: *asserting, requesting,* and *ordering.* These categories focus on how the speaker is using language rather than on the specifics of what was said. Assertions are almost as varied as topics of communication, whereas requests are usually for some kind of action or information. Others have elaborated on this focus with additional functions that language serves. Lahey (1988) provided a description of many functions that children's language serves. Some examples include:

1. Comment (I did it!)
2. Rejection (No anchovies!)
3. Pretend (Barbie goes in her dreamhouse . . .)
4. Obtain information (What's that?)
5. Routine (I pledge allegiance to the flag . . .)

As young children grow, so does their verbal repertoire, enabling the use of language forms that meet the demands of a particular situation. Children learn to communicate (verbally and nonverbally) one way to their peers, another way to their parents, and another way to the teacher or the doctor. The child learns that the situation or context of the communication has much to do with how things are phrased. The specific decision about what to say and how and when to say it is shaped by the success the child experiences in conversation. For example, the child

soon learns that he can call his cousins by their first names but he'd better use "Aunt" or "Uncle" with their parents, even though the adults address each other by first name alone. Furthermore, the child soon understands that Grandmother likes to use baby talk and that Grandfather uses a very adult language form. In Chapter 3, we saw the use of "child-directed-speech" by Abraham's parents when addressing their infant son. However, it is unlikely that these parents speak to their bosses or co-workers in this style of speech. Instead, they adjust the register of their speech to match the age and social status of their listener.

APPROACHES TO THE STUDY OF LANGUAGE ACQUISITION

During the first year of life, infants all over the world hear the languages spoken around them and eventually organize what they hear into some kind of meaning. Toward the end of the first year, babies respond to their name. They are able to respond to simple verbal commands and make simple motor responses using the objects in their immediate environment. As we saw in Chapter 3, their vocalizations toward the end of the first year have become a complex vocal pattern that resembles the patterns of the spoken languages they have been hearing. The first spoken words are followed by the orderly acquisition of one- and two-word utterances; these first words have primary value to the baby, such as *ma* and *mi(lk)*. These first words are also relatively easy to say and phonetically simple. As language is acquired during the second year, children are able to produce (and understand) longer and increasingly complex language constructions. Children acquire a grammar (rules of structure and sequence) of the language through its everyday use. As children put two or three words together, they use the rules of the grammar to keep the words in the form and sequence needed to facilitate comprehension by the listener. Children learn that to be understood by the listener, the verbal message must be said in a way that is reasonably similar to the language code of the listener.

There appears to be some uniformity across cultures regarding the acquisition and form of language. In contrast, there is great diversity in theories of language acquisition. In addition to speech-language pathologists and audiologists, many scholars from different backgrounds have studied language over the years. The philosopher and the psychologist have examined the relationship between language and thought. The linguist has studied the origins and forms of language. The psychologist and biologist have viewed language from its neurogenic origins. The neurologist and psychologist have studied the neurological foundations of both normal and disordered language. The child development specialist, the linguist, and psychologist have looked at cognition and language. Although some of the diversity of opinion about language is related to the particular discipline, some of it is related to the chronology or history of studying language. Over the years there have been major shifts in focus and viewpoint. The historical time at which language acquisition was studied (such as in 1950, as opposed to 1970 or 1990) has a influential role in one's approach to the topic. It would be convenient and encouraging to identify a sequential and progressive theme in the study of language

over the years, but it appears that there is some randomness, perhaps even circularity in our study of normal language. Among the many theoretical approaches to the acquisition of language that are available, let us select four and cite a few of the theorists who have advocated each point of view.

It must be recognized that any selection or listing of theoretical approaches to language acquisition is an oversimplification. Further, there is considerable overlap of view between particular approaches, as well as single proponents advocating several theories. Cruttenden (1979) advocated a "balanced viewpoint" in consideration of various approaches to language acquisition, recognizing that there is some truth in each. In this introductory work, our intent is to present each approach briefly, with no attempt to advocate any one theory of language acquisition.

The Behavioral Approach

According to the behavioral approach, language is a learned, conditioned behavior. This approach to language acquisition stresses the influence of environment rather than any innate abilities of the child. The origins of behavioral therapy perhaps started with the classical conditioning study of Pavlov, who conditioned dogs to salivate (Watson, 1970). Observing that dogs salivated when looking at meat, Pavlov presented a tuning-fork sound when the meat was presented. The dogs were soon *conditioned* to salivate when they heard the tuning fork (whether the meat was present or not). Like most automatic reflexes (such as salivation), many forms of human behavior (Skinner, 1957) can be conditioned.

Behavioralists assert that language can be taught as well. For example, the 9-month-old baby learns to attend to the voice of her caregivers; when she hears these voices and looks closely at these people, she discovers that she can derive various forms of comfort. She then repeats the comfort-producing behavior. The 12-month-old baby says "ma" when his mother is about to feed him. His *ma* production is followed by feeding, accompanied by many animated expressions of love from his mother. The positive response he received makes *ma* an attractive word to say. Every time he sees his mother (if there is enough positive reinforcement), he is likely to repeat it. He may also generalize the use of *ma* for all feeding situations regardless of who the caregiver may be. Such inappropriate stimulus generalization will eventually be extinguished through the reactions and feeding situations the baby experiences.

Skinner (1957) developed a behavioral theory of verbal learning. Language is conditioned as a child's early vocal behaviors receive positive reinforcement. As the child develops, correctly pronounced words and combinations of words are rewarded by approval or sometimes by the basic pleasure of verbalization (Cruttenden, 1979). Incorrect utterances are met with no approval and are subsequently replaced by correct (good) verbalizations. In this way, the caregiver becomes the teacher, providing reinforcements for the child's utterances, in effect *shaping* the child's productions to approximate those of the adult language model.

A behavioral approach to language learning strongly emphasizes shaping and reinforcement of speech attempts in the child's acquisition of language. In the first

two years of life, when the child is in close proximity to a caregiver, one can appreciate that the latter has a primary role in reinforcing the child's utterances. However, the caregiver role may be as much modeling and interacting as it is reinforcing, per se. Once the child reaches the age of 2, it is difficult to see how a heterogeneous society can provide a consistent model for shaping verbalizations. Young children encounter a great variety of linguistic models (baby talk, fragmented sentences, and sentences spoken in a way they do not understand) and varied reactions to their utterances (anger, annoyance, laughter, ignoring, and friendliness).

Despite its limitations for fully explaining normal language acquisition, the behavioral theory has been applied to teaching language in cases of language disorders. The behavioral approach to language acquisition was much utilized in the 1960s and 1970s as a clinical training model for children with deficient language. These approaches often involved repeated practice with reinforcement for correct productions. Although therapy approaches have become more naturalistic over the years, operant principles continue to be used for stimulating language in children with language disabilities of various kinds.

The Nativist (Innateness) Approach

In some respects, the nativist approach was a reaction to the behavioral theory of language acquisition. Proponents of the nativist approach (e.g., Chomsky, 1988; Pinker, 1984) noted that children rarely receive explicit feedback about the grammatical correctness of their speech (e.g., "That's not right. You say it this way."). The "learning by shaping" tenet of the behaviorist approach seemed unrealistic in the absence of evidence of explicit teaching by adults. In fact, nativists felt that children's relatively rapid and seemingly effortless acquisition of language suggests that knowledge of the rules of language is part of their biological endowment. Children are presumed to have an innate knowledge of how words are organized into sentences, even before hearing all the types of sentences possible in their native language.

Early proponents of the nativist approach (e.g., Chomsky, 1965; McNeill, 1970) argued that children come equipped with a Language Acquisition Device (LAD). All the language a child hears (the language "corpus") passes through the LAD, and this mechanism processes the structure of language so that the child becomes competent in his native language. McNeill provided a simple diagram of the LAD model as

Language Corpus → LAD → Grammatical Competence

The inner workings of how the LAD produces grammatical competence are not understood well, leading some to refer to it as a "black box" model. Explaining exactly what this black box does has occupied linguists for the past fifty years. Chomsky (1988) suggested that the LAD imparts knowledge of invariant features that characterize all languages (e.g., all languages use sentences that are constructed in rule-governed ways). These are referred to as language "universals." According to

the theory, the child need only be exposed to his or her native language to recognize the specific rules that govern that particular language.

The nativist approach makes certain claims that set it apart from other theoretical approaches. The first is that language is not explicitly taught to children; rather, they acquire it because they are biologically predisposed to do so. Second, the child possesses a biological mechanism that is responsible for acquisition. This mechanism is thought to be independent of brain systems that handle other aspects of cognition. This theory has focused on language form and has not addressed aspects of communication that involve language content or use. The narrow scope of the nativist approach has prompted the development of other theoretical positions that encompass aspects of communication in addition to language form.

The Cognitive Approach

The cognitivist approach assumes that language skills represent the application of general cognitive skills for the purpose of communication. This theoretical approach has its early roots in the work of Piaget, who proposed that children's developing facility with language is a reflection of their progression through hierarchical stages of cognitive development (1963). The acquisition of words and sentences is thought to reflect the child's increasing ability to represent thoughts and experiences in the abstract form of language.

Like the nativist approach, the cognitive approach assumes that language acquisition is mediated by the brain. In contrast to the nativist approach, the brain systems that support language are not independent of those that support other aspects of cognitive development. The cognitive approach also contrasts with the behaviorist approach because it emphasizes the contribution of the child's abilities rather than the external feedback the child may receive. The types of abilities that cognitivist researchers have explored are perceptual skills that allow children to discern the sounds of speech and cognitive skills like pattern recognition that allow them to note the regularities of how sounds are arranged into words and words into sentences. Note that basic skills, like perceptual capabilities and pattern recognition, are not only used for language, but can be used to acquire nonlinguistic skills as well (e.g. recognizing faces, learning sequenced activities).

According to the cognitivist approach, language acquisition is dependent on the child's experiences with communication. The child learns about his language from the patterns available in the environment. For example, let us suppose a child hears words associated with actions, like *jump* and *jumped*, *cry* and *cried*. He or she might learn the association between *–ed* and the ends of verbs. This child may even overextend this association to verbs that do not take the *–ed* ending (e.g., *runned, sitted*) for a while (as some children do). However, after he or she hears enough examples of the irregular forms (e.g., *ran, sat*), the child will use these forms correctly as well. If these irregular words occur quite frequently in the speech he or she hears, the child might learn these "exceptions to the rule" quite quickly. And in fact, irregular verbs are quite common in conversational speech.

This line of thinking led to the development of the cue-competition theory of language acquisition (Bates & MacWhinney, 1987). This theory is based on the premise that all native languages provide the child with cues as to its underlying structure. The effectiveness, or strength, of these cues is related to how frequently they occur in the language and how reliably they lead the child to the correct conclusion about communication. For example, English-speaking children hear "subject-verb-object" sentences quite frequently. Therefore, interpreting the initial noun of a sentence as the subject is quite reliable for understanding the sentence. This makes the "first-noun-as-subject" cue strong for English-speaking children. However, this same rule would not have high cue strength in other languages. This language-to-language variation in cues accounts for many of the differences in the age at which speakers of different languages acquire the specific components of their language.

A recent evolution in the cognitivist tradition has been the application of computer models to the problem of language acquisition (e.g., Cartwright & Brent, 1997; Huiskens, Coppen, & Jagtman, 1991; McClelland & Rumelhart, 1986). In some ways, the computer models are a reaction to nativist claims that specialized, language-specific mechanisms underlie language acquisition. Instead, these models use general associative processes that are not language specific. Few researchers would claim that a successful computer model proves how children acquire language. Instead, these models serve to broaden thinking about the possibilities that could account for acquisition. Simply put, the fact that a computer can mimic aspects of acquisition indicates that it is possible that those skills could be acquired without a language-specific mechanism.

Cognitive approaches have the advantage of being broad enough to account not only for language form, but also content and use. Because cognitive theories acknowledge the role of a child's experiences in shaping language acquisition, it is easy to see how the environment can dictate the types of words a child acquires and the social conventions the child uses when communicating. In fact, some theorists have suggested that the social function of language (why the child wants to say something) drives much of early language acquisition. This focus on the communication interaction also separates it from the other theoretical approaches discussed so far.

The Biological Approach

The modern biological approach to language actually has its roots in nineteenth century Europe. At a time that preceded direct methods to study brain-behavior relations, physicians and anatomists developed theories that have persisted centuries later. The concept of localization of function (see Chapter 2) was championed by Francis Gall. Gall was an anatomist who dedicated his career to study of the human brain. He received both international fame and later considerable derision for his ideas that individual variation in brain structure could account for individual differences in behavior. He developed maps that assigned different skills, attitudes, and personality traits to small regions of the brain. Given that there were

no methods for directly measuring variations in these areas in the living brain, he inferred brain differences by mapping the topography of the skull. Although time has refuted his methods and brain maps, his concept of localization of function has proved an important and powerful concept even today.

The localizationist perspective was further reinforced by the work of Paul Broca and Carl Wernicke, whose case studies with specific types of language loss lead to assignment of particular language functions to the left hemisphere of the brain. They began a tradition, that continues today, of examining the language deficits that occur after stroke, disease, or injury to infer function of the damaged area. With the advent of neuroimaging techniques in the mid-twentieth century, researchers were able to locate the area of damage in living patients, allowing greater specificity to the ability to localize function and document individual variations in brain-behavior relations.

At the same time, others were using both the time-tested methods of autopsy work and modern brain imaging techniques to discover if structural variations in the intact brain might explain the propensity of the left hemisphere to support language. Geschwind and Levitsky (1968) were the first to discover that the one area serving language was larger in the left hemisphere than in the right. Later work established that these asymmetries are present at birth (Chi, Dooling, & Gilles, 1977), supporting the idea that they provide an anatomical substrate for developing left hemisphere language representation. These discoveries in many ways were the twentieth century legacy of Gall's ideas two centuries earlier.

Today, researchers are fortunate to have a variety of tools to study the living brain's structure and function in amazing detail. These tools are being applied to the study of language acquisition during childhood (e.g., Holland, Plante, Weber, et al., 2001; Molfese, 1990), normal language in adults (e.g., Bookheimer, 2002; Kutas & Hillard, 1983), and the deficits and recovery patterns in those with neurological disorders (e.g., Hertz-Pannier et al., 2002; Rosen et al., 2000). New discoveries are modifying our view of language in the brain. We now know that language is better described as lateralized (more on the left than the right) rather than strictly localized to the left hemisphere. There are indications that the language areas of the right hemisphere might be one mechanism of recovery in some cases of left hemisphere brain damage. We are also developing a better appreciation of how the language systems interact with other regions that support memory and attention (e.g., Plante, Creusere, & Sabin, in press; Shaywitz et al., 2001). These investigations are guided by the three-hundred-year legacy of brain-language discoveries and by modern theories on the nature of language. Ultimately, the biological approach may provide evidence to support or refute the tenets of other approaches to language acquisition discussed in this text.

Summary

In many ways, the approaches described differ more in their focus than in their substantive claims. Indeed, writers frequently combine aspects of various positions or switch between them over time. Cognitive approaches tend to emphasize the

importance of the communicative function of language. Nativist approaches are frequently designed to account for language form. Cognitive and behavioral approaches often address language content as it is mapped to the child's experiences. Biological approaches concentrate on anatomical and physiologic correlates of language. The differences in focus reflect, in part, the different disciplines that have contributed to the field of language. As the study of language becomes increasingly interdisciplinary, we can look forward to a greater integration of such approaches.

Several of these perspectives on language acquisition reflect a nature versus nurture argument. For example, nativist theories have historically emphasized the child's innate endowment (nature) for language. In contrast, behavioral theories have emphasized the role of the environment (nurture). Recent advances in the neurosciences demonstrate that strict nature-nurture dichotomies are unrealistic. We now know that experience shapes the structure and function of the brain at very basic levels. The pattern of neuron activation is shaped and changed by sensory input and experiences. Activation, in turn, promotes neuronal survival and outgrowth. These changes in the brain's basic organization make the brain a ready and increasingly efficient processor of experience, including experience with language.

This type of dynamic interaction between children's biological nature and their experiences forces a redefinition of innate versus experience-based skills. The word *innate* typically means "present from birth," although this definition no longer means that experience has had no effect. Many brain systems rely heavily on sensory input to develop normally, and such input may begin prenatally. For example, the auditory system becomes functional during the third prenatal trimester. Some aspects of spoken language, such as its prosodic patterns and certain sound contrasts, are audible in the womb. As we saw in Chapter 3, infants hear and respond differentially to sounds they were exposed to while in the womb (e.g., DeCasper & Spence, 1986). Thus, infants are born with some knowledge of acoustic characteristics of their language community, and this knowledge appears to be experience-based. These types of discoveries force a reevaluation of the assumptions that underlie traditional approaches to language acquisition. As Locke (1990) suggested, language may be both innate and learned as certain biological characteristics may predispose a child to attend to language-relevant information, prompting the child to learn more about it. From this perspective, it is more productive to explore the interactions between the child and his or her experiences than to divide them artificially.

LANGUAGE DEVELOPMENT FROM SOUNDS TO SENTENCES

In Chapter 3, we followed the development of a young boy named Abraham. We saw his communicative development progress from his first exposures to the sounds of language to the point where he was able to produce sounds recognizable as single words. This is a truly remarkable accomplishment. It signals coordination of the range of biological systems (respiratory, vocal, articulatory, hearing, and cognition) to support spoken language. Once the first words appear, others soon

follow. A child learns words that characterize his environment. The family dog's name is learned and the word *dog* itself will follow. If there is no neighborhood cat, however, that word will take longer to appear. Sometimes these first words are highly context specific. For example, Abraham could name animals from his Noah's ark book that he did not name at the zoo. Nonetheless, with each day and every new experience, there were opportunities to learn new words and refine his understanding of words recently acquired. Let us continue to look at Abraham's communication from the perspective of his emerging language skills.

Twenty-One Months

Abraham visited us at the language clinic at 21 months of age. When he entered the large playroom, he was immediately attracted to the crayons and paper that we had set out on a child-sized picnic table. He loved to color, which at this point consisted of light marks scribbled mostly on the page, and occasionally on the table. Of course, at this age, Abraham's attention span for any one activity was fairly short, as we will see. When he began to color, his mother conducted the following conversation with him:

> **Mother:** You like to color, huh?
>
> **Abraham:** Gah!
>
> **Mother:** Yeah, you like to color, huh?
>
> **Abraham:** Ah deh. Out.
>
> **Mother:** Want to get out? (She lifts him out from between the table and bench.) You want to go look in that bag? Bring your bag. Bring the bag over here. (Abraham brings the bag.) All right! (Laughs.) What's in there?
>
> (Abraham and Mother look into the bag.)
>
> **Abraham:** Bribee (baby).
>
> **Mother:** Yeah.
>
> **Abraham:** Beebee (baby).
>
> **Mother:** That's your baby. (Takes it out.)
>
> **Abraham:** Night night. Deh coo.
>
> **Mother:** Blanket for the baby.
>
> **Abraham:** Deh yi gah.
>
> **Mother:** Yeah, that's your grrrr bear. (Takes it out.)
>
> (Abraham wanders off . . .)
>
> **Mother:** Where are you going, hun?
>
> **Abraham:** Ow meh.
>
> **Mother:** You're coming here?
>
> **Abraham:** Eeehhh. (yes).

> **Mother:** What else is in the bag?
>
> **Abraham:** Ehhh off. (Abraham pulls at the vest he is wearing.)
>
> **Mother:** Oh, we're gonna leave it on. Look how nice you look.
>
> **Abraham:** Ah hah.
>
> **Mother:** Very handsome.

This short conversation illustrates many aspects of Abraham's current stage of language acquisition. The first thing we notice is that, although he is now using words, we don't always understand what he is saying. Even his parents do not always understand everything he says. However, when the context gives clues to the meaning of the words (e.g., pulling objects out of a bag), his mother can translate his attempts into actual words. In fact, parents provide indirect feedback about the form of their children's language by repeating and expanding on their children's utterances (Demetras, Post, & Snow, 1986).

At this age, most of Abraham's language consists of single words. He is just beginning to use two-word combinations and an occasional three-word utterance as well. Clinicians often describe the stage of a child's early language development with reference to the average, or mean, length of utterance. In fact, this metric is so commonly used, it is typically referred to by the initials MLU. MLU is calculated by counting the number of morphemes in the child's utterances and calculating the average or mean number of morphemes used per utterance within the speech sample. At this age, Abraham's production of single words, with few multi-word combinations, is reflected by an overall MLU of 1.49. These utterances consist almost exclusively of content-rich words (e.g., nouns, verbs). Completely absent are any of the grammatical morphemes (e.g., articles, plurals, verb tense markers). In contrast, Abraham can comprehend much longer utterances than he is able to produce. For example, his mother's request ("Bring your bag.") and her direction to him ("Oh, we're gonna leave it on.") are longer than what he produced.

Abraham has between 50 and 100 different words in his language repertoire. However, his understanding of the meanings of words may be different than those of an adult. This is the age when toddlers point to strange men in grocery stores and exclaim "Daddy!" For them, the word *Daddy* may be broadly defined as including all adult males. The narrower meaning of "my male parent" will develop later. Conversely, other words may have too narrow a definition. *Doggie* may be used only with the household pet, and not for other dogs. Other words are actually social routines (e.g., *Night night*) or parts of songs, which may not be used outside of that specific context. As children grow in both experience and cognitive maturity, their understanding of the meaning of words will become more refined and adult-like.

Despite the fact that most of his language consists of single words, Abraham gets a lot of "mileage" out of those single words. He is actually able to convey a range of meanings with similar utterances, depending on the situational context and his intonation. When we look at his utterances from the perspective of language content and use, we can see this flexibility of expression.

Mother: We got a bunch of different books here.
Abraham: Elmo book! Elmo book!   (Content: Item name)
                                          (Use: Requests an action [reading])
Mother: You want to read the Elmo book?
Abraham: Elmo book.   (Content: Item name)
                                          (Use: Confirmation)

.

.

.

Mother: Who's that?
Abraham: Gower.   (Content: Character name)
                                          (Use: Labeling; reply to mother)
Mother: Grover.
Abraham: Gower coffee.   (Content: Possession)
                                          (Use: Comment)

Twenty-Eight Months

At 2 years of age, Abraham is quite the conversationalist. At this point, Abraham can be understood well by both family members and those who hear him speak less frequently. We can see an example when Abraham talks about his toddler gymnastics class.

Mother: What did you get to do at class?
Abraham: Jump!
Mother: You get to jump. On what?
Abraham: Trampoline.
Author: Did Mommy get to jump on the trampoline?
Abraham: Yeah.
Mother: Did I jump on that trampoline?
Abraham: No.
Mother: No.
Author: No? Why not?
Abraham: She want to get off.
Mother: Who else got to jump on it?
Abraham: Other boy turn.
Mother: Yeah. You guys shared, didn't you?
Abraham: Yeah. (Abraham crouches and makes a funny face.) Went
   nnnnngggggggggg.
Mother: Is that what he said?
Abraham: Yeah. I say that.

As this conversation illustrates, Abraham is talking in single words and short sentences. We hear the major content words (e.g., nouns, main verbs). We also hear the earliest acquired grammatical morphemes (e.g., "coming our house!" "Flowers."). However, most other grammatical units tend to be missing. In this early stage of language development, it is common to hear such "telegraphic speech" (Brown, 1976). Abraham's MLU on the day this conversation took place was 2.03, which is about average for children at this age.

We sometimes have difficulty understanding what Abraham says, not because the words themselves are mispronounced, but because he does not always provide enough information or background to convey the general context. For example, the word "jump" does not necessarily bring to mind bouncing on a trampoline when it is first said. In this case, Abraham's mother was filling in the background information and structure of the conversation by cueing him as to what information should be given next. In addition, children at this stage are likely to agree with what adults say, regardless of its actual truth, as we see here. Pragmatically, they understand that a positive response will continue the conversation, without appreciating that the listener's understanding has diverged from their own. Although Abraham's mother gets the conversation back on track, we can see that this tendency in young children can also lead to miscommunications.

Despite these limitations in form and content, Abraham is exhibiting a range of language use. During a play visit to the author at the clinic, we observed various pragmatic functions. The following is a small sample of these:

What that?	(request for information)
Mommy do it!	(request for action)
A doll.	(labeling)
Now him sad.	(commenting)
No! No!	(negating)

Thirty-Nine Months

Children's speech changes rapidly between the ages of 2 and 4. In twelve months, we can already see changes in the form of Abraham's language. We recorded this interaction between Abraham and his mother when Abraham was 39 months.

Mother: Oh, you know what? I should have brought your pictures of you and Christopher to show. They were so pretty. Remember?

Abraham: You forgot?

Mother: I forgot to bring them. They were really neat.

Abraham: The pictures that I made and colored?

Mother: Yep.

Author: You colored them by yourself?

Abraham: Mmmhmm. I made 'em mixed with for the sky.

Mother: Yep, you mixed the color of the sky.

Abraham: And I made the clouds inside.

Mother: You sure did.

Abraham: But the 'nuther one was messed up.

Mother: Well, yeah. You did make one that you didn't like much.

Abraham: It was messed up.

Mother: It was. But you really liked it because you put legs and feet and arms and hands.

Abraham: There wasn't enough room for the legs.

Although we still see a few form errors (e.g., *the 'nuther one'* for *'another one'*) we see noteworthy gains as well. Abraham increased the length of his utterances. His MLU on this day was 5.28. This is actually above average for his age. MLUs for children at this age typically range between 2.71 and 4.23 (Miller, 1981). Abraham's MLU fluctuates from day to day as well. In a sample collected one month later, his MLU was 4.03. Other aspects of language form are entirely appropriate for Abraham's age. Most of his utterances now are complete sentences with nouns and verbs serving as subjects and predicates. Notice that Abraham now uses both content words and a number of grammatical morphemes (e.g., past tense *-ed*; plural *s*, articles *the* and *a*). Occasionally, we see complex sentences (e.g., "The pictures that I made and colored?").

Compared with the conversation we saw at age 28 months, Abraham's contributions carry much more content. Instead of just providing input when prompted, he is now contributing new information spontaneously. There are still instances in which his meaning is not entirely clear (e.g., "And I made the clouds inside."), but most of the time others can follow his conversations with little effort.

We can clearly see how form, content, and use have developed and interact by revisiting some of the pragmatic functions we saw at 28 months and looking at the form and content now being used to code those functions at 39 months.

What does mine do?	(request for information)
Buy some at the store.	(request for action)
It is a tool.	(labeling)
That looks like a robot.	(commenting)
Mickey doesn't have shoes.	(negating)

At this age, Abraham is not just using language for communication with others, but for imaginative uses as well. He talks about what he is doing even when there is no one to hear or respond to him. The following excerpt was recorded while Abraham played alone with a large doll house and a family of dolls. What we hear is a verbal monologue of his ongoing thoughts as he plays. In this case, he is using language as a tool to organize and encode his thoughts and experiences in a pretend situation.

Oh, wow, oh man, I need all these guys. There's a bunch of people. I don't want the bunch of people, just a little bit. A little bit means, this is a little bit. Yeah, this is a little bit. (Looks at one figure.) Gross. I don't want you. Well, get your mom and dad. I'll get the mom. I'll get the dad. (Talks for the boy doll.) Mom, could we go to the park? Dad, could we go to the park? This is the park already. Okay, I want to sit right. Let's go over . . . let's take . . . take a nap. Our bed. Oh wow. Your bed is . . . my bed is right down . . . your bed is right down there. That's right. These are not the big people's. No, these are ours. The baby's is right there where his is. Mommy and Daddy are busy down there. You guys, you can't wait to go to the nap like that. You need someone to help you get into bed. You guys already got back into bed and get the baby.

Forty-Four Months

At age 4, children's language is adult-like in many respects. We rarely hear violations of language form, although we do hear false starts and revisions (even adults produce these periodically). At 44 months, Abraham's MLU is now 5.35, which indicates no increase in utterance length compared to five months before. In fact, Abraham has now passed the age where MLU is sensitive to gains in language acquisition. This is because his sentences are becoming more complex rather than becoming simply longer. We hear complex verb phrases ("He *wants to get* in there.") and conjoined sentences ("But not the boy, *'cause* he's hiding in a hiding place up there.").

The content of language continues to be dictated by experience. Children must hear new words to learn them (later, reading will contribute significantly to vocabulary growth). When children read a new book, play with others, go new places, or watch television programs, they are exposed to new words. Therefore, the words that children know depend, in large part, on their range of experience, which provides a context for new words to be learned. Once words are acquired, they are available to the child to help frame his or her future experiences and to support further learning. We can see the role of experience in building vocabulary when Abraham's preschool class made a trip to a local fire station. Although he had never been to one before, it was clear that he already had some very specific concepts about what a fire station is like and vocabulary to go along with the experience. In his case, a likely source of this vocabulary was a book that had been read to him many times. A home video captured the following conversation:

(The children enter the fire station.)

Abraham: What is . . . What's that? A fire truck. An old fire truck.

(The children go through the living areas.)

Abraham: We don't have one right here? We don't have a pole here?

Firefighter: We don't have a pole. There's only one or two left in the country that still has a pole and we don't . . .

Abraham: Whoa! Look at this. This is where the firefighter sleeps.

(The children look at the ambulance.)

Abraham: I have a question.

Firefighter: I have an answer. What can I do for you?

Abraham: These are the people that drive the ambulance?

Firefighter: That's right. Do you know I can drive this ambulance? That's my job.

In this conversation, we can see that Abraham is quite confident talking to others, although other children at this age may be shy. He is also beginning to show some of the subtleties of language use. For example, he uses the indirect "I have a question" before asking the actual question. We also see that his use of conversational conventions is still not perfect. Earlier, he asked a question and interrupted the adult before receiving the full answer. He will continue to refine skills within the domain of language use as he grows.

At 4 years of age, Abraham is developing skills in a second language modality—written language. His parents have been looking at books with him and reading to him since his first weeks. Through these activities, he has gained various preliteracy skills. These include awareness of print and the fact that information is carried by it. He also knows a set of social routines associated with reading: looking at a page and listening to the words, turning pages when the reading pauses, and even helping to fill in sentences for books he has heard over and over again. He enjoys both the books themselves and the attention he gets when he sits in his parent's lap to hear a book read. Abraham can identify the individual letters of the alphabet, although he makes some mistakes. He can print his name; typically with a giant A, a backwards b, and a letter or two that wanders above or below the horizontal plane on occasion. By this time next year, he will also recognize a handful of written words as well. All these skills are precursors to successful reading as he enters school. Within a few years of learning to read, this form of language will become an important tool for learning, exchange of ideas, and vocabulary growth.

In four short years, Abraham has gone from an infant, whose only means of expression was crying, to a preschooler whose language contains many of the features one would see in an adult speaker. In this chapter, we have seen the development of language *form* as he progressed from word attempts that were only approximations of the adult phonological form to fully intelligible speech. We saw single words progress to multiword phrases to sentences that contained clauses and complex verbs. We saw increased use of morphology as phrases and sentences emerged. We saw language *content* grow from the restricted meanings of the first few words to the multitude of words whose meanings approximate adult versions. Finally, we saw improvement in the *use* of language for a variety of communication functions. Although certain aspects of language form, content, and use will continue to expand as he grows, his language is, by age 4, already a remarkable tool for communication.

CLINICAL PROBLEM SOLVING

Here are two language samples obtained from Abraham at two different ages.

Twenty-eight months:
Mother: Is that a taco that you're making?
Abraham: Yeah.
Mother: Where do you eat tacos?
Abraham: With a mat.
Mother: On a placemat?
Abraham: (Pours beans into a bowl.) Put all in.
(They start to fall on the floor.)
Mother: Hey, honey, honey . . .
Abraham: Oh no, mommy!
Mother: Do you want help with the beans?
Abraham: It's a cooking beans!

Forty-four months:
Abraham: I ate eggs for breakfast.
Author: Did mommy make it?
Abraham: I got a gargoyle and I got a Casper today.
Author: What was the gargoyle on?
Abraham: They're just on my underwear.
Author: Oh, you have gargoyle underwear on.
Abraham: I have them not on today!
Author: You have Caspers on today?
Abraham: Yeah.

Look at the transcripts above and consider them from the perspective of language form, content, and use:

1. How has Abraham's language changed from 28 to 44 months?
2. Do you think that his content is typical of other children at each age? Why or why not?
3. What evidence can you find that Abraham has not yet reached adult-like competence in form, content, and use at each age?

REFERENCES

Bates, E. (1976). Pragmatics and sociolinguistics in child language. In D. Morehead & A. Morehead (Eds.), *Normal and deficient child language*. Baltimore: University Park Press.

Bates, E., Benigni, L., Bretherton, I., Camaioni, L., & Volterra, V. (1977). From gesture to the first word: On cognitive and social prerequisites. In M. Lewis & L. Rosenblum (Eds.), *Interaction, conversation, and the development of language*. New York: Wiley.

Bates, E., & MacWhinney, B. (1987). Competition, variation, and language learning. In B. MacWhinney (Ed.), *Mechanisms of language acquisition* (pp. 157–193). Hillsdale, NJ: Lawrence Erlbaum Associates.

Bloom, L. (1988). What is language? In M. Lahey, *Language disorders and language development*. New York: Macmillan.

Bookheimer, S. (2002). Functional MRI of language: New approaches to understanding the cortical organization of semantic processing. *Annual Review of Neuroscience, 25,* 151–188.

Brown, R. (1973). *A first language: The early stages.* Cambridge, MA: Harvard University Press.

Brown, R. (1976). *A first language.* New York: Penguin.

Bruner, J. S. (1975). The ontogenesis of speech acts. *Journal of Child Language, 2,* 1–19.

Cartwright, T. A., & Brent, M. R. (1997). Syntactic categorization in early language acquisition: Formalizing the role of distributional analysis. *Cognition, 63,* 121–170.

Chi, J. C., Dooling, F. C., & Gilles, F. H. (1977). Gyral development of the human brain. *Annals of Neurology, 1,* 86–93.

Chomsky, N. (1965). *Aspects of the theory of syntax.* Cambridge, MA: MIT Press

Chomsky, N. (1988). *Language and problems of knowledge: The Managua lectures.* Cambridge, MA: MIT Press.

Clark, E. (1979) What's in a word? On the child's acquisition of semantics in his first language. In V. Lee (Ed.), *Language development.* New York: Wiley.

Cruttenden, A. (1979). *Language in infancy and childhood.* New York: St. Martin's.

DeCasper, A. B., & Spence, M. B. (1986). Prenatal maternal speech influences newborns' perception of speech sounds. *Infant Behavior and Development, 9,* 133–150.

Demetras, M. J., Post, K. N., & Snow, C. E. (1986). Feedback to first language learners: The role of repetitions and clarification questions. *Journal of Child Language, 13,* 275–292.

Geschwind, N., & Levitsky, W. (1968). Human brain: Asymmetries in temporal speech region. *Science, 7,* 5097–5100.

Hertz-Pannier, L., Chiron, C., Jambaque, I., Renaux-Kieffer, V., Van de Moortele, P. F., Delalande, O., Fohlen, M., Brunelle, F., & Le Bihan, D. (2002). Late plasticity for language in a child's nondominant hemisphere: A pre- and postsurgery fMRI study. *Brain, 125,* 361–372.

Holland, S. K., Plante, E., Weber, A. M., Strawsburg, R. H., Schmithorst, V. J., & Ball, W. S. (2001). Functional MRI of brain activation patterns associated with normal language development. *NeuroImage, 14,* 837–843.

Hubbell, R. (1985). Language and linguistics. In P. Skinner & R. Shelton (Eds.), *Speech, language, and hearing* (2nd ed.). New York: Wiley.

Huiskens, L., Coppen, P. A., & Jagtman, M. (1991). Developing a tool for the description of language acquisition. *Linguistics, 29,* 451–479.

Ingram, D. (1981). Transitivity in child language. *Language, 47,* 888–910.

Kutas, M., & Hillyard, S. A. (1983). Event related brain potentials to grammatical errors and semantic anomalies. *Memory and Cognition, 11,* 539–550.

Lahey, M. (1988). *Language disorders and language development.* New York: Macmillan.

Lenneberg, F. (1967). *Biological foundations of language.* New York: Wiley.

Locke, J. (1990). Structure and stimulation in the ontogeny of spoken language. *Developmental Psychobiology, 23,* 621–643.

McClelland, J., & Rumelhart, D. (1986). A PDP model of the acquisition of morphology. In B. MacWhinney (Ed.), *Mechanisms of language acquisition.* Hillsdale, NJ: Lawrence Erlbaum.

McNeill, D. (1970). *The acquisition of language.* New York: Harper & Row.

Miller, J. (1981). *Experimental procedures: Assessing language production in children.* Baltimore, MD: University Park Press.

Molfese, D. L. (1990). Auditory evoked responses recorded from 16-month-old infants to words

they did and did not know. *Brain and Language, 38,* 345–363.

Oller, D. (1980). The emergence of speech sounds in infancy. In G. Yeni-Komshian, J. Kavanaugh, & C. Ferguson (Eds.), *Child phonology.* Vol. 1. *Production.* New York: Academic Press.

Piaget, J. (1963). *The origins of intelligence in children.* New York: Norton.

Pinker, S. (1984). *Language learnability and language development.* Cambridge, MA: Harvard University Press.

Plante, E., Creusere, M., & Sabin, C. (2002). Dissociating sentential prosody from sentence processing: Activation interacts with task demands. *NeuroImage, 17,* 401–410.

Rosen, H. J., Petersen, S. E., Linenweber, M. R., Snyder, A. Z., White, D. A., Chapman, L., Dromerick, A. W., Fiez, J. A., & Corbetta, M. D. (2000). Neural correlates of recovery from aphasia after damage to left inferior frontal cortex. *Neurology, 55,* 1883–1894.

Searle, B. (1969). Speech acts. London: Cambridge University Press.

Shaywitz, B. A., Shaywitz, S. E., Pugh, K. R., Fulbright, R. K., Skudlarski, P., Mencl, W. E., Constable, T., Marchione, K. E., Fletcher, J. M., Klorman, R., Lacadie, C., & Gore, J. C. (2001). The functional neural architecture of components of attention in language-processing tasks. *NeuroImage, 13,* 601–612.

Skinner, B. F. (1957). *Verbal behavior.* New York: Appleton-Century-Crofts.

Watson, B. B. (1970). *Behaviorism.* New York: Norton.

DISORDERS OF LANGUAGE IN CHILDREN

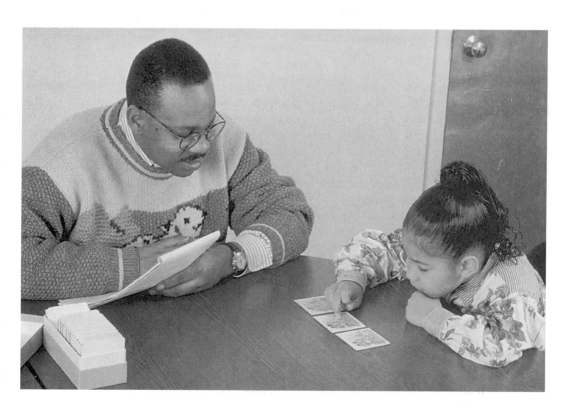

■ ■ ■ ■ ■

PREVIEW

When normal language acquisition is impeded because of a developmental disorder or childhood illness, language may become impaired. Language disorders in children may occur secondary to childhood illness or injury, but they often arise without identifiable cause.

For the young child, impaired oral language may interfere with the ability to express needs or understand what others say. As children progress through school, weak language skills may also impact reading, writing, and academic success. Because developmental language disorders result from a variety of causes and are associated with diverse skill profiles, assessment and intervention methods are tailored to the needs of the individual child.

As we discussed in Chapters 3 and 7, the development of language follows a fairly predictable sequence. Infants begin with an awareness of sound and quickly develop a preference for the sounds and patterns of their native language(s). Sounds, first produced reflexively, are soon produced intentionally and take on the characteristics of speech. Across cultures and languages, first words appear around the child's first birthday. By age 2, most children know many words and are combining them into short phrases. By age 4, children sound remarkably adult-like in their spoken language.

Not all children are so fortunate as to experience normal language acquisition. Language disorders may affect up to 13 percent of children (Tomblin, Records, & Zhang, 1996). A variety of conditions can lead to a language disorder. Genetic conditions may disturb the development of the brain and alter its capacity for normal language development. The presence of a hearing impairment can have a profound effect on language development. Injury or illness can arrest language development after a period of normal development. Finally, there is a wide variety of developmental syndromes that include impaired language as part of the presenting signs.

Although many conditions can lead to a language disorder, the types of skills affected may vary considerably. A language disorder includes any impairment of the ability to understand or use language—spoken, signed, or written—as well as same-age peers of the same community. Severity can vary widely among types of language disorders and even among children who are identified as having the same type of language disorder. Language disorders can affect language in any modality. In fact, it is often the case (although there are exceptions) that all modalities are affected to some extent when language is impaired. Language disorders are often first suspected because the child's language development lags behind the expected norms for children of the same age. The nature of the language disorder may change as age-expected language skills expand as the child grows. For example, language impairment will not affect reading until the child has reached an age

at which reading skills would be expected. Finally, language form, content, and use all vary from region to region and culture to culture. Therefore, language disorders must be distinguished from these regional and culturally derived differences.

LANGUAGE DIFFERENCES

There are children from particular cultural and social groups whose speech may differ in some respect from standard English. However, these differences do not, in themselves, constitute a language disorder. Such children have learned the language code of their community and may be quite competent in their use of the native language.

Some linguistic variation reflects regional differences in language, known as dialects. We recognize dialectal differences in how certain sounds are produced in the Northeast, or the Deep South, or the Midwest. Other differences may affect the choice of words that are used within a region. Carbonated drinks may be "soda" in one region and "pop" in another. Large-scale sandwiches on long rolls are "submarines," "hoagies," or "po' boys" depending on the region. Dialects can vary with social or cultural groups within a particular region. Communities with strong Hispanic roots may use a variant of English that includes influences from Spanish. Residents of both inner cities and rural districts may speak one or more versions of a dialect known as Black English (sometimes called Ebonics). Although these dialects are culturally influenced, speakers do not necessarily have to be members of the particular minority group to speak the dialect. Furthermore, any given speaker of a dialect may not use it at all times. Social rules may dictate when a dialect, or even which variant of a dialect, is appropriate to the situation. So, an individual who uses one version of Black English among friends may use another with parents and switch to standard English when addressing a teacher. This situational shifting of speech and language patterns is referred to as **code switching**.

The variations in language *form* observed in dialects are rule governed, meaning that there are strict conventions that dictate correct use of these forms. However, for the listener who is unfamiliar with the conventions of a dialect, it may seem as if the speaker is making linguistic errors. For example, residents of Maryland may "go down the shore for the weekend," omitting the preposition "to" that speakers in other parts of the country would typically use in that sentence. Forms of Black English may include omissions of certain grammatical forms (e.g., the contracted "is" or "are"; the infinitive "to") and changes in grammatical form (e.g., "hisself" for "himself"; "be" for "has been [continually]") in certain sentence contexts. These are normal forms within some versions of this dialect. However, not all speakers of Black English and other dialects use all the linguistic or pragmatic elements associated with the dialect. For example, Washington and Craig (1994) reported that young children within the same region may vary in their frequency and types of Black English forms in their speech. Speech-language pathologists must be able to distinguish between linguistic variation that reflects a dialect and

variation that signals a disorder and to treat those aspects that are attributable to the disorder alone. However, if a dialect speaker, who shows no sign of a language disorder, wishes to improve his or her use of standard English, a speech-language pathologist may provide such assistance (ASHA, 1983).

Children who speak more than one language may also show language differences that may be mistaken for a disorder. For example, the Navajo child in northeastern Arizona may be bilingual, using Navajo at home and English at school. Vocabulary development in each language may be restricted to the environment in which it is used. These children may appear to have limited lexical knowledge when tested in only one of their languages, but often have a large and rich vocabulary when both languages are considered. If a Navajo child moves to Los Angeles, his or her language *use* might be judged faulty by the non-Navajo listeners in the new city. Children in many parts of the world are multilingual, using a particular language for a specific situation. For most children, learning two or more languages (or dialects) in the preschool years is relatively easy given adequate experience with those languages. Some children, however, are unable to use any of the languages of their community proficiently.

EARLY SIGNS OF A LANGUAGE DISORDER

Infants at Risk

Some infants are born with genetic conditions, illnesses, or disabilities that interfere with their development (Clark, 1994; Sparks, 1984). In Chapter 11, we will see that a great many genetic and acquired conditions may affect hearing and consequently alter the course of language development. Many other conditions, such as drug exposure (Johnson, Seikel, Madison, Foose, & Rinard, 1997), infection (Bent & Beck, 1994), low birth weight, and premature birth (Byrne, Ellsworth, Bowering, & Vincer, 1993), increase the risk that a child will experience language and learning difficulties. In some cases, prolonged serious illness itself may interfere with language development. Infants who require hospitalization will not receive the same stimulation from their parents as a healthy baby. Babies who are confined to a hospital nursery will have limited opportunities to explore and interact with the people and objects around them. Other infants have physical disabilities that interfere with normal development, including speech and language development.

A speech-language pathologist may work with an infant's family and the hospital staff to provide experiences that facilitate language development. In these cases, speech and language intervention often must be integrated with medical treatments, physical therapy, and occupational therapy. The speech-language pathologist and audiologist are members of a multidisciplinary team, which may also include medical staff, rehabilitation staff, and social services. The team works closely with the infant's family to ensure understanding of the child's needs and how to best address them. When a child is born with an obvious disability, parent counseling and intervention for the child can begin right away. However, the im-

pact of prematurity on language and academic disorders can appear years later as the child develops (e.g., Halsey, Collin, & Anderson, 1996). Therefore, parents and professionals may need to monitor progress throughout childhood.

Late Talkers

One group of children at risk for language disorders are toddlers who lag behind their peers in the ability to understand or produce words. These children have been referred to as "late talkers." In the research literature, late talkers are typically defined as young children (between approximately 16 and 30 months) whose language skills fall below 90 percent of their age peers. These children are slow to acquire their first fifty words and slow to combine words into phrases. For example, Rescorla, Roberts, and Daahlsgard (1997) reported their group of late talkers had an average of twenty words at age 26 months, compared with their normal peers who had an average of 226 words. Furthermore, only one of thirty-four late talkers was combining words into phrases. The parents of late-talking toddlers may also report that their children seem to understand fewer words than would be expected for their age. These children lack a history of hearing loss, cognitive impairment, or medical factors that would otherwise place them at risk for poor language development.

Investigators who have followed the development of late-talking children have demonstrated that these children are at risk for continued language problems. Toddlers who are identified as late talkers tend to remain behind their peers over time (Rescorla et al., 1997; Thal, Bates, Goodman, & Jahn-Samilo, 1997). However, what is true for the group is not necessarily true for all its members. In fact, some late talkers do "catch up" with their peers (Ellis Weismer, Murray-Branch, & Miller, 1994; Rescorla et al., 1997; Thal, et al., 1997). There is currently no clear consensus concerning what factors present at early ages might predict which children prove to be "late bloomers" and which will continue to experience language difficulty. Some studies have suggested factors that predict language outcome include poor comprehension skills (Thal & Tobias, 1992), limited use of gestures for communication (Thal et al., 1997; Thal & Tobias, 1992), limited vocabulary (Fischel et al., 1989; Thal et al., 1997), and initial severity (Rescorla et al., 1997; Rescorla & Schwartz, 1990). In addition, the older a child is when identified as a late talker also appears to be predictive, with the younger children in the groups faring better than slightly older late talkers (Paul, 1993; Rescorla & Schwartz, 1990; Thal et al., 1997).

Late-talking toddlers are typically first identified by their impoverished vocabularies. However, for those late talkers who do not move into the normal range, a variety of language signs emerge over time. As we saw in Chapter 7, normally developing children acquire a corpus of single-word utterances that they then begin to combine into two-word utterances. From this point, children lengthen their phrases and eventually begin to produce more complex sentences. However, by age 3 or 4, children who were late-talking toddlers produced much shorter and morphologically and syntactically simpler phrases than their normally developing peers (Paul & Alforde, 1993; Rescorla et al., 1997). Interestingly, many of these

late-talking toddlers moved into the normal range for their vocabulary skills (Rescorla et al., 1997). Kindergarten children who were late talkers were less proficient in relating a story in logical order than their normally developing peers (Paul, Hernandez, Taylor, & Johnson, 1996). By second grade, however, these children appeared to have caught up in terms of narrative ability. However, there were still other differences in expressive language skills between the late-talking group and their peers (Paul, Murray, Clancy, & Andrews, 1997).

These studies demonstrate the long-term sequelae associated with late-talking status as a toddler. However, we also saw that not all late-talking toddlers have a poor language outcome. Despite our imperfect ability to predict outcome, status as a "late talker" is sufficient to indicate risk for language disorder. The long-term risk warrants close monitoring of late-talking children so that those who go on to show clear signs of a language disorder may receive the earliest possible intervention (Thal et al., 1997).

DEVELOPMENTAL LANGUAGE DISORDERS

For many children with language problems, there is no obvious cause for the impairment. They do not have the physical characteristics that would signal the presence of a developmental syndrome. Likewise, their cognitive abilities are good, ruling out mental retardation as a cause for poor language skills. They hear normally and lack any sign of brain damage or disease that might lead to impaired language, but their language skills lag behind those of their peers. These children are said to have a **developmental language disorder**.

Developmental language disorder is actually an umbrella term that encompasses children with a wide range of language-related problems. Although the exact cause of these disorders is unknown, parents are often relieved to know that it does not appear to be related to rearing practices or the way they have talked to their child. Instead, the underlying cause appears to be biological. Current information suggests that the brains of language-disordered children develop differently from most people (Cohen, Campbell, & Yaghmai, 1989; Gauger, Lombardino, & Leonard, 1997; Plante, Swisher, Vance, & Rapcsak, 1991). This altered brain development may underlie altered language development. Evidence of altered brain anatomy can also be found among the parents and siblings of these children (Jackson & Plante, 1997; Plante, 1991). Likewise, when one member of the family has a developmental language disorder, it is common that others do also (e.g., Tallal, Ross, & Curtiss, 1989; Tomblin, 1989). The fact that both the biological and behavioral aspects of this disorder tend to cluster in families suggests that it may be inherited in some cases.

Children may have developmental problems with receptive language, expressive language, or both. Language deficits may encompass any or all of the components of language *form*, *content*, or *use* (see Chapter 7 for a review) and any individual child's language difficulties may change over time. When language deficits occur in the absence of other handicapping conditions (e.g., cognitive, motor, sensory, emo-

tional), the child is said to have a **specific language impairment**. To understand this disorder, let us look at the development of one child diagnosed with specific language impairment.

> Troy had difficulty with communication from a very early age. He was reportedly about 20 months of age before he used his first word. His parents became concerned when at age 2 he used few words, communicating instead largely by grunting and pointing. Despite his limited expression, both parents felt that he understood speech well for his age. Troy's pediatrician also noticed his slow language development and arranged for him to be evaluated by a speech-language pathologist.
>
> During his initial evaluation, Troy passed a hearing screening. His parents completed a questionnaire that surveyed cognitive, motor, self-help, and social skills. Their responses placed him well within normal limits for each of these areas. Troy was then given a formal evaluation of language skills that involved a series of simple activities to test receptive and expressive skills. He correctly pointed to pictures and followed commands appropriately for his age. Test scores for receptive language confirmed relatively normal skills in that domain. In contrast, his expressive score placed him in the first percentile, or below 99 percent of other children his age. He had great difficulty naming pictures and imitating words on request. He often used the same "word" /da/, to refer to a variety of pictures and objects. In addition, Troy had a limited number of sounds that he used spontaneously, relying mostly on stop consonant-vowel combinations in the words he attempted.

In Troy's case, early deficits involved vocabulary and phonology. These delayed communication skills were present despite the fact that he was developing normally in other areas. As we saw in our discussion of late talkers, such delay is a risk factor for a developmental language disorder. However, not all children with a developmental language disorder are noticeably different from other children at this young age. For some, the first words emerge right on schedule for normal development, and the disorder only becomes apparent as the child fails to progress from words to sentences.

> Troy was enrolled in a preschool program for children with specific language impairment at age 3. His parents reported remarkable improvement from that time forward. In addition to his preschool class, his parents implemented a home program of language stimulation. This involved techniques for introducing new vocabulary and encouraging him to produce longer utterances. Troy's vocabulary expanded rapidly from fourteen words to well over 100 words in five months. His phonological repertoire also expanded, so that he was producing many more of the sounds appropriate for his age. At age 3, he was occasionally combining words to form two-word utterances as well. His mother reported that Troy was showing fewer signs of frustration in his attempts to communicate and that people outside of the family were having much less difficulty understanding his speech.
>
> At age 4, Troy was using many two- and three-word phrases, with an occasional four-word phrase in spontaneous speech. However, he used few grammatical morphemes (e.g., verb tense markers, prepositions), which is unusual for a child

his age. At age 4 years, 7 months, the following conversation was recorded while he played with a toy fire station:

> **Troy:**   This the fireperson. This the bell (indicating the fire alarm).
> **Mother:**   Does the bell ring in an emergency?
> **Troy:**   No. The bell, it has . . . the car come out.
> **Mother:**   The cars come out when the bell rings?
> **Troy:**   (nods) The telephone do that too!

Not surprisingly, formal tests documented below-normal expressive language skills at this time, including morphology and syntax. Although language form was still delayed, Troy showed marked improvement in language content and use. He spoke readily in a variety of contexts and was able to use language for a variety of purposes (e.g., requesting, explaining, directing).

This pattern of differential impairment across language domains is fairly common during the preschool years. In Troy's case, we observed a shift from the initial vocabulary deficit, which was apparent at age 2, to morphosyntactic deficits at age 4. This phenomenon is known as "growing into a deficit." We did not see morphosyntactic deficits early on simply because English-speaking children do not use syntax or morphology until words are combined into phrases. Therefore, we had to wait until Troy reached a developmental stage where these skills could be expected before determining whether they were impaired.

Some children with early language disorders ultimately achieve parity with their normally developing peers. For some, this marks the end of their language difficulties. However, for others, this period is temporary and is referred to as a period of "illusory recovery" (Scarborough & Dobrich, 1990) because these children who appear to recover once again fall behind their peers as they progress through grade school. In addition to these children are others who continue to show signs of language deficits as they enter the school years. We saw this pattern with Troy.

Troy's speech and language skills were reevaluated by the school speech-language pathologist when he entered first grade at 5 years 9 months. At that time, his early problems with phonology were almost completely resolved. His speech could be easily understood. The only remaining errors were occasional mispronunciations in conversation, and these involved only the late-acquired sounds of speech (see Chapter 3). However, his conversations consisted primarily of short, simple sentences. He continued to have difficulty with grammatical morphemes, making substitutions like "the paint guy" for "painter" and "the more big one" for "bigger" or omissions like "He run" for "He runs." Once again, formal testing documented poor language expression despite good overall comprehension. Both receptive and expressive vocabulary remained strong.

The school speech-language pathologist continued to see Troy twice a week to work on morphology. She also coordinated activities with the classroom teacher and Troy's parents to reinforce correct use of the morphological items that Troy was learning. This intervention was quite successful, and by the middle of second grade, Troy's conversational speech no longer contained obvious morphological errors. He was retested at this time because the school was considering his dismissal from

therapy. However, his standardized test scores continued to indicate that his expressive language skills lagged behind his peers. Because he was keeping up in the classroom and was doing well socially, it appeared that his weak expressive language skills were not a handicapping factor at this time. The school decided to monitor his progress, but to discontinue direct services.

The school staff's decision to discontinue services for Troy is consistent with their mandate to provide services to children with *educationally handicapping conditions*. The public law (P.L. 94-142) that first mandated services in 1975 guaranteed a free and appropriate education for all children with educationally handicapping conditions. Speech and language disorders are among the disorders covered under this law and subsequent legislation (P.L. 99-457, Individuals with Disabilities Education Act [IDEA], see also Chapter 11). Because Troy was functioning well in the educational system, the school staff decided he was best served in the regular classroom with monitoring and consultative support by the speech-language pathologist. For Troy, this educational plan places him in the *least restrictive environment* in which he is capable of functioning.

Other children with more serious handicaps may require greater educational support. This may include "pullout" services, in which the child leaves the classroom for brief periods of direct therapy, placement in special classrooms within the regular school, or even in specialized schools for severely handicapped children. Each of these modes of intervention involves increasing restrictions on the child's environment because less time is spent with normally developing peers. The type and frequency of service each child receives may change over the years as the degree to which the child's disorder impacts educational progress changes. The type and frequency of the child's services are determined by a multidisciplinary team that includes parents, teachers, therapists, and others who can provide insight into a particular child's learning difficulties. This team develops an *individualized educational plan* (IEP) that specifies the level of services, who will provide the services, and what the goals will be.

Three years later, at age 10, Troy's skills were reevaluated. This testing session revealed a shift in his language profile. Although his comprehension skills were previously a relative strength, comprehension skills had fallen below the average range at this time. This may well be another instance of "growing into the deficit" because these problems emerged at an age at which comprehension demands increase. This pattern of worsening comprehension, seen in Figure 8.1, was maintained into the teenage years. In fact, by age 14, his expressive skills exceeded his receptive skills. This impairment was significant because comprehension skills become increasingly important in later school years. The sentences spoken by teachers are often longer and more syntactically complex than those heard in casual conversation. Students are expected to conduct multiple language tasks simultaneously: listening to the teacher lecture, extracting the principal concepts, and encoding them as written notes. Comprehension becomes a learning tool, not just in listening but also in reading. Reading comprehension is a major source of vocabulary growth and academic learning throughout the school years.

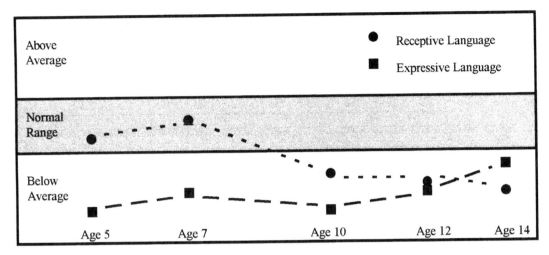

FIGURE 8.1   For children with developmental language disorders, the components of language can change over time. Here we can see receptive and expressive language skills shift over time in a single child (Troy) relative to typically developing peers.

Troy's expressive skills showed only slight improvement relative to others his age on standardized tests (see Figure 8.1). Once again, as children reach an age where more complex use of language is expected, new deficits may appear. Consider his attempt to relate the plot of a movie during a conversation, recorded when Troy was 12 years old:

> "It was hilarious. He didn't put the . . . um . . . 'owies.' He only put the best 'owie.' No, that was the second best 'owie.' The first was when the rope that he went down was soaked in some kind of thing . . . that it makes fire go on . . . makes it go faster and they were on the rope and say 'Hey Harry, are you there?' No, that's Clorox, or something like that. (Speaks for a movie character.) 'Oh guys.' (sound effect of guys falling) 'Get up! Get up!' (sound effect of guys yelling and hand gestures.) Then there's like a bridge and they fall right through and they get covered with all kinds of . . . sticky stuff.

We can see a number of problems in this short sample. First, the story he is telling lacks the structure of a identifiable beginning, middle, and end. Characters are referred to without first being introduced to the listener (e.g., He didn't put the . . . um . . . "owies"). We hear pauses and revisions throughout. In addition, the use of sound effects and gestures suggested that he may have been having difficulty retrieving specific words to communicate his thoughts.

The ability to organize and sequence verbal information becomes increasingly important as a child progresses through school. In fact, Troy's written work shows many of the same characteristics that we see in the verbal sample above. In

addition, he often made the same morphological errors in written language that we saw in his spoken language at age 5. For example, at age 12 he wrote:

Mom caned the riped vejedetables.

I don't wan't any.

But the two dog eat it.

At this point, Troy's language difficulties were again interfering with his academic progress. His reading was slow, and he did not always glean as much meaning from reading as he should. His writing was messy, with many spelling errors, and the flow of thoughts did not always follow a logical sequence. Because his weak language skills were having the greatest impact on educational skills, the school staff considered providing services for a **learning disability**. Children with learning disabilities often have difficulties in listening, speaking, reading, or writing. Their poor language skills can hold them back in any academic subject in which language is used as a tool for learning or problem solving.

The long-term outcome of children with developmental language disorders is quite variable. Some will overcome the handicap of an early language disorder. Others may struggle with language in either the oral or written modalities for years. Even as adults, individuals with a history of language therapy may still show subtle, residual deficits on standardized measures (Tomblin, Records, & Freese, 1992). However, these language difficulties may or may not prove handicapping in the individual's everyday life. In fact, adults with a childhood history of language disorders appear no less satisfied with their quality of life than those without such a childhood history (Records, Tomblin, & Freese, 1992).

Reading Impairments

Reading and writing require a child to apply what he or she already understands about oral language to visual-manual modalities. Just as oral language skills begin to develop before the child says his or her first words, literacy skills begin to develop far before the child can read his or her first words. When a young child is read to, he or she learns critical skills that will support later reading. As early as the first year of life, we have seen that a child who is read to learns the "routines" of reading. These include your holding a book so that its pages are easy to see. The child hears a few lines spoken and then pages are turned. The child views pictures that go along with the words, and these pictures give cues to the story's content. Later, the child will realize that the printed words on a page relate to the words that the reader says. A child who is read to frequently may even be able to recognize a few words that recur in favorite books, even before formal reading instruction takes place. These preliteracy skills give children who have been read to a head start on formal reading instruction because they already know quite a bit about books and what they are for. Conversely, children who come from households where books are scarce may already be at a disadvantage for reading because

they have missed these early literacy experiences. One role that a speech-language pathologist may play in fostering literacy is to encourage parents (and sometimes train them) to read to their young children to facilitate both oral language skills and later literacy skills (Dale, Crain-Thoreson, Notari-Syverson, & Cole, 1996).

As children move from informal experiences with books to formal instruction, they bring to bear preexisting oral language skills to the task of reading. When language skills are poor, as in the case of a developmental language disorder, reading and writing skills may also be impaired. Let us consider the case of Jimmy.

> Jimmy had received therapy for a speech and language impairment as a preschool child. Therapy was successful in that Jimmy's oral language was comparable to his peers by the time he left kindergarten. Therapy was discontinued at that time. In second grade, however, his teacher asked the reading resources specialist to assess Jimmy's reading skills. The specialist gave Jimmy a short passage from a second-grade book to read. At first, Jimmy attempted to avoid reading by calling the specialist's attention to a number of other things in the room. When he finally picked up the book, he announced that "he didn't know any of these words." When asked to sound out the first word, Jimmy named the first letter but was unable to say what sound it made. For other words, he would attempt the first sound, but could not go on to other sounds in the word.

Jimmy shows a marked deficit in the ability to sound out words from their letters. This skill, known as **phonological decoding**, is a skill that we all use when we encounter an unfamiliar word. However, some children have a great deal of difficulty associating the different letters with their sounds and have difficulty recognizing words when they string together sequences of phonemes. Jimmy had slid by until second grade because he was able to memorize the words in his first-grade reader by sight. Although developing a **sight word vocabulary** of memorized words is helpful for quickly reading words that occur frequently in text (e.g., *the, a, is*), this strategy could not carry Jimmy's reading beyond a preliminary level. Jimmy had also applied this memorization strategy to spelling as well. Although he received As on his weekly spelling quizzes of words he had studied, he was unable to apply the rules of spelling (e.g., *ph* sounds like *f, i* before *e* except after *c* . . .) to new words. His attempts at unfamiliar words were nearly random.

Children who have difficulty with phonological decoding, but not other aspects of reading, are sometimes referred to as having **dyslexia**. However, problems with phonological decoding are only one reason for poor reading skills. Let us consider the case of Carlos. Like Jimmy, Carlos also had a history of speech and language difficulties and had therapy from the age of 4.

> Carlos was a participant in a longitudinal research study that tracked children with early language disorders. His initial deficits, when enrolled in the study at age 5, included expressive problems with grammar and vocabulary. As he matured, it became apparent that he also had comprehension problems. His preliteracy skills at age 5 were good, because he came from a home in which both his mother and older brother read to him frequently. By third grade, Carlos' mother reported that he

was a good reader when made to do it, but he did not read for enjoyment. However, his reading assessment indicated a different profile. When asked to read a fairy tale, he read aloud with good pronunciation of the words and at a normal speaking rate. When he encountered an unfamiliar word, he successfully sounded it out. His oral reading was entirely consistent with his mother's report that he was a "good reader." He then went on to answer questions about the story. Although his answers were vaguely related to the story, it was apparent that Carlos had misunderstood key elements of the plot. For example, the story's main character had attempted to break into the grounds of a zoo, but Carlos reported that this character was trying to escape from the zoo. When asked to retell the story in his own words, it was apparent that Carlos understood very little of what he had read. When pressed for information he did not know, he simply made up an answer that seemed plausible based on what he did understand.

This case illustrates that phonological decoding is not enough to assure good reading. Comprehension is also key. When children have difficulty in comprehending oral language, they frequently also have difficulty with comprehension of written language as well. However, it is also possible to have comprehension problems in reading when oral language comprehension is within normal limits. Let us reconsider the case of Jimmy. When children struggle to sound out word after word as they read, they often have difficulty building any mental representation of what those words are intended to convey. Therefore, children may show poor comprehension because they have exhausted all their cognitive resources in phonological decoding at the expense of comprehension.

In addition to his reading, Carlos' writing also had limitations. His written stories for school tended to be short with very simple sentences. He rarely used adjectives to make his writing more colorful or conjunctions to integrate more than one thought into one sentence. Occasionally, his writing contained grammatical errors; these frequently involved verb errors. In contrast, his spelling was good.

These cases illustrate that children with early problems with oral language can go on to have problems in reading and writing. Although there are exceptions to this pattern, the relation is strong enough that early speech and language problems are considered a significant risk factor in predicting later reading ability (Bishop & Adams, 1990; Lewis & Freebairn, 1992; Menyuk & Chesnick, 1997; Snyder & Downey, 1997). Because of this link, speech-language pathologists may be called to serve a role in literacy instruction for these children (ASHA, 2001). The speech-language pathologist's knowledge about the links between oral and written language skills can help parents and teachers understand why particular deficits arise and can often provide suggestions to facilitate literacy instruction for these children.

The role of language disorders in reading goes beyond our introduction here. Readers interested in further information can consult texts by Bain, Bailes, and Moats (2001), Kamhi and Catts (1999), Paul (1995), or Butler and Silliman (2002).

OTHER DISORDERS THAT IMPACT LANGUAGE

Children experience difficulty with language for a variety of reasons. In the 1950s, the audiologist and speech-language pathologist tended to emphasize the cause, or etiology, of the child's language disorder. With the growth of behavioral and operant psychology in the 1960s, however, emphasis switched from etiology per se to changing the child's behavior regardless of etiology. However, knowledge of etiology presents at least two primary advantages. The first is being able to address parents' desires to know "why" their child has a disorder (Aram, 1991). The second involves clinical management. The initial diagnosis can serve to orient the clinician to the likely behavioral strengths and weaknesses. Given a diagnosis of seizure disorder, for example, a clinician is alerted by the diagnostic category to examine receptive language skills. The same clinician, faced with a case involving dyslexia would be prepared to evaluate the potential impact of language on reading abilities. Although the diagnostic "label" does not predict with 100 percent accuracy an individual's true profile, it can orient the clinician to what the most salient problems may be. Let us take a look at a small selection of the many conditions associated with impaired language to see how language may vary with different developmental conditions.

Attention Deficit Disorder

Children with Attention Deficit Disorder (ADD) are characterized by inattention and impulsivity, with hyperactivity occurring in a subset of children with ADD. Children with ADD are highly distractable, finding it difficult to focus, sustain their attention, and direct their activities toward the task at hand. These signs occur in the absence of any frank neurological deficit or acquired disorder. Parents often report that the first signs appear in the preschool years, although children may not be referred for services until their difficulties cause them problems in school. Their difficulties with attention and impulse control are a significant handicap in the classroom, interfering with the ability to listen to directions and complete work assignments. It is not surprising, therefore, that most children with ADD have difficulty learning. The signs of ADD can persist throughout the childhood years, with an estimated one-half to two-thirds of individuals continuing to show signs in late adolescence (Claude & Firestone, 1995; McGee, Partridge, Williams, & Silva, 1991).

The distractibility and impulsivity that interfere with school work are equally disruptive in games and conversations. Other children may view the ADD child as a troublemaker who breaks both rules and toys. Children with ADD often interrupt others who are trying to talk, shift from topic to topic without warning, and otherwise appear to have difficulties with the social aspects of language use. Other language problems may be a side effect of inattention. For example, children whose attention fluctuates may miss parts of what is said to them, mimicking a comprehension deficit. A subset of children with ADD also have coexisting speech and language disorders that are independent of attentional problems. For this reason, the American Speech-Language-Hearing Association (ASHA, 1997) rec-

ommended that speech-language pathologists and audiologists serve on multidisciplinary teams for the assessment of children with ADD.

The signs of ADD may be managed medically and behaviorally. Stimulant medications help some children by increasing attention and decreasing impulsive and hyperactive behaviors. Medication, even when beneficial, does not cure the disorder. Behavioral intervention is designed to provide the child with methods for staying on task and minimizing the effects of ADD in daily life. Some intervention techniques involve modifying the child's environment by providing routine and structure to support on-task behaviors. Rewards or recognition may also be effective in promoting appropriate behaviors. For older children, helping them develop plans for monitoring their own conduct may be appropriate.

Autism

The term *autism* describes a developmental disorder that profoundly affects the child's interactions with other people and with the world. The earliest signs of the disorder include disturbed social interaction between the infant and its parents. Even as infants, these children do not seem to bond with or take comfort from others. They may seem content watching the movements of their hands or performing repetitive actions. A majority of children with autism fall into the mentally retarded range of intellectual functioning. However, not all cognitive domains are equally affected. Minshew, Goldstein, and Siegel (1997) tested autistic individuals whose IQ scores fell within normal limits (although many were lower than average) and found that these individuals' greatest deficits involved the ability to handle complex information processing in many forms (e.g., high-level language tasks, complex memory). Simple information processing systems and visual-spatial memory were relatively spared.

As children with autism grow, other aspects of disturbed communication become apparent. Some of these children acquire some early language skills, only to lose them during the preschool years. For others, language development is disturbed from the start. Dunn (1997) reviewed the characteristics of autistic language, which can include deficits in language form, content, and use. Common characteristics include poor language comprehension and poor pragmatic skills. In more severe forms of the disorder, expressive language characteristics may become more apparent. A complete lack of speech, or mutism, is most likely to occur when the signs of autism are most severe (Miranda-Linne & Merlin, 1997).

The language signs most typical of this disorder involve disturbances of language *use*. Individuals with autism frequently have disturbed prosody in spoken language. They may repeat the words of others (a characteristic called *echolalia*) or use stereotyped speech routines rather than the original and context-appropriate speech of normally developing children. For example, one child repeated the phrase "want juice please" over and over again as he spun in a circle. However, this was not an actual request for juice, but continued use of a phrase beyond the setting in which it was appropriate. The bizarre elements of their communication also extend to nonverbal pragmatics. For example, children with autism often have

a flat facial affect and aberrant patterns of attention to people and objects and abnormal gaze during conversations (Lord & Pickles, 1996; Shields, Varley, Broks, & Simpson, 1996).

The bizarre social interactions of these children led early investigators to hypothesize that autism was the product of uncaring parents who failed to provide the emotional support children require (Kanner & Eisenberg, 1955). Later, more biological explanations of the disorder were offered (e.g., Rimland, 1964). Today, we have evidence of abnormal brain development in autistic individuals (e.g., Courchesne, Yeung-Courchesne, Press, Hesselink, & Jernigan, 1988) and preliminary evidence of a genetic role in the disorder (Petit, Herlault, Martineau, et al., 1995).

Mental Retardation

Language is complex and depends, in part, on other cognitive and social-adaptive skills. Children who are slow in all aspects of development are frequently also slow in the acquisition of language skills. The *Diagnostic and Statistical Manual of Mental Disorders* (DSM-IV; APA, 1994) defines **mental retardation** by an intelligence quotient (IQ) of less than 70 on a standardized IQ measure along with significant deficits in adaptive functioning. Even when IQ is low, an individual who shows no difficulty functioning in everyday life would not be considered to have mental retardation. The degree of mental retardation can vary considerably. DSM-IV recognizes four broad severity levels: mild, moderate, severe, and profound, which reflect a range from individuals considered "educable" to those few who require lifelong assistance.

There are many developmental conditions associated with mental retardation. Some of these are genetic (e.g., Down syndrome, Noonan syndrome, fragile X syndrome), some are due to exposure to toxins (e.g., fetal alcohol syndrome, lead poisoning), and for others the cause is unknown (idiopathic mental retardation). Given the range of conditions associated with mental retardation, it is not surprising that the language correlates can be quite variable. In general, however, children with mental retardation are slow to acquire communication skills. Even at the prelinguistic stage, some toddlers with retardation are less interactive and use fewer nonverbal forms of communication than normally developing children at these ages. The onset of spoken words may occur at a later chronological age. General language ability in retarded children is frequently reported to be like that of younger, normally developing children.

As noted, however, this general profile may not apply to all conditions associated with mental retardation. Children with different types of mental retardation have more difficulty with certain areas of language development than others. For example, some children with Down syndrome appear to have particular problems with syntax and morphology (Stoel-Gammon, 1990). In contrast, children with Williams syndrome are unusually proficient in syntax and morphology, despite having poor semantic skills (Bellugi, Marks, Bihrle, & Sabo, 1988). Children with fragile X syndrome tend to have particular problems with verbal and nonverbal pragmatic skills (Scharfenaker, 1990). Within any group of retarded children, there

is much individual variability in the acquisition of language skills. With guidance, retarded children can learn to maximize their communication skills.

Childhood Aphasia

Children who were developing normally can lose language skills because of brain damage. This acquired language disorder is known as childhood aphasia. Aphasia in children can be caused by the same disease processes that cause adult aphasia (see Chapter 9). These include relatively focal trauma to the head, stroke, infectious disease, tumor, or seizures. Also similar to the adult form of aphasia, language deficits typically occur after damage to the left hemisphere of the brain (Aram, Ekelman, Rose, & Whitaker, 1985; Cranberg, Filley, Hart, & Alexander, 1987). We see one such case with Daniel:

> Daniel was 4½ years old when he began having daily headaches, which were soon accompanied by behavioral problems and vomiting. He was taken to the hospital and received a brain scan. This revealed a large tumor in the temporal-parietal area of his left hemisphere. He was immediately scheduled for surgery to remove the tumor. On the morning following surgery, Daniel was unable to speak and showed signs of weakness on the right side of his body. A second brain scan showed that he had had a stroke, caused by bleeding of the middle cerebral artery, which damaged the language areas of the left hemisphere (see Chapter 2 for a review).
>
> Within days, Daniel began talking, but his speech and language were not at the level they had been before he was hospitalized. Initially, his speech was slow and effortful, and he drooled intermittently. He had great difficulty attending to what was said and could only follow simple directions. A preschool test of general language abilities indicated low language skills compared with others his age. He had difficulty naming pictures on a vocabulary test. Many times when speaking, he would substitute nonspecific pronouns for specific nouns (e.g., "push thing" for wagon; "the one" for any object). In addition, Daniel had difficulty on a test that required him to produce grammatical sentences to describe pictures. The speech-language pathologist worked with him three times a week until Daniel was released from the hospital. She also arranged to have Daniel enrolled in a preschool program for children with language disorders after he left the hospital.

An estimated three in 100,000 children each year experience a stroke (NIDCD, 1991). When the stroke leads to aphasia, children show difficulty comprehending or using spoken language, despite normal intelligence. As in Daniel's case, children may initially be mute following brain damage, and as they recover, begin to show signs of fluent or nonfluent aphasia types (we will look at adult aphasia types in Chapter 9). Children with fluent aphasia may use sentences with appropriate rate and intonation, but with the use of nonsense words (Van Dongen, Loonen, & Van Dongen, 1985). Nonfluent aphasia is more commonly reported in children. These children use short, simple phrases and sentences. Like Daniel, they omit grammatical morphemes, creating the impression of telegraphic speech. Children may also have difficulty with reading and writing. Since reading, listening,

and following directions are frequent school activities, it is not surprising that children with aphasia have academic difficulties (Cranberg et al., 1987). In contrast, language use is often well preserved. Language difficulties may resolve with time, so that the casual listener may be unaware that the child had experienced aphasia. However, language problems can persist and be documented with standardized testing years after the aphasia first appeared (Vargha-Khadem, O'Gorman, & Watters, 1985; Woods & Carey, 1979).

Traumatic Brain Injury

Each year, approximately 200 of every 100,000 children experience a traumatic brain injury (TBI) (NIDCD, 1991). TBI can be focal, as occurs after a penetrating or "open-head" injury (e.g., a gunshot wound), or diffuse, as the result of force applied without penetration of the skull (i.e., a "closed-head" injury). Most commonly, it involves some combination of focal and diffuse injury. TBI can be caused by any number of events, including motor vehicle accidents, in which the injury includes both diffuse damage from the brain moving within the skull as well as focal contusions where the brain contacts the skull. Other events that can produce a combination of diffuse and focal injury include rough shaking (e.g., shaken baby syndrome), falls, sports injuries, assaults, and pedestrian-motor vehicle collisions.

There is considerable heterogeneity among individuals with TBI. Some of this can be accounted for by differences in the nature and severity of the injury (Chapman, 1997). Other sources of heterogeneity are related to preinjury intelligence, health, and personality, as well as family and cultural factors. Among those at highest risk for severe injury are teenaged males, primarily due to driving accidents. Because of the widespread nature of the brain damage, the behavioral consequences range far beyond language skills. This is illustrated by the following case:

> Gerard was a 17-year-old high school junior when he had his car accident. He was ditching his afternoon classes with three friends when he lost control of his truck and it went off the road, flipping over several times. The two boys in the back were killed and the third was paralyzed by the crash. Gerard was in a coma for two weeks with severe head injuries. When Gerard emerged from his coma, cognitive and linguistic deficits were apparent. He was highly distractible and easily overwhelmed by new information or situations. Memory testing indicated that his postinjury abilities were in the fifth percentile, or below the performance of 95 percent of the normative sample for the test. He also had great difficulty understanding both written and spoken language, needing substantial amounts of time to process information and not always arriving at the correct interpretation. In contrast, his spoken language form and content appeared unaffected by his injury.
>
> His most noticeable communication deficit involved language use. Gerard's affect was flat and he failed to use prosodic variation to convey emotion in his speech. Likewise, he did not seem to pick up on the nonverbal cues of others in conversations. His thinking had a concreteness that did not allow him to interpret jokes or sarcasm. This concrete thinking had pervasive effects on his daily life as well. He was unable to conceptualize the future or plan for it effectively.

Language difficulties after TBI are different from those associated with developmental language disorders. For example, many children with TBI may do comparatively well on standardized tests of vocabulary, morphology, and syntax (Biddle, McCabe, & Bliss, 1996; Chapman, Watkins, Gustafson, et al., 1997; Ylvisaker, 1993). These tests tap knowledge gained prior to the injury. Communication breakdowns are more likely to occur in conversational or discourse contexts (Chapman et al., 1997; Chapman, Levin, Matejeka, Harward, & Kufera, 1995) or on language tasks that place particular demands on attention, information processing, and memory (Turkstra & Holland, 1988). Survivors also may have profoundly handicapping impairments in abilities referred to collectively as executive functions (Ylvisaker, Szekeres, & Feeney, 1998). These functions include the ability to plan and organize behavior, make decisions taking multiple factors into account, and regulate one's own behavior. An important difference between those with TBI and those with developmental language disorders is that individuals with TBI are likely to have had a period of normal development and must begin a new life with an uncertainty about their post-injury skills and limitations (Ylvisaker, 1998). This may have a profound effect on their attitude toward therapy.

For Gerard, therapy began in the hospital as soon as he was conscious and medically stable. Therapy was a multidisciplinary effort, with a speech-language pathologist, physical therapist, and psychologist helping Gerard address the physical, cognitive, and emotional aftermath of his injuries. By the time he was well enough to resume school, he had missed most of his junior year. The school provided a full-time classroom aide who took notes for him in class, organized his program of study, and helped him with assignments. The school's speech-language pathologist focused on improving Gerard's basic reading, helping him learn strategies for working within the limits of his impaired memory. Other activities included role-playing practice for various social and vocational situations to improve his poor pragmatics in these communicative contexts. Therapy was a challenge because Gerard did not acknowledge his language deficits and therefore did not see the point of the activities. Gerard also participated, although grudgingly, in a once weekly meeting with other teens who had sustained brain injuries.

The long-term profile of individuals with TBI is dependent in part on which abilities were already acquired and which were still developing at the age when the injury occurred. The full affects of the injury may not be apparent until months or years later (Chapman, 1997). It has been said that after traumatic brain injury "time reveals all wounds" (DePompei, Blosser, Savage, & Lash, 1997). For example we do not expect coherent, logical stories from 4-year-olds, but by 10 years of age incoherent storytelling would signal a deficit. When a brain injury is mild, the child may eventually return to normal or near normal functioning. However, when injuries are severe, the long-term outlook may be less positive.

Two years after his injury, Gerard was finishing high school, although his graduation was uncertain. His involvement in the school's TBI program focused on vocational training to prepare him for postgraduation life. However, he had been

through four jobs in as many months, quitting each time because he was bored or felt the job was beneath him in some way. He drifted away from the teens who were his friends before the injury, and his social and pragmatic problems made it difficult for him to make new social contacts.

Seizure Disorder

Childhood **seizures** can have many different underlying causes, or have no known cause at all. For many, a childhood seizure episode may cause considerable concern at the time, but have no long-lasting consequences. However, when seizures are severe and persistent, behavioral deficits, including impaired language, may follow. We saw one such case with Anita, who was diagnosed as having aphasia with convulsive disorder:

> Anita had been having seizures since 6 months of age. Management of those seizures included drug therapy and periodic monitoring of brain electrical activity. However, this was only partially successful. Anita spoke her first words at 18 months and speech-language development had been slow but steady since then. Following a particularly long generalized seizure at age 4, Anita lost her ability to speak and communication was reduced to slurred sounds and gestures. Although she regained some language skills after that episode, her language remained markedly impaired.
>
> At age 5, she was evaluated at a university clinic. She failed to respond to sounds when her hearing was tested and seemed only somewhat aware of when people were talking to her. A parent questionnaire revealed a significant delay in all areas of development, including motor, social, and self-help skills. Formal language assessment was discontinued because Anita was unable to maintain her attention to the tasks and became frustrated. However, during an hour-long session with her mother, Anita used fewer than 120 words total. Most of her utterances were one or two words in length, and she often used gestures in place of words. Speech was slow and effortful; words were sometimes slurred. Anita established attention very slowly and had difficulty maintaining it. This affected her comprehension, which was poor overall. Her mother used a number of techniques to facilitate attention and comprehension. She maintained close proximity to her daughter. The mother touched her own lips before speaking to draw Anita's attention. The mother physically directed Anita's attention first to her face as she spoke and then to the objects under discussion. She used short sentences and many repetitions to support the conversation. Occasionally, Anita echoed those repetitions back to her mother.

As we see in Anita's case, a prolonged period of seizure activity can lead to a deterioration of skills that were once evident. In fact, a change in language status, such as seen here, is a leading sign of an underlying neurological disturbance. For Anita, both language comprehension and expression were affected by seizure activity, as well as general functioning in nonverbal domains. In other cases of seizure disorder, receptive language abilities are far more impaired than expressive skills (Rapin, Mattis, Rowan, & Golden, 1977; Worster-Drought, 1971). Receptive abilities can be so severely impaired that the child behaves as if deaf. However,

these children have normal hearing acuity, as established by an audiometric evaluation. No longer able to understand his or her own speech, the child may stop talking altogether or speech may become garbled. However, language expression can continue if the child is introduced to signed language.

One subtype of seizure disorder is particularly associated with loss of language skills. Landau-Kleffner syndrome was first described as involving loss of language skills in children who had seizures (Landau & Kleffner, 1957). The seizure activity of these children typically involves both temporal lobes and is easily managed with medication. However, language difficulty may persist even after the seizures are brought under control. Recovery of language is quite variable, ranging from a few weeks to many years (Mantovani & Landau, 1980).

EVALUATION OF LANGUAGE DISORDERS

Evaluation of children with suspected language disorders takes many forms in order to accommodate the wide range of disorders that involve impaired language. The evaluation may address a number of questions of interest to the clinician and the parents. Does the child have a language disorder? Are there any factors that might account for the presence of a language disorder? How do the child's skills in various language domains compare to peers? If intervention is warranted, what aspects of language should be addressed? As we will see, components of the diagnostic process are tailored to address these types of questions.

Language Screening

Language screenings are designed to determine whether a child's language skills warrant a full evaluation. Screenings are relatively quick to administer and often sample a range of language skills that could potentially be impaired. They may be formal measures that have been administered to large groups of children who serve as a **normative sample**. Normative samples permit comparison of a single child's performance to a group of children who are of the same age. These children serve as a reference for the range of normal performance that can be expected. Other screenings may be informal in order to accommodate regional variations in language or dialect or to target skills of particular interest for a certain setting (e.g., conversational speech, reading readiness). Frequently, language screening is used as a cost-effective method of evaluating large numbers of children, most of whom will not have any difficulties with language skills. For example, a school district may routinely screen the language of all of their incoming kindergarten children. Only those children who fail the screening are referred for a full evaluation.

The Case History

The case history is a way to gather background information that may be used for many purposes. It may be obtained through conversation with those who know

the child best (usually the parents). In other cases, it may consist of a form that is completed prior to or during the initial evaluation. Many case histories include information concerning pregnancy, birth, and medical background. This information can be important for identifying potential causes for a language disorder. For example, if a mother reports having had rubella during her pregnancy, the clinician would be alerted to the possibility of hearing loss, which sometimes occurs under those conditions. The clinician can then plan for either a hearing screening during the evaluation or arrange a referral to an audiologist for a full hearing assessment if the child's hearing has not already been tested. Information concerning developmental and family history can help determine the degree of risk for a language disorder. As we saw in earlier sections, children who have developmental language disorders are likely to have a family member who also has a language or learning disorder. In other cases, a parent who reports a change or cessation of language skills during the child's development would alert the clinician to explore the possibility of autism, seizure disorders, or disease processes that would impact previously normal development.

Sometimes a case history will probe for more subjective information. Parents may be asked what led them to become concerned about their child's language development. They may report what they see as their child's overall strengths and weaknesses. The parents' input may help identify those skills that, if remediated, would make the biggest improvement in their child's daily life. They may even be able to provide information on strategies that they have developed that seem to help their child. This type of information is invaluable for guiding subsequent therapy.

Observation

Important diagnostic information can be gathered simply through observation. Let us consider the following case:

> Charise was a speech-language pathologist who worked at a community clinic that handled referrals from the state's program for children with disabilities. She always made a point of meeting her clients in the lobby because, as she said, "I can always tell a lot about the way things are going to go on the walk from the front door to my office." One particular morning, she had a new referral of a child with a reported language delay. The child, a 2-year-old boy, came in hand-in-hand with his mother. He was a little overweight, and his belly peeked out beneath his t-shirt. When Charise dropped down to his eye level, he greeted her with a smile as she explained who she was. He had a round, pleasant face, with widespread, almond-shaped eyes, a broad nose, and full cheeks and lips. Overall, his face appeared soft, as if the underlying muscle tone might be low. He seemed social and he pointed and made short one- or two-word comments about the children's paintings that hung along the hallway. There was one moment of difficulty when it came time to turn the corner and his eye caught something interesting in the opposite direction. He stamped his foot and sat down defiantly in the middle of the hallway. With a bit of cajoling, his mother got him back up and back on track. Once in the office, Charise confirmed

the presence of a language delay with formal diagnostic measures. She also made a referral to a medical geneticist. The facial features, low tone, and high weight, combined with a general immaturity, made her think that a genetic syndrome might be playing a role in this child's language problems. In fact, two months later, a follow-up report was received that confirmed a diagnosis of Prader-Willi syndrome, which involved a genetic abnormality involving chromosome 15.

In this case, the speech-language pathologist's initial observations contributed to this child's diagnosis. Observation is important at all stages of the diagnostic process. The speech-language pathologist may visit the child's home in order to get an idea of typical communication style within the family. A gross assessment of language functioning can be obtained by listening to a child's conversations. How the child plays can provide insight into the level of cognitive and social functioning. Classroom observations of school-age children can provide insight into the specific conditions that precipitate communication problems for the child. The speech-language pathologist may notice simple things that can greatly enhance a child's chances of success.

Formal Measures

There are literally hundreds of commercially available, formal measures for assessing children's language. These tests vary remarkably in their focus, quality, and suitability for a specific diagnostic purpose. One method that clinicians use to select among formal measures is to consider the information that they hope to gain by administering the test. Different formal measures are developed for different purposes. For example, clinicians who wish to compare a child's performance to that of other children of the same age will select one type of test. If they wish to establish whether a child can use certain syntactic structures in various speaking tasks a different type of test would be needed. The former purpose would require a **norm-referenced test**, and the latter would require a **criterion-referenced test**.

Norm-referenced tests allow comparisons between a child's performance and that of a group of children of similar age. Beyond this common feature, there is great variation among norm-referenced tests. Some measure narrow domains of language functioning. For example, one norm-referenced test may examine the number of words that a child recognizes; another will evaluate broader knowledge of word meanings. Some consist of a collection of subtests compiled into a battery that examines various components of language functioning. These may sample across the language domains of phonology, morphology, syntax, and semantics in both receptive and expressive modalities.

Criterion-referenced tests are typically more narrowly focused than norm-referenced tests. These tests are used to compare a child's performance against a standard, or criterion, for behavior. Most college examinations, for example, are criterion-referenced tests, in that the instructor compares each student's performance against a standard for knowledge of the course content. Criterion-referenced tests

may be informal, as when a clinician develops a series of "probes" that are meant to assess whether a child is able to use structures trained in therapy. Others are commercially available measures that sample language skills to determine a child's proficiency.

Once the purpose for administering a test has been determined, the clinician will examine the test's qualities. Specifically, the clinician must determine whether administering a particular test will result in valid conclusions about the child's language. Let us consider an example of why this is important.

> Brendon was just $3\frac{1}{2}$ when he was first enrolled in therapy for a language delay. At that point, his mean length of utterance (MLU) was moderately low for his age (see Chapter 7 for a review of MLU). A standardized test of expressive language placed him below the first percentile for his age, which means that 99 out of 100 children his age could be expected to score higher than Brendon on that particular test. A single-word vocabulary test was also administered, and he did not pass enough items to show that he understood even the most simple words. By contrast, his hearing, motor, and cognitive development tested well within normal limits. Based on these results, he was enrolled in a preschool program for children with specific language impairments. A little over a year later (age 4 years, 10 months), his skills were retested using a different battery of tests. At that time, all skills were well within normal limits according to the test norms. It was concluded that Brendon had overcome his earlier difficulties and was dismissed from the preschool program.
>
> Two months later (age 5 years, 0 months), his mother, still concerned about her son's language skills, enrolled him in a university-based research project for children with specific language impairment. His language was retested with a third battery of tests. This time, Brendon received expressive language scores and receptive vocabulary scores that were once again below the first percentile for his age. How could the appearing-disappearing-reappearing language deficits be explained? The lead researcher, a speech-language pathologist, consulted the normative tables for the tests Brendon received at age 4. She discovered that the test items were so difficult that most normal 4-year-old children could not pass them. Therefore, failure to pass any items on that test battery placed a child within normal limits of performance!

The test given at age 4 years lacked **validity**. Validity refers to the degree to which test results lead to correct conclusions concerning the skills measured (Messick, 1989). Another technical feature that clinicians will consider is a test's **reliability**. This refers to the degree to which a test provides consistent information. An unreliable test is never valid, in that it gives different information each time it is given. However, high reliability does not ensure validity. A ruler whose inch markings are too closely spaced will provide the same mismeasurement every time—highly reliable, but not at all valid! Standards for the assessment of test reliability and validity have been detailed by the combined efforts of the American Educational Research Association, American Psychological Association, and National Council on Measurement in Education (AERA/APA/NCME, 1985). Despite such standards, many tests of child language fall short of minimal criteria for va-

lidity and reliability (e.g., McCauley & Swisher, 1984; Plante & Vance, 1994). Unfortunately, use of a psychometrically weak test can lead to erroneous conclusions.

A final consideration in test selection is the context in which the skill domains are tested. The same items can be passed on one test and failed on another, just based on the context in which those items appear (e.g., Merrell & Plante, 1997; Wiig, Jones, & Wiig, 1996). Sabers (1996) pointed out that "the way a test measures behavior may introduce measurement aspects not intended for the test." In fact, if the simplest linguistic elements are presented in strange or difficult contexts, children will fail those items long after they are able to use and understand the elements in everyday life. For example, a child who has been using "me" since the age of 2 years will not use it in the context "You would have liked me to see the painting" until many years later. Test items designed to measure language, for example, may in fact be a stronger test of memory if the child is required to hold multiple words in memory before composing an answer using those words. Sometimes, the way test items are presented is enough to influence the child's performance. Wiig and colleagues (1996) demonstrated this when they developed a computerized version of one of their tests. They found that teens' performance differed significantly on the traditional and computer-based versions of the test, even though the items were identical. For these reasons, test content and context influence how a clinician interprets the test results.

Hearing Evaluation

As we will see in Chapter 11, hearing impairment can be an underlying cause for poor language development. Therefore, a pure-tone hearing screening is typically part of a language evaluation. If a child fails to respond during the hearing screening, a full audiological evaluation should be scheduled to rule out hearing loss as a contributing factor in the child's language difficulties.

LANGUAGE THERAPY

Approaches to language intervention are as diverse as the children who receive services. There is no "recipe book" of procedures or one-size-fits-all method that will work with all children. In fact, therapy methods that are successful with one child may not work well with another. As we saw above, children with different types of language disorders can vary considerably in terms of their language profiles. Furthermore, the child's age, cultural background, and family situation may greatly affect the type of intervention that is best for them. Therefore, language therapy tends to be highly individualized.

When we examine different intervention methods, we first consider what the therapy approach is intended to do for the child. Wilcox (1994) reviewed major approaches to intervention: prevention, remediation, and compensation. *Preventive* services may be provided to children at risk for language disorders. These children may be at risk because they are born with conditions associated with language

disorders (e.g., mental retardation, genetic disorders). Other children may receive preventive services because they are showing early signs of communication delay (e.g., late talkers). In this case, services are intended to maximize the child's potential early in development so that the impact on language can be lessened or avoided. Examples of preventive services include preschool "head start" programs and other programs designed to enrich a child's early language and educational experiences.

Remediation involves correction of current deficits and is perhaps the most frequent form of therapy for children. When therapy is oriented toward remediation, the clinician typically has very specific goals (e.g., increase use of target syntactic structures, morphemes, vocabulary). The clinician then devises a program to teach these linguistic targets. Let us look at an example of a therapy program designed to remediate expressive language deficits in a young boy.

> Davin is a 20-month-old boy who receives therapy in his home from Sue, a clinician in private practice. When therapy began recently, Davin had six word approximations that he used occasionally, although he understood about fifty words. Therefore, both his comprehension and expression were well below what is typical for a child his age. Sue decided that the top priority for Davin would be expressive language, specifically expanding the number of words he could use to express his needs. More words would help reduce the frustration Davin was displaying because of his poor ability to communicate. Furthermore, the fact that he had some word approximations suggested he was ready to communicate with words.
>
> On her first visit to Davin's home, she taught him signs for "eat," "drink," "want," "more," and "help." Sue elected to incorporate signs into Davin's therapy because children can often produce the more gross hand movements for words before they are able to produce the very precise oral-motor movements needed for intelligible speech. For many children, successful use of signs provides an immediate means for successful communication and a bridge to spoken language. Sue modeled the signs, then demonstrated them to Davin by placing her hands over his while forming the signs with him. By the second visit, it was apparent that Davin was using these first signs on his own.
>
> A critical part of Davin's therapy program is the involvement of his parents. Sue points out that it would be unrealistic to expect Davin to catch up with his peers in the hour a week she sees him at home. It is much more effective for language therapy to be continuous throughout the week. Therefore, a large part of the therapy program involves assuring that both parents develop techniques that they can use to continue Davin's progress after Sue leaves. Davin's mother requested that Sue come when both parents were available to participate in the therapy sessions. They learn signs along with Davin and also learn how to create opportunities for Davin to use the words he has and learn new words as well. Sue thus teaches the parents how to teach their child and gets feedback on their efforts of the previous week.

It seems obvious that parental involvement in therapy programs can be a positive thing. However, successfully bringing parents into the therapy process can be one of the biggest challenges for the clinician. Sue points out that Davin's

parents were anxious to be involved in the therapy process. They were also both highly educated, with college degrees, and came from middle class backgrounds. Davin is their only child, and his mother is able to stay at home with him full time. "You don't want to overwhelm parents, and parents need to be honest with me when I suggest something that is just not possible," says Sue. For example, Sue suggested to Davin's parents that they allow him to make some choices of his own at mealtimes as a way to encourage requests. This same suggestion would not work for a working mother trying to get five young children, one with a disability, dressed and off to school on time. Sue comments, "You can tell you have gone too far when you make a suggestion and their eyes glaze over."

Compensation involves the introduction of strategies that assist the child to manage the effects of the disorder, rather than eliminating its signs. Compensation is often used with conditions that are not completely correctable, such as brain injury or hearing loss. For example, in our case of seizure disorder, the mother's use of visual cues provided a strategy to aid comprehension. For older children and teens, the child may be responsible for use of the strategy. A child with a learning disability, for example, may be taught how to use diagrams to summarize information from his lecture notes. For a teen, compensation may involve strategies to support academic learning. Let's look at one such example.

> Mary works as a speech-language pathologist in a school system. Her role there is to support the children whose language deficits impact their educational progress. Jack is one of her students. In eighth grade, he still struggles with reading. It takes him a long time, and he doesn't always comprehend what he has read. Therefore, he does not learn as much from reading his textbooks as his peers do. Mary has worked with Jack on strategies that are designed to maximize his comprehension of text materials. She teaches him to recognize the cues that are used in textbooks to signal important information. These include strategies like reading the chapter and subheading titles to gain a broad idea about the content area that will be covered. Jack learns that bolded words are important, and if he doesn't fully understand them, he should look in the glossary found at the back of his book. Mary also has trained Jack on how to distinguish between a main point and the details that support them and how to spot these in text. Finally, Mary has worked with Jack's teacher to modify his homework load so that he can keep up with the content without falling behind because of the amount of time it takes him to complete assignments.

As we saw with the cases presented in this chapter, children with language disorders often have many areas of difficulty that could benefit from therapy. However, working on everything at once would be overwhelming for both the clinician and child. Therefore, the clinician may need to prioritize the areas of need and target these sequentially. Some goals receive priority because they offer the greatest potential for positive improvement in the quality of the child's life. For example, a program that provides a nonverbal child with more communicative functions (e.g., requesting, commenting) can reduce frustration for parent and child. A school-age child may benefit most from therapy that allows him or her to participate more fully in classroom activities. Occasionally, the goal that would make the

greatest difference in the child's language is not necessarily one selected. For example, one mother of a severely handicapped child was interested in her child learning social routines (e.g., greetings, "please," and "thank you"), even though other more functional aspects of communication could have been targeted. Social communication was important to the mother because she saw it as a way for her child to have positive interactions with others.

Certain therapy goals may receive priority because they help the child progress to a higher developmental stage. Wilcox (1992) developed an intervention program designed to move infants and toddlers from preverbal gestures and vocalizations to the verbal stage of communication. For a late-talking toddler, increasing the number of vocabulary words is a prerequisite for acquiring phrases and sentences. For older children, the developmental sequence for morpheme acquisition may guide selection of therapy targets. A developmental focus can combine both remediation and preventive components. For example, Dale and colleagues described a treatment method that used storybook activities to facilitate language in preschoolers (Dale et al., 1996). The immediate goal of this program was language facilitation. However, the treatment context of reading introduced preliteracy skills that are thought to contribute to reading success in later years.

Once the language goals are selected, the therapist must consider the structure used to train those goals. Naturalistic contexts have become very popular over the last decade. As a result, there has been an emphasis on home programs, classroom-based programs, and other intervention techniques that are incorporated into the child's daily life. For example, many programs have demonstrated that parents can be effectively trained to facilitate language development at home. Various programs have been used to teach parents to modify their speech and change how they respond to the child's attempts at communication (e.g., Eiserman, Weber, & McCoun, 1995; Gibbard, 1994; Girolametto, Pearce, & Weitzman, 1996). In fact, parent-administered programs can be as effective as clinician-administered programs, at least in the early stages of intervention (Eiserman et al., 1995; Fey, Cleave, & Long, 1997). Other programs emphasize remediation in naturalistic contexts (e.g., conversation, play) during which a clinician, parent, or teacher facilitates the learning of new linguistic forms as opportunities arise to do so within the interaction (Figure 8.2). This technique is sometimes called "incidental teaching" because language instruction follows from natural interactions with the child. For example, a child may learn to use questions by learning to request toys, food, and other items encountered in his or her daily life. The effectiveness of naturalistic intervention can vary depending on the specific techniques used to facilitate language (e.g., Camarata, Nelson, & Camarata, 1994; Kaiser & Hester, 1994; Warren, Gazdag, Bambara, & Jones, 1994) and the characteristics of the child (Yoder, Kaiser, & Alpert, 1991).

Some children need more structure than is afforded by naturalistic contexts because of the nature of their disorder. For example, a child with attention deficit disorder may prove too distractible in a completely naturalistic context to benefit from incidental teaching techniques. A teenager with a traumatic brain injury may not have deficits that involve conversational language per se, but may need help

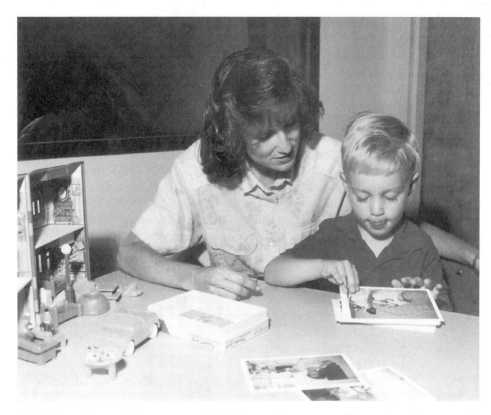

FIGURE 8.2   **A speech-language pathologist works on storytelling using picture cards to help the child sequence information. (Courtesy of The University of Arizona, Department of Speech & Hearing Sciences)**

with aspects of communication that do not necessarily lend themselves to naturalistic intervention. Students who need assistance with language skills in the academic domain may use strategies that are explicitly taught. Finally, what is "natural" to one child may be completely unfamiliar to another. For example, in some cultures, a conversation between a child and an adult who is not a close relative is not at all natural. A clinician who uses such a "natural" context may be confronted with a child who will not talk at all under those conditions. In contrast, the use of computers as a tool for therapy may be natural for children who have been interacting with educational software programs from early ages. For these children, the high level of structure in a computer-based program may feel as natural as conversationally based therapy.

Effective therapy takes into account all of these considerations and makes adjustments to fit the needs of each child. The clinician may use a highly structured, compensatory-based approach with one child and a parent-administered, conversationally based approach with another. For a third child, the clinician may simply

serve as a consultant to a classroom teacher who assists the language-disordered child with modifications of teaching activities and materials. This kind of flexibility allows therapy approaches to be tailored to each child's developmental stage and communicative needs.

CLINICAL PROBLEM SOLVING

Becky is a 30-month-old girl who was brought to the clinic by her parents. They were concerned about her language development because she did not seem to use as many words as the other children at her preschool. Although Becky seemed quite interested in the toys and books in the clinic play room, she said few words and often seemed to substitute gestures for words. All of her verbal utterances consisted of single words, with no multiword combinations. She was in good health and, other than language, the parents did not have any other concerns about her development.

1. Is this child at risk for a language disorder? Why or why not?
2. What should be included in the initial evaluation of this child? What is the purpose for including each of these components?
3. Given the child's age and language level, what approach might therapy take?
4. What do we know about the long-term outlook for young children whose language lags behind their age-mates?

REFERENCES

American Educational Research Association, American Psychological Association, and National Council on Measurement in Education. (1985). *Standards for educational and psychological testing.* Washington, DC: Author.

American Psychiatric Association. (1994). *Diagnostic and statistical manual of mental disorders* (4th ed.). Washington, DC: Author.

American Speech-Language-Hearing Association (ASHA). (1983). Social dialects. *Asha, 25,* 23–27.

American Speech-Language-Hearing Association (ASHA). (1997). Position statement: Roles of audiologists and speech-language pathologists working with persons with attention deficit hyperactivity disorder. *Asha, 39,* 14.

American Speech-Language-Hearing Association (ASHA). (2001). *Roles and responsibilities of speech-language pathologists with respect to reading and writing in children and adolescents.* Rockville, MD: Author

Aram, D. (1991). Comments on specific language impairment as a clinical category. *Language, Speech, & Hearing Services in Schools, 22,* 84–87.

Aram, D. M., Ekelman, B. L., Rose, D. F., & Whitaker, H. A. (1985). Verbal and cognitive sequelae following unilateral lesions acquired in early childhood. *Journal of Clinical and Experimental Neuropsychology, 7,* 55–78.

Bain, A. M., Bailes, L. L., & Moats, L. C. (2001). *Written language disorders: Theory into practice* (2nd ed.). Austin, TX: Pro-Ed.

Butler, K. G., & Silliman, E. R. (2002). *Speaking, reading and writing in children with language learning disabilities.* Mahwah, NJ: Lawrence Erlbaum.

Bellugi, U., Marks, S., Bihrle, A., & Sabo, H. (1988). Dissociation between language and cognitive functions in Williams syndrome. In D. Bishop & M. Mogford (eds.), *Language development in exceptional circumstances.* New York: Churchill Livingstone.

Bent, J. P., & Beck, R. A. (1994). Bacterial meningitis in the pediatric population: Paradigm shifts and ramifications for otolaryngology-head and neck surgery. *International Journal of Pediatric Otorhinolaryngology, 30,* 41–49.

Biddle, K. R., McCabe, A., & Bliss, L. S. (1996). Narrative skills following traumatic brain injury in children and adults. *Journal of Communication Disorders, 29,* 447–470.

Bishop, D., & Adams, C. (1990). A prospective study of the relationship between specific language impairment, phonological disorders and reading impairment. *Journal of Child Psychology and Psychiatry, 31,* 1027–1050.

Byrne, J., Ellsworth, C., Bowering, E., & Vincer, M. (1993). Language development in low birth weight infants: The first two years of life. *Journal of Developmental and Behavioral Pediatrics, 14,* 21–27.

Camarata, S. M., Nelson, K. E., & Camarata, M. N. (1994). Comparison of conversational recasting and imitative procedures for training grammatical structures in children with specific language impairment. *Journal of Speech and Hearing Research, 37,* 1414–1423.

Chapman, S. B. (1997). Cognitive-communication abilities in children with closed head injury. *American Journal of Speech Language Pathology, 6,* 50–58.

Chapman, S. B., Levin, H. S., Matejka, J., Harward, H. N., & Kufera, J. (1995). Discourse ability in head injured children: Consideration of linguistic, psychosocial, & cognitive factors. *Journal of Head Trauma Rehabilitation, 10,* 36–54.

Chapman, S. B., Watkins, R., Gustafson, C., Moore, S., Levin, H. S., & Kufera, J. A. (1997). Narrative discourse in children with closed head injury, children with language impairment, and typically developing children. *American Journal of Speech Language Pathology, 6,* 66–76.

Clark, D. A. (1994). Neonates and infants at risk for hearing and language disorders. In K. G. Butler (Ed.), *Early intervention I: Working with infants and toddlers.* Gaithersburg, MD: Aspen Publishers.

Claude, D., & Firestone, P. (1995). The development of ADHD boys: A 12-year follow-up. *Canadian Journal of Behavioral Science, 27,* 226–249.

Cohen, M., Campbell, R., & Yaghmai, F. (1989). Neuropathological abnormalities in developmental dysphasia. *Annals of Neurology, 25,* 567–570.

Courchesne, E., Yeung-Courchesne, R., Press, G., Hesselink, J. R., & Jernigan, T. L. (1988). Hypoplasia of the cerebellar vermal lobes VI and VII in infantile autism. *New England Journal of Medicine, 318,* 1349–1354.

Cranberg, L. D., Filley, C. M., Hart, E. J., & Alexander, M. P. (1987). Acquired aphasia in childhood: Clinical and CT investigations. *Neurology, 37,* 1165–1172.

Dale, P. S., Crain-Thoreson, C., Notari-Syverson, A., & Cole, K.(1996) Parent-child book reading as an intervention technique for young children with language delays. *Topics in Early Childhood Special Education, 16,* 213–235.

DePompei, R., Blosser, J. L., Savage, R., & Lash, M. (1997, November). *Effective long-term management for youths with TBI.* Miniseminar presented at the annual conference of the American Speech-Language-Hearing Association, Boston, MA.

Dunn, M. (1997). Language disorders in children with autism. *Seminars in Pediatric Neurology, 4,* 86–92.

Eiserman, W. D., Weber, C., & McCoun, M. (1995). Parent and professional roles in early intervention: A longitudinal comparison of the effects of two intervention configurations. *Journal of Special Education, 29,* 20–44.

Ellis Weismer, S., Murray-Branch, J., & Miller, J. F. (1994). A prospective longitudinal study of language development in late talkers. *Journal of Speech and Hearing Research, 37,* 852–867.

Fey, M. E., Cleave, P. L., & Long, S. H. (1997). Two models of grammar facilitation in children with language impairments. *Journal of Speech and Hearing Research, 40,* 5–19.

Fischel, J. E., Whitehurst, G. J., Caulfield, M. B., & Debaryshe, B. (1989). Language growth in children with expressive language delay. *Pediatrics, 82,* 218–227.

Gauger, L. M., Lombardino, L. J., & Leonard, C. M. (1997). Brain morphology in children with specific language impairment. *Journal of Speech, Language, and Hearing Research, 40,* 1272–1284

Gibbard, D. (1994). Parental-based intervention with pre-school language-delayed children. *European Journal of Communication Disorders, 29,* 131–50.

Girolametto, L., Pearce, P. S., & Weitzman, E. (1996). Interactive focused stimulation for toddlers with expressive vocabulary delays. *Journal of Speech and Hearing Research, 39,* 1274–1283.

Halsey, C. L., Collin, M. F., & Anderson, C. L. (1996). Extremely low-birth-weight children and their peers. A comparison of school-age outcomes. *Archives of Pediatrics and Adolescent Medicine, 150,* 790–794.

Jackson, T., & Plante, E. (1997). Gyral morphology in the posterior sylvian region in families affected by developmental language disorder. *Neuropsychology Review, 6,* 81–94.

Johnson, J. M., Seikel, J. A., Madison, C. L., Foose, S. M., & Rinard, K. D. (1997). Standardized test performance of children with a history of prenatal exposure to multiple drugs/cocaine. *Journal of Communication Disorders, 30,* 45–72.

Kaiser, A. B., & Hester, P. P. (1994). Generalized effects of enhanced milieu teaching. *Journal of Speech and Hearing Research, 37,* 1320–1340.

Kamhi, A. G., & Catts, H. W. (1999). *Language and reading disabilities.* Boston: Allyn and Bacon.

Kanner, L., & Eisenberg, L. (1955). Notes on the followup studies of autistic children. In P. H. Hoch & J. Zubin (Eds.), *Psychotherapy of childhood.* New York: Grune & Stratton.

Landau, W. M., & Kleffner, F. R. (1957). Syndrome of acquired aphasia with convulsive disorder in children. *Neurology, 7,* 523–530.

Lewis, B. A., & Freebairn, L. (1992). Residual effects of preschool phonology disorders in grade school, adolescence, and adulthood. *Journal of Speech and Hearing Disorders, 35,* 819–831.

Lord, C., & Pickles, A. (1996). Language level and nonverbal social-communicative behaviors in autistic and language-delayed children. *Journal of the American Academy of Child and Adolescent Psychiatry, 35,* 1542–1550.

Mantovani, J. F., & Landau, W. M. (1980). Acquired aphasia with convulsive disorder: Course and prognosis. *Neurology, 30,* 524–529.

McCauley, R. J., & Swisher, L. (1984). Psychometric review of language and articulation tests for preschool children. *Journal of Speech and Hearing Disorders, 49,* 34–42.

McGee, R., Partridge, F., Williams, S., & Silva, P. A. (1991). A twelve-year follow-up of preschool hyperactive children. *Journal of the American Academy of Child and Adolescent Psychiatry, 30,* 224–232.

Menyuk, P., & Chesnick, M. (1997). Metalinguistic skills, oral language knowledge, and reading. *Topics in Language Disorders, 17,* 75–87.

Merrell, A. W., & Plante, E. (1997). Norm-referenced test interpretation in the diagnostic process. *Language, Speech, & Hearing Services in Schools, 28,* 50–58.

Messick, S. (1989). Meaning and values in test validation: The science and ethics of assessment. *Educational Researcher, 18,* 5–11.

Minshew, N. J., Goldstein, G., & Siegel, D. J. (1997). Neuropsychologic functioning in autism: Profile of a complex information processing disorder. *Journal of the International Neuropsychological Society, 3,* 303–316.

Miranda-Linne, F. M., & Merlin, L. (1997). A comparison of speaking and mute individuals with autism and autistic-like conditions on the Autism Behavior Checklist. *Journal of Autism and Developmental Disorders, 27,* 245–264.

National Institute on Deafness and Other Communication Disorders (NIDCD). (1991). *National strategic research plan for balance and the vestibular system and language and language impairments* (NIH Publication No. 91-3217). Bethesda, MD: Author.

Paul, R. (1993). Patterns of development in late talkers: Preschool years. *Journal of Childhood Communication Disorders, 15,* 7–14.

Paul, R. (1995). *Language disorders from infancy through adolescence.* St. Louis, MO: Mosby.

Paul, R., & Alforde, S. (1993). Grammatical morpheme acquisition in 4-year-olds with normal, impaired, and late-developing language. *Journal of Speech and Hearing Research, 36,* 1271–1275.

Paul, R., Hernandez, R., Taylor, L., & Johnson, K. (1996). Narrative development in late talkers: Early school age. *Journal of Speech and Hearing Research, 39,* 1295–1303.

Paul, R., Murray, C., Clancy, K., & Andrews, D. (1997). *Journal of Speech and Hearing Research, 40,* 1037–1047.

Petit, E., Herlault, J., Martineau, J., Perrot, A., Barthelemy, C., Hameury, L., Sauvage, D., Lelord, G., Muh, J. P., (1995). Association study with two markers of a human homeogene in infantile autism. *Journal of Medical Genetics, 32,* 269–274.

Plante, E. (1991). MRI findings in the parents and siblings of specifically language-impaired boys. *Brain and Language, 41,* 52–66.

Plante, E., Swisher, L., Vance, R., & Rapcsak, S. (1991). MRI findings in boys with specific language impairment. *Brain and Language, 41,* 52–66.

Plante, E., & Vance, R. (1994). Selection of preschool language tests: A data based approach. *Language, Speech, & Hearing Services in Schools, 25,* 15–23.

Plante, E., & Vance, R. (1995). Diagnostic accuracy of two tests of preschool language. *American Journal of Speech-Language Pathology, 4,* 70–76.

Rapin, I., Mattis, S., Rowan, A. J., & Golden, G. G. (1977). Verbal auditory agnosia in children.

Developmental Medicine and Child Neurology, 19, 192–207.

Records, N. L., Tomblin, J. B., & Freese, P. R. (1992). The quality of life of young adults with histories of specific language impairment. *American Journal of Speech-Language Pathology, 1*, 44–53.

Rescorla, L., Roberts, J., & Dahlsgaard, K.(1997). Late talkers at 2: Outcome at age 3. *Journal of Speech and Hearing Research, 40*, 555–566.

Rescorla, L., & Schwartz, E. (1990). Outcome of toddlers with expressive language delay. *Applied Psycholinguistics, 11*, 393–407.

Rimland, B. (1964). *Infantile autism*. New York: Appleton-Century-Crofts.

Sabers, D. L. (1996). By their tests we will know them. *Language, Speech, and Hearing Services in Schools, 27*, 102–108.

Scarborough, H. S. (1990). Very early language deficits in dyslexic children. *Child Development, 61*, 1728–1743.

Scarborough, H. S., & Dobrich, W. (1990). Development of children with early language delay. *Journal of Speech and Hearing Research, 33*, 70–83.

Scharfenaker, S. K. (1990). The fragile X syndrome. *Asha, 32*, 45–47.

Shields, J., Varley, R., Broks, P., & Simpson, A. (1996). Social cognition in developmental language disorders and high-level autism. *Developmental Medicine and Child Neurology, 38*, 487–495.

Snyder, L. S., & Downey, D. M. (1997). Developmental differences in the relationship between oral language deficits and reading. *Topics in Language Disorders, 17*, 27–40.

Sparks, S. N. (1984). *Birth defects and speech-language disorders*. Boston: College Hill.

Stoel-Gammon, C. (1990). Down syndrome: Effects on language development. *Asha, 32*, 42–44.

Tallal, P., Ross, R., & Curtiss, S. (1989). Familial aggregation in specific language impairment. *Journal of Speech and Hearing Disorders, 54*, 287–295.

Thal, D. J., Bates, E., Goodman, J., & Jahn-Samilo, J. (1997). Continuity of language abilities: An exploratory study of late- and early-talking toddlers. *Developmental Neuropsychology, 13*, 239–274.

Thal, D. J., & Tobias, S. (1992). Communicative gestures in children with delayed onset of oral expressive vocabulary. *Journal of Speech and Hearing Research, 35*, 1281–1289.

Tomblin, J. B. (1989). Familial concentration of developmental language impairment. *Journal of Speech and Hearing Disorders, 54*, 287–295.

Tomblin, J. B., Records, N., & Freese, P. (1992). Diagnosing specific language impairment in adults for the purpose of pedigree analysis. *Journal of Speech and Hearing Research, 35*, 832–843.

Tomblin, J. B., Records, N. L., & Zhang, X. (1996). A system for the diagnosis of specific language impairment in kindergarten children. *Journal of Speech and Hearing Research, 39*, 1284–1294.

Turkstra, L. S., & Holland, A. L. (1998). Working memory and syntax comprehension after adolescent traumatic brain injury. *Journal of Speech, Language, and Hearing Research, 41*.

Van Dongen, H. R., Loonen, M. C. B., & Van Dongen, K. J. (1985). Anatomical basis for acquired fluent aphasia in children. *Annals of Neurology, 17*, 306–309.

Vargha-Khadem, F., O'Gorman, A. M., & Watters, G. V., (1985). Aphasia and handedness in relation to hemisphere side, age at injury, and severity of cerebral lesion in childhood. *Brain, 108*, 677–695.

Warren, S. F., Gazdag, G. E., Bambara, L. M., & Jones, H. A. (1994). Changes in the generativity and use of semantic relations concurrent with milieu language intervention. *Journal of Speech and Hearing Research, 37*, 924–934.

Washington, J. A., & Craig, H. K. (1994). Dialectal forms during discourse of poor, urban, African American preschoolers. *Journal of Speech and Hearing Research, 37*, 816–823.

Wiig, E. H., Jones, S. S., & Wiig, E. D. (1996). Computer-based assessment of word knowledge in teens with learning disabilities. *Language, Speech, and Hearing Services in Schools, 27*, 21–28.

Wilcox, M. J. (1992). Enhancing initial communication skills in young children with developmental disabilities through partner programming. *Seminars in Speech and Hearing, 13*, 194–212.

Wilcox, M. J. (1994). Delivering communication-based services to infants, toddlers, and their families: Approaches and models. In K. G. Butler (Ed.), *Early intervention I: Working with infants and toddlers*. Gaithersburg, MD: Aspen Publications.

Woods, B. T., & Carey, S. (1979). Language deficits after apparent clinical recovery from childhood aphasia. *Annals of Neurology, 6*, 405–409.

Worster-Drought, C. (1971). An unusual form of acquired aphasia in children. *Developmental Medicine and Child Neurology, 13*, 563–571.

Ylvisaker, M. (1993). Communication outcome in children and adolescents with traumatic brain

injury. *Neuropsychological Rehabilitation, 3,* 321–340.

Ylvisaker, M. (1998). Traumatic brain injury in children and adolescents: Introduction. In M. Ylvisaker (Ed.), *Traumatic brain injury rehabilitation in children* (2nd ed. pp. 1–10.). Boston: Butterworth-Heinemann.

Ylvisaker, M., Szekeres, S. F., & Feeney, T, J. (1998). Cognitive rehabilitation: Executive functions.

In M. Ylvisaker (Ed.), *Traumatic brain injury rehabilitation in children* (2nd ed. pp. 221–270). Boston: Butterworth-Heinemann.

Yoder, P. J., Kaiser, A. P., & Alpert, C. L. (1991). An exploratory study of the interactions between language teaching methods and child characteristics. *Journal of Speech and Hearing Research, 34,* 155–167.

READINGS FROM THE POPULAR LITERATURE

Dorris, M. (1996). *Broken cord.* Boston: G. K. Hall & Co. (fetal alcohol syndrome)

Geraldi, C. (1996). *Camille's children.* Kansas City, KS: Andrews and McMeel. (foster mother of multiply handicapped children)

Gerlach, E. (1999). *Just this side of normal: Glimpses into life with autism.* Eugene, OR: Four Leaf Press. (family and autism)

Grandin, T., & Scariano, M. M. (1996). *Emergence: Labeled autistic.* New York: Warner Books. (personal account of autism)

Greenfield, J. (1980). *A place for Noah.* New York: Holt, Rinehart and Winston. (family with autistic child)

Jablow, M. (1982). *Cara: Growing up with a retarded child.* Philadelphia, PA: Temple University Press. (mental retardation)

Kaufmann, B. (1976). *Son-rise.* New York: Warner Books. (autism)

Kaufmann, S. (1995). *Retarded isn't stupid, Mom!* Baltimore: P.H. Brookes. (mental retardation)

Lane, G., & Sagmiller, G. (1996). *Dyslexia my life.* Waverly, IA: Doubting Thomas Pub. (dyslexia)

Maurice, C. (1994). *Let me hear your voice: A family's triumph over autism.* New York: Fawcett Columbine. (family and autism)

Papazian, S. (1997). *Growing up with Joey: A mother's story of her son's disability and her family's triumph.* Santa Barbara, CA: Fithian Press. (cerebral palsy and the family)

Rogers, D. E. (1992). *Angel unaware*: Westwood, NJ: Fleming Revell Press. (Down syndrome)

Stallings, G., & Cook, S. (1998). *Another season: A coach's story of raising an exceptional son.* New York: Broadway Books. (Down syndrome)

Williams, D. (1994). *Nobody nowhere.* New York: Perennial. (personal account of autism)

DISORDERS OF LANGUAGE IN ADULTS

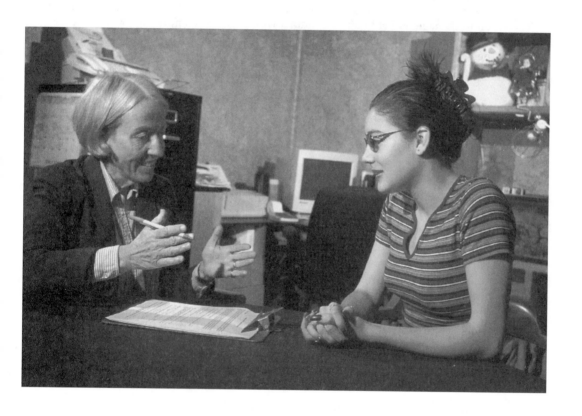

PREVIEW

Language is well established by the adult years. Most adults have mastered the syntax and morphology of their primary language in both the spoken and written form, and language formulation and speech production occur with relatively little effort. Adult vocabularies continue to grow as life experience is gained, and adults typically become more adept at the subtleties of language use. With advanced age, language knowledge and use remain relatively stable with the exception of some minor word retrieval problems. In some adults, however, sudden or progressive damage to portions of the brain that are important for language and thought significantly disturb the ability to communicate. The extent and location of brain damage influence the resulting behavior so that various syndromes are associated with certain patterns of brain damage. Rehabilitation of adults with acquired communication disorders is challenging and rewarding work typically accomplished in partnership with the patient, clinician, caregivers, and other professionals.

Normal language and cognition are dependent upon a healthy nervous system. Damage to portions of the brain that support language may result in an impairment of language referred to as **aphasia**. Because language centers are in the left hemisphere in most people, aphasia typically is associated with left hemisphere damage. Acquired language impairments may occur in children, as reviewed in Chapter 8, but aphasia is most often observed in adults. When the right hemisphere is damaged rather than the left, the resulting syndrome of cognitive and communication impairment is quite different from aphasia. In other cases, widespread or diffuse damage to both hemispheres may occur, as is frequently observed following traumatic brain injury (TBI). As discussed in Chapter 8, teenagers and young adults are at greatest risk for TBI, but older adults may suffer the cognitive and behavioral consequences of head injury as well. With advanced age, there is increased likelihood of progressive intellectual and linguistic decline associated with various types of dementia.

APHASIA

Aphasia is an acquired impairment of language. It results from damage to the language centers of the brain, that are typically located in the left hemisphere, as reviewed in Chapter 2. The areas of damage or injury are called **lesions**. In the case of aphasia, an individual who had normal language suddenly finds those abilities lost or degraded. Speech-language pathologists in medical settings frequently participate in the evaluation and rehabilitation of individuals with aphasia.

Mr. Wallace was a right-handed man who had a bachelor's degree in engineering and had retired after a distinguished career in the army. At age 67, he had a stroke

in the left cerebral hemisphere. He did not suffer any physical impairment after the stroke, but his ability to communicate was markedly impaired due to aphasia. A conversational exchange with Mr. Wallace went as follows:

PB: Tell me about the work that you did.

Mr. Wallace: When I grew up in the army, this was my whole *fife, lar . . . light.* I was in the army, the army, and the war and everything else under the sun. Everything. And various *coun, coun, coun,* countries, and things in different places we went and in the armies. I was a colonel in the infantry. And I liked it. I was very fond of . . . I knew everybody in Westpoint. We all grown in our lives, grown up, and we were children. And we knew a lot of people and I think we were useful. And the people we work with. And so we did.

Mr. Wallace did not have trouble pronouncing words, nor was his speech hesitant or effortful, but his language certainly was lacking content. He seemed to have difficulty coming up with the words he needed to explain his thoughts. For example, it was obvious that Mr. Wallace intended to say, "When I grew up in the army, this was my whole *life.*" But he did not say the word *life.* He first said the word *fife,* then he said a nonword *lar,* and finally he said an incorrect word, *light.* Mr. Wallace retained his lifelong memories and did not have an impairment of his intellect, he had an impairment specific to language—he had aphasia.

It is important to appreciate that aphasia is an impairment of language, not simply a problem with speech production. Recall from Chapters 3 and 7 that language is a symbol system used to convey thoughts, whereas speech refers to the meaningful sounds produced by articulatory movements. Language includes the words we speak and the rules that govern how words are combined to make utterances. Mr. Wallace had trouble coming up with the appropriate words and also had difficulty combining them into meaningful sentences. Although some of Mr. Wallace's words were pronounced incorrectly, this was not due to a speech problem; it was part of his language impairment. Some individuals with aphasia *do* have difficulty articulating words, that is, they have speech problems that co-exist with their aphasia. We discussed those acquired speech disorders in Chapter 4.

Language is distinguished not only from speech, but also from thought. Patients with severe aphasia often demonstrate that they have relatively well-preserved thought processes. They retain their world knowledge, remember their life histories, and learn new things about what is going on in the world. Therefore, aphasia is not an impairment of general intellect as is observed in dementing diseases. It would be an oversimplification to suggest that individuals with aphasia possess all the cognitive abilities they had before the onset of their aphasia (see, e.g., Beeson, Bayles, Rubens, & Kaszniak, 1993; Murray, 2002), but it is the language impairment that is central to their communication problem.

Characteristics

The difficulty in coming up with words that was evident in Mr. Wallace's conversation is called **anomia**, which refers to a failure to retrieve a name. Anomia is the

hallmark of aphasia, that is, all people with aphasia complain of difficulty coming up with the names of things. The rambling emptiness of Mr. Wallace's conversation resulted from his anomia. He overused pronouns such as *we*, *thing*, and *it* rather than giving specific names of people, places, or things. Individuals with aphasia may identify instances of anomia by saying something like, "oh, I can't think of the word for it," or they may describe the item that they cannot name. For example, to refer to the Veteran's Affairs hospital, a patient said, "you know, the place where I met you . . . with all the soldiers and where we did those things with the tests." This sort of "talking around the word" is called **circumlocution**. Although circumlocution is an indicator of word retrieval problems, it is also a very useful communication strategy to compensate for anomia. Not all individuals with aphasia can detect or correct their own errors.

Sometimes incorrect words or nonwords are produced in place of the desired word. Such errors are called **paraphasias**. Mr. Wallace's incorrect attempts to produce the word *light* resulted in several paraphasias. They can be whole word substitutions, such as *world* for *life*, single-sound substitutions such as *fife* for *life*, or nonwords that are close or totally unrelated to the target word, such as *lar* for *life*. Such nonwords are also called **neologisms**, meaning "new words," but they have no meaning to the listener.

Fluent versus Nonfluent Aphasia

Mr. Wallace's speech output was considered "fluent" in that it had relatively normal prosodic variations of pitch, loudness, and stress. Although there were some hesitations due to word finding difficulties, the words flowed in a manner that sounded fairly normal so that it is referred to as **fluent aphasia**. It was also articulated without excessive effort. The utterances were generally of normal length in terms of the number of words and there was some syntactic structure, such as the use of articles, prepositional phrases, and appropriate word endings, such as -ed.

Not all individuals with aphasia speak fluently. Those with **nonfluent aphasia** produce utterances characterized by effortful, hesitant speech that may be poorly articulated. Mr. Brown provides an example of nonfluent aphasia. He was a 36-year-old man who had a congenital malformation of his vascular system that required surgery when he was 31. The surgery was complicated by a hemorrhage that occurred in the region of the left middle cerebral artery and caused extensive damage to the language areas of his left hemisphere. He had weakness of the right side of his body and a significant nonfluent aphasia. Two years after his stroke we had the following conversation.

> **PB:** What can you tell me about the stroke?
>
> **Mr. Brown:** Um . . . (sighs) . . . um . . . (sighs) . . . left . . . (gestures to right side of body) . . . right side . . . (shakes his head and sighs).
>
> **PB:** And before your stroke, what did you do?
>
> **Mr. Brown:** Um . . . resale sales (holds up 6 fingers).

PB: Six years?

Mr. Brown: No. Six . . . store . . . chain . . . California.

PB: Did you do sales?

Mr. Brown: No. No. This time . . . general . . . manager.

Mr. Brown's utterances were quite different from those of Mr. Wallace. He spoke mostly in single words and short phrases. Whereas Mr. Wallace had an excess of vague, empty words, Mr. Brown's words were almost all meaningful content words. This type of output has been called telegraphic speech because it is lacking the little functor words, like *is* or *the*, that are typically omitted when one sends a telegram. (In the old days people sent telegrams rather than e-mails, and you had to pay by the word.) The pauses and interjection of "um" give the impression that Mr. Brown is struggling to find and produce the words he wanted to say, and he had difficulty constructing complete sentences with appropriate grammatical structure. The overall speech pattern is lacking normal prosodic variation, that is, there is not the normal melodic variation of pitch, loudness, and stress. The term **nonfluent** is used to capture the essence of this effortful, **telegraphic speech** pattern. It should not be confused with the term **disfluent**, which refers to the disruption of speech fluency that is observed in stuttering (see Chapter 5).

The differences in fluency noted between Mr. Wallace and Mr. Brown are consistent with differences in the location of brain damage that caused their respective aphasias. To understand the relationship between fluency and lesion location, we need to briefly review brain anatomy relevant to aphasia. Aphasia typically results from damage to the left hemisphere in an area that surrounds the major horizontal fissure called the Sylvian fissure. This region is shaded in Figure 9.1 (p. 212), and is called the perisylvian region (peri = around). A brain scan of an individual who had a stroke in this area and persistent aphasia is shown in Figure 9.2 (p. 212). The scan was taken several years following the stroke and the dark regions of brain damage are clearly visible in the two images. It should be apparent from image 9.2A that the damage falls within the left perisylvian region shown schematically in Figure 9.1.

The relatively large perisylvian region is often divided into anterior and posterior regions relative to another major fissure, the Rolandic fissure (also called the central sulcus) that runs roughly perpendicular to the Sylvian fissure as seen in Figure 9.1. The primary motor area and the areas important for motor planning are located in the frontal lobe, which is anterior to the Rolandic fissure. Broca's area is a frontal lobe region important for the motor planning of speech movements (see Figure 9.1). Therefore, it makes sense that brain damage to those anterior regions of the left hemisphere are likely to affect motor control and planning, and thus contribute to a disruption of speech production like that observed in nonfluent aphasia. As observed with Mr. Brown, anterior lesions often damage the motor areas for the right arm and leg as well, so that individuals with nonfluent aphasia often have right-sided weakness or paralysis, which is called right **hemiparesis**. Conversely, lesions that spare the anterior motor regions (i.e., that are posterior to the Rolandic fissure) are typically associated with fluent aphasia and no hemiparesis, as

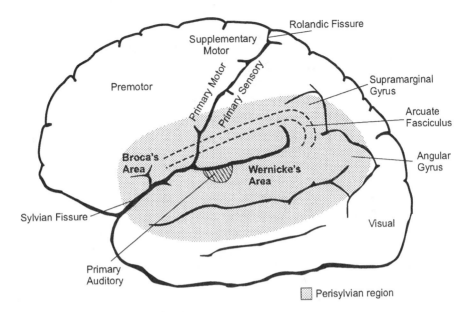

FIGURE 9.1   A schematic drawing of the left hemisphere indicates the language centers in the perisylvian region. Note that the primary auditory area is actually hidden from view inside the Sylvian fissure; the arcuate fasciculus is a white matter pathway that is deep within the hemisphere. [Reprinted from Beeson, P. M., & Rapcsak, S. Z. (1998). The aphasias. In P. J. Snyder & P. D. Mussbaum (Eds.), *Clinical Neuropsychology: A Pocket Handbook for Assessment* (pp. 403–425), with permission from American Psychological Association.]

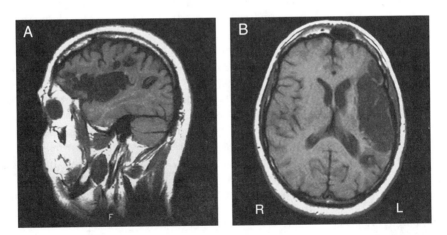

FIGURE 9.2   An MRI (magnetic resonance imaging) scan of the head showing a large perisylvian lesion in the left hemisphere that resulted in significant aphasia. Image A shows the dark region of damage from a lateral perspective (in a vertical plane), with the patient looking to the left. Image B shows an image in a horizontal plane near the Sylvian fissure. Note that the lesion is on the right side in image B because radiologic films are often flipped so that right and left are reversed.

observed in Mr. Wallace. In general, anterior lesions are associated with nonfluent aphasia, and posterior lesions are associated with fluent aphasia. Large lesions that encompass both anterior and posterior regions would result in nonfluent aphasia because damage includes the critical anterior motor regions.

Beyond the distinction between fluent and nonfluent aphasias, classification systems have been used over the past century to distinguish identifiable aphasia subtypes. The Boston classification system is commonly used in North America (Goodglass, 1993; Helm-Estabrooks & Albert, 1991). In general, the aphasia types reflect performance profiles that indicate (1) whether the aphasia is fluent or nonfluent, (2) whether auditory comprehension is relatively good or impaired, and (3) whether the ability to repeat sentences is preserved or impaired. Just as fluency characteristics offer some insight regarding lesion location, some inferences can be drawn from the status of auditory comprehension and verbal repetition abilities. An understanding of those processes is helpful before examining some aphasia types in more detail.

Auditory Comprehension

Auditory comprehension requires the extraction of meaning from spoken words and the processing of grammatical structures in connected utterances. Auditory comprehension problems are common in aphasia, but the degree of impairment can vary considerably. Some individuals have trouble understanding the meaning of single words and simple commands, such as when they are asked, "Show me the table." Others can respond to such simple requests, but have trouble when understanding is dependent upon careful processing of each word in relation to other words in the utterance. For example, the following verbal request would challenge most individuals with aphasia, "Do you want chicken or steak for dinner? Because if you want chicken, you need to get it out of the freezer."

Auditory comprehension is dependent upon information processing in the posterior, superior temporal lobe in the region called Wernicke's area, which is adjacent to the primary auditory region (Figure 9.1). Damage to Wernicke's area does not impair the ability to hear, but interferes with the understanding of spoken language. Lesions to Wernicke's area are considered "posterior," because they are posterior to the Rolandic fissure and do not include the frontal motor regions. Mr. Wallace's stroke damaged Wernicke's area, and he had trouble understanding what was said in conversation. He also made errors on yes/no questions such as, "Do you eat a banana before you peel it?" Mr. Wallace's comprehension was assessed using a variety of tasks that included pointing to items in response to their name, simple and complex commands, yes-no questions, and more difficult tasks such as comprehending a paragraph read aloud.

Repetition

Although the ability to repeat what other people say is not a particularly important or meaningful use of language, it is a useful diagnostic task when examining for aphasia. The ability to repeat words, phrases, and sentences requires auditory

processing by posterior regions of the left hemisphere as well as verbal formulation by the anterior regions of the left hemisphere. So, the ability to repeat sentences is a good test of the integrity of the entire left perisylvian region. Difficulty with verbal repetition can arise for several reasons. The attempts to repeat sentences by Mr. Wallace (with fluent aphasia) resulted in errors because of his auditory comprehension problems and his many paraphasic errors. Mr. Brown (with nonfluent aphasia) had trouble repeating sentences because he omitted the little grammatical words, just like he did in his conversational speech. Repetition can also be disrupted by damage to fibers that connect the posterior and anterior perisylvian regions. The **arcuate fasciculus** is a collection of nerve fibers that originate in the superior temporal lobe, course up and around the Sylvian fissure, and project to the frontal lobe (Figure 9.1). Damage to these fibers, as well as other posterior regions in the left hemisphere, disrupt repetition abilities even when Broca's and Wernicke's areas are spared (Damasio & Damasio, 1980). Such lesions appear to disconnect the posterior and anterior language regions so that auditory input processed in Wernicke's area does not get conveyed to Broca's area for speech production.

Relatively good verbal repetition is observed in some aphasias that result from brain damage that is on the periphery of the left perisylvian region, or from isolated lesions within the perisylvian region that do not disturb the input and output processes necessary for repetition. In such cases, it is somewhat surprising to observe a patient who can repeat full sentences, but cannot formulate a sentence on his or her own.

Summary of Neuroanatomical Principles Related to Aphasia

Several neuroanatomical principles have been introduced that highlight the relation between brain regions and language behaviors. Before summarizing those principles, it is important to remember that successful communication requires participation of many parts of the brain and that damage to a particular area does not mean that *only* the damaged area is responsible for the impaired function. Also, it is known that people vary in terms of their precise brain organization, so that identical lesions in two people may result in slightly different profiles. With those caveats in mind, the following generalizations can be made:

1. Large anterior lesions interfere with fluent speech production, so that nonfluent aphasia is associated with anterior lesions and fluent aphasias are associated with posterior lesions.
2. Lesions in and around Wernicke's area interfere with auditory comprehension, so that posterior lesions tend to be associated with poor auditory comprehension and anterior lesions may leave auditory comprehension relatively well preserved.

3. Lesions within the perisylvian region disrupt the ability to repeat sentences, but lesions on the periphery of the perisylvian region result in relatively preserved ability to repeat.
4. Lesions throughout the left hemisphere can disrupt naming abilities resulting in anomia, so that the presence of anomia is not predictive of lesion location.

Aphasia Types

We have noted the general predictability of language performance based on lesion location and have suggested that patients with similar lesions tend to have similar language characteristics. Aphasia classification systems are useful for identifying such clusters of language behaviors. We will review some of the more common aphasia types. The syndromes are labeled according to the Boston classification system, which indicates aphasia type on the basis of fluency, auditory comprehension, and repetition abilities. Such classification systems are clinically useful, but not all individuals with aphasia will fit a specific type. In a large aphasia recovery study, Wertz and colleagues (1981) found that about 75% of the individuals with aphasia were classifiable by aphasia type, leaving 25% who were considered unclassifiable. In those cases, it is still useful to characterize the aphasia in terms of fluency, auditory comprehension, and repetition abilities.

Figure 9.3 shows the decision process for classifying four of the more common aphasia types: Broca's, global, conduction, and Wernicke's. The classification of aphasia type is based on the observed fluency of spontaneous speech (fluent versus nonfluent) and the status of auditory comprehension (good or poor). The figure also includes schematic drawings intended to depict a typical lesion location for each aphasia type. As indicated in Figure 9.3, the aphasia types differ with regard to observable language characteristics and likely lesion location. The nonfluent aphasias include damage to anterior portions of the brain, and the fluent aphasias are restricted to posterior lesions. As mentioned, however, there is considerable variation from person to person, so the predicted relations between lesion location and language behavior are not without many exceptions.

Broca's Aphasia. Broca's aphasia is a nonfluent aphasia characterized by slow, hesitant, telegraphic speech. We saw an example of **Broca's aphasia** in Mr. Brown, the 36-year-old with nonfluent aphasia. As noted in his conversational sample, utterances are of reduced length, typically fewer than four words, and have little syntactic complexity. The utterances are mostly isolated productions of nouns with some adjectives and verbs, and they are notably lacking articles, prepositions, and other functors. Broca's aphasia is sometimes referred to as "motor aphasia" or "expressive aphasia," terms that highlight the observed production problems. Auditory comprehension is relatively well preserved for conversation, but breaks down when comprehension is dependent upon correct understanding of complex grammar or understanding of the little functor words. Repetition is limited to a few words. When asked to repeat full sentences, individuals with Broca's aphasia may

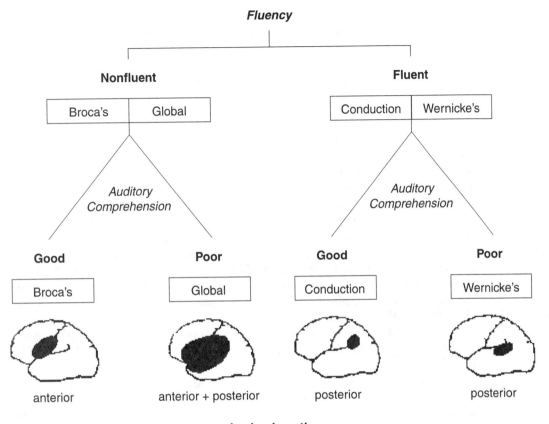

FIGURE 9.3   A decision tree used to guide the classification of four common aphasia types based upon fluency of spontaneous speech (fluent vs. nonfluent) and auditory comprehension (good vs. poor). Schematic drawings depict typical brain lesions associated with each aphasia type and indicate whether the lesion extends anterior or posterior to the Rolandic fissure.

simply repeat the content words. Reading and writing are also impaired in individuals with Broca's aphasia because the aphasia affects all language modalities.

Broca's aphasia results from lesions affecting the posterior portion of the left inferior frontal lobe. These are considered anterior lesions because they lie anterior to the Rolandic fissure (see Figure 9.3). When the lesions are small and restricted to Broca's area, the individual may have Broca's aphasia for only a short time following the brain damage, and then recover to a more fluent aphasia. Persistent Broca's aphasia typically results from larger lesions that affect not only Broca's area but extend posteriorly to the anterior parietal lobe. An extensive anterior lesion often results in right hemiparesis as noted with Mr. Brown.

Wernicke's Aphasia. In contrast to Broca's aphasia, **Wernicke's aphasia** is characterized by fluent speech that is difficult to understand because it contains numerous paraphasias (incorrect or nonwords) and is relatively devoid of content. Mr. Wallace, the man who was introduced as an example of fluent aphasia, had Wernicke's aphasia that was improving to the extent that it increasingly contained portions of conversation that were somewhat understandable. Immediately following his stroke, however, his profile was highly characteristic of Wernicke's aphasia. His utterances were heavily sprinkled with paraphasias in place of meaningful words, so that he made comments such as, "Oh, and there is a *kusbit* and a *wuzman.*" Other individuals with more severe Wernicke's aphasia produce full strings of neologisms (nonwords) so they may sound like they are speaking a foreign language. They have a normal flow of speech with variations in prosody, but few real words. This type of output is sometimes called **jargon aphasia**, and it sounds similar in some ways to the jargon of a young child learning language.

In addition to their fluent, paraphasic speech, individuals with Wernicke's aphasia have significant impairment of auditory comprehension (Figure 9.3). They have difficulty understanding spoken sentences and even have trouble comprehending many single words. This was the case for Mr. Wallace. When asked to point to the table, he blankly repeated, "table, table, I should know what that is." Another patient with more severe Wernicke's aphasia responded to the task by pointing to the door, and saying something that sounded like "*illotime.*" Another sign of the impaired auditory processing is the failure of individuals with Wernicke's aphasia to attempt to correct their production errors. They often show a lack of awareness of their many errors. When asked to repeat words or sentences spoken by the clinician, their performance is no better. Repetition abilities are impaired due to the poor auditory processing and production problems. Reading and writing are typically impaired in much the same way as auditory comprehension and speech production.

As might be expected, Wernicke's aphasia is associated with lesions in what is known as Wernicke's area (Figure 9.1). This region in the posterior, superior portion of the temporal lobe is adjacent to the primary auditory cortex and is thought to be critical for auditory comprehension of language. Such posterior lesions typically spare the cortical areas important for motor control of the body, so that individuals with Wernicke's aphasia rarely have hemiparesis.

Conduction Aphasia. **Conduction aphasia** is somewhat similar to Wernicke's aphasia in that the verbal output is fluent and paraphasias are common. Individuals with conduction aphasia have better auditory comprehension than those with Wernicke's aphasia, presumably because much of Wernicke's area is spared (Figure 9.3). It is not uncommon for individuals with conduction aphasia to attempt to self-correct their own errors, and frequently they are successful after several attempts. The self-corrections and hesitations associated with word-finding problems cause some disruption of the flow of speech, but the verbal output retains a sense of fluency in that articulation is accomplished with relative ease. Because the

lesion spares the anterior motor regions, conduction aphasia typically is not associated with hemiparesis.

Conduction aphasia is associated with lesions in the left temporal-parietal region, particularly in an area that is immediately posterior to the Sylvian fissure called the supramarginal gyrus. As mentioned earlier, such a lesion disrupts the connection between the anterior and posterior language regions so that poor repetition of spoken utterances is a hallmark of this aphasia type.

Global Aphasia.   **Global aphasia** refers to severe language impairment affecting all domains. It is associated with large left hemisphere lesions that essentially damage the entire perisylvian region (Figure 9.3). In global aphasia, meaningful verbal output is typically extremely limited. In some cases, it is limited to repetitive utterances such as "one, two, three" or "I can see." In other cases, the utterances are repetitive jargon such as "nanna nanna nanna." Utterances that are repeated are called **perseverations**. It is worth mentioning that even individuals with significant global aphasia are capable of communicating wants, needs, and opinions if the listener provides a supportive communication environment.

Anomic Aphasia.   A common aphasia type that is not shown in Figure 9.3 is called **anomic aphasia**. This syndrome is characterized by word retrieval difficulty in conversation and in the context of naming tasks, with relative preservation of auditory comprehension and repetition abilities. Whereas all aphasia types exhibit word-finding difficulty, in the case of anomic aphasia, it is the primary deficit. Anomic aphasia can result from relatively isolated lesions in the posterior temporal-parietal region, but has also been associated with lesions throughout the left hemisphere. Some of the other aphasia types may evolve to anomic aphasia after a period of recovery if the extent of brain damage is not extensive. Therefore, the presence of anomic aphasia does not provide information about the location of the aphasia-producing lesion.

Causes of Aphasia

There are about one million Americans with aphasia, and about 80,000 new cases of aphasia every year (National Aphasia Association, 1999; National Institute on Deafness and Other Communication Disorders, 1997). It is a disorder most often associated with older age, with the average age for people with aphasia being about 67 years (Hier, Yoon, Mohr, et al., 1994). Stroke is the most common cause of brain damage resulting in aphasia. A **stroke**, also called a cerebrovascular accident, is an interruption of blood flow to the brain caused by blockage of an artery or the bursting of an artery (hemorrhage). When blood flow to brain cells is interrupted, they are deprived of oxygen, which ultimately results in cell death. Those brain cells do not regenerate, so the functions subserved by the damaged cells are impaired. Other causes of brain damage can also result in aphasia, such as traumatic accident, brain tumor, or infection.

It has long been known that in right-handed people, language problems tend to occur after damage to the left rather than the right hemisphere. It is damage to the left perisylvian region that typically results in aphasia. The major blood vessel that serves the perisylvian region is the middle cerebral artery; therefore, stroke affecting the left middle cerebral artery is the most common cause of aphasia (Benson & Ardila, 1996).

The onset of aphasia is typically abrupt but some etiologies may be associated with a slowly progressive onset. Brain tumors can cause slow onset of aphasia as they either infiltrate or compress critical language areas. **Progressive aphasia** is a relatively rare syndrome in which aphasia slowly develops in the absence of a documented neurological event (Duffy & Petersen, 1992; McNeil & Duffy, 2001).

Assessment

The initial evaluation of a person with aphasia may take place at the bedside while in an acute care hospital. Informal interaction with the patient allows observation of some aspects of verbal fluency, auditory comprehension, and word retrieval. A few structured tasks can further inform the speech-language pathologist of the patient's ability to understand spoken and written language, to repeat sentences, and to communicate by writing. The initial assessment goal is typically to characterize the nature of the impairment to appraise the functional abilities of the patient. A more comprehensive language assessment is typically deferred for a few days or weeks when the patient is able to sit at a table and tolerate the demands of sustained, structured interaction. However, the speech-language pathologist can be of considerable assistance to the patient and family during the first few days after the onset of aphasia as they seek to understand this strange disorder. Most importantly, the speech-language pathologist can facilitate successful communication with the patient and begin the process of training useful compensatory strategies to be used on a temporary or long-term basis.

Mrs. Victor awoke one morning and fell as she tried to get out of bed. She realized that her right side was weak and that she felt odd. After dragging herself to the nightstand, she dialed her daughter's phone number using her left hand. As she tried to respond to her daughter's "hello," Mrs. Victor realized that she could not speak. Her daughter recognized the unintelligible sounds as her mother's voice and assured her that she would be right over. Later that day, after a trip to the emergency room and admission to the medical center, Mrs. Victor lay in the hospital bed with her daughter at her side. It had been a hectic five hours of medical examinations, a brain scan, and admissions paperwork. When the hospital speech-language pathologist arrived for her first bedside visit, she found Mrs. Victor's daughter upset and confused about her mother's condition.

After ten minutes of informal interaction with Mrs. Victor, it was apparent to the speech-language pathologist that Mrs. Victor had global aphasia. In order to support Mrs. Victor in her attempts to communicate, the speech-language pathologist provided a pad of paper and began to write single words as possible responses

to questions she was asking. For example, to help Mrs. Victor respond to the question, "Where are you from?," the speech-language pathologist wrote (and said) *Tucson?* When Mrs. Victor shook her head no, the speech-language pathologist offered *Green Valley?* To which Mrs. Victor smiled and said, "yes." After several successful exchanges of information using the written support, Mrs. Victor and her daughter were obviously showing some relief. This initial visit ended with the speech-pathologist explaining to the daughter about aphasia and providing some written information about the nature of the communication impairment. Over the next several days, the daughter and nursing staff became adept at supporting Mrs. Victor's communication by offering written words, pictures, and objects as needed to clarify her intentions. Mrs. Victor was then transferred to a rehabilitation facility where she would receive aphasia treatment for several months. During her initial session with the speech-language pathologist at the rehab facility, she received a relatively extensive evaluation of her language abilities.

Comprehensive language assessment is frequently accomplished by the use of standardized tests for aphasia. Most of the tests take an hour or less to administer. They sample language behaviors of varying difficulty and allow the examiner to create a summary profile of aphasia type and severity. There are many supplemental tests that may also be used to characterize patient performance, as well as informal measures constructed by the speech-language pathologist. Some protocols are specifically designed to examine the impact of the language impairment on everyday communication situations and are considered functional communication measures. The overall goal of assessment is to document the current status of the patient and provide direction for the treatment plan.

Treatment

Individual Therapy.   The goal for aphasia treatment is to maximize the recovery of impaired language functions, to assist in the development of alternative and compensatory communication strategies, and to help the patient adjust to the residual deficits (Rosenbek, LaPointe, & Wertz, 1989). There are countless approaches to achieving such goals. It is the responsibility of the speech-language pathologist to select an existing treatment approach or to design a unique approach that is appropriate for the specific patient. The treatment plan should take into consideration the nature and extent of the language impairment as well as the residual language and cognitive abilities. Treatment plans are influenced by additional factors such as the time post onset of aphasia, the patient's functional needs, motivation, and desires. Although the classification by aphasia type is useful to characterize the overall aphasia profile, it does not offer specific direction for treatment because individuals with the same aphasia type may differ in many ways.

There is a large body of literature to guide speech-language pathologists to appropriate treatment approaches for a particular set of symptoms (see, e.g., Chapey, 2001; Helm-Estabrooks & Albert, 1991; Holland & Forbes, 1993; Rosenbek et al., 1989); however, it is the patient's response to treatment that is the ultimate

test of its effectiveness. The experienced clinician knows that a given treatment can be effective for patients with different impairments and that patients with similar impairments may respond differently to the same treatment approach (Hillis & Caramazza, 1994).

When selecting or designing a treatment plan, the speech-language pathologist may approach treatment from several different perspectives. One approach is to stimulate the return of language abilities that are impaired but appear to have potential to improve or be restored. For example, the stimulation approach pioneered by Hildred Schuell employed the repetition of phrases and sentences to improve auditory comprehension and verbal production (Jenkins, Pabon-Jimenez, Shaw, & Williams Sefer, 1975). Many treatment protocols are designed to stimulate language by following a task hierarchy that elicits responses that are progressively more difficult for the patient to produce (some are reviewed in Helm-Estabrooks & Albert, 1991). The speech-language pathologist may determine what support or cues are necessary to help the patient respond correctly and then systematically withdraw the support as the patient progresses. This approach incrementally shifts the burden from the clinician to the patient to achieve the desired response. When implementing a treatment plan, the speech-language pathologist is challenged to find the appropriate tasks that help the patient improve to a higher level of functioning. Whereas patients or family members may initially set their goals for completely normal language without any intermediate steps, the speech-language pathologist charts a realistic path that moves toward normal language but has many intermediate goals.

Some treatment approaches take advantage of residual abilities that can be used to substitute or compensate for impaired abilities. For example, a patient may be able to write a word, or part of a word, that he or she is unable to say. The use of writing to supplement spoken output may be an effective strategy; however, another possibility is that the written word may facilitate the spoken production of the word.

> After several months of language therapy, Mrs. Victor showed significant improvement of her comprehension of spoken and written language. Her spoken language remained severely impaired, however. She had several words and phrases that she typically uttered, such as, "yes, but I don't know," and "oh my, oh my." The speech pathologist implemented treatment to improve Mrs. Victor's ability to write meaningful single words to communicate her thoughts. Mrs. Victor was able to relearn the spellings of many words, so that after several months of treatment, she was able to write more than fifty words. It was noteworthy that on occasion, Mrs. Victor was able to say the word that she was writing, despite the fact that she rarely spoke meaningful words in other contexts.

Individual treatment plans may include several goals that variously address auditory comprehension, speech production, reading, writing, and gestural communication. The treatment for Mrs. Victor focused on written rather than spoken language due to the severity of her aphasia. Figure 9.4 (p. 222) shows another patient who responded well to a writing treatment (Beeson, 1999; Beeson, Hirsch, &

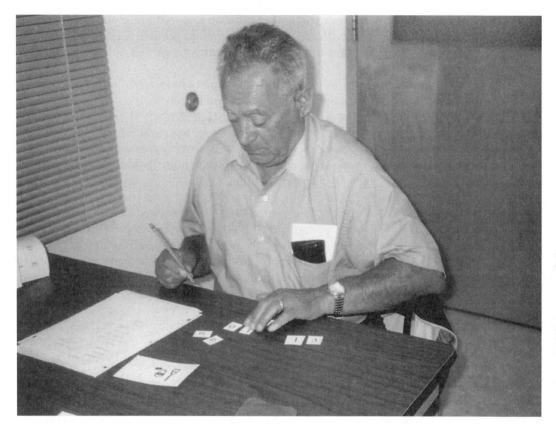

FIGURE 9.4   **Individual therapy to improve writing for single words that includes arrangement of letters to spell the word and copy of the word. (Courtesy of The University of Arizona, Department of Speech & Hearing Sciences)**

Rewega, 2002). Obviously, the return of spoken language is the treatment goal whenever possible. A variety of treatment approaches to improve spoken language have been shown to be effective (for examples, see Chapey, 2001; Helm-Estabrooks & Albert, 1991). Many individuals with aphasia are able to say a word if they hear the first sound or syllable of the word. This responsiveness to phonemic cueing (as it is called) can be particularly useful if the patient can learn to provide his or her own phonemic cue for the word (Nickels, 1992). Therapy goals are selected so that they are appropriate for the particular patient and have immediate or eventual impact on their functional communication abilities.

Group Therapy.   Aphasia may result in social isolation and reduced opportunity to engage in conversation. Group therapy for individuals with aphasia provides a setting where conversation is facilitated and supported by the clinician, and patients can learn to maximize their communication skills (see Figure 9.5). In a small

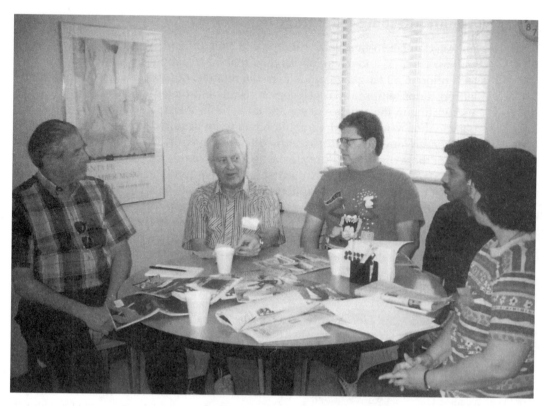

FIGURE 9.5 Group therapy for aphasia focuses on conversational language supplemented by writing and gestures. (Courtesy of The University of Arizona, Department of Speech & Hearing Sciences)

group of three to five individuals with aphasia, the speech-language pathologist can work with the patients to (1) facilitate successful communication despite their residual language impairment; (2) encourage communication using all modalities; and (3) teach and elaborate specific communication strategies (Holland & Beeson, 1998). In the small group setting, patients can learn from the clinician and from each other how to compensate for language difficulties. Alternative communication strategies including gestures, drawing, and writing are encouraged to supplement the spoken utterances of group members. Groups also can offer considerable psychological and social support for members as they adjust to their impairment. Many examples of structured and informal conversational activities have been reported in recent literature regarding group therapy (Elman, 1998; Kearns, 1994; Marshall, 1993; Springer, 1991), and there is evidence that some individuals with aphasia can continue to improve language abilities long after the time of their strokes (Holland & Beeson, 1998).

Acquired Reading and Writing Impairments

As noted, most individuals with aphasia have difficulty reading and writing as well as listening and speaking, so that aphasia treatment frequently includes intervention in all language modalities. On relatively rare occasions, damage to the left posterior temporal-parietal region results in isolated impairments of reading and writing in the absence of significant aphasia. Alexia refers to an acquired impairment of reading, and agraphia refers to an acquired impairment of writing. The speech-language pathologist is often involved in the assessment and treatment of these disorders. Pure **alexia**, also known as **alexia without agraphia**, is an unusual syndrome wherein the patient is able to write but cannot read. It is thought to result from a disruption of the transfer of visual information to the part of the brain that recognizes the word as a meaningful unit. The individual with pure alexia can see the words, and may even be able to identify the letters of the word, but fails to recognize the word as a whole. Many individuals with pure alexia compensate for their lack of word recognition by reading the individual letters aloud; when they hear the word spelled aloud, they can recognize it. This letter-by-letter reading approach is useful, but painfully slow.

> One day Mr. Lincoln answered the telephone and wrote down a message from the caller for his wife. Later, when his wife called home, Mr. Lincoln picked up the note to read her the message. To his surprise, the letters made no sense to him. He told his wife that there was something wrong with his eyes and that he thought he should go see his eye doctor. He told his doctor that he could not read his own handwriting! The eye doctor found that there was nothing wrong with Mr. Lincoln's eyes, but recognized that he probably had had a stroke affecting his ability to recognize written words.
>
> Within a week, Mr. Lincoln was in treatment with a speech-language pathologist to improve his reading. He could recognize single letters and "figure out" most words by spelling them letter-by-letter, but Mr. Lincoln had great difficulty recognizing written words as a whole unit. The speech-language pathologist implemented a reading treatment that involved reading written passages multiple times in order to increase his reading rate for the practiced text (Beeson & Hillis, 2001). Over the course of treatment, Mr. Lincoln showed improved reading rate for the practiced text, and, more importantly, his reading rate and accuracy improved for new reading material. In other words, the treatment appeared to improve his ability to recognize written words. Ultimately, Mr. Lincoln was able to read with adequate accuracy and speed to meet his daily needs.

Some individuals with acquired alexia also have difficulty spelling. They experience a syndrome called **alexia with agraphia**. As expected, the term **agraphia** refers to an acquired impairment of spelling. Individuals with acquired agraphia vary with regard to their residual writing abilities (Rapcsak & Beeson, 2002). Some may be able to sound out the spellings of words they cannot recall, relying on their preserved knowledge of the relations between sounds and letters. In such cases, it is not uncommon to make errors on irregularly spelled words. For example, "school" might be spelled *skool*. Given that individuals vary with regard to the na-

ture of their reading or writing difficulties, treatment approaches for acquired alexia and acquired agraphia are tailored to the specific nature of the impairment (Beeson & Hillis, 2001).

RIGHT-HEMISPHERE COMMUNICATION DISORDERS

Damage to the right hemisphere may result in some word retrieval difficulties similar to that observed in left-hemisphere damage. However, the prominent features of right-hemisphere damage (RHD) tend to be quite different from those associated with left hemisphere damage. Individuals with RHD may have a host of subtle impairments in their thought organization, mental flexibility, and their use of language that affect their ability to understand and communicate effectively (Myers, 1997; Tompkins, 1995). Although individuals with RHD typically understand the content of individual sentences, they often fail to understand the gist of the conversation; may not appreciate humor, figures of speech, facial expressions, and other nonverbal communication cues; and simply fail to keep up with natural give-and-take and shift of topic in conversation. These functions are referred to as extralinguistic aspects of communication, meaning that they are features other than the actual words used to speak. These problems sound rather vague and, in fact, individuals with RHD simply may be perceived as odd, or rude, or inattentive, rather than brain-damaged. Their change in cognitive and communication abilities is clearly evident to friends and family who know them well. One of the patients at our clinic, Mr. Rice, explained his perception of one of the effects of his right hemisphere stroke as follows:

> Taking turns in talking in conversation was very difficult . . . because I would interrupt and have something to say in the middle of the conversation and interrupt everything. Train of thought and everything else. I thought I had to jump in otherwise I'd lose what I was trying to say.

Mr. Rice was 66 years old when he experienced a right hemisphere stroke. One year after his stroke he still had weakness of his left arm and leg, but he could walk without assistance and communicated effectively. His speech was easy to understand but the prosody sounded somewhat flat, as if lacking emotion; even when he joked, his voice and facial expression were difficult to interpret. It was notable that Mr. Rice was able to provide some insight into the nature of his problem because many individuals with RHD do not recognize their problems.

Mr. Rice also experienced **left neglect**, in that he tended to orient his gaze away from the left and was relatively unaware of sensory input on the left side of his body and the left side of his visual field. Left neglect is relatively common following right-hemisphere damage, and it occurs even when there is no loss of sensory or motor function on the left side and no loss of vision on the left (Heilman, Watson, & Valenstein, 1993). In other words, the visual images are getting to the brain, but they are essentially ignored.

These effects of brain damage have shown that the right hemisphere plays a special role in maintaining attention to the space around us and our intrapersonal space as well. Left neglect may interfere with communication in that people to the patient's left are ignored, just as the left half of the page may be ignored when reading and writing. Myers (1997) suggested that neglect may be a significant contributor to the cognitive-communication impairment in a more general sense. Future research may help to clarify the relation between neglect and the behavioral profile associated with right-hemisphere damage.

Incidence of Right-Hemisphere Damage

Given the relatively subtle nature of the cognitive-communication problems associated with RHD, it is not surprising that the incidence and prevalence are not well documented. The American Heart Association (1992) reported that there were about 500,000 new strokes each year in the United States, with about half affecting the right hemisphere. Tompkins (1995) estimated that about half of RHD adults will have communication impairments, so we would estimate 125,000 new cases of right hemisphere-related communication impairments caused by stroke per year. Stroke is the most common cause of damage isolated to the right hemisphere, but other causes include traumatic injury or tumor.

Assessment and Treatment

Assessment of the patient with RHD typically includes sampling language in conversational and picture description tasks, assessing the extralinguistic aspects of communication, and examining for evidence of neglect or attentional problems (Myers, 1997; Tompkins, 1995). Examination of extralinguistic deficits includes tasks such as interpretation of a story or a pictured scene that requires integration of the component parts into one main idea. Patients may be asked to give the meaning of figures of speech or to produce the appropriate prosodic variation for expressions to convey different emotions. They may also be asked to produce and understand narrative stories. All of these tasks share the common goal of probing comprehension and use of language in a flexible, abstract manner that comes naturally to most adults, but may be problematic for those with RHD. Numerous tasks can be used to examine for neglect, including a very simple request for patients to put a mark on a line to divide it in half. Individuals with left neglect often bisect the line to the right of the midline because they do not perceive the leftmost part of the line. The ability to sustain attention is also assessed using tasks that increase from focused attention on one stimulus to divided attention to two stimuli. Some standardized tests are available to structure the examination of the RHD patient.

Treatment for cognitive and communication deficits associated with RHD is challenging. It may be directed toward facilitating recovery of the underlying impairment or toward the development of compensatory strategies to overcome the problems. Greater understanding of the underlying causes of the communication

deficits observed in RHD is needed, but it is currently assumed that the extralinguistic deficits are related to the features of neglect and inattention (Myers, 1997). For that reason, some treatment tasks are directed toward improving performance on attention tasks. For example, patients may be asked to listen or look for specific stimuli such as a particular number or word in the midst of other numbers or words (Sohlberg & Mateer, 2001). These types of attention tasks are also used with individuals with traumatic head injury because they also may have problems with attention. Tasks that are directed toward improving extralinguistic abilities may be similar to those used for assessment. After observing the patient's deficits, the speech-language pathologist may structure the language tasks in such a way that a hierarchy of cues provides support for the patient. As discussed in aphasia therapy, the clinician's goal is to assist the patient to make small sequential gains in the direction of normal performance. This may require providing feedback when the patient fails to produce or comprehend the extralinguistic features, such as prosodic variation to mark emotion, followed by a model of the appropriate response. The treatment goals are directed toward improved performance in a variety of settings and communication environments, not simply in the therapy room. This is true for all treatments for speech, language, and hearing disorders, but is especially relevant for the problems associated with RHD because they are often most evident during real-life communication.

DEMENTIA

Dementia refers to an acquired, progressive impairment of intellectual function that is chronic and affects several aspects of mental activity including memory, cognition, language, and the processing of visual-spatial information (Cummings & Benson, 1992; Kaszniak, 2002). Dementia may also result in changes in emotion or personality. It is distinguishable from temporary conditions that impair mental function such as confusional states that may last for a few hours or a few days, at most. The progressive intellectual decline in dementia is distinct from isolated, specific impairments such as aphasia due to focal brain damage. Numerous disease processes can cause the diffuse brain damage that results in dementia. The characteristics of the dementia vary to some extent depending on the disease process.

Types of Dementia

The most common type of dementia is **Alzheimer's disease** (AD) (Cummings & Benson, 1992). With about 4 million Americans affected by AD, it accounts for more than half of all dementias (Alzheimer's Association, 1995). It is characterized by language, memory, and cognitive impairments that include poor judgment, difficulty with calculation, reasoning, and higher level thinking. Caregivers note that the early signs of dementia include memory and concentration problems including forgetting the location of things, poor recall for recent events, and trouble

handling finances and performing complex tasks. Speech is typically well articulated and fluent and may have good grammatical structure, but the content is increasingly empty as the disease progresses. In the early stages, the language impairment may appear similar to anomic aphasia in that there are many instances of word-finding difficulties. In later stages, it may resemble the empty ramblings observed in some individuals with Wernicke's aphasia. At the end stages, there may be little verbal output at all.

Alzheimer's disease can be confirmed after death by the presence of specific brain changes observed if an autopsy is performed. For that reason, the diagnosis of AD prior to death is tentative, referred to as "probable" AD, based on the presenting symptoms and the exclusion of other causes of dementia. The criteria for the behavioral diagnosis of Alzheimer's disease and other types of dementia are described in detail in a manual published by the American Psychiatric Association (1994).

In addition to Alzheimer's disease, there are some forty or fifty other causes of dementia. One of the more common causes is vascular disease resulting in multiple strokes that produce diffuse brain damage. Whereas Alzheimer's disease tends to have a steadily progressive course, the cognitive decline associated with vascular, or **multi-infarct**, dementia may cause a stair-step decline as subsequent strokes occur. Other types of dementia are associated with Pick's disease, Parkinson disease, and Huntington's disease. **Pick's disease** is characterized by brain abnormalities in the frontal and temporal lobes and typically results in marked changes in personality. Parkinson disease is a relatively well-known progressive disorder of movement that is accompanied by dementia in about 35 to 40 percent of cases (Kaszniak, 2002). Huntington's disease is a genetic disorder that results in progressive onset of movement disorder and eventual dementia.

Memory impairment is often the initial symptom of dementia; however, in some cases the language decline may be the first sign. At our clinic, Mr. Dean brought his 67-year-old wife for an evaluation because her language "was becoming more and more confused," he said. Her speech was well-articulated and easy to understand, but it was devoid of meaningful content and contained many perseverative thoughts. A report of a head scan indicated there was a generalized loss of brain substance, but there was no evidence of a stroke.

When shown a toy gun and asked to name it, Mrs. Dean said:

Mrs. Dean: This is to put. Um, you can put a thing inside the . . .

PB: Can you tell me the name of it?

Mrs. Dean: Well, it's supposed to be, to do. But that, that's musty. It's hard, when you're on the table and the table is dirty, I take the longer thing, like this this, and get the end. I don't, don't go by this thing. No, this I, see it always in my house. Oh here I can do this, I can do this. It goes if you go.

Mrs. Dean's verbal output sounded in many ways like an individual with aphasia. However, there were some features of her behavior that were unlike those

observed in aphasia. She showed anxiety and perseverative thoughts as she re-peatedly asked where her husband had gone and how was she going to get home. Mr. Dean indicated during a private interview that his wife had become paranoid about her money. She no longer used the bank, but had begun stuffing money under the mattress at home. Six months following the interview, Mrs. Dean's neu-rologist observed that her behavior became increasingly bizarre, showing signs as-sociated with frontal lobe damage, such as lack of inhibition and modesty. The neurologist rejected a diagnoses of progressive aphasia and Alzheimer's disease in favor of a working diagnosis of Pick's disease. Like AD, Pick's disease is a cortical dementia. In Pick's disease, brain changes occur primarily in the frontal and tem-poral lobes resulting in changes in personality that accompany the changes in in-tellect, memory, and language. Like Alzheimer's disease, the diagnosis of Pick's disease is not actually confirmed unless the brain is studied after death.

Prevalence

Although the exact prevalence of dementia is not known, there is a clear increase with age. It has been estimated that the syndrome affects approximately 5 to 8 per-cent of individuals over 65 years, 15 to 20 percent of individuals over 75 years, and 25 to 50 percent of those over 80 years (American Psychiatric Association, 1997). The prevalence of dementia is expected to increase as the older segment of our population continues to grow in number.

Assessment and Intervention

A comprehensive neuropsychological examination of cognitive function is critical to the diagnosis of dementia and may be performed by a neuropsychologist. Several standardized rating scales are used to screen for dementia. These scales include tasks that look at general knowledge, memory, communication, and visual-spatial skills (such as drawing). Other scales rate the severity of dementia using observa-tional criteria, rather than direct testing. Comprehensive tests of cognitive function evaluate attention, initiation, visual-spatial construction, conceptualization, lan-guage, and memory. In many settings, a speech-language pathologist is involved in the assessment of language and communication abilities and contributes to the un-derstanding of language function relative to other cognitive abilities. Individuals with dementia may also have concomitant hearing impairment that interferes with daily function and performance on cognitive assessments, so that an audiological evaluation is an important component of the diagnostic process.

Speech-language pathologists are taking an increasingly active role in the care of individuals with dementia. Although dementia is an irreversible process, therapeutic approaches may be employed that maximize communication and cog-nitive performance (Mahendra, 2001). There are numerous sources of information regarding environmental and linguistic manipulations that positively influence the behavior of individuals with dementia (Bayles & Tomoeda, 1995; Glickstein, 1988; Hopper, 2001; Lubinski, 1991). For example, communication performance

can be improved by minimizing distractions and using familiar objects or pictures to stimulate recollections. Auditory comprehension may be improved with the use of simplified syntax and vocabulary. Memory demands can be minimized by making use of a memory book that contains biographical information, pictures of family and friends, and schedule information (Bourgeois, 1992).

The patient's performance profile on a test battery can be examined to determine the relative strengths and weaknesses of the individual with dementia. This information combined with observation and experimentation may help clinicians discover the cognitive, language, and environmental manipulations that minimize the effects of the dementia (Bayles & Tomoeda, 1995). It is often the role of the speech-language pathologist to develop a program that outlines strategies for communicating with specific dementia patients. The speech-language pathologist works with caregivers including family members and nursing home staff to implement the plan and thus provide consistent support to maximize the performance of the dementia patient. In the case of Mrs. Dean, it was apparent that her husband was exhausted by his failure to communicate successfully with his wife. He stated, "She can't even tell me what she wants to eat for dinner." One easy solution to that problem was discovered: If Mr. Dean wrote down three choices for dinner as he asked his wife what she would like, she was able to respond by pointing to one of the options. Other suggestions were made to Mr. Dean to adapt his communication style in such a way as to maximize his wife's ability to communicate.

In closing this chapter, we want to emphasize that acquired impairments of language and cognition may have profound implications for the lives of the affected individuals and their families. Patients may experience significant limitations on their daily activities and may greatly restrict their participation in society. Thus, speech-language pathologists who work with adults with acquired language disorders are not simply concerned with the acquired impairment, but with the consequences of that impairment. Evaluation and treatment approaches are sensitive to the specific needs of a given individual in their unique life situation.

CLINICAL PROBLEM SOLVING

Mrs. Anderson was a 55-year-old woman who suffered a left-hemisphere stroke that resulted in aphasia. She was administered the Western Aphasia Battery (Kertesz, 1982) to sample her language abilities. As part of the test, she was asked to describe what was happening in a pictured scene of a man and a woman having a picnic near a lake. Her spoken response follows:

> Is family, um, picnic. And fish, and man is, um, oh, um reading, and, and, um lady is pouring and set, um, son is, is, ha . . . is, um, is, um, flying kite. And neighbor is fishing and neighbor is um, sailing, and boy is, um, playing in water, and man, and lady in, listen to radio. And daughter, I mean, dog, oh . . . oh . . . stave, is lady, is man, is stave, oh, stay. I don't know.

1. Would you classify Mrs. Anderson's aphasia as fluent or nonfluent?
2. In what lobe of the brain is the lesion most likely to be located? Why?
3. Mrs. Anderson had trouble repeating sentences longer than four words. Would you expect her lesion to be in the perisylvian region or outside the perisylvian region? Why?
4. Would you guess that Mrs. Anderson had right hemiparesis? Why, or why not?

REFERENCES

Alzheimer's Association. (1995). *The changing face of Alzheimer care: Proceedings of the 4th National Alzheimer's Disease Education Conference.* Chicago: Author.

American Heart Association. (1992). 1992 heart and stroke facts, quoted in medical news and perspectives. *Journal of the American Medical Association, 267,* 335–336.

American Psychiatric Association. (1994). *Diagnostic and statistical manual on mental disorders* (4th ed.). (DSM-IV). Washington, DC: Author.

American Psychiatric Association. (1997). Practice guidelines for the treatment of patients with Alzheimer's disease and other dementias of late life. *American Journal of Psychiatry, 154,* 1–33.

Bayles, K., & Tomoeda, C. (1995). *The ABCs of dementia.* Tucson, AZ: Canyonlands Publishing.

Beeson, P. M. (1999). Treating acquired writing impairment: Strengthening graphemic representations. *Aphasiology, 13,* 367–386.

Beeson, P. M., Bayles, K. A., Rubens, A. B., & Kaszniak, A. W. (1993). Memory impairment and executive control in individuals with stroke-induced aphasia. *Brain and Language, 45,* 253–275.

Beeson, P. M., & Hillis, A. E. (2001). Comprehension and production of written words. In R. Chapey (Ed.), *Language intervention strategies in adult aphasia* (4th ed., pp. 572–595). Baltimore, MD: Lippincott, Williams & Wilkins.

Beeson, P. M., Hirsch, F., & Rewega, M. (2002). Successful single-word writing treatment: Experimental analysis of four cases. *Aphasiology, 16,* 473–491.

Benson, D. F., & Ardila, A. (1996). *Aphasia: A clinical perspective.* New York: Oxford University Press.

Bourgeois, M. S. (1992). *Conversing with memory impaired individuals using memory aids: A memory aid workbook.* Gaylord, MI: Northern Speech Services.

Chapey, R. (Ed.). (2001). *Language intervention strategies in adult aphasia* (4th ed.). Baltimore: Lippincott, William & Wilkins.

Cummings, J. L., & Benson, D. F. (1992). *Dementia: A clinical approach.* Boston: Butterworth.

Damasio, H., & Damasio, A. (1980). The anatomical basis of conduction aphasia. *Brain, 103,* 337–350.

Elman, R. (1998). *Group treatment of neurogenic communication disorders: The expert clinician's approach.* Boston: Butterworth-Heinemann.

Glickstein, J. K. (1988). *Therapeutic interventions in Alzheimer's disease.* Rockville, MD: Aspen Publishers.

Goodglass, H. (1993). *Understanding aphasia.* San Diego, CA: Academic Press.

Heilman, K. M., Watson, R. T., & Valenstein, E. (1993). Neglect and related disorders. In K. M. Heilman & E. Valenstein (Eds.), *Clinical neuropsychology* (3rd ed., pp. 279–336). New York: Oxford University Press.

Helm-Estabrooks, N., & Albert, M. L. (1991). *Manual of aphasia therapy.* Austin, TX: Pro-Ed.

Hier, D. B., Yoon, W. B., Mohr, J. P., Price, T. R., & Wolf, P. A. (1994). Gender and aphasia in the stroke data bank. *Brain and Language, 47,* 155–167.

Hillis, A. E., & Caramazza, A. (1994). Theories of lexical processing and rehabilitation of lexical deficits. In M. J. Riddoch & G. W. Humphries (Eds.), *Cognitive neuropsychology and cognitive rehabilitation* (pp. 449–484). Hillsdale, NJ: Lawrence Erlbaum Associates.

Holland, A. L., & Beeson, P. M. (1998). Aphasia groups: The Arizona experience. In R. Elman (Ed.), *Group treatment of neurogenic communication disorders: The expert clinician's approach.* Boston: Butterworth-Heinemann.

Holland, A. L., & Forbes, M. (Eds.). (1993). *Aphasia treatment: World perspectives*. San Diego, CA: Singular.

Hopper, T. (2001). Indirect interventions to facilitate communication in Alzheimer's disease. *Seminars in Speech and Language, 22*, 290–304.

Jenkins, J. J., Pabon-Jimenez, E., Shaw, R. E., & Williams Sefer, J. (1975). *Schuell's aphasia in adults: Diagnosis, prognosis and treatment* (2nd ed.). Hagerstown, MD: Harper & Row.

Kaszniak, A. W. (2002). Dementia. In V. S. Ramachandran (Ed.), *Encyclopedia of the human brain*. San Diego: Elsevier Science.

Kearns, K. P. (1994). Group therapy for aphasia: Theoretical and practical implications. In R. Chapey (Ed.), *Language intervention strategies in adult aphasia* (3rd ed., pp. 304–318). Baltimore: Williams & Wilkins.

Kertesz, A. (1982). *Western Aphasia Battery*. New York: Grune & Stratton.

Lubinski, R. (1991). (Ed.). *Dementia and communication*. Philadelphia: B. C. Decker.

Mahendra, N. (2001). Direct interventions for improving the performance of individuals with Alzheimer's disease. *Seminars in Speech and Language, 22*, 275–290.

Marshall, R. (1993). Problem focused group therapy for mildly aphasic clients. *American Journal of Speech-Language Pathology, 2*, 31–37.

Murray, L. L. (2002). Attention deficits in aphasia: Presence, nature, assessment, and treatment. *Seminars in Speech and Language, 23*, 107–116.

Myers, P. S. (1997). Right hemisphere syndrome. In L. L. LaPointe (Ed.), *Aphasia and related neurogenic language disorders* (2nd ed., pp. 210–225). New York: Thieme.

National Aphasia Association. (1999). Aphasia fact sheet. New York: Author.

National Institute on Deafness and Other Communication Disorders (NIDCD). (1997). *NIDCD fact sheet: Aphasia* (NIH Publication No. 97-4257). Bethesda, MD: Author.

Nickels, L. (1992). The autocue? Self-generated phonemic cues in the treatment of a disorder of reading and naming. *Cognitive Neuropsychology, 9*, 155–182.

Rapcsak, S. Z., & Beeson, P. M. (2002). Neuroanatomical correlates of spelling and writing. In A. E. Hillis (Ed.). *Handbook on adult language disorders: Integrating cognitive neuropsychology, neurology, and rehabilitation.* (pp. 71–99). Philadelphia: Psychology Press.

Rosenbek, J. C., LaPointe, L. L., & Wertz, R. T. (1989). *Aphasia: A clinical approach*. Austin, TX: Pro-Ed.

Sohlberg, M. M., & Mateer, C. A. (2001). *Cognitive rehabilitation: An integrative approach*. New York: Guilford.

Springer, L. (1991). Facilitating group rehabilitation. *Aphasiology, 6*, 563–565.

Tomkins, C. A. (1995). *Right hemisphere communication disorders: Theory and management*. San Diego, CA: Singular Publishing Group.

Wertz, R. T., Collins, M. J., Weiss, D., Kurtzke, J. F., Friden, T., Brookshire, R. H., Pierce, J., Holzapple, P., Hubbard, D. J., Proch, B. E., West, H. A., Davis, L., Matlvitch, V., Morley, G. K., & Resurreccion, E. (1981). Veteran's Administration cooperative study on aphasia: A comparison of individual and group treatment. *Journal of Speech and Hearing Research, 24*, 580–594.

READINGS FROM THE POPULAR LITERATURE

Bauby, J-D. (1997). *The diving bell and the butterfly*. New York: Random House. (locked-in syndrome)

Bayley, J. (2000). *Elegy for Iris*. New York: St. Martin's Press. (Alzheimer disease)

Bryant, B. (1992). *In search of wings: A journey back from traumatic brain injury*. South Paris, ME: Wings Press. (traumatic brain injury)

Crimmins, C. (2000). *Where is the mango princess?* New York: Random House. (traumatic brain injury)

Davidson, A. (1997). *Alzheimers, a love story. One year in my husband's journey*. Secaucus, NJ: Carol Pub. Group. (Alzheimer disease)

DeMille, A. (1981). *Reprieve*. New York: Doubleday. (famous dancer's account of her stroke)

Douglas, K. (2001). *My stroke of luck*. New York: W. Morrow. (actor's experience with stroke, aphasia, and dysarthria)

Ellison, B., & Ellison, J. (2001). *Miracles happen: One mother, one daughter, one journey*. New York: Hyperion. (spinal cord injury)

Fishman, S. (1988). *A bomb in the brain: A heroic tale of science, surgery and survival*. New York: Scribner. (brain hemorrhage, subsequent epilepsy)

Harper, M. S. (2001). *The worst day of my life, so far*. Athens, GA: Hill Street Press. (Alzheimer's disease)

Klein, B. S. (1998). *Slow dance: A story of stroke, love and disability*. Berkeley, CA: Page Mill Press. (stroke and aphasia)

McCrum, R. (1999). *My year off: Recovery from stroke*. Canada: Random House. (stroke and aphasia)

McGowin, D. F. (1994). *Living in the labyrinth: A personal journey through the maze of Alzheimer's disease*. New York: NY: Dell Publishing. (early Alzheimer's disease from patient's perspective)

Newborn, B. (1997). *Return to Ithaca: A woman's triumph over the disabilities of a severe stroke*. Rockport, MA: Element. (young woman with aphasia)

Osborne, C. (1998). *Over my head: A doctor's own story of head injury from the inside looking out*. Kansas City, MO: Andrews McMeel Pub. (traumatic brain injury)

Quinn, D. (1998). *Conquering the dark: One woman's story of recovering from a brain injury*. St. Paul, MN: Paragon House. (traumatic brain injury)

Rife, J. M. (1994). *Injured mind, shattered dreams: Journey from severe head injury to a dream*. Cambridge, MA. Brookline Books. (traumatic brain injury)

Shiplett, J. L. (1996). *A glass full of tears*. Aurora, OH: Writer's World Press. (dementia)

Swanson, K., & Chrunka, M. (1999). *I'll carry the fork*. Los Altos, CA: Rising Star Press. (traumatic brain injury)

Talavaro, J. (1998). *Look up for yes*. New York: Kodansha International. (locked-in syndrome)

Wulf, H. (1973). *Aphasia, my world alone*. Detroit, MI: Wayne State University Press. (aphasia)

THE BIOLOGICAL
FOUNDATIONS OF HEARING

THEODORE J. GLATTKE

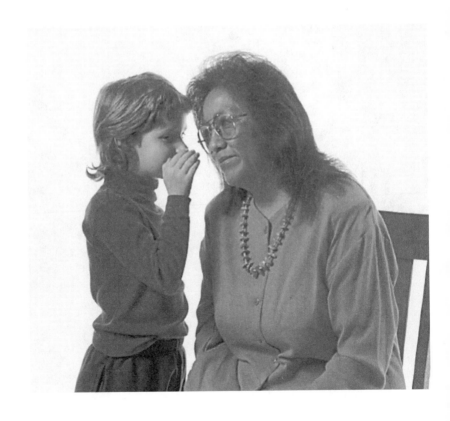

■ ■ ■ ■ ■ ▬▬▬▬▬▬▬▬▬▬▬▬▬▬▬▬▬▬▬▬▬▬▬▬▬▬▬▬▬▬

PREVIEW

Sound is a form of energy that is present everywhere in our environment. In Chapter 3, we learned that sound can be described in terms of frequency and intensity and the characteristics of the sounds associated with speech. In this chapter, we consider how the sounds around us are received and processed by the auditory system. We will see how the structures of the outer and middle ear transmit sound to the inner ear. We will learn how the structure of the inner ear contributes to our ability to hear sounds of different pitches and how the nervous system further shapes sound perception.

STRUCTURE AND FUNCTION OF THE EAR

The Outer Ear

The ear usually is described as having three distinct divisions: outer, middle, and inner. As illustrated in Figure 10.1 (p. 236), the outer ear consists of a visible portion, the **auricle** or **pinna**, and a canal that leads from the pinna to the eardrum or tympanic membrane. The canal between the pinna and tympanic membrane is the **external ear canal**.

The shape of the pinna is created by pieces of cartilage that form ridges and depressions that are peculiar to each person. In fact, pinna configurations are so unique that we could identify people using "pinna prints" instead of fingerprints. In adults, the pinna is about 3.5 inches in height and about 1.5 inches wide. It is a sound collector and also serves to enhance the sound pressure of certain frequencies. You can exaggerate this effect by cupping your hand behind your pinna and thus increasing the dimension of the sound collector. For most people, the pinna acts to increase high frequency sounds by about 5 dB SPL. It also helps us to locate the sources of high-frequency sounds that are overhead, such as those produced by flying insects.

The external ear canal is about 1 inch long and about 0.4 inch in diameter. Cartilage forms the foundation of the canal near the pinna. The inner portion of the canal is framed by hard bone. If you place you finger slightly into the canal and move your jaw, you can feel your jawbone moving against the flexible portion of the external ear canal. The canal protects the tympanic membrane from physical trauma due to nearly everything except for cotton swabs pushed into the canal by the owner! Specialized cells in the floor of the ear canal produce a waxy substance called **cerumen** that helps to keep the skin of the canal moist and traps debris that might normally fall against the tympanic membrane. Like the pinna, the length and shape of the ear canal also serves to enhance sound pressure. The canal produces a boost in SPL of about 15 dB for sounds in the frequency region of 2500 to 3500 Hz and for multiples of those frequencies. Taken together, the effects of the

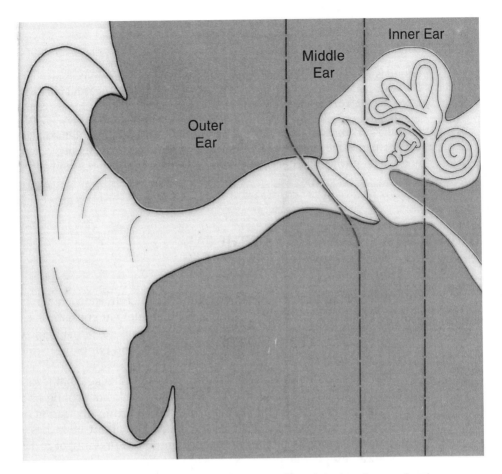

FIGURE 10.1   **A schematic drawing of the divisions of the hearing mechanism.**

pinna and external ear canal provide a helpful boost in the mid and high frequency region of the sound spectrum. Without those structures, we would have a slight loss of hearing.

The Middle Ear

The **middle ear** consists of a cavity, a ventilating tube that connects the cavity to the pharynx, and several moving parts that work together to boost the pressure created by the sound energy that arrives at the eardrum or tympanic membrane. The middle ear apparatus is called a **transformer** because of the change in pressure that it creates. You probably use transformers every day: The small adapters that are connected to electric outlets to power recorders, CD players, computer accessories, and video cameras are transformers that change the voltage (pressure) sup-

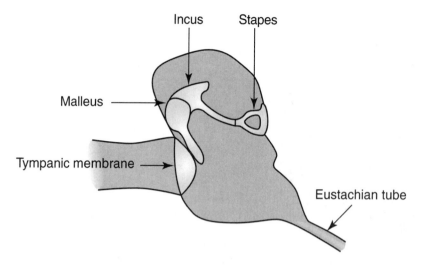

FIGURE 10.2   The middle ear.

plied by the power company to a value that is required by the device. By analogy, the middle ear provides a boost in pressure to drive the inner ear system.

The principal parts of the middle ear are illustrated in Figure 10.2. The middle ear cavity is formed of bone that is covered by thin mucosa that is similar to the lining of the nasal cavities. The volume of the cavity is small, less than about 2 cc. The eardrum, or **tympanic membrane**, is stretched across the opening of the external canal so that nearly all of the sound energy entering the canal pushes on the eardrum. It is thin, flexible, and yet strong enough not to burst when humans dive 100 or more feet below the surface of the ocean. The eardrum is roughly circular in shape and has a diameter of about 1 cm, a little less than 1/2 inch. It is connected to three bones, or **ossicles** that span the middle ear cavity between the eardrum and the inner ear. The names of the ossicles were inspired by their shapes. The hammer, or **malleus**, is the first of the ossicles. It is about 9 mm long and its long arm is attached firmly to the eardrum. The anvil, or **incus**, is the second ossicle and is about 7 mm in size. The head of the incus and head of the malleus are covered by tissue that holds them together so that they move together. In this way, they form two arms of a lever. The difference in the length of the two bones helps to create the transformer effect of the middle ear. The third ossicle is the stirrup, or **stapes**. The footplate of the stapes looks like the bottom of a stirrup. The footplate is oval, and it is about 3 mm in length and about 1 mm in width. It fits into an opening called the oval window of the inner ear system.

The principles by which the middle ear transformer works are illustrated in Figure 10.3 (p. 238). The transformer boosts the pressure by a significant amount. The largest boost is due to the differences in the areas of the eardrum and stapes footplate. The part of the eardrum that moves in response to the incident sound

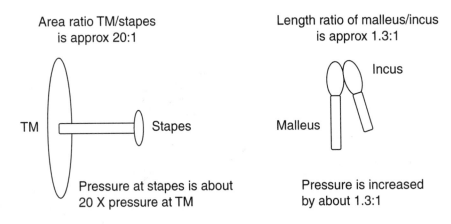

Area ratio TM/stapes
is approx 20:1

Length ratio of malleus/incus
is approx 1.3:1

TM   Stapes   Incus   Malleus

Pressure at stapes is about
20 X pressure at TM

Pressure is increased
by about 1.3:1

Combination of area ratio and lever
system = pressure boost of 26:1

FIGURE 10.3   Mechanisms that create the transformer effect of the middle ear.

has an area that is about twenty times the area of the stapes footplate. The force that collects on the eardrum is transmitted directly to the footplate and so the force per square mm of area at the stapes is boosted by a factor of about 20 to 1. This boost in pressure, or *force per unit of area*, is the same effect that occurs when a thumbtack is used. The force applied to the large head is sufficient to enable the tack to penetrate a piece of wood because the area of the point of the tack is much smaller than the area of the head.

The second mechanism that helps to boost the pressure is found in the lever action resulting from the difference between the lengths of the malleus and incus. The ratio of 9 mm (malleus) to 7 mm (incus) is equivalent to about 1.3 to 1. Force applied to the long arm of the lever is increased by an amount equal to the ratio of the lengths of the long and short arms, or about 1.3 to 1. The combination of the ratio of the areas of the eardrum and stapes (20:1) and the lever action of the ossicles (1.3:1) provides a boost of about 26 to 1, or about 28 dB. The combined effects of the outer and middle ear systems allow us to hear sounds that are about 30 to 60 dB below the intensities that would be needed if our outer and middle ear apparatus did not exist or was destroyed. Individuals born without an external ear canal or middle ear apparatus or persons who have an ear infection that leaves the middle ear full of thick fluid will experience a loss of hearing of about 60 dB for airborne sounds.

This middle ear transformer will work properly only *when the eardrum is intact* and when the *cavity is filled with air*. The **Eustachian tube** connects the middle ear cavity with the pharynx, and it opens each time a swallow occurs. When the tube opens, air passes from the back of the throat into the middle ear, and fluid that is secreted by the lining of the middle ear is allowed to drain into the throat. If the

tube is blocked, the exchange of air and drainage of fluid will be affected. The tube may become blocked if someone has upper respiratory allergies, a cold, or other condition that causes an increase in secretion or swelling of the tissue that lines the middle ear, Eustachian tube, or pharynx. If the air is not refreshed, then the air in the middle ear cavity will be absorbed by the tissue and the eardrum will be pushed inward by the difference in air pressure between the atmosphere and the middle ear cavity. A clinician looking at the eardrum will say that it is "retracted." Many people experience a temporary retraction of the eardrum when they are passengers in an airplane that descends rapidly for a landing. The increase in air pressure associated with the loss of altitude must be matched by the middle ear—this usually is accomplished by swallowing. If an air passenger has a cold, it may be difficult to balance the pressure. The result may be a painful experience and a temporary loss of hearing. The pain is a signal that the eardrum is pushed inward or retracted, and the loss of hearing is due to the fact that the stiffness of the eardrum is increased when the pressure in the middle ear does not match the pressure in the ear canal. The increased stiffness resulting from a pressure imbalance will cause the eardrum to respond poorly to low-frequency sounds and the result may be a loss of hearing in the low-frequency region.

If the Eustachian tube remains blocked for a long period of time, the clear fluid that is secreted by the lining of the middle ear cavity will collect in the cavity. The fluid replaces the air and the fluid level can rise to a point where it can be seen by a clinician using an otoscope to examine the eardrum. The addition of the fluid increases the stiffness of the eardrum considerably because of the reduction of the volume of air in the middle ear cavity and the incompressibility of the fluid. This produces a greater hearing loss that may eventually include both low and high frequency sounds if the cavity fills completely. The disorder caused by fluid in the ear is called *otitis media* (see also Chapter 11). It not only creates a hearing problem, but it also is a serious medical problem that requires attention. If the fluid remains for a long period of time, it serves as a fertile medium for infection that can lead to serious consequences, including spontaneous rupture or perforation of the eardrum. A middle ear that is filled with fluid combined with a perforated tympanic membrane loses its ability to work as a transformer.

The middle ear ossicles are attached to two small muscles. The tensor tympani muscle pulls the malleus inward, toward the center of the head. The muscle is named because it tenses or stiffens the eardrum or tympanum. The tensor tympani muscle is innervated by the Vth cranial nerve (trigeminal), which is the principal sensory nerve of the face and controls the muscles that are involved in chewing. The tensor tympani contracts when we swallow, yawn, and chew, and it also responds to tactile stimulation of the skin of the face. The second muscle is the stapedius. When it contracts, it pulls the stapes outward. The stapedius muscle is innervated by the VIIth cranial nerve (facial), which controls the muscles of facial expression. The stapedius muscle contracts in response to sounds that are about 60 to 80 dB SPL in persons with normal hearing thresholds.

When the stapes contracts in response to sound, it adds stiffness to the middle ear transformer system. The change in stiffness can be measured by a clinical

instrument known as a tympanometer. The change in stiffness resulting from contraction of the stapes is known as the *acoustic reflex*. The reflex is bilateral, which is to say that it appears on both sides during stimulation of either ear. In this way it is like the change in pupil diameter that occurs when a bright light is presented to either eye. Traditionally, the acoustic reflex was thought to serve to protect the ear from intense sound. However, few sounds found in nature (such as thunder, the roar of waterfalls, rockslides, an imminent predator) are of sufficient intensity to activate the acoustic reflex. It is noteworthy that our world became very noisy long after middle ear muscles were created. Therefore, it is unlikely that these muscles were designed to protect against the industrial noises of gunpowder, steam, internal combustion, and jet engines.

A modern view of the action of the acoustic reflex is that, although it may help to protect the ear from intense sounds, its principal role is to alter the transmission characteristics of the middle ear to enable us to hear important sounds, such as speech, in noisy situations. The tensor tympani muscle may serve the same role when we are creating noise by eating, swallowing, or talking. Neither muscle can react with sufficient speed to protect us from the most dangerous sounds in our world: the explosive reports of firearms.

In Chapter 2, we considered how the biological systems that support speech and language were affected in a child with Down syndrome. This genetic disorder also affects the hearing mechanism as well. We can see how the outer and middle ear mechanisms are affected in the case of Alicia.

> Alicia underwent a full audiologic evaluation to determine hearing function. Like most children with Down syndrome, she has small and irregular pinnas. The audiologist used an otoscope in order to examine the appearance of the ear canal and tympanic membrane. For some children with Down syndrome, the ear canal is narrower than usual. In the case of Alicia, the ear canals have a normal appearance and are open and clear. However, she appears to have some fluid in the middle ear. This is common in children with Down syndrome, who have a high rate of middle ear infections. Alicia's mother reports that her child has been plagued by these infections. On this day, the presence of middle ear fluid was accompanied by a mild degree of hearing loss because the fluid changed the mechanical workings of the tympanic membrane and ossicles. The fluid caused an increase in the stiffness of the moving parts of the middle ear apparatus.

The Inner Ear

The inner ear converts energy to a code that can be interpreted by the brain. In this way, it serves the same role as the retina of the eye, touch receptors in the skin, and olfactory receptors in the nose and taste buds. The process of conversion is called *transduction*. The inner ear has three separate transduction systems: (a) the vestibule, (b) the semicircular canals, and (c) the cochlea. Transducers in the vestibule help us to maintain our orientation with respect to gravity, or the center of the earth. The semicircular canal systems provide us with information about head position and help us to maintain a fix on visual targets when we are moving.

The cochlea contains the transducers for hearing. The three parts of the inner ear share important features. The first is that the inner ear is filled with fluid. Forces acting on the inner ear due to gravity, acceleration of the head or body, or sound ultimately create motion of the fluid in the inner ear system. The fluid couples the energy of the stimulus to the transducers that convert the stimulus to responses of neurons. The second shared feature is that the transducer mechanisms are similar in all three parts of the inner ear. They consist of a mechanical receptor, called a *hair cell*, and a *covering membrane* that causes or otherwise enhances the motion of the hairlike cilia found on the top of the hair cells. The remainder of the chapter will focus on how these principles apply in the cochlea—the end organ for hearing.

Cochlear Structure and Function

The fundamental arrangement of several important parts of the cochlea is illustrated in the series drawings in Figure 10.4 on page 242 (after Kiang, 1975). The cochlea is a hard-walled chamber that is filled with fluid (Figure 10.4A). There are two flexible "windows." The **oval window** is the location at which the stapes footplate connects to the inner ear. The **round window** is a second opening on the body of the cochlea, and it is also covered with a flexible membrane. When the stapes forces the oval window inward, the round window is forced outward by the pressure of the fluid in the chamber. In Figure 10.4B the stapes has been added and a "basilar" (basement) or supporting membrane is stretched across the cavity. The inward motion of the stapes causes the **basilar membrane** to move in response to fluid displacement because it lies in the pathway of the fluid.

Sensory cells are added in Figure 10.4C. These are hair cells that sit on the basilar membrane. An opening called the helicotrema allows the fluid in the top channel to flow directly into the bottom channel. (Note that the helicotrema is located at the top, or apex, of the cochlea in its true, coiled shape.) Fluid will flow through the opening only when the stapes moves very slowly, such as in the case in which a change in air pressure within the middle ear causes the oval window to be pushed inward or pulled laterally. When stapes vibrations occur rapidly, such as at the lower limit of our range of hearing, then the basilar membrane responds to the forces applied by the stapes.

There are about 12,000 hair cells in the cochlea of humans with healthy ears. The structure is designed to accommodate the hair cells along a length of about 36 mm (from the end close to the stapes to the opposite end, called the apex). To illustrate this point, Figure 10.4D extends the length of the fluid chamber. Figure 10.4E shows the fluid chamber coiled into a shell shape, approximating the true configuration of the cochlea.

Sitting on the basilar membrane is the **organ of Corti**, named for the anatomist who provided an early description of its structure. In Figure 10.5 (p. 243), we see its components, which include supporting structures, hair cells, and an overlying membrane called the tectorial membrane (tectum = roof). This is the view you would have if you unrolled the cochlea as in Figure 10.4D and then sliced it as if you were slicing salami. There are two sets of hair cells—a single row

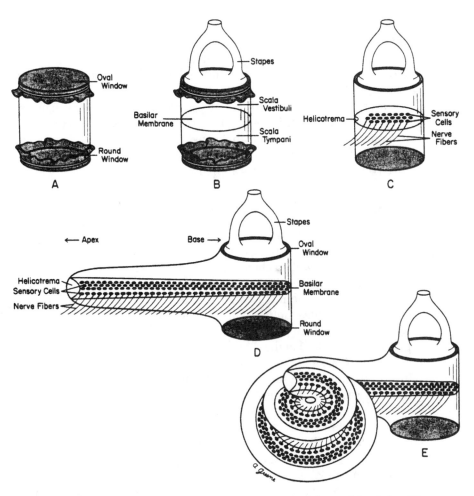

FIGURE 10.4 Schematic drawing of the components of the cochlea (after Kiang, 1975). As shown in drawings A and B, the cochlea is likened to a hard-walled container with flexible membranes on the top and bottom and another membrane stretched across the middle (C). Drawings D and E elongate the container to better represent the structure of the true cochlea.

of inner hair cells and three rows of outer hair cells. These cells are so named because they contain hairlike projections called **cilia**. Hair cells are delicate and can be easily damaged through aging, disease, exposure to certain drugs, or by prolonged exposure to loud noise. Once damaged, the hair cells can regenerate in some species, such as birds, but they do not repair themselves in mammals. Movement of the basilar membrane sets off a shearing motion of the hair cell cilia. This motion is translated by the receptor cells into a chemical-electrical signal that is carried to the brain via auditory nerve fibers.

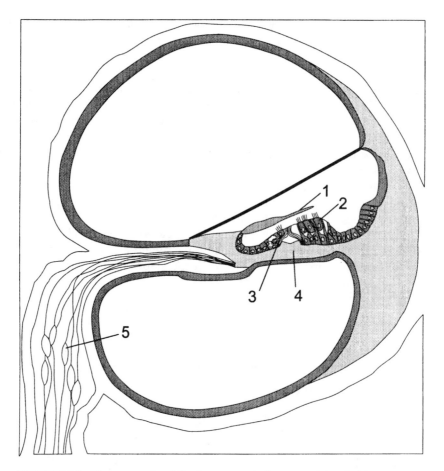

FIGURE 10.5   Components of the inner ear and organ of Corti: (1) tectorial membrane, (2) outer hair cells, (3) inner hair cells, (4) basilar membrane, (5) cell body within the acoustic nerve.

The shape of the basilar membrane influences how sound energy is analyzed by the cochlea. The membrane is relatively narrow at the base, the end near the stapes. It is about ten times wider at the apex. A change in stiffness accompanies the change in width of the basilar membrane so that the base end is about 100 times stiffer than the apex end. The gradation in stiffness is important because it helps to determine how sounds are represented in the cochlea. The stiffness of the basilar membrane near the base of the cochlea creates an efficient response for high-frequency sounds. The more flaccid region near the apex cannot respond to high frequency energy, so its responses are limited to low frequencies.

The stiffness change from the base to the apex of the cochlea allows the cochlea to analyze the sounds transmitted by the stapes, much like a spectrum

analyzer discussed in Chapter 3. The basis of the analysis was described by Georg von Békésy in 1928. He examined the behavior of the cochleas of several species of animals. The bone containing the cochlea was removed from the animal's skull and drilled to expose the membranes in the fluid spaces of the ear. The preparation was placed under a conventional light microscope and then driven mechanically by a sound source. Von Békésy described the motion patterns of the basilar membrane and noted that a *traveling wave* developed along the membrane in response to sound. When high frequency sounds were employed, the disturbance traveled only a few millimeters from the base of the cochlea. When low frequencies were used, the traveling wave spread from the base to the apex. The place of maximum vibration of the traveling wave was determined by the frequency of the sound. Because each frequency was associated with a specific place of stimulation, the cochlea was said to be *tonotopically organized*.

The illustrations in Figure 10.6 are based on von Békésy's observations (Békésy, 1960). Three sketches of the basilar membrane are shown. The membrane is "unrolled" as in Figure 10.4D, with the stapes on the base on the right and

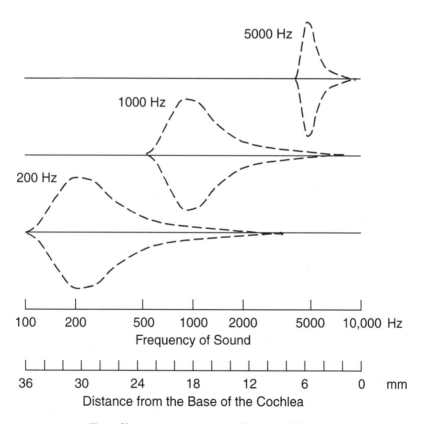

FIGURE 10.6 **Traveling waves corresponding to different sound frequencies as described by von Békésy.**

the apex at the left. The dashed lines represent the gross patterns of the traveling wave disturbances for 5000, 1000, and 200 Hz, respectively. The numerical scales below the three schematics provide an indication of the distance along the basilar membrane in millimeters and the places where individual frequencies would create the maximum disturbances. The traveling waves described by von Békésy appeared to move from base to apex. Frequencies between about 1000 and 20,000 Hz are represented along the 18 mm of the membrane closest to the base of the cochlea. Frequencies between about 100 and 1000 Hz are represented in the "upper" half of the cochlea, between about 18 and 36 mm from the base. Frequencies below about 100 Hz probably result in a wave that sweeps the basilar membrane from end to end without developing a peak in the disturbance pattern.

Von Békésy's work ushered in a new understanding of how the inner ear analyzed sound. His continuing efforts over the next thirty years led to the Nobel Prize in Medicine and Physiology, which was awarded to him in 1961. Two physicists, Gold and Pumphrey, examined the von Békésy studies and studies of human threshold sensitivity and frequency discrimination and concluded that there had to be some active amplifier process that actually added energy to the signal arriving via the stapes footplate (Gold, 1948, 1989). They reasoned that this amplifier might occasionally become unstable and develop a shrill whistle, like one hears when a public address system produces "feedback." They also reasoned that the amplifier elements must be highly tuned. Gold and Pumphrey presented their ideas to scientific experts about 1948, twenty years after von Békésy's report, but they were unable to convince anyone of the merit of their theory and so they pursued other scientific ventures.

About twenty years after Gold and Pumphrey's brief visit to auditory science, evidence for the leakage of energy from the ear back into the air was discovered by David Kemp, who also had a background in physics. Kemp was listening to low-intensity sounds and realized that some unknown source of sound was interacting with the external sound. When he placed a miniature microphone in the ear of a listener, he was he was able to record the "whistle" that reflects the "feedback" predicted by Gold and Pumphrey (Kemp, 1978). The tones recorded by Dr. Kemp, and from thousands of other subjects since 1978, must reflect an energy source within the inner ear and some disturbance that is transmitted backward through the fluid of the inner ear and middle ear cavity to the eardrum. In this case, the eardrum works like a loudspeaker diaphragm, producing vibrations in the air rather than responding to them! These sounds are called **otoacoustic emissions**. Emissions occur spontaneously and in response to stimulation and are present in virtually every healthy ear. Kemp found the evidence needed to support the notion that an active "amplifier" exists inside of the cochlea.

For a power source, we must look at the details of the organ of Corti. Recall that there are three rows of outer hair cells and only a single row of inner hair cells. Therefore, the outer hair cells outnumber the inner hair cells by about 3:1 (9000 to 3000 in humans). There are also a number of other differences between these two types of cells (see Table 10.1, p. 246). The hair cells also differ in shape—the outer hair cells are relatively cylindrical in shape whereas the inner hair cells are jug-

TABLE 10.1   **Differences between Inner and Outer Hair Cells**

OUTER HAIR CELLS	INNER HAIR CELLS
Three rows of cells	One row of cells
Cylindrical shape	Jug-shaped
Contact tectorial membrane	No contact with tectorial membrane
Sit on flexible basilar membrane	Sit on bony shelf
Support cells at hair cell base	Support cells surround hair cells
Receive efferent nerve fibers from the brain	Send afferent nerve fibers to the brain

shaped. The position and structural support of the two types of cells also differs. The outer hair cells are in contact with the tectorial membrane, but the cilia of the inner hair cells are free of attachments above their cell bodies. Outer hair cells are also situated over the flexible basilar membrane, whereas the inner hair cells sit on a rigid bony shelf. The inner hair cells are firmly encased in supporting structures that surround each inner hair cell, but the outer hair cells are situated on supporting cells at their base. Finally, the inner hair cells receive nearly all of the afferent or sensory nerves leading from the ear to the brain. In contrast, the outer hair cells receive nearly all of the efferent or control nerves leading from the brain back to the ear.

These differences point to important functional differences between the outer and inner hair cells. Today, most theories of inner ear function argue that the inner hair cells are the actual "sensory" transducers. The nerve supply attached to the inner hair cells and measures of their electrical properties during stimulation of the ear are compatible with this notion. The outer hair cells are thought to contribute to the amplification of motion in the inner ear in response to low intensity sounds. No one has actually "seen" the outer hair cells in operation inside of the ear, but we do know several things about how they work. If outer hair cells are missing, hearing loss occurs in that region. When outer hair cells are compromised or destroyed, the inner hair cells do not function normally. However, if the outer hair cells return to normal function, the inner hair cells do so as well. Likewise, otoacoustic emissions disappear when outer hair cells are compromised, only to reappear if the outer hair cells are restored to normal function.

Outer hair cells have been studied *in vitro*, that is to say, in artificial environments after being removed from an ear. Studied this way, Brownell and his coworkers (1983) discovered a startling fact in the early 1980s: They demonstrated that the outer hair cells changed their lengths in response to chemical stimulation. Other investigations have demonstrated that changes in cell length of 5 to 10 percent of the original length can occur in response to electrical, chemical, or mechanical (acoustic) stimulation. When the cell is activated, or depolarized, by a stimulus, *it becomes shorter*! If the cell is returned to its resting electrical (chemical) state, then *its length is restored*! Finally, if the cell is hyperpolarized, the opposite of depolarization, then *its length increases*! As illustrated in Figure 10.7, depolarization

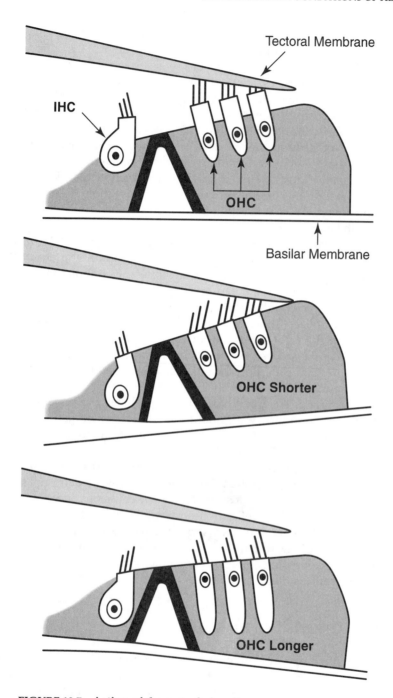

FIGURE 10.7 Action of the outer hair cells.

of the outer hair cells occurs when the cilia are tilted toward the tallest row. Hyperpolarization would occur if the cilia are forced to move in the opposite direction beyond their normal resting positions. In a sense, the outer hair cells act like small biological motors or muscles, changing length with each cycle of the stimulus that is effective in driving them. If the *in vitro* observations predict what is occurring in the living ear, then it is possible that the outer hair cells enhance the motion of the organ of Corti structures by alternately compressing and then expanding. During upward motion of the basilar membrane, as illustrated in Figure 10.7, the outer hair cells become shorter, effectively pulling the tectorial membrane and other structures closer together and forcing endolymph to stream across the inner hair cell cilia. Basilar membrane motion in the opposite direction is associated with a lengthening of the cells, exaggerating the motion and amplifying the motion of the fluid across the inner hair cell cilia.

It is clear that the analysis of incoming sounds performed by the cochlea is very precise and sensitive to exquisitely low levels of stimulus intensity. A leading scientist and physician of the nineteenth century, Helmholtz (1885) predicted today's theory about 140 years ago by suggesting the cochlea contained highly tuned resonators that could vibrate to enhance the response of the basilar membrane. The earlier observations of von Békésy (1860), based on dead ears, took auditory theory in the right direction, toward recognition of the importance of a traveling wave in the analysis of sounds by the inner ear. When the highly tuned devices (the outer hair cells) become unstable, spontaneous otoacoustic emissions are created in a way that is probably similar to the creation of feedback in a conventional hearing aid. The inner hair cells are probably the actual sensory transducers that provide information about sound. The outer hair cells appear to enhance the performance of the cochlea so that minute amounts of energy can create a sensation of sound! The outer hair cells work very hard to help us to hear, and they are very vulnerable to noise, certain medications, and systemic problems that compromise their energy supply. When outer hair cells are damaged temporarily by loud noise, we experience a loss of otoacoustic emissions and a temporary loss of hearing. When outer hair cells are destroyed, the losses of emissions and hearing become permanent. No other sensory system comes with its own built-in amplifier. If it did, you would find energy leaking from the system back to the environment (like emissions): Eyes would emit light, noses would emit odorants, temperature receptors might emit heat!

AUDITORY CONNECTIONS IN THE BRAIN

We hear with our brains, not our ears. Each ear communicates with the central nervous system (CNS) through afferent (ascending) and efferent (descending) connections. The outer hair cells receive nearly all of the efferent connections from the brain to the ear. The inner hair cells are connected to nearly all of the afferent neurons. The afferent neurons travel from the ear to the CNS in the VIIIth cranial nerve, referred to as the auditory nerve. The auditory nerve also contains the neu-

rons from the vestibular system. The neurons from the auditory portion of the VIIIth cranial nerve end when they reach the brain stem. They make connections with neurons in the cochlear nucleus.

As illustrated in Figure 10.8, the neurons that leave the cochlear nucleus travel to other places in the CNS, where they make connections. In the figure, ascending pathways from the right and left ears are shown as solid and dashed lines, respectively. The ascending nerve fibers connect with several groups of neurons (called nuclei) within the brainstem, where auditory information is processed. These are shown in light gray. There are two sets of nuclei in the brainstem, where some of the ascending auditory information crosses from one side of the brain to the other. Neurons in the brainstem project to the cerebrum, first through subcortical nuclei (dark gray), and from there neurons radiate diffusely to the primary auditory cortex, which is found in the temporal lobe of the brain.

It is important to note that the right and left ear inputs are mixed together in the brain stem and that each of the nuclei and fiber tracts above the cochlear

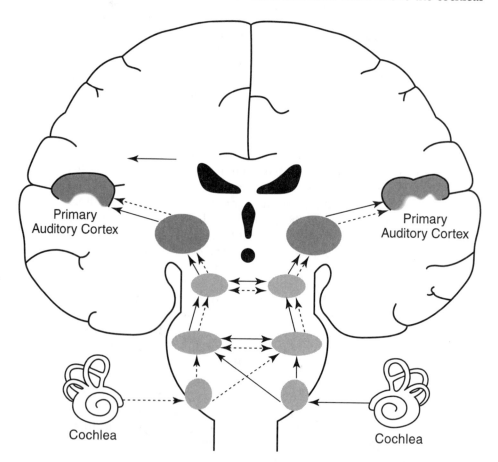

FIGURE 10.8 The central auditory pathways (components not to scale).

nucleus contains neurons that can be traced to both ears. This *binaural* representation helps us to locate sounds in space by comparing the information received from one ear with the information received from the other. The function of each of the major structures in the CNS that contain auditory neurons is not understood completely. However, we know that all of the structures maintain the tonotopic organization that was established in the cochlea. In other words, individual frequencies in simple and complex sounds are represented at specific places within the nervous system from ear to cortex. Much of what we know about the function of individual parts of the auditory nervous system comes from studying humans who have experienced damage to structures due to physical trauma or disease. Mr. Viner provides one such example.

> Mr. Viner suffered a small stroke (blockage of blood flow within the brain). This damaged the tissue of the primary auditory cortex on the left side of his brain. However, the surrounding language areas within the left hemisphere were left intact. Because the auditory cortex in his right hemisphere was intact, he could still process sounds and his hearing was normal. Two years later, he suffered a second stroke, this time in the right hemisphere. It was much more extensive, damaging the primary auditory cortex and surrounding cortical regions. Suddenly, Mr. Viner's hearing changed drastically. He could detect when sounds occurred, but he could not "make sense" of them. His wife now had to write notes to communicate, because when she spoke he heard jibberish. In fact, his own speech sounded so abnormal to him, he soon stopped talking as well, resorting to the use of a writing pad to communicate with others.

In Mr. Viner's case, the blood supply to the auditory cortex was eventually interrupted on both sides of the brain. When damage affects only one side, the patient may not experience a hearing loss and may reveal only subtle problems associated with understanding speech in noisy situations. If the auditory cortex is destroyed on both sides, then the patient may have a loss of hearing but will not be deaf. Rather, he or she may have difficulty finding the sources of sounds in space, understanding speech, and making sense of musical sequences. At the lower end of the system, damage to the auditory nerve will affect hearing in the ear served by that nerve. The amount of hearing loss due to damage to the nerve is not easy to predict exactly. Persons with auditory nerve damage often have difficulty understanding speech, even without a significant hearing loss for pure tones. In addition, they may not hear intense sounds with appropriate loudness. In contrast, persons who lose outer hair cells reveal a hearing loss and an abnormal growth of loudness when sounds become intense! Reports of subtle symptoms by patients will help a clinician arrive at a clearer picture of the causes of the patient's problems.

In summary, the auditory system is exquisitely designed to help us become aware of and to use the sounds that occur in our environment. The design enhances our ability to hear by virtue of three important features: (1) resonance properties of the outer ear, (2) transformer action of the middle ear, and (3) active amplification of the energy that arrives at the inner ear. The cochlea analyzes sounds into the individual frequencies that are present in a way that is similar to a

spectrum analyzer. Individual inner hair cells are responsive to very narrow ranges of frequencies in the spectrum through a process that creates *tonotopic organization* in the cochlea. Neurons carrying information from the inner hair cells to the CNS maintain the tonotopic organization. The CNS is also organized so that information about individual tones projects to specific places. All of the elements of the auditory system operate constantly, because we are never free of auditory stimulation. At a primitive level, the auditory system helps us to ward off danger and to find sources of survival. At a more advanced level, the visual system connects us with the objects in our world and the auditory system connects us with the people in our world through speech, music, and other sounds that we associate with them.

Our most important link with people is language and our most important link in language that develops normally is hearing. The auditory system is uniquely designed to allow us to be aware of sounds, locate them, and recognize them. Its acoustical, physical, and psychological features are unique, sensitive, and structured to enhance our listening abilities. The most vital parts can be permanently injured by intense stimulation. Once gone, they cannot be repaired. The best hearing aids that we have today cannot restore normal quality to sound, though they provide remarkable assistance to persons with hearing impairments. The best action to take is to avoid situations that are dangerous to your hearing so that you can preserve the unique human link that is associated with the auditory system.

CLINICAL PROBLEM SOLVING

Mr. Johnson is 65 years old and has worked in a newspaper press room for forty years. Although he has been using ear plugs to protect his hearing for ten years, he did not think about protecting his hearing when he was much younger. Today, he has a permanent hearing loss, mainly in the high frequency region.

1. What region of the basilar membrane (base, middle, apex) is likely to be damaged in Mr. Johnson's ears?
2. Which cells in the organ of Corti are likely to be affected by a forty-year history of noise exposure?
3. Give some examples of speech sounds that Mr. Johnson might not be able to recognize because of his hearing loss.

REFERENCES

Békésy, G. von (1960). *Experiments in hearing*. New York: McGraw Hill.

Brownell, W. E. (1983). Observations on a motile response in isolated hair cells. In W. Webster & L. Aitkin (Eds.), *Mechanisms of hearing*. (pp. 5–10). Clayton, Australia: Monash University Press.

Gold, T. (1948). Hearing: II. The physical axis of the action of the cochlea. *Proceedings of the Royal Society, 135*, 492–498.

Gold, T. (1989). Historical background to the proposal 40 years ago of an active model for cochlear frequency analysis. In J. P. Wilson &

D. T. Kemp (Eds.), *Cochlear mechanisms: Structure, function and models* (pp. 299–306). London: Plenum Press.

Helmholtz, H. L. von (1885). *On the sensations of tone as a physiological basis for the theory of music. (Translated by Alexander Ellis.)* London: Longmans, Green. (Reprinted by Dover Publications, 1954.)

Kemp, D. T. (1978). Stimulated acoustic emissions from within the human auditory system. *Journal of the Acoustical Society of America, 64,* 1386–1391.

Kiang, N. Y-S. (1975). Stimulus representation in the discharge patterns of auditory neurons. In D. B. Tower (Ed.), *The nervous system: Volume 3: Human communication and its disorders* (pp. 81–96). New York: Raven Press.

CHAPTER ELEVEN

DISORDERS OF HEARING
IN CHILDREN

ANNE MARIE THARPE

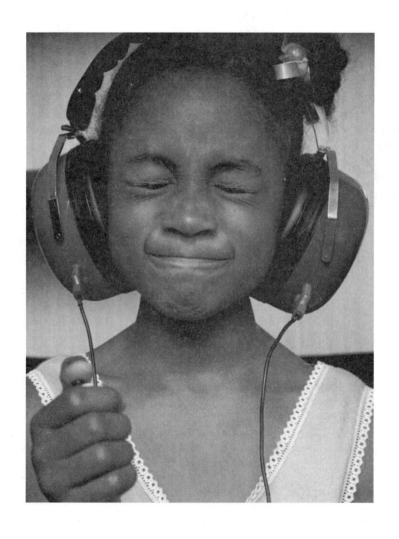

■ ■ ■ ■ ■

PREVIEW

For the vast majority of children, listening and learning through the auditory modality is a passive and natural process. However, some children experience a hearing loss that impairs their ability to communicate and may require some level of habilitation. Audiologists are uniquely trained professionals with the skills to evaluate the hearing of children of any age, even newborns. Audiologists are also prepared to initiate intervention, provide support and counseling to families, and work with educators and other professionals to design habilitation and educational programs for children with hearing loss. This chapter will begin with a discussion of the various causes, types, and degrees of hearing loss in children. We will investigate the identification and impact of hearing loss on the receptive and expressive communication of children.

Between 1 and 6 per 1000 children experience a hearing loss that impairs their ability to communicate and may require some level of habilitation (Parving, 1993; Watkin, Baldwin, & McEnery, 1991). The presence of a hearing loss can create challenges for the developing child related to communication, education, and socialization. To understand the potential impact for the child, the following questions must be addressed: How severe is the hearing loss? Is it permanent or temporary? Which frequencies are affected by the hearing loss? A hearing test will begin to answer these, and other, questions. To test hearing, we use an electronic instrument called an **audiometer**. It generates pure-tone frequencies at different levels of intensity. The goal of hearing testing is to determine the lowest intensity level at which various pure tones are detected. The person's responses are plotted on an **audiogram**. A sample audiogram of a person with normal hearing can be seen in Figure 11.1. It shows the test frequencies marked along the horizontal row at the top of the audiogram, with the lowest pure tone representing 125 cycles per second or 125 Hz and the highest 8000 Hz. The intensity is represented in decibels and is marked in the column on the left margin. A typical normal threshold is zero, and the most intense signal that can be produced by most audiometers is 120 dB. The right-ear response is plotted with a circle (red, if color is used). We can remember this with the mneumonic "red, right, round." The left-ear response is plotted with an X (blue, if in color).

When a person has normal hearing, the audiogram shows thresholds at or around 0 dB. Recall that 0 dB reflects the softest sounds detectable by most healthy young listeners. In Figure 11.1, the audiogram shows thresholds for the right and left ear are between 0 and –5 dB, showing normal hearing.

Air conduction audiometry refers to the presentation of speech or pure-tone stimuli transmitted through earphones to the patient. The test signal travels through the ear canal, across the eardrum and middle ear space, to the inner ear, and is ultimately transmitted to the auditory centers in the brain. You can follow

Frequency (Hz)

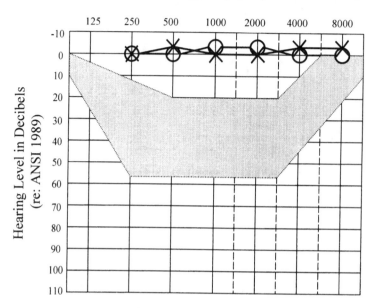

FIGURE 11.1   **An audiogram displays results of hearing testing. An individual's responses to pure tones of varying frequencies (labeled across the top of the audiogram) are plotted according to the lowest intensity level at which they heard those tones (labeled along the vertical axis). Round symbols correspond to responses to tones in the right ear; the *xs* correspond to responses to tones in the left ear. The gray region represents the range frequencies and intensities over which most speech sounds occur.**

the path of an air-conducted signal by viewing Figure 11.2A on page 256. As you can see, if someone has difficulty hearing a signal by air conduction, the problem could be in any of the areas through which the signal travels.

   Bone conduction audiometry refers to the transmission of sounds presented to the patient by a bone vibrator that is usually placed behind the ear on the mastoid bone. The vibrator causes the bones of the skull to vibrate, which in turn stimulate the inner ear or **cochlea**. The cochlea is a labyrinth carved into the skull that is lined with a membranous surface and filled with fluid. When a signal causes the skull to vibrate, the cochlea is stimulated directly, and hearing does not depend on the outer and middle ears. You can follow the path of a bone-conducted signal by viewing Figure 11.2B on page 256. If someone has difficulty hearing by bone conduction, the damage must be in the inner ear or auditory nerve. Such hearing losses result in fairly equal air and bone conduction thresholds, and the condition is known as a sensorineural hearing loss (Figure 11.3A).

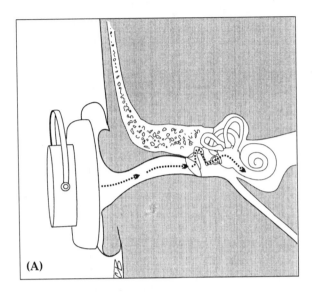

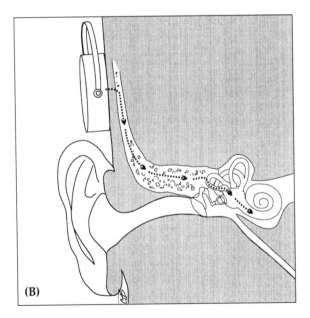

FIGURE 11.2   The two pathways of sound in the ear. Broken arrows demonstrate the route of (A) air conduction hearing and (B) bone conduction hearing.

When someone demonstrates normal hearing by bone conduction, but has difficulty hearing signals presented by air conduction, the problem must be in the outer or middle ears. This condition is known as a conductive hearing loss (Figure 11.3B). The difference between the air and bone conduction responses is referred to as an air-bone gap. When an individual has both a sensorineural and a conductive hearing loss it is referred to as a **mixed hearing loss** (Figure 11.3C).

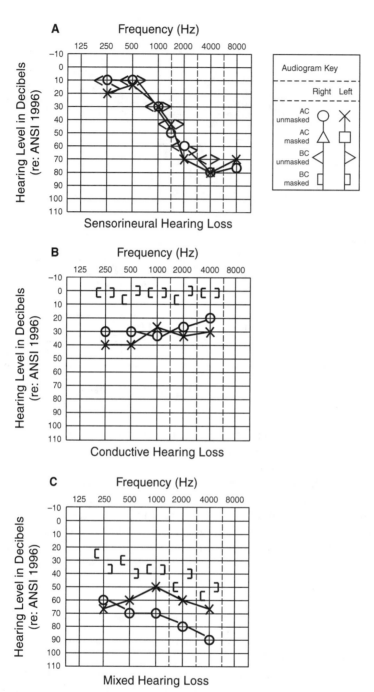

FIGURE 11.3   Pure tone air and bone conduction audiograms. (A) Severe high-frequency sensorineural hearing loss. (B) Mild conductive hearing loss. (C) Moderate to severe mixed hearing loss.

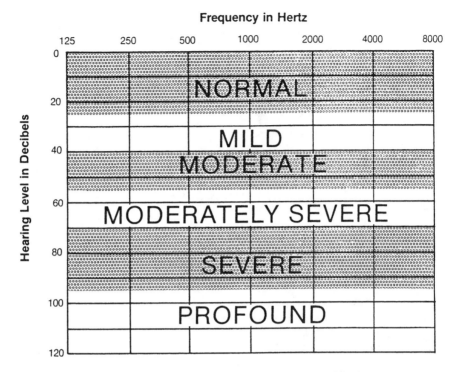

FIGURE 11.4   Classification of pure tone hearing loss by degree.

In addition to classifying the type of hearing loss, the audiogram is also used to classify the degree of hearing loss. Figure 11.4 illustrates a widely accepted classification of the degree of hearing loss.

As valuable as the audiogram is for describing the type and degree of hearing loss, it is important to note that we cannot predict academic, social, or communicative success or limitations from the audiogram alone. It simply defines the line between hearing and not hearing at various frequencies. It does not describe the quality of what is heard or the difficulties that the hearing loss may impose on an individual. Those issues will be addressed later in this chapter.

AUDITORY PATHOLOGIES

Disorders associated with hearing loss in children can be genetic, **congenital** (present at birth), or acquired at any point in development. It is important to note that these categories can overlap. That is, not all genetic disorders are congenital and not all congenital disorders are genetic. For example, mucopolysaccharidoses syndrome (MPS) is a genetically inherited metabolic disorder but children with MPS are healthy at birth. Over time, the genetic effect of this disorder results in a progressive hearing loss with age. On the other hand, children whose mothers abuse

alcohol during pregnancy may incur damage to the auditory mechanism in utero as one of several symptoms of fetal alcohol syndrome. The resulting hearing loss is congenital, acquired during prenatal development, but not genetic. We will review a variety of disorders using the following categories: *genetic without associated abnormalities, genetic with associated abnormalities, acquired prenatally, acquired perinatally,* and *acquired postnatally.*

Genetically Inherited Hearing Loss

Over the last decade, our knowledge of genetic hearing impairment has increased dramatically. Approximately thirty auditory genes have been identified, and hereditary hearing impairment occurs as a result of mutations in these genes (Morton, 1991). It is estimated that 50 percent of all hearing loss is genetically transmitted (or **endogenous**). Approximately two-thirds of genetic hearing losses occur as the only abnormality, and one-third occurs in association with additional abnormalities or as part of a *syndrome*. Pediatric audiologists frequently must draw on knowledge of genetics to counsel families. We see this in the following case:

> Caesar's parents were taken totally by surprise when they were told that he had a moderate sensorineural hearing loss in both ears. After several weeks of thinking and talking with each other about the hearing loss, they returned to Caesar's audiologist and asked him whether their future children were at risk for hearing loss. Although not a geneticist, their audiologist knew that because Caesar had no other risk factors for hearing loss, there was a high likelihood that the hearing loss was the result of a recessive mode of genetic inheritance. After explaining the possible causes of hearing loss to Caesar's parents, they were referred for further genetic counseling.

Genes occur in pairs and are located on twenty-three pairs of **chromosomes**. One member of each gene pair is inherited from each parent. Each egg and sperm carries one-half of the chromosomes from each parent so that when the egg is fertilized by the sperm, a child inherits half of the genes from the father and half from the mother. There are three primary patterns of inheritance: *autosomal dominant, autosomal recessive,* and *x-linked.*

Autosomal Dominant.   Approximately 20 percent of genetic hearing loss is the result of dominant inheritance (Morton, 1991). With this type of inheritance, only one copy of the gene is required to transfer the trait to the next generation. As illustrated in Figure 11.5 (p. 260), one parent typically exhibits the trait and each offspring has a 50 percent chance of inheriting the gene for hearing loss.

This does not mean that half of the children of a parent with an autosomal dominant gene will be affected. It does mean, rather, that each child has a 50 percent chance of being affected. Furthermore, a dominant type of hearing loss may present a different clinical picture from one child to the next. If different children exhibit different features of the same genetic disorder, the disorder is said to have a *variable expression.* In other cases, some children who inherit the gene may not

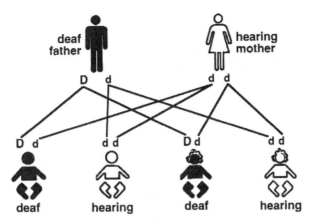

FIGURE 11.5 Persons with dominant deafness have one dominant gene (D) and a corresponding normal gene (d). Each child has a 50/50 chance to inherit the deafness gene (D) from the parent who has this trait. (From Shaver, 1988. Reprinted with permission.)

exhibit any features of the syndrome, or the disorder may be very mild. This is known as *reduced penetrance*.

The first autosomal dominant gene localization was identified in 1992 (Leon, Raventos, Lynch, et al., 1992). Since then, approximately forty autosomal dominant gene loci for nonsyndromic hearing loss have been identified. Typically, these losses have onset between 11 and 30 years of age, are progressive, and sensorineural in nature. Some of the most common types of dominantly inherited syndromes associated with hearing loss can be found in Table 11.1.

Autosomal Recessive. Recessive inheritance accounts for the vast majority (approximately 80%) of genetic hearing loss (Shaver, 1988). A child must receive two copies of the gene for **hearing impairment** in order for the trait to be expressed. This means the parents of a child with recessive hearing loss each carry one normal and one abnormal gene in the pair so both have normal hearing. However, if their child receives both copies of the abnormal gene, a hearing loss will occur. As shown in Figure 11.6, when both parents are carriers of the recessive gene for hearing loss, each child of that union has a 25 percent chance of being affected. If only one abnormal gene is inherited, the child will be a carrier for that trait but will not be affected.

Although approximately one in eight individuals carries a gene for hearing loss, there are so many different types of recessive genes for hearing loss that it is extremely rare for two individuals carrying the same gene for hearing loss to mate. When blood relatives mate, referred to as a **consanguineous** union, however, it is more common for recessive hearing loss to appear because of the increased likelihood that parents have inherited the abnormal gene from a common ancestor.

To date, ten autosomal-recessive genes for nonsyndromic hearing loss have been discovered. Nearly all genes for autosomal recessive genetic hearing

TABLE 11.1 Genetic Disorders Associated with Hearing Loss

DISORDER	CLINICAL SIGNS
AUTOSOMAL DOMINANT DISORDERS	
Waardenburg's syndrome	Pigment abnormalities including a white forelock and different colored irises; unilateral or bilateral sensorineural hearing loss.
Alport's syndrome	Nephritis; ocular lesions; progressive hearing loss.
Stickler syndrome	Ocular anomalies; cleft palate; progressive hearing loss.
Treacher Collins syndrome	Facial malformations including depressed cheek bones, deformed pinna, receding chin; conductive or mixed hearing loss.
Branchio-oto-renal syndrome	Ear malformation; renal anomalies, mixed hearing loss.
Neurofibromatosis	Tumor disorder; variable audiological findings.
AUTOSOMAL RECESSIVE DISORDERS	
Usher syndromes	Retinitis pigmentosa; congenital sensorineural hearing loss.
Friedrich's ataxia	Nervous system disorder; ocular abnormalities; abnormal movement; progressive sensorineural hearing loss.
Hurler's syndrome	Growth failure; mental retardation; progressive hearing loss.
X-LINKED DISORDERS	
Hunter's syndrome	Growth failure; mental retardation; mixed or conductive hearing loss.
Norrie's syndrome	Progressive visual impairment; mental retardation, progressive sensorineural hearing loss.
Alport's syndrome	Renal disorder; ocular abnormalities; progressive sensorineural hearing loss.

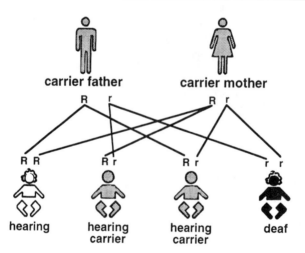

FIGURE 11.6 Persons with recessive deafness have a double dose of the deafness gene (r), one inherited from each of the parents. The parents are hearing carriers and have a 25 percent chance to produce a deaf child with each pregnancy. (From Shaver, 1988. Reprinted with permission.)

impairment identified thus far cause **prelingual** (before the development of speech) severe-to-profound hearing loss (Sundstrom, Van Laer, Van Camp, & Smith, 1999). By far the most important gene identified is commonly referred to as the connexin gene. The connexin gene is believed to be responsible for almost 40 percent of nonsyndromic, autosomal recessive hearing loss (Steel & Bussoli, 1999). Family studies have revealed that hearing loss associated with this gene abnormality is quite variable, ranging from mild-moderate to profound (Cohn & Kelley, 1999). Some of the more common examples of recessively inherited syndromes that include hearing loss are provided in Table 11.1.

X-Linked (also known as sex-linked).   In the x-linked mode of inheritance, traits are determined by genes located on the one pair of 23 chromosomes referred to as the sex chromosomes. Genes for hearing loss can be located on the X chromosome. Females inherit two X chromosomes (one from each parent) and males inherit one X chromosome from their mother and one Y chromosome from their father. As exhibited in Figure 11.7, a female with a recessive gene for hearing loss on one of her X chromosomes will not exhibit hearing loss but each son has a 50 percent chance of having the trait, and each daughter has a 50% chance of being a carrier. If an affected male's wife is not a carrier, all of their daughters will be carriers and all of their sons will have normal hearing because they inherit the Y chromosome from their father. Approximately 2 to 3 percent of hearing loss is the result of x-linked transmission.

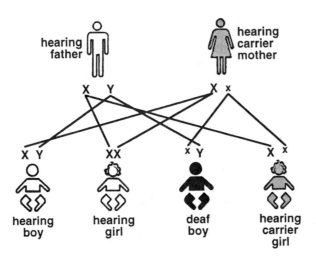

FIGURE 11.7   X-linked recessive deafness is caused by a gene on the X chromosome and occurs only in males. The sons of a woman who is a carrier of x-linked deafness have a 50 percent chance to be deaf and the daughters have a 50 percent chance to be carriers. (From Shaver, 1988. Reprinted with permission.)

Acquired Hearing Loss

Acquired hearing losses are those that are caused by factors that are **exogenous** (outside the genes), such as disease, toxicity, or accident. These factors can occur during pregnancy (**prenatally**), shortly before, during, or shortly after delivery (**perinatally**), or after birth (**postnatally**). In the case of prenatal insult, gestational age of the fetus is an important factor in the effect on hearing. For example, if the infection occurs during the development of the organs, or during the first trimester, the fetus is more likely to incur damage than when the fetus is exposed later in the gestational period. It is important for pediatric audiologists to be familiar with the consequences of conditions or events of these infections in order to appropriately counsel families regarding expectations for their children. For example, some infections result in hearing losses that are progressive and audiologists should prepare families for that eventuality. Other prenatal infections result in hearing losses that are not present at birth but appear later in childhood. Many of the pre- and perinatal diseases have come to be known as part of the STORCH complex of infections. **STORCH** is an acronym for (S)yphilis, (T)oxoplasmosis, (O)ther, (R)ubella, (C)ytomegalovirus, and (H)erpes simplex. All of these diseases put infants at high risk for hearing loss. The pediatric audiologist is alert to these possibilities and can arrange for periodic audiological monitoring of these children.

Prematurity. Approximately 11 percent of all births are less than 37 weeks gestation and are considered preterm. Low birthweight due to preterm birth is a strong predictor of developmental problems and mortality. Imagine the concerns of a new mother who has delivered her infant two months early.

> Maya weighed only 1450 grams (approximately 3.2 lbs.) at birth and could be held in the palm of one hand. Maya's mother knew from her prenatal classes that premature babies are about thirty times less likely to survive than are full-term infants, and those who survive are at high risk for health and developmental problems. Immediately after birth, Maya had her first test—the APGAR. Fortunately, she scored within normal limits on this measure.

The **APGAR** scoring system was devised in 1953 to identify infants who are severely stressed and in need of resuscitation (Apgar, 1953). The five signs used to score the baby's condition can be remembered easily using the mnemonic (A)ppearance, (P)ulse, (G)rimace, (A)ctivity, and (R)espiration. Immediately prior to birth and during the delivery process, an infant may receive insufficient oxygen across the placenta from her mother. This results in reduced oxygen and increased carbon dioxide in the blood and tissues, or *asphyxia*. Because asphyxia commonly occurs in premature infants who have other medical conditions, it is difficult to pinpoint asphyxia as a cause of hearing loss. Simmons (1980), however, identified asphyxia as the most common high risk factor in the medical histories of babies with hearing loss.

> Maya's mother noticed her daughter's skin was a yellowish color. She was told by her nurse that this was caused by jaundice or hyperbilirubinemia, the result of

excessive *bilirubin* (a bile pigment in the blood). Maya seemed to enjoy lying naked under warm lights for her phototherapy (treatment by exposure to light) and in a few days, the yellow tinge to her skin was gone.

If Maya had had a more serious case of jaundice, she would have required a blood transfusion and may have been at risk for hearing loss. Although some researchers have reported that up to 80 percent of infants surviving hyperbilirubinemia demonstrate some degree of sensorineural hearing loss, others have reported no such relationship (Bergman, Hirsch, Fria, et al., 1985; de Vries, Lary, & Dubowitz, 1985; Sabo, Brown, & Watchko, 1992; Salamy, Eldredge, & Tooley, 1989). In addition to these medical concerns, preterm infants are susceptible to bleeding within the skull or *intracranial hemorrhage*. Mental retardation and hearing loss are common sequelae of intracranial hemorrhage (Krishnamoorthy, Shannon, DeLong, Todres, & Davis, 1979).

In Maya's case, a brain scan showed no evidence of intracranial hemorrhage. Other than being very small, Maya was in good health overall. Once it was clear that Maya's health was not in any danger, her physician recommended that she receive a hearing evaluation by the audiologist. The results of her evaluation were normal. (Later in this chapter, information on hearing testing techniques for infants will be described.) Maya was required to stay in the hospital until her weight was increased, and then she went home with her mother to begin her new life.

Other premature infants are not as lucky as Maya. Some infants, because they are born before their immune systems are fully developed, are susceptible to a variety of infections. Because of this, they are given medications to help them fight off the bacteria. Some antibiotics (e.g., streptomycin, kanamycin) are known to cause sensorineural hearing loss by damaging structures of the inner ear. In addition, diuretics, commonly used with neonates with chronic lung disease, have been shown to have a negative effect on hearing (Sabo et al., 1992), and when used with other ototoxic drugs, the effects may be multiplied (Salamy et al., 1989). The typical hearing loss associated with ototoxicity is bilateral, sensorineural, and high frequency.

The precise risk of hearing loss associated with each of the factors we have discussed is difficult to establish since premature infants generally have multiple risk factors simultaneously. Consequently, researchers have had heated debates regarding the contributions of each of these risk factors to subsequent hearing loss. As a general rule, however, all premature infants requiring a stay in the neonatal intensive care unit are considered at risk for hearing loss and should have their hearing screened prior to discharge (Davis, Wood, Healy, et al, 1995).

Postnatal Infections.   In contrast to Maya, Cole had an uneventful pre- and postnatal course.

Cole was the product of a full-term gestation and normal delivery. After 24 hours in the hospital, he and his mother went home. Cole continued to develop normally, babbling and sitting up around 6 months of age, walking and producing his first

words around 1 year of age. By the time Cole was in kindergarten, he was quite a precocious child. He seemed to be into everything and was always full of stories about his latest adventures to tell his mother. One day during his first year of kindergarten, Cole had flulike symptoms. He ran a fever and slept a great deal. After several days with no break in his fever, Cole's mother took him to the doctor. Following a brief examination, his pediatrician instructed Cole's mother to take him to the emergency room at the hospital. A test at the hospital confirmed that Cole had *bacterial meningitis*.

The age at which children are most likely to contract meningitis is 6 to 12 months, however, it is possible for older children to contract the disease as well. Approximately 15 percent of meningitis survivors have neurologic sequelae that may include seizures, paresis, learning or developmental disabilities, and hearing loss (Kallio, Kilpi, Anttila, & Peltola, 1994). The hearing loss is usually bilateral, sensorineural, mild to profound in degree, and permanent.

With this knowledge in mind, when Cole was feeling better, his physician ordered a hearing test. A pediatric audiologist found that Cole demonstrated a profound hearing loss in both ears.

Audiologists should be seeing fewer cases like Cole in the future. The recent release of a preventive vaccine should result in a marked decline in hearing loss secondary to meningitis (Klein, 1994; Stein & Boyer, 1994).

Viral infections can also lead to hearing loss. A common viral cause of unilateral sensorineural hearing loss in children is *mumps*. The associated hearing loss occurs suddenly and can range in severity from mild to profound. Approximately 5 percent of mumps patients acquire hearing loss (Vuori, Lahikainen, & Peltonen, 1962). *Measles* is another viral cause of sensorineural hearing loss in children. Approximately 10 percent of those with measles have resulting hearing loss. The pattern is typically a bilateral severe-to-profound, high-frequency hearing loss (Bergstrom, 1984).

Other Hearing High-Risk Factors

Fetal Alcohol Syndrome (FAS). One of the most common birth defects today, FAS has been estimated to occur in one of every 750 live births (Streissguth, Landesman-Dwyer, Martin, & Smith, 1980). FAS, and the milder version called fetal alcohol effects (FAE), result from drinking during pregnancy because alcohol affects the developing fetus. FAS is characterized by mental retardation, low birthweight, and abnormal facial features (Clarren & Smith, 1978). Only a few investigations of hearing status in this population have been conducted; however, they suggest a high incidence of recurrent otitis media and bilateral sensorineural hearing loss (Church & Gerkin, 1988; Streissguth, Clarren, & Jones, 1985).

Persistent Pulmonary Hypertension of the Newborn (PPHN). Also known as persistent fetal circulation, PPHN is a cardiac abnormality exhibiting persistence of

the fetal vessel joining the pulmonary artery to the aorta, which results in deficient oxygenation of the blood, or severe hypoxemia. Twenty to 40 percent of infants diagnosed with PPHN have sensorineural hearing loss (Leavitt, Watchko, Bennett, & Folsom, 1987; Sell, Gaines, Gluckman, & Williams, 1985; Walton & Hendricks-Munoz, 1991). The onset of hearing loss is thought to be related to the combined effects of the very medical procedures (e.g., drug therapy, ventilation) used to keep these babies alive (Hendricks-Munoz & Walton, 1988; Walton & Hendricks-Munoz, 1991). Hearing loss associated with PPHN has been described as bilateral, progressive, and sensorineural, with variability in degree and the possibility of delayed onset (Hendricks-Menoz & Walton, 1988; Naulty, Weiss, & Herer, 1986).

Otitis Media.   Inflammation of the middle ear space, or **otitis media**, is the most frequent cause of hearing loss in young children. Approximately one-third of children in the United States have recurrent and severe middle ear disease by age 3; the peak age for acute otitis media is 7 to 12 months (Klein, 1992). Hearing loss associated with otitis media when fluid is present in the middle ear (called otitis media with **effusion** [OME]) is conductive, unilateral, or bilateral. This loss typically fluctuates. The average hearing loss caused by otitis media is between approximately 25 and 30 dB (Brookhouser, Worthington, & Kelly, 1993; Fria, Cantekin, & Eichler, 1985). Several factors contribute to the likelihood of the occurrence of otitis media (Table 11.2). These include placement in day care centers (Alho, Koivu, Sorri, & Rantakallio, 1990; Pukander, 1982; Sipila, Karma, Pukander, et al., 1988), parental smoking (Sipila et al., 1988; Stahlberg, Ruuskanen, & Virolainen, 1986), and the autumn season (Alho, Oja, Koivu, & Sorri, 1995). Antibiotic therapy is the most common form of treatment for OME. The insertion of tubes into the eardrums for treatment of OME usually eliminates the conductive hearing loss by allowing drainage of middle ear fluid and is the most common operation for children in the United States (Kleinman, Kosecoff, DuBois, & Brook, 1994).

TABLE 11.2 High Risk Factors for Middle Ear Disease in Children

1. First episode of acute otitis media prior to 6 months of age
2. Infants who are bottle-fed
3. Children with craniofacial anomalies, stigmata, or other findings associated with syndromes known to affect the outer and middle ear
4. Ethnic populations with documented increased incidence of outer and middle ear disease (e.g., Native American and Eskimo populations)
5. Family history of chronic or recurrent otitis media with effusion
6. Children in group day care settings or crowded living conditions
7. Children exposed to excessive cigarette smoke
8. Children diagnosed with sensorineural hearing loss, learning disabilities, behavior disorders, or developmental delays and disorders

From Bluestone & Klein (1996).

DEGREE OF HEARING LOSS AND ITS EFFECT ON COMMUNICATION

The classification of hearing loss is usually a bit different for children than for adults. Hearing loss in adults has been defined as an average of greater than 25 dB thresholds at the frequencies 500, 1000, 2000, and 3000 Hz (American Academy of Otolaryngology and American Council of Otolaryngology, 1979). In children, how-ever, hearing loss is frequently regarded as an average threshold of greater than 20 or even 15 dB over the same range of frequencies (Northern & Downs, 1991). After all, young children are in the process of learning speech and language and cannot always "fill in the gaps" of conversation the way that adults can. If some words or sounds are missed in conversation, an adult can often determine what was said by the context. For example, if an adult hears "The ole of my shoe needs repairing," he or she will figure out that the misunderstood word must be "sole" based on the other key words in the sentence. Children, on the other hand, do not have the extensive vocabularies, linguistic experiences, or strategies to assist them in interpreting mis-understood words. This means that even a slight hearing loss can result in speech perception that is missing critical consonant or vowel sounds. Some of the un-voiced consonants (e.g., th, f, k, t) are produced with intensities that fall at or below normal hearing thresholds for soft conversational speech (see Figure 11.8).

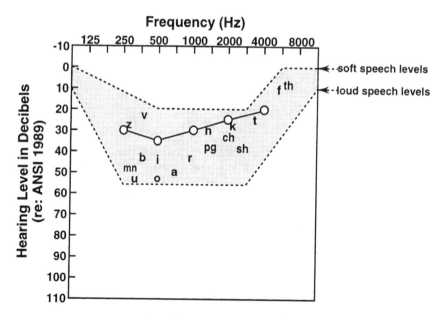

FIGURE 11.8   Effects of a mild hearing loss on ability to hear conversational levels of speech. The connected circles reflect the air conduction thresholds. For simplicity, only the right ear is shown.

An audiogram will provide a good starting place for understanding the impact of a hearing loss, because greater degrees of loss are typically associated with more severe consequences to the individual. We can see this relationship in Table 11.3. However, it is impossible to characterize the type or severity of communication problems an individual child with hearing impairment will have from the audiogram alone. Many factors contribute to communication ability such as severity, configuration, and age of onset of hearing loss. Additional factors such as intelligence, extent and quality of intervention, and family support also influence a child's communication development. With those factors in mind, we will attempt

TABLE 11.3   Impact of Hearing Loss

BILATERAL HEARING LOSS	
Minimal Hearing Loss (16 to 25 dB HL)	At 15 dB a student can miss up to 10 percent of the speech signal when a teacher is at a distance greater than 3 feet and when the classroom is noisy.
Mild Hearing Loss (26 to 40 dB HL)	With a 30 dB loss, a student can miss 25 to 40 percent of a speech signal. Without amplification, the child with 35 to 40 dB loss will miss at least 50% of class discussion.
Moderate Hearing Loss (41 to 55 dB HL)	Child understands conversational speech at a distance of 3 to 5 feet (face-to-face) only if structure and vocabulary are controlled. Without amplification, the amount of speech signal missed can be 50 to 75 percent with a 40 dB loss, and 80 to 100 percent with a 50 dB loss.
Moderate to Severe Hearing Loss (56 to 70 dB HL)	Without amplification, conversation must be very loud to be understood. A 55 dB loss can cause a child to miss up to 100 percent of speech information.
Severe Hearing Loss 71 to 90 dB HL)	Without amplification, may hear loud voices about 1 foot from ear. When amplified optimally, children with hearing ability of 90 dB or better should be able to identify environmental sounds and detect all the sounds of speech.
Profound Hearing Loss ($\geq$ 91 dB HL)	Aware of vibrations more than tonal patterns. May rely on vision rather than hearing as primary avenue for communication and learning.
UNILATERAL HEARING LOSS (Normal hearing in one ear with the other ear exhibiting at least a mild permanent loss.)	May have difficulty hearing faint or distant speech. Usually has difficulty localizing sounds and has greater difficulty understanding speech in background noise.

to describe general effects of hearing loss on communication in the following scenarios.

> Julia, age 7, has a mild conductive hearing loss (15–30 dB) bilaterally. Julia's hearing loss is the result of otitis media with effusion. This temporary loss should disappear as the middle ear fluid resolves. As can be seen in Figure 11.8, Julia has a mild hearing loss that is "flat" in that all frequencies are affected to a similar degree. She can hear vowels clearly but has some difficulty hearing voiceless consonants. For example, Julia cannot hear the fricatives f, th, v, z because they are below her threshold. This type of hearing loss would be similar to trying to listen with cotton balls in your ears. Her teachers noticed that Julia seemed to have difficulty paying attention in class and frequently appeared to daydream.

☞ Numerous studies suggest that some children with recurrent bouts of otitis media are at risk for language delays or disorders. However, the research has not been clear regarding the long-term effects of otitis media on speech and language, that is, the impact after the otitis media has cleared up.

> Suzanne, age 10, has a mild to moderate hearing loss (30–50 dB) bilaterally. As illustrated in Figure 11.9, without her hearing aids, Suzanne misses almost all of the speech sounds at normal conversational loudness levels. She can hear vowels better than consonants and has difficulty discriminating between consonants. Therefore, she misunderstands similar-sounding words such as *sue, shoe, two, coo.* In

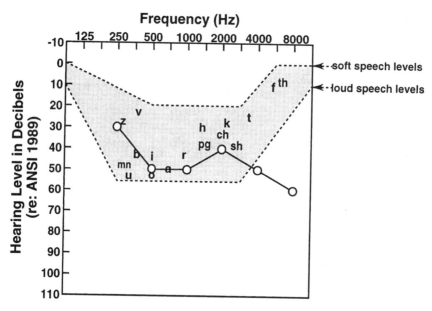

FIGURE 11.9   Effects of a mild to moderate hearing loss on ability to hear conversational levels of speech. The thresholds fall below the intensity of many speech sounds.

addition, her speech is sometimes difficult to understand because she frequently distorts or omits consonants. Suzanne is considered at risk for academic problems even though her hearing loss is relatively mild (Tharpe & Bess, 1991).

Catherine, age 2 years, has a severe to profound sensorineural hearing loss (80 sloping to 100 dB) bilaterally. Catherine's parents initially requested a hearing test because they were concerned about her lack of speech and language development. As illustrated in Figure 11.10, she cannot hear conversational level speech or many environmental sounds. Catherine can hear loud environmental sounds and loud speech if the speaker is close by. Without the use of hearing aids, Catherine will not develop speech. Even though she now uses hearing aids, she still exhibits severe speech and language deficits. Her speech is characterized by excessive nasality, substitutions, omissions, restricted range of voice pitch, and extended duration of phonation.

Roy, age 9 years, has a profound hearing loss (90 dB or greater) in his right ear with normal hearing in his left ear. Roy's parents never noticed that he had difficulty hearing until age 4 when they observed that he would always switch the telephone to his left ear when his grandparents called him. When he started school at age 5, Roy's teacher reported problems of inattention and daydreaming. Figure 11.11 illustrates Roy's unilateral hearing loss. It was once believed that such losses would result in little if any problems as long as a child was seated preferentially in the classroom, with the normal hearing ear toward the teacher. Unilateral hearing losses, however, have been found to put children at risk for communication and

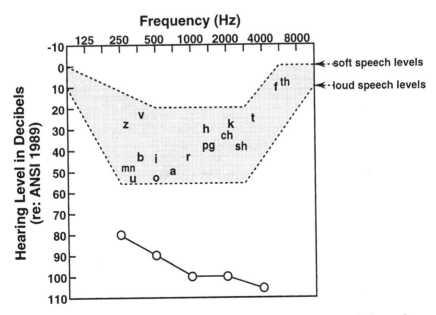

FIGURE 11.10   Effects of a severe to profound hearing loss on ability to hear conversational levels of speech. Note that the thresholds fall well below the level of even loud speech.

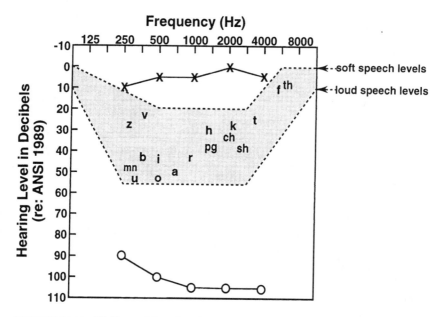

FIGURE 11.11 Unilateral hearing loss of the right ear. Note the normal hearing thresholds for the left ear as indicated by the xs.

academic problems (Bess & Tharpe, 1986). In fact, approximately 30 percent of children with unilateral hearing loss have been found to need grade repetition or resource assistance in school (Bess & Tharpe, 1986; Oyler, Oyler & Matkin, 1988).

AUDIOLOGICAL TESTING

In the last decade, several organizations and lawmakers have called for earlier identification and intervention of infants with hearing impairment (Healthy People 2000, 1990; Joint Committee on Infant Hearing, 2000; NIH, 1993). As a result, audiologists are identifying and evaluating younger children than ever before. This evaluation of infants and children requires the use of behavioral and electrophysiological test procedures.

Behavioral Testing

Even with the widespread use of advanced technological evaluation tools, behavioral testing remains a valuable part of hearing assessment for children. The behavioral technique employed depends largely on the age and developmental level of the child. Some general principles hold across all behavioral tests. Testing is conducted in sound-treated rooms that meet the requirements for accurate measurements set forth by the American National Standards Institute (1991). Test signals

are increased and decreased systematically until the softest level at which the infant or child responds (usually 50% of the time) is reached. This level is called the *threshold* or *minimum response level* (MRL) in the case of young infants because they may actually hear a sound at a lower level than that to which they are able or willing to respond. Thresholds or MRLs can be determined via earphones for air conduction testing, via a bone vibrator for bone conduction testing, or via loud speakers for soundfield testing.

When testing is conducted via earphones or a bone vibrator, one problem that must be addressed is *cross-over* of sound presented to the opposite ear. This refers to the fact that the two ears are not totally isolated, and sometimes a sound going to one ear can cause the skull to vibrate and actually stimulate the other, or nontest, ear. The audiologist must eliminate participation of the nontest ear during testing. To do so, noise is delivered to the nontest ear with a frequency spectrum similar to the test signal, but at a higher intensity, so that any sound crossing over from the test ear will not be heard. This is called masking noise, and responses obtained in this manner are referred to as *masked thresholds*.

For children, behavioral testing usually begins with the use of speech stimuli. A *speech reception threshold* is determined by asking the child to repeat two-syllable words that have equal stress on each syllable, called **spondaic words**. These are words such as *baseball*, *hotdog*, or *airplane*. For children whose speech is difficult to understand, or if they are shy, they may point to the picture of the word that they heard rather than say the word. If a child is unable to repeat words or identify pictures, a *speech awareness threshold* is obtained that simply identifies the softest intensity level at which a child responds. Pure tone air conduction testing is typically conducted next. Several techniques for obtaining pure tone thresholds from children of different ages are discussed below.

Behavioral Observation Audiometry (BOA). For infants from birth to approximately 5 months of age, *Behavioral Observation Audiometry* is typically employed. With this technique, the audiologist looks for gross body movements such as eye-widening, startles, breathing changes, facial grimaces, or cessation of movements that are time-locked with sound presented through speakers. Although BOA is a useful clinical procedure for infants, responses are highly variable and subjective (Moore & Wilson, 1978). One reason that BOA is so subjective is that the infant's responses to sound are variable and open to the observer's interpretation. Thus, BOA allows only a limited number of responses before the infant gradually adapts, or **habituates**, to the sound. With maturation, the child responds to lower and lower signal intensity levels until approximately 2 years of age (Thompson & Weber, 1974). These factors contribute to a wide range of results in typically developing infants, so it is impossible to define hearing loss as a change or deviation from this "norm" (Thompson & Weber, 1974). Rather than measuring the softest sound that infants can hear, audiologists measure the lowest level at which they respond to sound (the *minimum response level*). Therefore, BOA is probably best viewed as a hearing screening assessment procedure that allows one to conclude that an infant's hearing is grossly within or outside the range of normal hearing.

Visual Reinforcement Audiometry (VRA)> *Visual Reinforcement Audiometry* is a procedure that addresses many of the problems inherent in BOA. Used for infants and young children from approximately 6 months to 2 years of age, VRA depends on the child's natural inclination to turn toward a sound source. The schematic in Figure 11.12 illustrates the VRA test arrangement. An infant (I) is seated in a high chair or parent's lap facing forward toward an observation window. Examiner 1 (E_1) is in a darkened room and cannot be seen by the infant. When E_1 determines that the infant is in a quiet state, an auditory signal is delivered through earphones or speakers. When the infant turns in response to the signal, a toy in a Plexiglas box, the visual reinforcer (VR), is animated and lights up on the side where the sound emanated. Examiner 2 (E_2) (perhaps the infant's parent) serves as an assistant who is needed to keep the infant content and sitting quietly during the test.

    Figure 11.13 (p. 274) illustrates several aspects of the VRA procedure. In the first panel of Figure 11.13, note that the assistant who is in the booth with the baby is wearing earphones. Because the infant is being tested through speakers, the assistant is wearing earphones with music or masking noise to prevent unintentional cuing of the infant when a sound occurs. The middle panel demonstrates the use

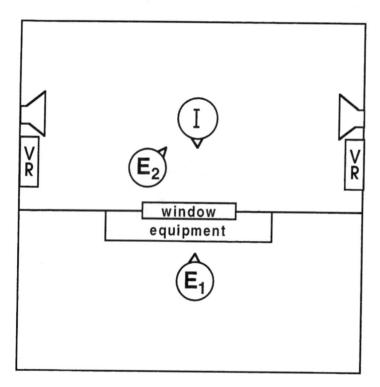

FIGURE 11.12   Typical two-room test suite arrangement for conducting VRA.
E1 = Examiner 1, E2 = Examiner 2, I = Infant, VR = Visual Reinforcer.

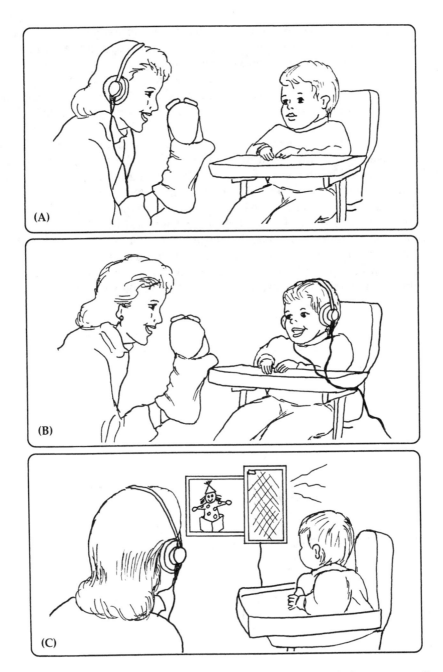

FIGURE 11.13   Illustration of various aspects of visual reinforcement audiometry (VRA). Panel A illustrates the assistant wearing masking earphones while the child is being tested through speakers. Panel B illustrates the VRA procedure with the infant wearing earphones. Panel C illustrates the infant head-turn in response to sound and the subsequent animation of the mechanical toy as reinforcement.

of earphones in the VRA procedure in order to obtain individual ear information from the infant. The bottom panel illustrates the infant head-turn to the sound being reinforced by the mechanical toy.

Conditioned Play Audiometry (CPA).   At approximately 2 to 2½ years of age, play audiometry becomes the behavioral technique of choice. *Tangible Reinforcement Operant Conditioning Audiometry (TROCA)* is one form of play audiometry developed by Lloyd and colleagues (Lloyd, Spradlin, & Reid, 1968). For this technique, the child is conditioned to push a button when a sound is heard. The button push is followed by the delivery of an edible reinforcement controlled by the examiner. The reinforcement is small, preferably sugarless, and quick to eat. The treat may be varied to keep a restless or experienced child's interest. More traditional conditioned play audiometry techniques include placement of a peg in a pegboard or a block in a box when the child hears the sound. The audiologist chooses tasks that are fun and interesting to the child.

Speech Discrimination Testing.   As discussed earlier in this chapter, the pure tone audiogram does not tell precisely how well a person understands the most important sound stimulus, speech. For that reason, *speech discrimination* testing is usually conducted after pure tone testing for children who are approximately 3 years of age or older. Unlike threshold tests, speech discrimination testing is conducted at a comfortable loudness level in an attempt to determine the child's ability to understand conversational speech. Typical materials for discrimination testing consist of monosyllabic words that can be repeated or pointed to on picture cards.

Auditory Brainstem Response Testing

Sometimes valid behavioral tests cannot be obtained from children. This may be because the child is too young (under 4 or 5 months of age) or uncooperative due to behavioral or developmental disabilities. For those children, alternative testing procedures that do not require voluntary responses are quite useful. You will recall from Chapter 10 that information about sounds must be transmitted from the inner ear to the brain via the brainstem pathways. The **auditory brainstem response** (ABR) reflects the electrical activity along the auditory pathway rather than testing hearing directly. A waveform can be recorded in response to acoustic stimuli with electrodes placed on the scalp and on the earlobes or mastoids of the patient. The normal waveform consists of five waves that occur at specific time intervals or latencies. At high intensity levels (approximately 80 dB), all five waves should be observable. One of these waves (V) is observable even with very soft intensity levels, within approximately 10 dB of true auditory threshold. It is this feature of the ABR that is useful for estimating hearing threshold. Since a child does not provide a voluntary response and can even be asleep for this test, the ABR makes a valuable contribution to the pediatric test battery, particularly for children who are unable or unwilling to cooperate for behavioral testing.

Immittance Audiometry

A standard component of the pediatric test battery is **immittance audiometry**, which includes *tympanometry* and *acoustic reflex thresholds*. Tympanometry is a measurement of the mobility of the middle ear system as air pressure is varied in the external auditory canal. It is a valuable tool for identifying the presence of middle ear fluid associated with otitis media and other middle ear pathologies commonly seen in children. The procedure is quick and painless, making it ideal for children. A rubber-tipped probe is inserted gently into the child's ear canal, and air pressure is pumped into the cavity formed between the end of the probe and the eardrum (tympanic membrane). As the air pressure in the cavity is varied above and below ambient air pressure, the middle ear mobility is measured and plotted on a graph called a *tympanogram*. In a normally functioning ear, maximum middle ear mobility should occur at or near ambient air pressure. This is an important measurement because pathology, such as otitis media, will influence the movement of the eardrum.

The acoustic reflex threshold is the lowest intensity required to elicit a contraction of the middle ear muscle (see Chapter 10). This contraction can be evoked by introducing a loud sound (usually a pure tone) to the ear canal either through the probe or through an earphone placed on the opposite ear from the probe. This test provides information about the functioning of the middle and inner ear as well as the auditory nerve. In a normal functioning ear, a reflex is elicited when the sound is between about 65 and 95 dB. A hearing loss may result in an elevation of the sound level needed to evoke the acoustic reflex or an absence of it altogether. If middle ear fluid is present or the acoustic nerve is damaged, it may also affect the acoustic reflex. The acoustic reflex thresholds, viewed in conjunction with the tympanogram and audiogram, can assist the pediatric audiologist in determining the type and degree of hearing loss.

Otoacoustic Emissions

Evoked otoacoustic emissions (OAEs) were discovered in 1978 (see Chapter 10) and were quickly incorporated into the audiologist's clinical armamentarium. Although there are several types of evoked OAEs, they are all produced by presenting sound to the ear and then examining the sound recorded by a miniature microphone in the ear canal. The presence of OAEs suggests a normal functioning cochlea; absent or reduced OAEs are the result of conductive or cochlear hearing loss. Like immittance audiometry, this tool is particularly useful for children because it is quick, painless, and requires no voluntary response.

It is important to note that no one test should be depended upon when testing infants or young children. Rather, a battery of tests is used by pediatric audiologists. Let us look at a typical evaluation.

Juan's mother brought him in for a hearing evaluation at age 2 years because of concern about his lack of speech and language development. Juan had several aunts

and uncles on his mother's side of the family with hearing loss so she was particularly concerned that his hearing might be a factor in his communication problems. His medical history included a normal gestation and delivery, a few colds and upper respiratory infections, and several episodes of otitis media that had been treated with antibiotics. When testing began, Juan refused to wear earphones by crying and yanking them off. As an alternative to the earphones, Juan was tested in soundfield through speakers utilizing visual reinforcement audiometry. Responses were consistent with a mild (35–45 dB) hearing loss for all of the test frequencies and speech. In an effort to determine if the hearing loss was conductive or sensorineural, the audiologist attempted to put a bone vibrator on Juan. Again, he resisted the placement of anything on his head so the audiologist had to abandon that tactic. By having an assistant blow bubbles to distract him while he sat on his mother's lap, the audiologist was able to place the probe for tympanometry in his ear canal and obtain a tympanogram. The results were consistent with the presence of middle ear fluid in both ears. Even though the audiologist was not able to obtain all of the test results that she wanted, the overall pattern of the test results (i.e., the mild hearing loss and abnormal tympanograms) suggested that the hearing loss was conductive. She then recommended that Juan be seen by his pediatrician for treatment of the middle ear fluid and then return for another hearing test to determine if his hearing loss resolved following medical treatment.

Hearing Screening

One of the many responsibilities of the pediatric audiologist is to organize and oversee the screening of neonates, infants, preschoolers, and school-age children for hearing loss and middle ear disease (otitis media). The process of screening involves identifying those at risk for hearing loss or ear disease so they can be referred for further evaluation. Screening tests provide a quick, simple, safe, valid, reliable, and cost-effective means of identification of risk status; they are not intended to diagnose hearing loss.

Guidelines for screening procedures are available for children at various ages. For infants, both brainstem response testing and evoked otoacoustic emissions are used for screening purposes. The Joint Committee on Infant Hearing (2000) and the American Speech-Hearing-Language Association (ASHA, 1997) recommend screening infants with identified indicators associated with sensorineural or conductive hearing loss if screening for all newborns is not available. As recently as 2002, thirty-seven states had mandated newborn hearing screening statutes or regulations (ASHA, 2002).

ASHA (1997) recommended screening preschoolers who have any indicators associated with late-onset or progressive hearing loss or parental or health care provider concerns regarding hearing, speech, language, or developmental delay. Play audiometric techniques are recommended, although visual reinforcement audiometry may be used if necessary. ASHA (1997) recommended screening school-age children upon initial entry to school, annually in kindergarten through third grade, and in seventh and eleventh grades. Furthermore, all children entering special education, those repeating a grade, or entering the school

system without evidence of having passed a previous hearing screening are typically screened. In addition, school-age children reporting exposure to high levels of noise should receive a hearing screening. The recommended screening procedure is play or conventional audiometry with earphones.

There has been considerable debate on the issue of *who* should be screened for middle ear disease. Some professionals feel that *all* children should be screened, while others believe only those considered at greatest risk for middle ear disease should be screened. ASHA has left that decision to each individual screening program (1997). ASHA recommended a middle ear screening protocol that includes a case history from the parent or guardian; visual inspection of the ears to identify risk factors for outer and middle ear disease, and any contraindications for performing tympanometry; examination of the external ear canal and tympanic membrane; and tympanometry with a screening or diagnostic tympanometer (ASHA, 1997).

MANAGEMENT OF CHILDREN WITH HEARING IMPAIRMENT

Once hearing loss has been identified and described in terms of type and degree, a decision regarding the most appropriate intervention, medical or audiological, or both, must be made. Consideration is given to possible medications, surgical interventions, or the fitting of hearing aids. As a general rule, conductive types of hearing loss are most likely to benefit from surgical approaches or amplification, whereas the options for sensorineural hearing losses are usually limited to amplification.

Amplification

The early identification of hearing loss in children has little value if intervention is not initiated in a timely manner. The first, and perhaps the most important, step in intervention is the fitting of appropriate sound amplification. It is the role of the pediatric audiologist to ensure that children receive a consistent and audible speech signal at intensity levels that are safe and comfortable. The Pediatric Working Group (1996) developed recommendations for fitting amplification on infants and children. Although no hard and fast rules exist regarding the specific degree of hearing loss at which amplification should be fit, the group concurred that any child with thresholds exceeding 25 dB HL should be considered a candidate for amplification. This includes children with unilateral or bilateral hearing loss.

There are several different types of hearing aids available today. These include the (1) *body aid*, (2) *behind-the-ear aid*, (3) *in-the-ear aid*, and (4) *in-the-canal aid*. These are worn by both adults and children (see Chapter 12 for a photograph of these types of aids). By far, the most common hearing aid type for children is the behind-the-ear (see Figure 11.14). All of these hearing aid types contain similar internal components and function similarly. The hearing aid microphone picks up

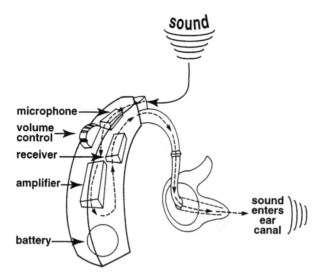

FIGURE 11.14   Schematic of a behind-the-ear hearing aid.

the acoustic signal and converts it to an electrical signal that is amplified (made louder), filtered, and converted back to an acoustic signal by a receiver. In behind-the-ears hearing aids, the amplified sound is routed to the child's ear by tubing that leads to an earmold. The earmold is made specifically for an individual child's ear, allows the sound to be directed to the ear canal, and keeps the hearing aid in place.

It is particularly important when fitting children to know exactly how much the sound is being amplified since it is difficult or impossible for an infant or young child to tell you when the amplified sound is too loud or not loud enough. Although initial hearing aid settings can be made with computerized prescriptive formulae, amplified sound levels are typically verified by an audiologist using *probe microphone measures*. A probe microphone is one that is small enough to be inserted into the ear canal of a child while the hearing aid is worn (see Figure 11.15, p. 280). A sound signal is presented from a small speaker and the probe microphone system records the intensity level of the test signal amplified through the hearing aid from within the child's ear canal. Several techniques are available for making needed measurements quickly from a child.

Sometimes, traditional hearing aids are not sufficient to overcome the hearing deficits of those with profound hearing losses. An alternative to traditional hearing aids for those children is the **cochlear implant**. The cochlear implant is a surgically implanted device with electrodes that are coiled into the cochlea to stimulate the auditory nerve with electrical current (see Figure 11.16, p. 281). A microphone is worn on the child's ear, in a casing that looks like a hearing aid, and converts the acoustic signal to an electrical signal. The electrical signal is modified

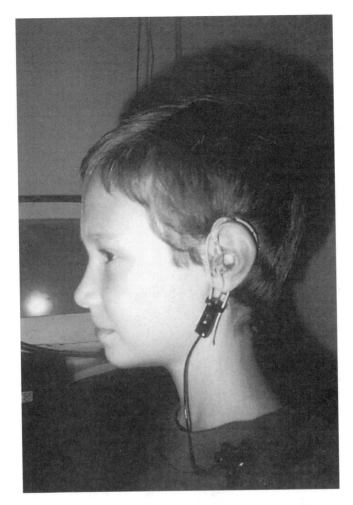

FIGURE 11.15   Probe microphone measurements with a cooperative child.

by a processor, which may be in a body-worn or behind-the-ear case, and is then sent to a receiver worn behind the child's ear. The signal is then transmitted through the skin to an internal receiver implanted in the mastoid bone where it is transmitted to electrodes implanted in the cochlea. Although cochlear implants do not restore normal hearing, children vary markedly in terms of the benefits received from the implant. Most children experience a minimum of sound awareness while others have excellent speech recognition ability. The pediatric audiologist assists in determining whether a child is an appropriate candidate for the cochlear implant, counsels families on the benefits and limitations of the implant, sets the stimulus levels of the speech processor after implantation, and works with the child to develop or improve listening skills.

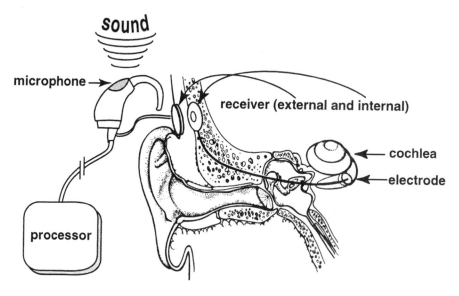

FIGURE 11.16   Schematic of a cochlear implant.

Communication and Education Approaches

One of the most difficult decisions facing parents of a child newly identified with hearing loss is how to communicate most effectively with their child. The most common communication options are *auditory-oral, total communication,* and *manual* modes. Auditory-oral communication emphasizes listening and oral communication. A total communication approach includes listening, speech reading, signing, finger spelling, and oral expression. A manual mode of communication uses one of the signed languages, typically without oral speech. The decision regarding which communication mode to adopt usually is highly influenced by the degree of the child's hearing loss. Children with mild or moderate hearing losses generally use an auditory-oral approach because they have a considerable amount of residual hearing. Children with severe-to-profound hearing loss, however, may have a more difficult time acquiring spoken language and may require the additional visual input afforded by a total or manual communication approach. It is not uncommon, however, for children or their parents to adopt communication modes for cultural reasons. For example, when a child with moderate hearing loss is born to parents who are deaf and who use a manual communication approach, the child is most likely to use a manual approach also. Many factors, audiological, educational, and cultural, are considered when choosing the communication mode that is best for an individual family. After all, the best communication mode is the one that will be most comfortable for the entire family to use.

Federal law has strongly influenced the education of children with hearing loss. Public Law 99-457, or Individuals with Disabilities Education Act (IDEA),

was intended to fulfill four primary purposes: (1) to ensure that all children with handicaps have available to them a *free, appropriate public education* that emphasizes special education and related services designed to meet their unique needs; (2) to ensure that the rights of handicapped children and their parents or guardians are protected; (3) to help states pay for education of all children with handicaps; and (4) to ensure and assess the effectiveness of educational programs. Children who are deaf or hard-of-hearing are covered by this legislation. Under PL 99-457, *deaf* means a hearing impairment that is so severe that the child is impaired in processing linguistic information through hearing, with or without amplification, which adversely affects educational performance. *Hard-of-hearing* means a hearing loss, permanent or fluctuating, that adversely affects a child's educational performance. Children with handicaps from birth to age 3 years and their families are provided with early intervention programs under Part H of PL 99-457. Part B provides free and appropriate public education and related services to children with disabilities 3 to 5 years of age.

In the past, children with hearing loss received their education in segregated schools and classrooms. Now most are enrolled in general education programs in their local schools with their normal hearing peers. This trend is referred to as *inclusion* and may occur on a full-time or part-time basis. If additional services are needed for these children, they may attend resource classrooms by leaving their general education classroom for short periods during the day. Another alternative is to receive additional support from an itinerant teacher who travels from class to class. Special services are designed to meet the unique needs of children with hearing loss and maximize the benefit they receive from their educational program. These special services may include speech-language pathology, audiology, psychology, counseling, or physical therapy, among others.

The role of the audiologist in the schools is an important one. Duties include developing and supervising the school's hearing screening program, monitoring the hearing of children identified with hearing loss, participating in the educational planning for children with hearing loss, monitoring individual hearing aids or other assistive devices to ensure their proper function, and educating teachers and other school personnel regarding hearing loss, hearing aids, and communication with children having hearing loss.

Counseling

Counseling is an important component of the overall services that audiologists provide to children and their families and, more specifically, a critical part of the management process. Counseling can range from explaining test results, to making recommendations for habilitation services, to assisting families as they work through feelings of confusion and disappointment about their child's hearing loss. Although not trained as professional counselors, audiologists can provide educational and supportive counseling to assist families in making practical life changes to ease the unexpected disruptions that hearing loss can cause.

Parents often look to professionals for answers and direction. The audiologist's goal in counseling, however, is to provide the information and guidance that families need to make their own decisions and solve their own problems. That is, not every child or family is the same and there is not one approach to communication and education that is right for every child. Parents must ultimately find the answers they are seeking; audiologists simply provide the tools to help that happen.

Most counseling takes place informally while discussing test results or responding to a parent's phone call. Support groups can provide a more structured setting where families share their feelings of fear, confusion, and perhaps guilt, with other parents of hearing-impaired children. It is through communication with other families that parents learn that they are not alone. Support groups may include parents, siblings, and even extended family members such as grandparents, aunts, and uncles.

CLINICAL PROBLEM SOLVING

The parents of 4-year-old Josh were shocked to learn that his articulation problems were the result of a moderate sensorineural hearing loss in both ears. After all, neither of them had a hearing loss nor did any of their parents or siblings. The pregnancy with Josh was normal as was his entire postnatal course.

1. What are some possible causes of Josh's hearing loss?
2. Is it more likely that Josh's hearing loss will be treated medically or with hearing aids?
3. What receptive communication difficulties might you expect with this degree of hearing loss?
4. What expressive communication difficulties might you expect with this degree of hearing loss?

REFERENCES

Alho, O. P., Oja, J., Koivu, M., & Sorri, M. (1995). Risk factors for chronic otitis media with effusion in infancy. *Archives of Otolaryngology Head and Neck Surgery, 121,* 839–843.

Alho, O. P., Koivu, M., Sorri, M., & Rantakallio, P. (1990). Risk factors for recurrent acute otitis media and respiratory infection in infancy. *International Journal of Pediatric Otorhinolaryngology, 19,* 151–161.

American Academy of Otolaryngology and American Council of Otolaryngology. (1979). Guide for the evaluation of hearing handicap. *Journal of the American Medical Association, 241,* 2055–2059.

American National Standards Institute (ANSI). (1991). *Maximum permissible ambient noise levels for audiometric test rooms* (ANSI S3.1-1991). New York: Acoustical Society of America.

American Speech-Language-Hearing Association Panel on Audiologic Assessment. (1997). *Guidelines for audiologic screening.* Rockville, MD: ASHA.

American Speech-Language-Hearing Association (ASHA). (2002, June 27). *Early hearing detection and intervention action center.* Retrieved June 27, 2002, from http://www.professional.asha .org/resources/legislative/ih_index.cfm

Apgar, V. (1953). A proposal for a new method of evaluation of the newborn infant. *Anesthesia and Analgesia, 32,* 260.

Bergman, I., Hirsch, R. P., Fria, T. J., Shapiro, S. M., Holzman, I., & Painter, M. J. U. (1985). Cause of hearing loss in the high-risk-premature infant. *Journal of Pediatrics, 106,* 95–101.

Bergstrom, L. (1984). Congenital hearing loss. In J. L. Northern (Ed.), *Hearing disorders* (2nd ed.). Boston: Little, Brown.

Bess, F. H., & Tharpe, A. M. (1986, Jan/Feb). Case history data on unilaterally hearing-impaired children. In F. H. Bess et al. (Eds.), Children with unilateral hearing loss. *Ear and Hearing Monograph.*

Bluestone, C. D., & Klein, J. O. (1996). Otitis media, atelectasis, and eustachian tube disfunction. In C. D. Bluestone, S. E. Stool, & M. A. Kenna (Eds.), *Pediatric otolaryngology* (3rd ed., vol. I, pp. 388–582). Philadelphia: Saunders.

Brookhouser, P. E., Worthington, D. W., & Kelly, W. J. (1993). Middle ear disease in young children with sensorineural hearing loss. *Laryngoscope, 103*(4), 371–378.

Church, M. W., & Gerkin, K. P. (1988). Hearing disorders in children with fetal alcohol syndrome: Findings from case reports. *Pediatrics, 82*(2), 147–154.

Clarren, S. K., & Smith, D. W. (1978). The fetal alcohol syndrome. *New England Journal of Medicine, 198,* 1063–1067.

Cohn, E., & Kelley, P. (1999). Clinical phenotype and mutations in connexin 26 (DFNB1/GJB2), the most common cause of childhood hearing loss. *American Journal of Medical Genetics, 89,* 130–136.

Davis, A., Wood, S. Healy, R., Webb, H., & Rowe, S. (1995). Risk factors for hearing disorders: Epidemiologic evidence of change over time in the United Kingdom. *Journal of the American Academy of Audiology, 6*(5), 365–370.

deVries, L. S., Lary, S., & Dubowitz, L. M. S. (1985). Relationship of serum bilirubin level to ototoxicity and deafness in high-risk low-birth-weight infants. *Pediatrics, 76,* 351–354.

Fria, T. J., Cantekin, E. I., & Eichler, J. A. (1985). Hearing acuity of children with otitis media with effusion. *Archives of Otolaryngology, 111,* 10–16.

Healthy People 2000. (1990). U.S. Department of Health and Human Services, Public Health Service, DHHS Publication No. (PHS) 91-50213. Washington, DC: U.S. Government Printing Office.

Hendricks-Munoz, K. D., & Walton, J. P. (1988). Hearing loss in infants with persistent fetal circulation. *Pediatrics, 81,* 650–656.

Joint Committee on Infant Hearing. (2000). Year 2000 position statement: Principles and guidelines for early hearing detection and intervention programs. *American Journal of Audiology, 9,* 9–29.

Kallio, M. J. T., Kilpi, T., Anttila, M., & Peltola, H. (1994). The effect of a recent previous visit to a physician on outcome after childhood bacterial meningitis. *Journal of the American Medical Association, 272*(10), 787–791.

Klein, J. O. (1992). Epidemiology and natural history of otitis media. In F. H. Bess & J. W. Hall, III (Eds.), *Screening children for auditory function.* Nashville, TN: Bill Wilkerson Center Press.

Klein, J. O. (1994). Antimicrobial therapy and prevention of meningitis. *Pediatric Annals, 23*(2), 76–81.

Kleinman, L. C., Kosecoff, J., DuBois, R. W., & Brook, R. H. (1994). The medical appropriateness of tympanostomy tubes proposed for children younger than 16 years in the United States. *Journal of the American Medical Association, 271*(16), 1250–1255.

Krishnamoorthy, K. S., Shannon, D. C., DeLong, G. R., Todres, I. D., & Davis, K. R. (1979). Neurologic sequelae in the survivors of neonatal intraventricular hemorrhage. *Pediatrics, 64*(2), 233–237.

Leavitt, A. M., Watchko, J. F., Bennett, F. C., & Folsom, R. C. (1987). Neurodevelopmental outcome following persistent pulmonary hypertension of the neonate. *Journal of Perinatology, 7*(4), 288–291.

Leon, P. E., Raventos, H., Lynch, E., Morrow, J., King, M. C. (1992). The gene for an inherited form of deafness maps to chromosome 5q31. *Proceedings of the National Academy of Sciences, 89*(11), 5181–5184.

Lloyd, L. L., Spradlin, J. E., & Reid, M. J. (1968). An operant audiometric procedure for difficult-to-test patients. *Journal of Speech and Hearing Disorders, 33,* 236–245.

Moore, J. M., & Wilson, W. R. (1978). Visual reinforcement audiometry (VRA) with infants. In S. E. Gerber & G. T. Mencher (Eds.), *Early diagnosis of hearing loss.* New York: Grune & Stratton.

Morton, N. (1991). Genetic epidemiology of hearing impairment. *Annals of the New York Academy of Sciences, 630,* 16–31.

Naulty, C. M., Weiss, I. P., & Herer, G. (1986). Progressive sensorineural hearing loss in survivors of persistent fetal circulation. *Ear and Hearing, 7*, 74–77.

NIH. (1993). *Early identification of hearing impairment in infants and young children.* NIH Consensus Statement online. March 1–3, *11*, 1–24.

Northern, J. L., & Downs, M. P. (1991). *Hearing in children* (p. 7), Baltimore: Williams & Wilkins.

Oyler, R. F., Oyler, A. L., & Matkin, N. D. (1988). Unilateral hearing loss: Demographics and educational impact. *Language, Speech, and Hearing Services in Schools, 19*, 201–210.

Parving, A. (1993). Congenital hearing disability: Epidemiology and identification; A comparison between two health authority districts. *International Journal of Pediatric Otolaryngology, 27*, 29–46.

Pediatric Working Group. (1996). Amplification for infants and children with hearing loss. *American Journal of Audiology, 5*(1), 53–68.

Pukander, J. (1982). Acute otitis media among rural children in Finland. *International Journal of Pediatric Otorhinolaryngology, 4*, 325–332.

Sabo, D. L., Brown, D. R., & Watchko, J. F. (1992). Sensorineural hearing loss in high-risk infants. In F. H. Bess & J. W. Hall (Eds.), *Screening children for auditory function.* Nashville, TN: Bill Wilkerson Center Press.

Salamy, A., Eldredge, L., & Tooley, W. J. (1989). Neonatal status and hearing loss in high-risk infants. *Journal of Pediatrics, 114*, 847–852.

Sell, E., Gaines, J., Gluckman, C., & Williams, E. (1985). Persistent fetal circulation. *Archives of the Journal of Disorders of Children, 139*, 25–28.

Shaver, K. (1988). Genetics and deafness. In F. H. Bess (Ed.), *Hearing impairment in children* (pp. 15–32). Parkton, MD: York Press.

Simmons, F. B. (1980). Patterns of deafness in newborns. *Laryngoscope, 90*, 448.

Sipila, M., Karma, P., Pukander, J., Timonen, M., & Kataja, M. (1988). The Bayesian approach to the evaluation of risk factors in acute and recurrent acute otitis media. *Acta Otolaryngology, 106*, 94–101.

Stahlberg, M. R., Ruuskanen, O., & Virolainen, E. (1986). Risk factors for recurrent otitis media. *Pediatric Infectious Disease Journal, 5*, 30–32.

Steel, K. P., & Bussoli, T. J. (1999). Deafness genes: Expressions of surprise. *Trends in Genetics, 15*, 207–211.

Stein, L. K., & Boyer, K. M. (1994). Progress in the prevention of hearing loss in infants. *Ear and Hearing, 15*(2), 116–125.

Streissguth, A. P., Clarren, S. K., & Jones, K. L. (1985). Natural history of the fetal alcohol syndrome: A 10-year follow-up of eleven patients. *Lancet, 2*, 85–91.

Streissguth, A. P., Landesman-Dwyer, S., Martin, J. C., & Smith, D. W. (1980). Teratogenic effects of alcohol in humans and laboratory animals. *Science, 209*, 353–361.

Sundstrom, R., Van Laer, L., Van Camp, G., & Smith, R. (1999). Autosomal recessive nonsyndromic hearing loss. *American Journal of Human Genetics, 89*, 123–129.

Tharpe, A. M., & Bess, F. H. (1991). Identification and management of children with minimal hearing loss. *International Journal of Pediatric Otolaryngology, 21*.

Thompson, G., & Weber, B. A. (1974). Responses of infants and young children to behavior observation audiometry (BOA). *Journal of Speech and Hearing Disorders, 2*, 140–147.

Vuori, M., Lahikainen, E. A., & Peltonen, T. (1962). Perceptive deafness in connection with mumps. *Acta Otolaryngologica, 55*, 231–236.

Walton, J. P., & Hendricks-Munoz, K. (1991). Profile and stability of sensorineural hearing loss in persistent pulmonary hypertension of the newborn. *Journal of Speech and Hearing Research, 34*, 1362–1370.

Watkin, P., Baldwin, M., & McEnery, G. (1991). Neonatal at risk screening and the identification of deafness. *Archives of Diseases in Children, 66*, 1130–1135.

READINGS FROM THE POPULAR LITERATURE

Bowers, T. (1999). *Alandra's lilacs.* Washington, DC: Gallaudet University Press. (hearing parents, deaf child)

Cohen, L. H. (1994). *Train go sorry: Inside a deaf world.* New York: Vintage Books. (deafness)

Greenburg, J. (1071). *In this sign.* New York: Henry Holt & Co. (novel about a deaf family)

Keller, H. (1961). *The story of my life: The autobiography of Helen Keller.* New York: Dell. (deaf-blind)

Kisor, H. (1990). *What's that pig outdoors: A memoir of deafness*. New York: Hill and Wang. (deafness)

Sidransky, R. (1990). *In silence: Growing up hearing in a deaf world*. New York: St. Martin's Press. (hearing child, deaf parents)

Walker, L. A. (1986). *A loss for words: The story of deafness in a family*. New York: Harper & Row. (hearing child, deaf parents)

DISORDERS OF HEARING IN ADULTS

LINDA NORRIX

FRANCES P. HARRIS

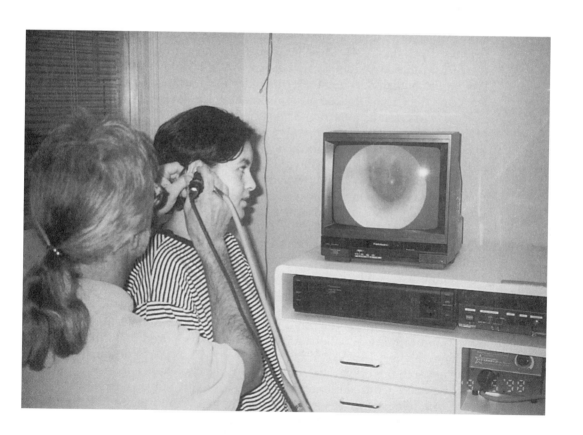

PREVIEW

About 29 million Americans report difficulties with their hearing. This is an increase from the 1984 estimate of 16.4 million, a number much greater than that expected from population growth. The increase can partly be explained by the aging of the population as well as higher levels of environmental noise that are present today compared with the past. Of those with hearing loss, the majority are adults. Hearing loss in adulthood can have devastating effects on one's ability to communicate and may significantly impact family relationships, social interactions, vocation, self-identity, and economic well-being. Because communication is such a vital part of human existence, hearing difficulties can decrease one's quality of life. The audiologist plays a critical role in the assessment and rehabilitation of adults with acquired hearing loss. This chapter focuses on causes, effects, and treatments of adult-onset hearing loss.

Approximately 29 million Americans, most of whom are adults, report difficulty hearing (Kochkin, 2001). Most individuals with hearing impairments develop these difficulties in adulthood, and our focus in this chapter will be on this group. It is important to understand the terminology that is associated with hearing problems, and the effects of those problems on individuals and society (ASHA, 1995). *Hearing impairment* is defined as a loss or abnormality in the structure or function of the auditory system. Impairments can be measured using laboratory techniques (Stephens & Hetu, 1991). Hearing-impaired individuals may have reduced sensitivity for detection of sound, may exhibit poor understanding of speech, or both. Although Giolas (1994) recommended that the term **hearing loss** be used to quantify the degree of the impairment (e.g., Frank has a 50 dB hearing loss), it is often used interchangeably with the term hearing impairment. **Hearing disability** refers to the restrictions in daily activities that a person may experience as a result of a hearing impairment; therefore, one's social environment must be considered in determining disability (Stephens & Hetu, 1991). A hearing impairment may or may not result in a disability. For example, an individual who is socially active and who has a high-frequency hearing impairment is likely to report difficulties understanding speech in noisy environments. In contrast, a person with the same impairment who has few social contacts may not report such problems.

Handicapping situations are sometimes experienced by individuals with hearing disabilities (ASHA, 1995). Environmental or social restrictions may be part of the nonauditory effects that a person experiences. These effects might include social isolation, reduced economic resources, and difficulty maintaining independence. Audiologists working with the adult population need to understand not only the hearing impairment but also the disability and handicapping situations that can be associated with the impairment. The World Health Organization has proposed that the terms *disability* and *handicap* be replaced by *activity limitations* and *participation restrictions*, respectively. Physical, social, and attitudinal environ-

mental factors are also considered in the proposed classification system (World Health Organization [WHO], 2001). The newer terms and classification system emphasize how individuals live with their health conditions, specify what an individual can and cannot do, and eliminate some of the negative connotations associated with the terms now in use. The focus is on how to optimize a person's ability to live a full life by remaining active in the workplace and society. By considering the hearing impaired individual's abilities, restrictions, and limitations in the context of his or her personal and environmental situations, an appropriate rehabilitation plan may be developed.

CONDUCTIVE HEARING LOSS

A small percentage of hearing losses in adulthood are conductive. A conductive hearing loss occurs when the sound cannot efficiently get to the inner ear to stimulate the sensory receptors for hearing (see Chapter 10). The audiogram for a conductive loss will exhibit elevated thresholds by air conduction and normal thresholds by bone conduction, so that an air-bone gap will be present (see Chapter 11). The hearing-impaired person typically has good word recognition provided that speech is loud enough to be heard. Causes of conductive impairments include excess *cerumen*, or ear wax, blocking the ear canal, fluid behind the eardrum within the middle ear space (see Chapter 11 for a discussion of middle ear fluid in children), a perforated eardrum, or damage to the ossicles within the middle ear. **Otosclerosis** is an example of a disorder that occurs in adulthood and causes a progressive, conductive hearing impairment. In otosclerosis, bony tissue is replaced by spongy or fibrous bone growth. The most common place for this abnormal bone growth to occur is in the area of the oval window resulting in reduced motion of the stapes and a conductive hearing loss. Otosclerosis is more commonly found in both ears than in one, in women than in men, and in Caucasians rather than Asian or African Americans. Genetics seem to play a role because a family history is often reported (Balloh, 1998).

> Ms. Garrett, age 35 years, reported that within the last several years she has had difficulties understanding speech when there is background noise, localizing sounds, hearing people talk when they are positioned to her left, and using the left ear on the telephone. Figure 12.1 (p. 290) illustrates Ms. Garrett's audiogram and word recognition ability. She has otosclerosis in the left ear. Notice that when tested in the left ear at a normal conversational level (45 dB HL) she only repeated 44 percent of the single-syllable words correctly. This was because the entire speech signal was not audible to her.

To appreciate the effect of hearing loss on the ability to understand speech, it is helpful to examine the relative contribution of the different frequency and intensity combinations for speech audibility, as shown in Figure 12.2 (p. 290). One hundred dots are displayed on the graph. The denser the distribution of dots, the

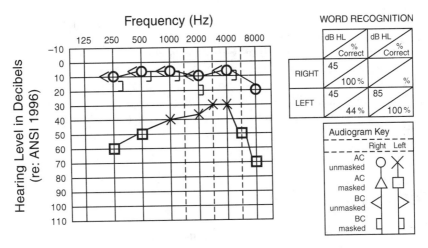

FIGURE 12.1   Audiogram illustrating a conductive hearing loss in the left ear due to otosclerosis.

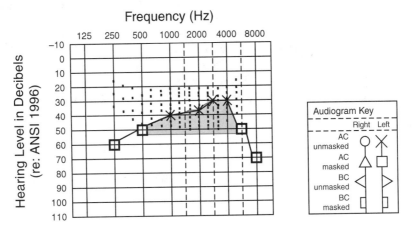

FIGURE 12.2   The left ear thresholds of an individual with unilateral otosclerosis superimposed on the Count-the-Dot audiogram for calculation of the articulation index (adapted from Mueller & Killion, 1990). The shaded portion of the graph indicates the frequency range and hearing levels that are audible when speech is presented at a normal conversational level. Note that it was necessary to use masking at levels of 50 dB and above to prevent cross-over of sounds to the opposite ear. Masked thresholds are represented by squares on the audiogram.

greater the amount of speech energy that falls within that frequency band. An **articulation** or **audibility index** is calculated by assigning 0.01 (one percent) to each dot that is within a person's audibility range. Ms. Garrett's left ear air conduction thresholds are superimposed on the graph.

Ms. Garrett's audiogram reveals approximately 36 dots that fall below her audiometric curve (between her thresholds and 110 dB HL), which results in an AI of 0.36. The AI can then be used in a formula to estimate syllable, word, or sentence intelligibility (Mueller & Killion, 1990). In Ms. Garrett's case, a left ear intelligibility score of approximately 56 percent would be predicted based on her AI of 0.36. This is close to the 44 percent that was measured directly during testing. When words were presented at a higher level (85 dB HL), Ms. Garrett's word recognition ability was excellent (100% correct).

Ms. Garrett's profile indicates that she is an excellent candidate for wearing a hearing aid because her hearing loss is primarily conductive, so there is little or no sound distortion. When provided with appropriate amplification, the individual with a conductive hearing impairment will have few if any limitations or restrictions. Depending on the cause of the conductive hearing loss, surgery or medical treatment may improve or restore an individual's hearing. Surgeries, however, are not risk free, as we will see when we continue to follow Ms. Garrett's history.

Ms. Garrett had surgery in an attempt to eliminate the conductive hearing loss due to otosclerosis. The surgery, performed by an Ear, Nose, and Throat (ENT) specialist, is known as a **stapedectomy** and often reduces or nearly eliminates the conductive component of a hearing impairment. During her surgery, the footplate of the stapes was removed and replaced with a wire prosthesis. Although initial results indicated almost complete elimination of the conductive hearing impairment, one month after the surgery she returned to the clinic because she was hearing a loud roaring noise in the left ear. Figure 12.3 illustrates the audiogram obtained

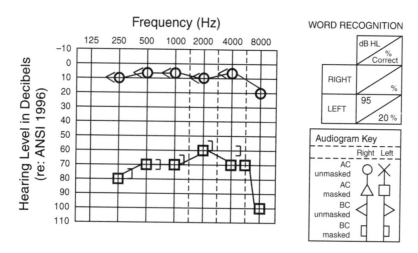

FIGURE 12.3   Audiometric results after an unsuccessful stapedectomy that resulted in a moderate-to-severe sensorineural hearing loss in the left ear. Word recognition was also very poor.

from this visit. Her left ear thresholds had deteriorated and her audiogram revealed a sensorineural hearing loss (note that the air and bone conduction thresholds are in the same place) with very poor word recognition ability (20% correct) when words were presented well above her thresholds for tones (95 dB HL). Because of the poor word recognition ability, she was no longer a candidate for amplification in this ear.[1] Amplification would make sounds audible but not very clear, possibly interfering with speech understanding in the good ear.

SENSORINEURAL HEARING LOSS

The majority of hearing impairments in adulthood are sensorineural. A sensorineural hearing impairment occurs when there is damage to the inner ear, the VIII nerve, or both (see Chapter 10).

Prior to the now widespread use of imaging and electrophysiological techniques, cochlear damage was not easily differentiated from damage within the auditory nervous system. Therefore, hearing impairments in which the audiogram does not exhibit an air-bone gap are generally described as sensorineural (Northern & Downs, 2002). A sensorineural hearing loss, as evidenced by the pure-tone audiogram, usually means cochlear damage. Pathology within the auditory nervous system, beyond the cochlea, is known as retrocochlear. Retrocochlear pathology generally does not affect pure-tone thresholds, unless the damaging agent has secondary effects on the cochlea (see VIIIth nerve tumor). Individuals with damage to the central auditory nervous system find it difficult to understand speech, especially in difficult listening environments. The three most common conditions in adulthood that are associated with sensorineural hearing impairments due to cochlear processes are aging, noise exposure, and Ménière's disease. A less common occurrence is a cochlear insult due to toxic influences. Additional problems may include tumors on the VIIIth nerve and diseases of the central auditory nervous system.

Aging Process

The proportion of people with hearing loss increases with age. It is estimated that 43 percent of the population with hearing loss are age 65 years or older (National Academy on an Aging Society, 1999). The decrease in hearing associated with the aging process is known as **presbycusis**. A lifetime of environmental noise exposure, disease processes, drug effects, and genetic predisposition to hearing impairment contribute to presbycusis. Although changes in the cochlea probably begin early in life, it is not until middle age that people most commonly begin to have difficulties understanding speech. Initial changes occur in the basal end of the cochlea, which is responsible for detecting high-frequency sounds. Because low-

---

[1]Only 1 to 3% of stapedectomies result in sensorineural hearing loss.

frequency hearing is relatively normal, individuals with early presbycusis typically report that they can hear people talk, but that they cannot understand what is being said. This is because the low-frequency, high-intensity vowels are audible, but the high-frequency, low-intensity consonants, which are most important for intelligibility, are inaudible. Figure 12.4 depicts the frequency and intensity characteristics of four classes of speech sounds: nasals, vowels, stops, and fricatives (Olsen, Hawkings, & Van Tasell, 1987). Notice that the cues for stops and fricatives are high in frequency compared to the cues for nasals and vowels (see Chapter 11). Stops and fricatives are, therefore, easily missed by the person with a high-frequency hearing loss. Cues to distinguish place of articulation (e.g., distinguishing /b/ from /d/ from /g/) are also dominated by energy in the high frequencies. Without using speechreading or contextual cues, a person with a high-frequency hearing loss might report hearing "ben" for "den" or "gay" for "day" or "bay." Another common complaint of individuals with high-frequency hearing loss is the inability to understand speech in the presence of background noise that masks the weaker components of the speech signal (e.g., the high-frequency consonants and place of articulation cues). Rooms with reverberation (echoes) are also difficult listening environments for those with hearing impairment.

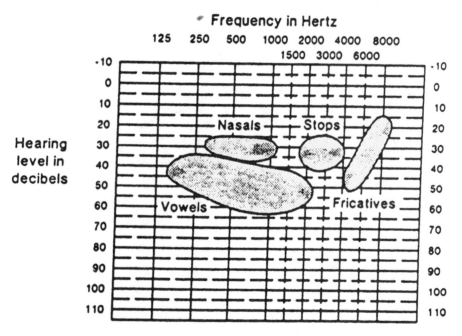

FIGURE 12.4 The frequency and decibel levels of several classes of speech sounds. (From Olsen, W., Hawkins, D., & Van Tasell, D. [1987]. Representations of the long-term spectra of speech. *Ear and Hearing, 8*(5), 1003–1085. Reprinted with permission of Lippincott Williams & Wilkins.)

Typical thresholds for individuals of various ages are illustrated in Figure 12.5. Notice that with increases in age, the low-frequency sounds also become more difficult to detect. Although not indicated on this graph, hearing thresholds decline at an earlier age and more quickly in men than in women (Pearson, Morrell, Gordon-Salant, et al., 1995). With advanced presbycusis, a loss of central auditory neurons may accompany the changes within the cochlea resulting in central presbycusis or a **central auditory processing disorder**. A sign of central presbycu-

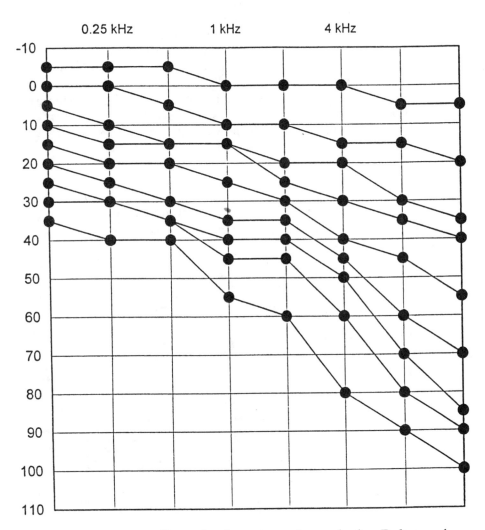

FIGURE 12.5 Audiogram illustrating the patterns of normal aging. Each curve from top to bottom represents groups of increasing ages. (From Goodhill, V., *Presbycusis in Ear Diseases, Deafness and Dizziness*. Hagerstown, MD: Harper and Row, p. 719 [1979]. Reprinted by permission of Lippincott Williams & Wilkins).

sis is **phonemic regression**. This refers to word recognition that is very poor and cannot be explained based on the amount of hearing loss for pure tones. A common report of individuals with central presbycusis is "I can hear fine but everyone mumbles."

Central auditory processing disorders associated with the aging process may be difficult to distinguish from the cochlear damage that almost always accompanies it.

> Mr. Robinson, age 70 years, came to the clinic to have his hearing evaluated. He was accompanied by his two daughters who reported that their father was answering questions inappropriately and saying "huh" constantly. Although Mr. Robinson admitted that he had some difficulty hearing, he commented that his hearing "was not all that bad" and that he would be able to hear better if people "would speak more clearly." Figure 12.6 illustrates Mr. Robinson's audiogram. He has central presbycusis. He shows signs of a central auditory processing disorder along with the cochlear impairment. This is evident because of his word understanding ability, which is poorer than expected given his pure-tone audiogram. His word recognition ability was 28 percent in his left ear and 32 percent in his right ear when presented at a level well above his thresholds.

In contrast to Mr. Robinson's test results, the same degree of hearing loss in a 44-year-old man tested at the same clinic was associated with 80 percent word recognition ability. Stach, Spretnjak, and Jerger (1990) estimated that by the age of 65 years, over 50 percent of the elderly will have a central auditory processing disorder. This population, compared to the hearing-impaired population without central auditory processing disorders, has greater difficulty extracting speech from

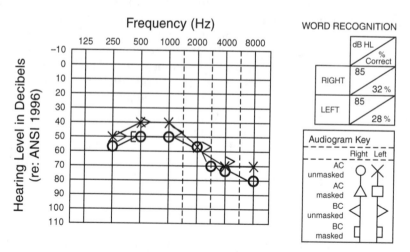

FIGURE 12.6   Audiogram illustrating a sensorineural hearing loss. The poor word-recognition scores suggest a central auditory processing disorder in addition to cochlear damage.

noise, understanding speech when reverberation is present, and successfully using amplification devices.

The increasing prevalence of central auditory processing disorders with increasing age is important to consider when working with individuals in retirement and nursing home facilities. As the baby-boomer population ages, an increasing number of elderly people will be living in retirement and nursing home facilities. It is estimated that by the year 2030 there will be 3 million residents of nursing homes (Sahyoun, Pratt, Lentzner, Dey, & Robinson, 2001). These living conditions impose different kinds of demands on hearing. Communicative difficulties for elderly individuals living in group facilities are likely to be experienced in areas such as meeting rooms, dining areas, and recreational rooms. For the nursing home resident, hearing loss may result in poor patient-staff relationships. Hearing-impaired residents are often labeled as being withdrawn, uncommunicative, or confused.

Hearing impairment can also be associated with poor performance on cognitive tests, especially if administered verbally. For example, Weinstein and Amsel (1986) tested hearing-impaired patients using a test of mental function. Patients were tested with and without their hearing aids. Results indicated that 33 percent of the patients were reclassified as less severely demented when amplification was used compared to no amplification. Thus, the use of amplification with nursing home residents may have profound implications for their perceived versus actual mental status. The impact that a hearing impairment can have on the nursing home resident is particularly important given that Schow and Nerbonne (1980) estimated that 48 percent of residents have a hearing impairment that interferes with communication. Although some residents may own personal hearing aids, many hearing aids are likely to be malfunctioning (Erber & Heine, 1996; Thibodeau & Schmitt, 1988). In addition, few health care providers have received formal training in the management of patients with communication disorders. Because of the high prevalence of hearing loss in this population, an audiologist might be employed to provide audiologic evaluations, fit hearing aids, and train staff members on how to use strategies to enhance communication and how to troubleshoot malfunctioning hearing aids. These services are important because isolation as a result of hearing loss can dramatically decrease the quality of life for those living their last years in a nursing home facility.

Many factors contribute to hearing impairment in the aged population; therefore, each person's hearing capabilities are unique, and therapies must be tailored to each individual's needs. Hearing rehabilitation for the elderly individual presents an exciting challenge for the audiologist.

Noise Exposure

Many Americans are exposed to potentially hazardous noise levels in the workplace, at home, as well as during recreational activities. The National Institute on Deafness and Other Communication Disorders (1999) estimated that 30 million Americans are exposed to dangerously high sound levels on a regular basis. They

also estimated that noise exposure has contributed to about one-third of the hearing impairments reported. Noise exposure can cause a "threshold shift" initially observed around 4000 Hz. That is, hearing a tone in the 4000 Hz frequency region will be more difficult after noise exposure than before.

> Mr. McGee, age 52 years, has been employed in a manufacturing plant for twenty-five years. He also enjoys carpentry work and snowmobiling as recreational activities. He reported that he hears ringing in his ears (**tinnitus**) and that speech sounds are muffled. The audiologist employed by his company evaluated his hearing (see Figure 12.7) and compared the results to previous evaluations. She noted a threshold shift—that is, his hearing for the frequencies 3000, 4000, and 6000 Hz had become poorer since his previous tests.

Thresholds that are poor around 4000 Hz (4k Hz) and improve at 8000 Hz are known as the "**4k notch**" because of the dip that appears on the audiogram (see Figure 12.7). This threshold shift is due to damaged sensory cells in the cochlea resulting in sensorineural hearing loss. Initially, the threshold shift may be temporary. After removing oneself from the high noise levels (or removing the noise from oneself, as in the case of portable tape player headphones), thresholds may return to normal. This is known as a *temporary threshold shift* or TTS. However, it is likely that some damage to the sensory cells has been done. Furthermore, with repeated exposures, exposure for a longer period of time, or in an individual with susceptibility to noise damage, the recovery may not be complete, resulting in *permanent threshold shift* or PTS. Like those with presbycusis, individuals with noise-induced hearing loss have difficulties understanding speech in noisy environments and in rooms with high levels of reverberation.

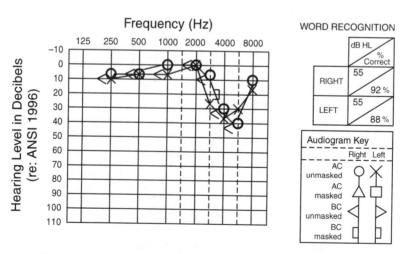

FIGURE 12.7 **Audiogram illustrating a sensorineural hearing loss centered around the 4000 Hz region as a result of excessive noise exposure.**

Mr. McGee received a complete audiometric evaluation and was counseled about the harm that noise exposure causes, as well as the effects of that high-frequency hearing loss on communication ability. He was shown how to wear earplugs appropriately, and instructed to limit his exposure to noise and wear hearing protectors at work and during recreational activities in the presence of high noise levels.

Ménière's Disease

Mrs. Hill, age 55 years, experiences episodic attacks of vertigo, nausea, tinnitus, and a sensorineural hearing loss in the right ear that is more severe in the low frequencies than in the high frequencies. A feeling of pressure in her right ear often precedes the attacks. The most distressing symptom for her is the vertigo that comes on suddenly with little warning. Because of the unpredictability of these attacks and the embarrassment she feels, Mrs. Hill is no longer employed and has stopped socializing with friends. She was diagnosed with **Ménière's disease** ten years ago. Figure 12.8 displays her audiogram. She has had Ménière's disease for ten years. The hearing loss has become slightly worse over the last five years.

Between 3 and 5 million people in the United States suffer from Ménière's disease (National Institute on Deafness and Other Communication Disorders, 1998). Although the exact cause of Ménière's disease is unknown, it is thought to be due to an excess buildup of inner ear fluid called *endolymph*. Ménière's disease is often unilateral and fluctuates. One-third of those with the disease will develop it in both ears. It is common for the first episode to occur from early- to mid-adulthood. As the disease progresses, the low-frequency hearing loss becomes more severe and permanent. The role of the audiologist with this population is to provide information about the disease and the available audiologic rehabilitation

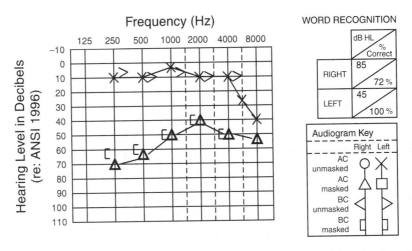

FIGURE 12.8 **Audiogram illustrating a right sensorineural hearing loss due to Ménière's disease.**

methods. Amplification may be necessary depending on whether a stable or deteriorating hearing impairment is present. Noise maskers may also be necessary to help the patient with Ménière's disease become less aware of the tinnitus.

Although sensorineural hearing impairments associated with the aging process, noise exposure, and Ménière's disease are the most prevalent causes of hearing impairments in the adult population, the audiologist will test and provide rehabilitation for adults with impairments due to other causes. The audiologist must know about toxins to and disorders of the auditory system such as ototoxicity, acoustic neuromas, and diseases of the central auditory system.

Ototoxicity

Ototoxicity results when certain drugs damage the inner ear resulting in sensorineural hearing loss. The damage is usually in the high frequencies and can be reversible or permanent. Examples of ototoxic drugs are the aminoglycosides used for treatment of many and often life-threatening infectious diseases, diuretics used to reduce edema or excessive fluid from renal failure, high doses of acetylsalicylic acid (i.e., aspirin), and cisplatin, a drug used to treat cancer. The audiologist's role is to obtain periodic audiograms prior to, during, and after drug therapy. For those individuals who develop hearing loss, the audiologist provides rehabilitation services that may consist of providing amplification, support, and encouragement. Education about hearing conservation is also important because individuals on drug therapies may be more susceptible to noise damage than those not receiving such therapies.

Acoustic Neuroma

Ms. Parker, age 56 years, came to the ENT clinic because she was having pain on the left side of her face, tinnitus in the left ear, and dizziness. Her audiogram (Figure 12.9, p. 300) revealed a sloping, mild-to-moderate sensorineural hearing loss in the left ear and mild high-frequency sensorineural hearing loss in the right ear. Her word recognition was excellent in the right ear when words were presented at normal and loud conversational levels (50 and 90 dB HL, respectively). Left ear results revealed good word recognition at 70 dB HL but poor recognition when words were presented at 90 dB HL.

This dramatic decrease in word recognition as the presentation level of the words is increased is known as **rollover** and is often associated with pathology in the auditory nervous system.

The audiologist evaluated Ms. Parker using the auditory brainstem response (ABR) test (see Chapter 11). Four electrodes were placed on the surface of her scalp and clicking sounds were presented to each ear. The electrodes detected the electrical activity that occurred in response to the clicks. Samples of the electrical activity that occurred after each click were averaged with a computer.

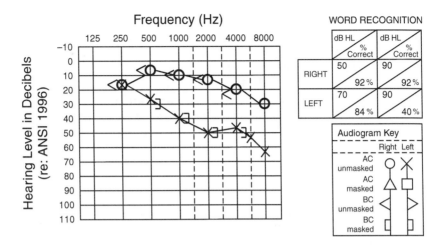

FIGURE 12.9   Audiogram illustrating a left sensorineural hearing loss associated with an acoustic neuroma. Note that the word recognition score for the left ear (seen at upper right) decreased when words were presented at 90 dB HL compared to 70 dB HL (rollover).

In neurologically normal individuals, several positive peaks can be identified that occur within a certain number of milliseconds following the clicks. Delayed peaks in the absence of a conductive hearing loss or delayed intervals between peaks are a strong indication that the pathology is located in the ascending pathways of the auditory system (see Chapter 10).

Figure 12.10 exhibits Ms. Parker's ABR results. The peaks for waves III and V for the left ear were at 5.16 ms and 7.44 ms, respectively. These were much longer than the latencies for waves III and V for the right ear (4.64 ms and 6.72 ms, respectively). Ms. Parker subsequently had an MRI (magnetic resonance image) of the internal auditory canal (the bony canal that extends from each cochlear nucleus to its corresponding cochlea) and an **acoustic neuroma** (tumor) on the left VIIIth nerve was confirmed. The tumor was surgically removed but the surgery, unfortunately, resulted in no measurable hearing in the left ear. Ms. Parker, being active in her vocation and community, found that the unilateral hearing loss restricted her participation in everyday activities. As is common with unilateral hearing loss, she had difficulties localizing sounds, understanding a talker when positioned on the side of the poorer ear, and understanding speech in noise. The audiologist fit her with a hearing aid that placed a microphone at the unusable left ear and a receiver on the good right ear. The microphone picked up the signal reaching the impaired ear and sent it to the good ear to allow detection.

A hearing aid arrangement in which a microphone is placed behind an unaidable ear and sends the signal to the good ear is known as *contralateral routing of signals* or a CROS hearing aid. Wearing a CROS hearing aid makes it easier for

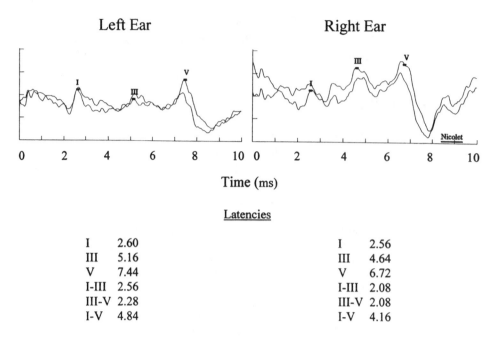

Latencies

I	2.60		I	2.56
III	5.16		III	4.64
V	7.44		V	6.72
I-III	2.56		I-III	2.08
III-V	2.28		III-V	2.08
I-V	4.84		I-V	4.16

FIGURE 12.10   The auditory brainstem response of a patient with a left acoustic neuroma. When clicks were presented to the left ear, waves III and V were abnormally delayed compared to the waves associated with right ear click stimulation.

the individual with a unilateral hearing impairment to hear sounds directed to the impaired ear. It also restores a sense of sound balance and an improvement in the signal-to-noise ratio when the signal is on the side of the poorer ear. Although acoustic neuromas only affect 1 out of 100,000 people, if undetected, they can result in death by exerting pressure on brainstem structures as they grow. If detected early and surgically removed, hearing may be preserved. Therefore, patients experiencing unilateral hearing loss or unilateral tinnitus should be tested to determine if an acoustic neuroma is the cause of their symptoms.

Diseases of the Central Auditory System

Audiologists may also test and participate in the rehabilitation of patients who have lesions to the brain or brainstem that affect hearing (see Chapter 10 for a discussion of the central auditory pathways). Such disorders include multiple sclerosis, strokes, and cortical and brainstem tumors. A central lesion can disturb the blood supply to the cochlea resulting in damage to the hair cells and a reduced ability to hear pure tones. However, most often a central auditory disorder will cause difficulties with speech processing without affecting pure-tone hearing sensitivity. Individuals with central auditory lesions report difficulties listening when there is background noise or reverberation, when visual cues are not available, and

when speech is spoken at a rapid rate. An elderly person with a central auditory lesion will likely have some difficulty hearing pure tones due to the effects of aging on the cochlea.

MIXED HEARING LOSS

Finally, a hearing loss can have both conductive and sensorineural components and is known as a *mixed hearing loss*.

Mrs. Leon, age 84 years, reported a sudden decrease in her hearing. Her family, who accompanied her to the evaluation, reported that for many years she had some difficulties understanding speech and had to turn the television to higher-than-normal loudness levels in order to hear most programs. Recently, her neighbors had complained about the loud noise coming from her apartment. Mrs. Leon reported a sudden hearing loss coincident with a cold that she developed approximately two months prior. She expressed much concern about her deteriorating hearing ability, as it was a sign of "getting old" and "one more thing going wrong."

Mrs. Leon's audiometric results are displayed in Figure 12.11. The audiogram showed that she had a mixed hearing loss. Notice the 30 to 40 dB air-bone gap, which reflects the conductive component of the hearing loss, in addition to a mild-to-moderate 30 to 50 dB sensorineural hearing loss (thresholds for bone conduction range from 30 to 50 dB HL). The conductive component of her hearing impairment was due to bilateral middle ear infection (otitis media, see Chapter 11). The sensorineural component was diagnosed as presbycusis. Pressure equalization tubes

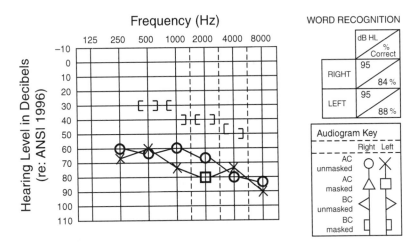

FIGURE 12.11 Audiogram illustrating a mixed hearing loss due to otitis media (which caused the conductive component) and presbycusis (which caused the sensorineural component).

were placed in her ears by an ENT specialist.[2] After medical intervention, the audiologist recommended hearing aids and assisted her in the rehabilitation process. Mrs. Leon adapted quite well to her new hearing aids and showed a renewed interest in communicating with her family and friends. Comforted by the knowledge that she was not rapidly going deaf, and assisted with amplification, she was better able to participate in community functions and in religious services.

PSYCHOSOCIAL IMPACT OF HEARING LOSS

Ramsdell (1960) distinguished three psychological levels of hearing: primitive level or the auditory background of daily living, signal/warning level, and symbolic or social level. Any or all of these levels can be affected by a hearing impairment. For example, an individual with a sudden and total hearing loss will have difficulties at all three levels. In contrast, a person with a mild hearing loss still feels connected to the world (still hears background noises) and is able to hear warning signals. However, the social level of hearing may be affected by a mild hearing loss if it impacts communication. When this happens, emotional difficulties can also arise.

> Mr. Cohen, a 42-year-old salesman, experienced a sudden, severe, and bilateral sensorineural hearing loss. Mr. Cohen had provided the sole financial support for his family that included three children. Because of the severity of the loss and the communication demands that his job required, he had to quit his job. His wife became employed and Mr. Cohen became more responsible for daily activities in the home. He often declined social invitations because he tired easily when trying to participate in the conversations. He relied on his wife to interpret for him and often pretended to understand what people were saying.

A hearing impairment also impacts the family and significant others. Often a hearing-impaired individual is seen in the clinic at the urging of a spouse or partner. Family members may become frustrated at continually repeating and interpreting for the hearing-impaired individual. The extra effort required to include the hearing-impaired individual in conversations and spectator activities such as plays, movies, and lectures can put stress on family relationships and result in exclusion of the hearing-impaired person. It is not uncommon to hear an elderly hearing-impaired person say, "If I don't do something about my hearing, my spouse will leave me." Even said in jest, the statement reflects the seriousness of communication breakdown and its impact on relationships. Likewise, hearing impairment can interfere with activities of daily living. Communicating on the telephone and asking a passerby for directions are just two examples of the many activities that may become more difficult with hearing impairment.

---

[2]Some audiologists work in an ENT clinic. Others work more autonomously as part of a rehabilitation unit in a hospital or in private practice. If the patient with a conductive hearing impairment has not been evaluated by an ENT, an ENT referral is made.

The audiologist must be knowledgeable and competent in assessing the effects of hearing loss on functional communication, including how it influences the psychosocial, educational, and occupational well-being of the client (ASHA, 2002). Training the hearing-impaired individual and significant others to use effective communication strategies and offering counseling for those adjusting to hearing loss are two very important services that an audiologist provides.

AUDIOLOGICAL EVALUATION

Hearing Screenings

The audiologist may screen for hearing loss or oversee such a screening program. The purpose of screening is to identify individuals who have a high probability of having a hearing loss (those who fail the screening) so that they can be referred for appropriate diagnostic testing (ASHA, 1995). ASHA recommends that adults be screened *at least* every ten years through age 50 and then at three-year intervals after that. Common settings for screenings include health fairs and medical facilities. High-noise industries are particularly important sites for screening because noise damage to the cochlea can be avoided. Nursing homes are also important screening sites because of the high prevalence of hearing impairments that exist in the elderly population. In these high-risk environments, screenings are needed on a regular basis.

Hearing screenings consist of presenting pure tones at a predetermined level. The American Speech-Language-Hearing Association (1997) recommends that if an individual responds to pure-tone air-conducted stimuli at 25 dB HL at 1000, 2000, and 4000 Hz in both ears, then he or she passes the screening. If no response is obtained at any frequency in *either* ear, then the individual fails the screening. The 25 dB HL level was recommended because even mild hearing loss can negatively influence a person's health and well-being.

In addition to pure-tone screening, a hearing disability index should be used to identify individuals who perceive themselves as having a disability (ASHA, 1997). One such self-assessment measure is displayed in Table 12.1. Use of a Hearing Disability Index, in conjunction with pure-tone screening, can help identify those individuals who believe that they have a disability. These individuals will be most motivated to attempt rehabilitation and actively utilize newly developed strategies for improved communication. Individuals who fail the pure-tone screening or the Hearing Disability Index should be counseled regarding hearing impairment and the need for a referral for a complete audiologic evaluation.

Hearing Assessment

A second task of the audiologist is to assess a client's hearing status. A complete audiologic evaluation will determine the need for medical referral, additional audiologic followup, or both. The test results will assist the physician in diagnosing

TABLE 12.1   Hearing Handicap Inventory for the Elderly—Screening Version (HHIE-S)

	YES (4)	SOMETIMES (2)	NO (0)
E-1 Does a hearing problem cause you to feel embarrassed when meeting new people?	___	___	___
E-2 Does a hearing problem cause you to feel frustrated when talking to members of your family?	___	___	___
S-1 Do you have difficulty hearing when someone speaks in a whisper?	___	___	___
E-3 Do you feel handicapped by a hearing problem?	___	___	___
S-2 Does a hearing problem cause you difficulty when visiting friends, relatives, or neighbors?	___	___	___
S-3 Does a hearing problem cause you to attend religious services less often than you would like?	___	___	___
E-4 Does a hearing problem cause you to have arguments with family members?	___	___	___
S-4 Does a hearing problem cause you difficulty when listening to TV or radio?	___	___	___
E-5 Do you feel that any difficulty with your hearing limits or hampers your personal or social life?	___	___	___
S-5 Does a hearing problem cause you difficulty when in a restaurant with relatives or friends?	___	___	___

A "yes," "no," and "sometimes" response scores 4, 0, and 2 points, respectively. Possible scores range from 0 to 40. Ventry and Weinstein suggest that scores of 0–8 indicate no perceived handicap, scores of 10–22 indicate mild to moderate handicap, and scores of 24–40 indicate severe handicap. (E-emotional, S-social)

From Ventry, I., & Weinstein, B. (1982). Identification of elderly people with hearing problems. *Ear and Hearing, 3,* 128–134. Reprinted with permission from Lippincott Williams & Wilkins.

and treating the patient. A complete evaluation also provides the basis for a rehabilitation plan.

The audiologic evaluation begins with a case history. The audiologist obtains information about the hearing difficulties that the person is experiencing, family history of hearing loss, medical history, and whether hearing aids were previously worn. Next, the audiologist examines the patient's external ears using a handheld **otoscope** or using **video otoscopy**. With video otoscopy, enlarged images of the tympanic membranes and ear canals can be projected on a video monitor. A photoprint of these structures can be made to document pathology and medical treatment outcomes. If excessive *cerumen* (wax) is observed in the ear canal, it must be removed prior to testing. Cerumen removal can be performed by an audiologist with specialized training or by appropriate medical personnel. Audiologic testing

is performed to determine if a hearing impairment exists, the type of impairment (conductive, sensorineural, or mixed), and the severity of the impairment for various frequencies and for speech. We can examine the stages of the audiologic evaluation by following the case of Mr. Peterson.

> Mr. Peterson came to the clinic because he was having difficulties hearing his co-workers. He reported having more difficulty hearing from his right ear than his left ear. After a case history was obtained and an otoscopic examination revealed the ear canals to be free of cerumen, immittance measures were obtained (see Chapter 11 for a discussion of immittance). Next, Mr. Peterson was seated inside a sound-treated booth and miniature earphones were inserted in his ear canals. The audiologist tested the hearing of each ear individually using an audiometer. The test began with the audiologist saying two-syllable words (such as "cowboy" and "armchair") to Mr. Peterson, who was not allowed to see the audiologist's face to prevent speechreading. The lowest level at which Mr. Peterson was able to repeat the two-syllable words 50 percent of the time was recorded for each ear. These were his speech reception thresholds (SRTs). Next, the pure-tone air-conduction and bone-conduction thresholds were obtained. Word recognition ability was then assessed. Single-syllable words were presented to Mr. Peterson in quiet at normal and loud conversational levels, and the audiologist recorded the percent of words he repeated correctly.

Audiologists also test some adults who are not able to respond verbally to the test stimuli, such as adults with developmental disabilities, severe head injury, or stroke. Written or picture-pointing responses can be used during word recognition testing. *Otoacoustic emissions* (see Chapter 10) can be used to screen for hearing loss in difficult-to-test adults because such tests do not require a volitional response. If a person fails the screening, then an auditory brainstem response threshold search can be obtained.

Assessing Participation Restrictions

For those hearing impairments that are not medically correctable, the audiologist has the task of developing and implementing a rehabilitation plan in conjunction with the patient. Results from the audiologic evaluation are useful in determining the appropriate rehabilitation plan. The audiologist must also obtain information about the individual's daily life in order to formulate an appropriate plan. Some individuals may be homebound with few visitors; others are involved actively in their vocation and other social activities. Because of the range of communicative needs and the lack of good correspondence between audiologic results and degree of perceived difficulties (Matthews, Lee, Mills, & Schum, 1990; Weinstein & Ventry, 1983), self-assessment tools have been used to gauge functional communication.

The audiologist must understand the individual's hearing abilities as they relate to communication demands. An understanding of the needs of the patient will assist the audiologist in jointly developing rehabilitation goals with the patient and the patient's family.

MANAGEMENT STRATEGIES

According to ASHA (2002), "Audiologic/aural rehabilitation (AR) is an ecological, interactive process that facilitates one's ability to minimize or prevent the limitations and restrictions that auditory dysfunctions can impose on well-being and communication, including interpersonal, psychosocial, educational, and vocational functioning" (p. 90). The audiologist achieves these goals with a variety of methods. One of the most important goals of rehabilitation is to facilitate accurate understanding of speech. This may involve the use of hearing aids.

Hearing Aids

Hearing aids are electronic devices that amplify sound. To provide maximum benefit to an individual client, they must be selected and fit appropriately. ASHA (1998) has defined several stages in the hearing aid selection and fitting process including *assessment*, *selection and fitting*, *verification*, *orientation*, and *validation*. By completing each of these stages carefully, the audiologist increases the likelihood that clients will not only receive amplification that is appropriate for them, but also that they will use it successfully. Hearing aids come in various styles (Figure 12.12). The

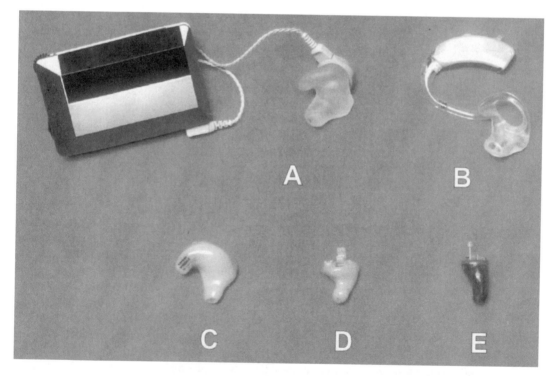

FIGURE 12.12   Types of hearing aids. From top to bottom, left to right: (A) body; (B) behind-the-ear; (C) in-the-ear; (D) in-the-canal; and (E) completely-in-the-canal.

ear-level hearing aids are the most commonly dispensed devices and include the behind-the-ear, in-the-ear, in-the-canal, and completely-in-the-canal styles. Special fittings, such as the CROS aid, described for Ms. Parker, are also available.

All hearing aids, no matter the style, have the same components: a microphone for sound input and conversion to an electrical signal, an amplifier to increase the level of sound, a receiver to convert the electrical signal to an acoustic signal, and a battery to power the device. The circuitry of a hearing aid or how it processes the electrical signal may vary across instruments. Many hearing aids in today's market are digital rather than analog. This means that the hearing aid uses a computer chip and special mathematical algorithms to manipulate the incoming signal after it is converted to a series of digits. The digital signal is adjusted so that it is tailored to the individual's audiometric configuration. For example, if a client has a loss of hearing for the high frequencies only, then the hearing aid's frequency response would reveal more amplification in that frequency range and little if any amplification in the lower frequencies.

Decisions concerning the circuitry of the hearing aid are determined primarily by the *assessment* of the degree of the hearing loss. Hearing aid *selection* depends on both the nature of the hearing impairment and the client's preferences and lifestyle. For example, the behind-the-ear hearing aid has the most flexibility for fitting any magnitude of hearing loss, but may not be as readily accepted by a client as a smaller style such as a completely-in-the-canal aid. However, this smaller hearing aid cannot compensate for more severe hearing losses and is difficult for many elderly clients to insert and remove. The use of two hearing aids (binaural amplification) is generally recommended because of the advantages for localizing sound and for understanding speech in background noise. Guidance and counseling are important to assist a client in realizing the advantages and disadvantages of each style so that an appropriate selection may be made. The advanced technology now available in hearing aids makes them more flexible; however, many of the limitations of using amplification for an individual with a sensorineural hearing loss remain. Two of these limitations include distortion of the signal that arises from within the cochlea and intolerance for loud sounds. Having realistic expectations improves satisfaction with a hearing aid.

Hearing aids are custom-fitted to the client's ear. After *fitting* the hearing aid, the audiologist must *verify* the fitting to assure that it is correct and appropriate for the client. One way is to insert a small probe microphone in the ear canal, near the tympanic membrane. The microphone measures the characteristics of sounds near the plane of the eardrum. These recordings are referred to as *real ear* or *probe microphone measurements*. Sounds of various frequencies are presented through a loudspeaker while the probe microphone measures the sound pressure level with the hearing aid in the ear and turned on (aided condition) and without the hearing aid in the ear (unaided condition). The difference in sound pressure level between the aided and unaided conditions tells the audiologist how much gain the hearing aid provides at different frequencies. Because probe microphone measurements require no response from the patient, they are reliable and can be used to verify hearing aid fittings even with a difficult-to-test patient. Although this is the pre-

ferred verification method, other means of verification are available if real ear measurements cannot be done.

During the *orientation* stage, the patient is instructed in the use and care of the hearing aids. Following the orientation, the patient is usually given a trial period with the devices during which time any problems with the fitting may be resolved. Let us examine this aspect of the rehabilitation process by following Mrs. Leon, the woman who received pressure equalization tubes to correct the conductive component of a mixed hearing impairment (see Figure 12.11 for a review of Mrs. Leon's audiogram).

> Written and oral instructions were provided to Mrs. Leon and her family regarding her hearing aids. A gradual listening program was recommended. Mrs. Leon was instructed to wear the hearing aids initially in quiet environments such as when watching television or having a conversation with one or two people. After she became comfortable using the hearing aids in quiet, she was instructed to wear them in noisier environments. Listening activities were also recommended. Mrs. Leon was instructed to make a list of common, everyday background sounds in her environment (e.g., water running, the refrigerator humming) and to listen to these sounds while wearing the hearing aids. She was informed that these exercises would assist her in relearning how to tune out or ignore the background noises that she may not have heard for quite some time due to her hearing loss.
>
> A needs assessment tool was administered to her both before and after a trial use period with her hearing aids. She indicated that she wanted to hear the minister in her church during the Sunday sermon. The needs assessment revealed that the hearing aids had achieved this goal for her, thus validating one aspect of the fitting.

Although hearing aids are the most common form of treatment for sensorineural hearing impairment, only 6.35 million people own them, while 22.3 million individuals with hearing impairments do not use them (Kochkin, 2001). The low percentage of hearing aid users is likely due to denial, embarrassment, or a belief that a hearing aid will not help. The statistics are unfortunate given the research that shows hearing aid use to be associated with improvements in social, emotional, psychological, and physical well-being (National Council on the Aging, 1999). These improvements in the quality of life are found not only for those with severe hearing loss but also for those with mild loss.

Technological advances as well as skillful counseling are likely to increase the number of adults who become successful hearing aid users. One of the greatest predictors of hearing aid success is a patient's motivation and perception of handicap. An individual who purchases a hearing aid because he or she is missing out on conversations during social interactions is much more likely to make a successful adjustment than is a person who has stopped socializing and purchases a hearing aid because of family pressure. Presbycusic listeners with severe central auditory processing disorders are also less likely to benefit from wearing hearing aids. Assistive listening devices (ALDs) are available to supplement what can be achieved with conventional amplification

Assistive Listening and Alerting Devices

An **assistive listening device** is any device, excluding hearing aids, designed to improve a hearing-impaired individual's ability to communicate and therefore function more independently than without the device. Closed-captioning of television broadcasts is one example of an assistive device that can be used in the home. A **closed caption decoder** displays the television dialogue in written form at the bottom of the television screen. Many public venues, like theaters or meeting halls, are equipped with frequency-modulated or **FM systems**. These systems use radio waves to send signals such as a speaker's voice or a movie sound track to a listener who is equipped with a receiver and earphones or a connection to his or her own hearing aid. Because an FM system is wireless, the hearing-impaired individual and the talker are able to move around freely within the listening environment. Other types of assistive listening devices are designed for one-on-one communication. For example, a simple amplified handset is often sufficient to allow the hearing-impaired individual to communicate over the telephone. For more profound hearing losses, the telephone message can be typed by a relay operator and transmitted to a special **telecommunication device for the deaf** (TDD) for the hearing-impaired individual to read.

In addition to assistive listening devices, **alerting devices** are also available for the hearing-impaired individual. These include devices that provide a visual signal for common environmental sounds (e.g., the ringing of a phone or a doorbell). Vibrotactile devices, such as an alarm clock that vibrates the pillow, are also available. Alerting devices can be used to indicate dangerous situations (e.g., the sounding of a smoke alarm). Finally, hearing-ear dogs are also trained to help alert their owners to auditory signals.

Not all hearing-impaired persons come to the audiologist's office with the intent to purchase hearing aids or assistive listening and alerting devices. Mrs. Lough is an example of a client who continued to deny that she had a hearing problem and had no intention of trying amplification.

> Mrs. Lough came in for testing urged by her husband, who was having difficulty communicating with her. He reported that when she does not hear him (which is most of the time) he raises his voice and then Mrs. Lough gets angry because she feels like he is yelling at her. Mrs. Lough's first comment to the audiologist was "I hope you're not going to fit me with hearing aids because I don't want them." She had tried hearing aids twice previously at other clinics and was very dissatisfied with them. The hearing evaluation was performed, and as Figure 12.13 indicates, Mrs. Lough had a moderate sensorineural hearing loss in both ears. Her word recognition ability was fair at a high presentation level. Once the testing was completed, the audiologist used a handheld amplifier to describe the hearing impairment and its implications for understanding speech. Oral and written information was provided to Mrs. Lough and her husband about hearing aids (what hearing aids could and could not do) and strategies that could facilitate the communication process. Assistive listening devices (ALDs) were also discussed as an alternative to hearing aids. Mrs. Lough was resistant to purchasing any type of amplification including ALDs.

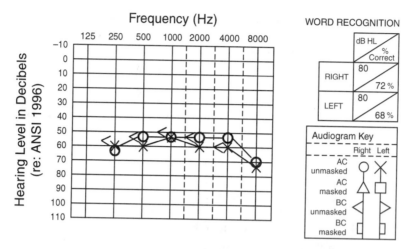

FIGURE 12.13 Audiogram of a moderate sensorineural hearing loss with fair word recognition ability. Although amplification would make more speech sounds audible to this client, she refused to try it.

Unfortunately, sometimes counseling cannot undo the negative impact of bad experiences with prior amplification or poor motivation to communicate more effectively. A patient must accept the hearing loss and be ready to work with the audiologist to improve his or her communication abilities.

Cochlear Implants

For those with severe to profound hearing loss who do not benefit substantially from amplification, cochlear implants might be recommended. To date, the cochlear implant has been more successful in adults who acquired a hearing loss compared with adults who have been deaf since childhood. As we saw in Chapter 11, the implant consists of multiple electrodes surgically placed within the cochlea. The electrodes conduct electrical current that directly stimulates auditory nerve fibers to produce hearing sensations. Audiologists play an important role in education and counseling of potential candidates for cochlear implants. Although surgically inserted into the cochlea by a surgeon, the audiologist activates and maps the implant approximately four weeks after surgery. Mapping involves determining the appropriate levels of electrical stimulation for each electrode. The audiologist also participates in the follow-up and long-term rehabilitation plan that involves teaching the client to use available auditory cues in conjunction with speechreading.

Auditory Training and Speechreading

Historically, **auditory training** and speechreading were used to teach children who were deafened before or shortly after birth to understand speech. However, techniques may be useful for adults who use amplification but still have difficulty

understanding speech. Auditory training involves teaching the individual to optimize use of available sound cues. Several approaches to auditory training exist. These range from drill on sound sequences (e.g., /ba/ vs. /da/) to teaching strategies that capitalize on knowledge of the topic of conversation to assist speech comprehension.

The short- and long-term effects of auditory training on speech perception in those with acquired hearing loss are not known. However, there is indirect evidence that auditory training in individuals learning a second language can facilitate speech discrimination (Logan, Lively, & Pisoni, 1991) and even make changes in the central auditory nervous system (Kraus, McGee, Carrell, King, & Tremblay, 1995; Tremblay, Kraus, Carrell, & McGee, 1997).

Adding visual information to auditory speech signals improves identification relative to auditory input alone (Hardison, 1998). **Speechreading** is a technique that capitalizes on this improvement. In face-to-face communication, listeners can improve their ability to understand speech considerably by watching the speaker's mouth as words are formed (Sumby & Pollack, 1954). Attending to the speaker's face provides information about the place of articulation (see Chapter 3). This provides a significant benefit because the acoustic cues are most severely affected by background noise and high-frequency hearing loss.

The ability to speechread varies widely across individuals. However, there are some factors that can increase the likelihood of success (see also Montgomery, 1993, for suggestions to maximize speechreading in combination with amplification). Training in speechreading might include strategies like making sure that a speaker's face is visible and well lit so that mouth movements can be seen. A client also learns to attempt to understand phrases and ideas, rather than phonemes and words.

Counseling and Communication Strategies

The audiologist provides critical information to the client and significant others. Individuals must understand the nature of their hearing impairment and its implications for day-to-day life. Furthermore, it is important for hearing-impaired individuals and their significant others to understand the limits of the technology and rehabilitative methods that can be offered to them. For example, the client should understand that hearing aids will not restore normal hearing. Strategies to improve the communication process are also discussed with the patient and significant other(s). Kaplan (1988) listed several strategies that can be used by both the hearing-impaired person and the person speaking. For example, the client with a hearing loss may be advised to ask a speaker to repeat or rephrase a statement that was not understood, or read reviews prior to seeing a movie to better follow the plot. Significant others might be advised not to talk to the client from other rooms and to face the client when speaking.

In addition to informational counseling, the audiologist must be sensitive to how an individual reacts to his or her hearing impairment and to any adjustment problems related to the impairment. Tanner (1980) provided an excellent article

about loss related to communication disorders and Kübler-Ross's (1969) five stages of the grieving process (i.e., denial, anger, bargaining, depression, acceptance). It is important to keep in mind that an individual may not only be grieving the loss of hearing but also the loss of independence, vocation, and group or self-identity. Hard-of-hearing support groups offer an excellent opportunity for those with hearing impairments to share their experiences and feelings with others experiencing similar problems.

Support Groups

Members of national and local support groups work together to improve communication and teach self-management skills. Information about hearing impairment is often provided at support group meetings, as are discussions about communication problems and solutions. The meetings provide an opportunity for the hearing-impaired individual to practice assertive communication strategies in a nonthreatening environment. The groups also offer an opportunity for members to be proactive in political issues related to the civil rights of those with a hearing loss. For example, members of Self-Help for the Hard of Hearing (SHHH) were actively involved in developing regulations for section 255 of the Telecommunications Act of 1996. This section requires telecommunication products and services to be accessible to people with disabilities. The group was also instrumental in developing regulations for the Americans with Disabilities Act (ADA) of 1990. The ADA was designed to ensure that those with disabilities are not discriminated against in employment, public accommodations, transportation, state and local government services, and telecommunications.

CLINICAL PROBLEM SOLVING

Mr. Westrich, age 76 years, reported that he has difficulty understanding his wife and grandchildren when they talk. He also has difficulty understanding speakers on television. He suggested that "all newscasters must go to the same school of mumbling." At family gatherings, he relies on his wife to repeat what people have said and often gets left out of conversations. He was a pilot in the military for thirty years and enjoyed hunting before he retired. Figure 12.14 (p. 314) displays his audiogram and word-recognition ability.

1. What type of hearing loss does Mr. Westrich have?
2. What factors are likely to have contributed to Mr. Westrich's hearing loss?
3. What class(es) of speech sounds will Mr. Westrich have most difficulty hearing?
4. Is Mr. Westrich a candidate for amplification? Why or why not?
5. What types of communication strategies might Mr. Westrich use when communicating? What might the speaker do to facilitate Mr. Westrich's speech understanding?

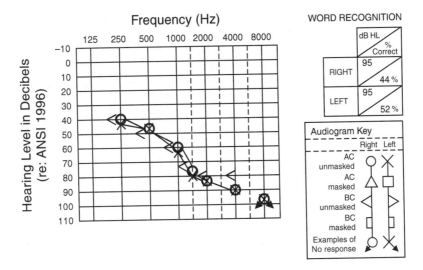

FIGURE 12.14   Audiogram of a client who came to the clinic because of difficulties communicating with his family.

REFERENCES

American Speech-Language-Hearing Association (ASHA). (1995, February). Report on audiological screening. *American Journal of Audiology, 4*, 24–40.

American Speech-Language-Hearing Association (ASHA). (1997). *Guidelines for audiologic screening* (pp. 49–59). Rockville, MD: Author.

American Speech-Language-Hearing Association (ASHA)(1998). Guidelines for hearing aid fitting for adults. *American Journal of Audiology, 7*, 5–13.

American Speech-Language-Hearing Association (ASHA). (2002). Knowledge and skills required for the practice of audiologic/aural rehabilitation: Executive summary. *ASHA Supplement, 22*, in press.

Americans With Disabilities Act of 1990, Pub. L. No. 101-336, § 2, 104 Stat. 328 (1991).

Balloh, R. W. (1998). *Dizziness, hearing loss, and tinnitus.* Philadelphia, PA: FA Davis Co.

Erber, N. P., & Heine, C. (1996). Screening receptive communication of older adults in residential care. *American Journal of Audiology, 5*, 38–46.

Giolas, T. G. (1994). Aural rehabilitation of adults with hearing impairment. In J. Katz (Ed.),

Handbook of clinical audiology (pp. 776–789). Baltimore: Williams & Wilkins.

Goodhill, V. (1979). *Presbycusis in ear diseases, deafness and dizziness* (p. 719). Hagerstown, MD: Harper and Row.

Hardison, D. M. (1998). Acquisition of second-language speech: Effects of visual cues, context and talker variability (Doctoral dissertation, Indiana University, 1998). *Dissertation Abstracts International, 59* (5-A), Z5053.

Kaplan, H. (1988). Communication problems of the hearing-impaired elderly: What can be done? *Pride Institute Journal of Long Term Home Health Care, 7*, 10–22.

Kochkin, S. (2001). The VA and direct mail sales spark growth in hearing aid market. *The Hearing Review, 8*, 16–24.

Kraus, N., McGee, T., Carrell, T. D. , King, C., & Tremblay, K. (1995). Central auditory system plasticity associated with speech discrimination training. *Journal of Cognitive Neuroscience, 7*, 25–32.

Kübler-Ross, E. (1969). *On death and dying.* New York: Macmillan.

Logan, J. S., Lively, S. E., & Pisoni, D. B. (1991). Training Japanese listeners to identify /r/ and

/l/: A first report. *Journal of the Acoustical Society of America, 89,* 874–886.

Matthews, L. J., Lee, F., Mills, J. H., & Schum, D. J. (1990). Audiometric and subjective assessment of hearing handicap. *Archives of Otolaryngology—Head and Neck Surgery, 116,* 1325–1330.

Montgomery, A. A. (1993). Management of the hearing-impaired adult, In J. Alpiner & P. McCarthy (Eds.), *Rehabilitative audiology: Children and adults* (pp. 311–330). Baltimore: Williams & Wilkins.

Mueller, H., & Killion, M. (1990). An easy method for calculating the articulation index. *Hearing Journal, 3,* 14–17.

Mulrow, C. D., Aguilar, C., Endicott, J. E., Tuley, M. R., Velez, R., Charlip, W. S., Rhodes, M. C., Hill, J. A., & DeNino, L. A. (1990). Quality-of-life changes and hearing impairment. *Annals of Internal Medicine, 113,* 188–194.

National Academy on an Aging Society. (1999). Hearing loss: A growing problem that affects quality of life. [online]. Available: http://www.agingsociety.org/profiles.htm. Accessed 5/02/02.

National Council on the Aging. (1999). *The consequences of untreated hearing loss in older persons.* Conducted by the Seniors Research Group [online]. Available: http://www.ncoa.org/news/hearing/01_intro.htm. Accessed 4/02.

National Institute on Deafness and Other Communication Disorders. (1998, July). *Because you asked about Meniere's disease* [online]. Available: http://www.nidcd.nih.gov/health/pubs_hb/meniere.htm. Accessed 4/02.

National Institute on Deafness and Other Communication Disorders. (1999, April). *Noise-induced hearing loss* (NIH Pub. No. 97-4233). Bethesda, MD [online]. Available: http://www.nidcd.nih.gov/health/pubs_hb/noise.htm#who. Accessed 4/02.

Northern, J. L., & Downs, M. P. (2002). *Hearing in children* (5th ed.). Baltimore, MD: Lippincott Williams & Wilkins.

Olsen, W., Hawkins, D., & Van Tasell, D. (1987). Representations of the long-term spectra of speech. *Ear and Hearing, 8*(5), 1003–1085.

Pearson, J. D., Morrell, C. H., Gordon-Salant, S., Brant, L. J., Metter, E. J., Klein, L. L., & Fozard, J. L. (1995). Gender differences in a longitudinal study of age-associated hearing loss. *Journal of the Acoustical Society of America, 97,* 1196–1205.

Ramsdell, D. (1960). The psychology of the hard of hearing and deafened adult. In H. Davis & S. Silverman (Eds.), *Hearing and deafness.* New York: Holt, Rinehart & Winston.

Sahyoun, N. R., Pratt, L. A., Lentzner, H., Dey, A., & Robinson, K. N. (2001). *The changing profile of nursing home residents: 1985–1997.* Aging Trends, No. 4. Hyattsville, Maryland: National Center for Health Statistics [online]. Available: http://www.cdc.gov/nchs/data/agingtrends/04nursin.pdf. Accessed 4/02.

Schow, R., & Nerbonne, M. (1980). Hearing level in nursing home residents. *Journal of Speech and Hearing Disorders, 45,* 124–132.

Stach, B. A., Spretnjak, M. L., & Jerger, J. (1990). The prevalence of central presbycusis in a clinical population. *Journal of the American Academy of Audiology, 1,* 109–115.

Stephens, D., & Hetu, R. (1991). Impairment, disability and handicap in audiology: Toward a consensus. *Audiology, 30,* 185–200.

Sumby, W. G., & Pollack, I. (1954). Visual contributions to speech intelligibility in noise. *Journal of the Acoustical Society of America, 26,* 212–215.

Tanner, D. (1980). Loss and grief: Implications for the speech-language pathologist and audiologist. *Asha, 22,* 916–928.

Thibodeau, L. M., & Schmitt, J. (1988). A report on condition of hearing aids in nursing homes and retirement centers. *Journal of the American Academy of Audiology, 21,* 99–112.

Tremblay, K., Kraus, N., Carrell, T. D., & McGee, T. (1997). Central auditory system plasticity: Generalization to novel stimuli following listening training. *Journal of the Acoustical Society of America, 102,* 3762–3773.

Ventry, I., & Weinstein, B. (1982). Identification of elderly people with hearing problems. *Ear and Hearing, 3,* 128–134.

Weinstein, B. E., & Amsel, L. (1986). Hearing loss and senile dementia in the institutionalized elderly. *Clinical Gerontology, 4,* 3–15.

Weinstein, B. E., & Ventry, I. M. (1983). Audiometric correlates of hearing handicapped inventory for the elderly. *Journal of Speech and Hearing Disorders, 48,* 379–384.

World Health Organization (WHO). (2001, November). WHO publishes new guidelines to measure health [online]. Available: http://www.who.int/inf-pr-2001/en/pr2001-48.html. Accessed 4/02.

READINGS FROM THE POPULAR LITERATURE

Biderman, B. (1998). *Wired for sound: A journey into hearing*. Toronto: Trifolium Books. (cochlear implant to restore hearing)

Lane, H., Bahan, B., & Hoffmeister, R. (1996). *A journey into the deaf world*. San Diego, CA: Dawn Sign Press. (deaf culture)

Lane, H. (2000). *The mask of benevolence: Disabling the deaf community*. San Diego, CA: Dawn Sign Press. (deafness)

Merker, H. (1999). *Listening*. Dallas: Southern Methodist University Press. (sudden adult-onset hearing loss)

Nieminen, R. (1990). *Voyage to the island*. Washington, DC: Gallaudet University Press. (deaf woman, teaching deaf children)

Niesser, A. (1990). *The other side of silence*. Washington, DC: Gallaudet Press. (deafness)

Padden, C., & Humphries, T. (1990). *Deaf in America: Voices from a culture*. Cambridge, MA: Harvard University Press. (Deaf culture)

Romoff, A. (1999). *Hear again: Back to life with a cochlear implant*. New York: League for the Hard of Hearing Publications. (adult restoration of hearing via implant)

Sacks, O. (1989). *Seeing voices: A journey into the world of the deaf*. New York: Harper Perennial. (deafness and Deaf culture)

Schaller, S. (1995). *A man without words*. Berkeley: University of California Press. (adult learning to talk)

PROFESSIONAL ISSUES

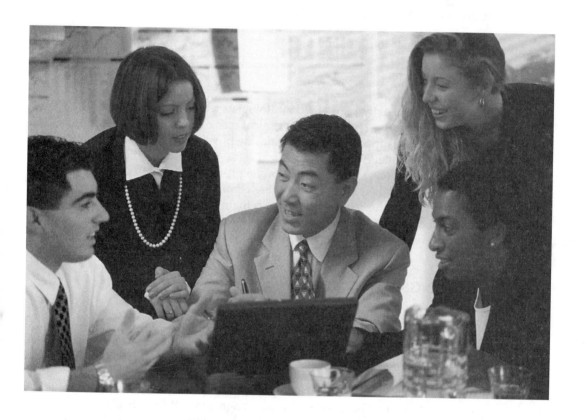

PREVIEW

In this book, we have reviewed normal communication processes and disorders of communication that require the professional services of speech-language pathologists and audiologists. Along the way, we have introduced various aspects of clinical practice. In this final chapter we will provide an overview of professional work settings, discuss interdisciplinary interactions, and address some professional issues such as standards, ethics, and certification requirements. Future advances in the understanding of communication processes and disorders will influence approaches to evaluation and treatment. In addition, professional practice patterns are likely to undergo change in response to social, political, and economic influences. We will touch on some forseeable future trends.

Speech-language pathologists and audiologists work in a variety of settings. Each work environment is shaped by the clinical caseload, professional colleagues, administrative and support personnel, and the physical and procedural characteristics of the work site. A change in clinical setting can mean a drastic change in the characteristics of one's employment. Some professionals enjoy the opportunity to shift the nature of their work by changing clinical environments over the course of their career. Even those who appreciate remaining in one type of setting are likely to experience considerable variety in their professional activities from day to day and year to year.

CLINICAL SETTINGS

Public Schools

The public schools employ 55 percent of all speech-language pathologists and 10 percent of all audiologists, making it the most common work setting for ASHA members (ASHA, 2002a). The initiation of speech and hearing programs in the schools dates as far back as 1910 in the Chicago public school system (Paden, 1970). Programs developed because educators recognized that speech and hearing problems affected performance in the classroom and deemed it appropriate to provide services onsite. The scope of public school services has expanded over the years to include any child who has a communication disorder that negatively affects his or her education. Services for "educationally handicapped children" became nationwide with the passage of Public Law 94-142, The Education for All Handicapped Children Act, in 1975. Other public laws were passed that govern services for children within the schools. Public Law 95-561 expanded remedial services by providing federal support to improve children's basic educational skills, including listening and speaking. Preschool children who appear to have a speech, language,

or hearing problem became eligible for assessment and remediation services through their local school system with the passage of Public Law 99-457. The public schools also conduct hearing screening programs at specified intervals that may involve the direct or indirect participation of the audiologist.

Speech-language pathologists in the public schools may work with children individually, in small groups, or in an entire classroom. The caseload can vary from multiply handicapped children to those with specific speech or language difficulties. Some professionals serve children in only one school, whereas others are itinerant, traveling to several schools. Audiologists provide a range of services to public school children that include screening, diagnostic, and aural habilitation programs. They also assist students with the wide variety of personal and classroom amplification systems. One notable feature of work in the public school setting is the academic calendar, which holds appeal for some professionals, particularly if their own children are of school age.

Medical Settings

Medical settings are second to schools as the most common employment site for speech, language, and hearing professionals. In 2001, 72 percent of audiologists and 37 percent of speech-language pathologists worked in medical settings (ASHA, 2002a). These worksites include a broad spectrum of health care delivery environments, including hospital-based acute care and rehabilitation units, in- and outpatient rehabilitation facilities, nursing homes, and medical clinics. Even within one hospital, there are a variety of settings where speech-language pathologists and audiologists work. In the past it was common for audiology and speech-language pathology to comprise their own department, but that is no longer standard practice. In relatively large hospitals, speech-language pathologists and audiologists tend to be members of various teams throughout the hospital. For example, audiologists may be associated with otolaryngology or physical medicine and rehabilitation. Speech-language pathologists may be allied, for example, with inpatient neurology or neurosurgery, pediatrics, or the dysphagia team. The particular demands of medical settings have been addressed in some excellent resources for medical speech-language pathology (Golper, 1992; Johnson & Jacobson, 1998).

Just as clinical practice in the public schools has been influenced by public laws, service delivery in medical settings is greatly influenced by forces such as health care legislation, managed care, and health insurance policies. Hospital stays have shortened considerably in recent years, and there has been an increase in service delivery in the home provided through home health care agencies. Patients tend to receive therapy for shorter durations than in the past, and clinicians must clearly justify their patients' need and benefits of their services. These changes have been accompanied by an emphasis on the functional outcomes of treatment, so that clinicians focus on very practical aspects of the patients' needs and how treatment will make a difference in their everyday life (Frattali, 1998).

Academic and Clinical Training Programs

Clinical training in the evaluation and treatment of communication disorders is conducted in many colleges and universities. The departments that provide coursework and professional preparation in speech-language pathology and audiology have various names, such as Speech and Hearing Sciences, Audiology and Speech-Language Pathology, and Communication Disorders. Clinical training involves academic coursework at the undergraduate and graduate levels and supervised clinical training. Most university programs include an on-campus clinic that offers student training opportunities and practicum training with cooperating clinical placement sites in the community. University clinics typically serve both children and adults who have hearing, language, articulation, voice, and fluency problems. The clinics may offer students the opportunity to observe evaluation and treatment procedures in communication disorders prior to beginning direct clinical work and provide supervised clinical training for graduate students. Many training programs confer bachelor's, master's, and doctoral degrees.

University programs also contribute to the knowledge base of the professions through the conduct of basic and applied research. The research endeavors within a particular department reflect the areas of interest to the faculty. Students may become involved in research in a variety of informal and formal ways through work-study programs, volunteering, independent study, and thesis options. Research doctoral degree programs (e.g., Ph.D., Sci.D.) are research-oriented and require completion of original research in the form of a dissertation. There are also doctoral programs that focus on the clinical aspects of the professions.

Community Speech and Hearing Centers

Many of the first speech and hearing services in the United States that were outside of the public schools were provided in community speech and hearing centers. Such clinics are often housed in free-standing buildings rather than within an educational or medical facility. Community clinics are not as common as they once were, but those that exist often derive some of their financial support from supplemental sources. For example, they may be funded by agencies such as United Way or county public health programs, philanthropic groups such as Scottish Rite, or national organizations such as the Easter Seal Society. The clientele may be specific to certain disorders, such as children with cerebral palsy, or may include a wide variety of disorders that affect individuals of all ages.

Private Practice

An increasing number of audiologists and speech-language pathologists are choosing careers in private practice. In 2002, almost 10 percent of certified speech-language pathologists were in full-time private practice, and another 14 percent worked part-time. In audiology, 21 percent of the certified professionals were in

full-time private practice and 15 percent worked in part-time private practice (ASHA, 2002a). These individuals may provide services in their own office setting or through contractual arrangements with other care providers (e.g., hospitals, schools, nursing facilities). Practitioners who work part-time in a private practice may spend the rest of the day in another clinical setting (such as a public school). Private practitioners treat a wide variety of disorders. Adults may seek a private practice speech-language pathologist to continue treatment for a chronic condition, such as aphasia or a motor speech disorder. Parents may contact a private practitioner to supplement the services their child receives through the schools or to treat conditions not otherwise covered in school-based programs (e.g., tongue thrust). Schools, hospitals, and other agencies may contract with private practitioners in order to relieve personnel shortages. In such cases, the private practitioner operates as an independent contractor to these businesses and organizations rather than as one of their employees. It is this autonomy that appeals to clinicians who choose to maintain a private practice.

INTERDISCIPLINARY INTERACTIONS

Almost all speech-language pathologists and audiologists work in conjunction with other professionals to some degree. Some of the cases presented earlier in this text provide examples of interdisciplinary interactions in the treatment of communication disorders. We can find out more about the nature of these interactions by reading about the experiences of clinicians who work on interdisciplinary teams. We will also consider the professions that comprise these teams and work with speech-language pathologists and audiologists in a variety of settings.

Team Approach in Public Schools

We begin with professionals who work with children in a public school setting. These individuals are jointly involved at all levels of case management, from the initial referral through the implementation of therapy goals on a daily basis.

Patty is a speech-language pathologist with ten years' experience in the public school setting. She currently works with Cheryl, an occupational therapist, and Jean, a physical therapist, along with psychologists and several regular preschool and special education teachers. "An obvious motor impairment or speech-language problem is usually the cause for referral at our center. But often, with years of experience, you can just watch a kid and know that this kid needs to be seen by other professionals," Cheryl reported. The initial screening team in this school consisted of the classroom teacher, the speech-language pathologist, and the psychologist, with additional professions brought in as needed.

Each of the team members participates in joint evaluation of the child. However, their participation fluctuates as activities are more or less appropriate for providing each of them with relevant information. For example, Patty may do

some formal language testing and come back to the evaluation during assessment of gross motor activities, because she knows that children are likely to use the most spontaneous language during that time. Cheryl reported that the group has come to work smoothly by getting to know what each other does. "Initially, it was intimidating, not knowing when it was my turn to do something. Then [over time] it just kind of smoothed out." "We pretty much follow the child's lead," added Patty. "When I'm preparing my next set of materials, Cheryl is already in there doing her next thing. The nice thing is it really speeds up the evaluation so the child doesn't really get bored."

The group pointed to several factors that made their work as an evaluation team effective. "First, it really helped that we all had experience with this population. Then, it was a matter of picking up on each other's pace," reported Jean. Patty added, "It's also a matter of knowing which activities of the others are going to provide me with language information. Or when I'm presenting information, Cheryl might say 'You want to hold that at an angle because you can tell he's got low vision,' which helps me get optimal performance." The group agreed that teams work well when there is a respect for other professions and some knowledge of what each can contribute. The members must understand that the domains represented by each profession really do affect each other. As Cheryl put it, "I think that if you go in thinking that your own profession is the only one that is going to make the difference for that child, you're missing out on an integrated picture of the whole child."

This group offered many examples of how the goals of different therapists interrelate for a particular child. For example, the positioning guidelines from the physical therapist may also be used by the occupational therapist and speech-language pathologist to provide the stability a child needs before learning can occur. To maximize their joint efforts, they often develop methods to address multiple goals at the same time.

Patty related, "If I am working on increasing requests by a child, I can have the child ask for materials during an art project. When the request is made, I hand the crayon or straw to the child. I can do that in a way that reinforces the reaching or grasping behaviors I know Cheryl is working on as well." Often, motor activities can serve as the reinforcement for training speech goals. One popular activity is an obstacle course that primarily serves OT and PT goals. Children are "allowed" to run the course after producing three correct articulation targets. Jean remarked that she often watches Patty to see at what level she is presenting language to the child. "It doesn't do me any good if a child can't perform a movement because he didn't understand my directions." In return, Patty has "borrowed" techniques from both Cheryl and Jean because she has noticed their effectiveness in helping children maintain their attention during various activities.

In the school setting, the speech-language pathologist may find himself or herself interacting with a variety of other professionals. In the example above, we have seen how some of these professionals may work together with preschool children. Let us now take a closer look at the professional interactions of a speech-language pathologist in a pediatric clinic.

Team Approach in a Pediatric Clinic

Lora is a speech-language pathologist who serves as the coordinator of her hospital's cleft palate team (see Chapter 4 for a discussion of this condition). This team consists of an audiologist, geneticist, nurse, otolaryngologist (ENT), pediatrician, plastic surgeon, dentist, orthodontist, prosthodontist, and social worker, who interact as a full team or as individuals with the parents and child.

"We get notified [that a child has been born with a cleft palate] from the birthing clinic. If it's feasible, we try to do a hospital visit within that first 24 to 48 hours," Lora reports. This visit usually involves a speech-language pathologist, a social worker, or a nurse. These individuals provide the parents with initial information concerning their child's condition, what can be done, and what to expect as the child develops. Lora also provides important information about feeding the child during this early visit. Lora commented, "We feel that this early visit provides a valuable service."

Soon after, the audiologist will see the child to evaluate hearing status and to counsel the parents about possible concerns with hearing health as their child develops. Other early appointments will be with the geneticist, ear-nose-throat doctor, and the plastic surgeon. "As the child grows," related Lora, "he or she will be seeing the ENT, plastic surgeon, and some of the other team members on a regular basis. Then our program requires that the child visit the entire team, which meets once a month, for certain procedures to be approved. They want [the treatment] to be a team consensus to be sure that it is the appropriate treatment for the child." Procedures that routinely involve team discussion are things like pharyngeal flap, bone graphs, and lip and nose revisions. The team may brainstorm ideas about the timing and course of treatment that takes into consideration the various aspects of each child's condition.

The team meeting starts with a pre-conference. "I type a summary of what surgeries have already been done, the diagnosis, presenting concerns and [histories of all other services] ahead of time," reported Lora. "One of the physicians will act as the presenting or attending physician, who will say what the main concerns are. If any questions come up right then, we will discuss them." Then the parents come into the meeting and the team members have an opportunity to examine the child. This is also an opportunity for the parents to provide all the professionals with input on treatment decisions and to ask questions about possible future intervention. "We really try to encourage the parents to consider themselves a member of the team," said Lora, "and I know that it can sometimes be a bit intimidating for some of them."

The team meeting is an opportunity for the parents and professionals to see how all the components of intervention that they each contribute are coming together for the child. Through these meetings, Lora has learned about state-of-the-art techniques for the management of cleft palate from the other professionals. In addition, she has provided the team with valued contributions. She provides this example: "I've had to sell the team on the usefulness of videoendoscopy (see Chapter 6), and they've pretty much bought into it now. We've had a couple of cases

where we discovered that the child didn't need surgery [based on the videoendoscopy results]. I feel really good about how that has developed." Lora concludes with this thought, "I know that I have grown tremendously being in this role professionally. I used to be so intimidated. I would dread that day and I would know inside 'Oh, it's three days away,' and now I've been doing it for six years. I've grown much more confident. Over time, I've earned the other team members' respect. And I had to earn it."

Team Approach in a Medical Setting

Tom is a speech-language pathologist with twelve years of professional experience. Most of his work has been in medical settings with adults with acquired communication disorders, typically related to stroke or head injury. Tom currently works in a hospital in a skilled nursing unit, which provides subacute care. The patients in the subacute program are medically stable, but in need of rehabilitation and nursing care. Many of them were transferred to the unit after a stay in the acute care unit of the hospital, where they were admitted following a medically significant event, such as a stroke. Other patients were admitted directly to the subacute unit for a period of diagnostic and rehabilitative care to improve their independent living skills. Although Tom works in a hospital setting, many skilled nursing facilities are not located on a hospital campus.

Tom is part of a multidisciplinary rehabilitation team that includes a physical therapist, occupational therapist, dietician, nurse, and medical director. His workspace is part of a common rehabilitation area where the physical therapist and occupational therapist also work with patients. Interdisciplinary interaction is completely natural and occurs in both planned and spontaneous ways. For example, Tom had a patient who fatigued easily and had a limited amount of time when he was awake, alert, and able to participate in therapy. In order to maximize the patient's optimal treatment time, Tom conducted speech and language therapy at the same time that the PT was working with the patient on balance. The simultaneous attention to two tasks, balance and speech, offered an additional challenge to the patient that was more representative of real life than treating each in isolation. In other cases, therapy goals may be common across several disciplines and may be referred to as *conjoint treatment goals*. Tom told of a patient with a hip fracture who could not remember the precautions he was given by the physical therapist to protect his healing hip; therefore, part of the cognitive training that Tom implemented with this patient included strategies to assist him in learning the hip precautions. In this case, all of the therapies had common treatment goals that related to safety and achieving independent living.

Team interaction is a big part of what Tom enjoys about his current job. In fact, he selected his current worksite because the team approach appealed to him. He said that "it is important to go beyond what you have been taught" to be successful in a given setting. Working side by side with other professionals is one important way to continually expand and integrate professional knowledge.

THE PROFESSIONAL ASSOCIATION: THE AMERICAN SPEECH-LANGUAGE-HEARING ASSOCIATION

History and Purpose

The professions of speech-language pathology and audiology emerged and grew over the course of the twentieth century. In the early 1900s the focus was on speech disorders, particularly articulation and stuttering. In 1925, a group of professionals devoted to the treatment of communication disorders started an association called the American Academy for Speech Correction (Paden, 1970). The profession of audiology developed after World War II, owing to the needs of many soldiers who returned home with acquired hearing loss (Cherry & Giolas, 1997). As the audiology profession was established, audiologists were included among the ranks of professionals dealing with communication disorders. In 1948, the professional organization became the American Speech and Hearing Association (ASHA). As clinical attention to language impairments was increasingly evident in both children and adults, the profession changed the name again in 1978 to the American Speech-Language-Hearing Association, although the ASHA acronym was retained. In 1998, over 93,000 speech-language pathologists, audiologists, and speech, language, and hearing scientists belong to the organization. Information about this organization can be found at the ASHA website at www.asha.org. Additional discussion concerning professional issues is found in Lubinski and Frattali (1994).

ASHA is the primary professional organization for speech, language, and hearing professionals, although there are other related professional organizations to which audiologists and speech-language pathologists belong. The mission of ASHA is to promote the interests of the professions and to advocate for people with communication disabilities. The purposes are reflected in the Association by-laws (ASHA, 1997a), which are paraphrased here:

1. To encourage basic research and scientific study of human communication and its disorders.
2. To promote appropriate academic and clinical preparation for individuals preparing to enter the professions, and to promote continuing education within the discipline.
3. To promote investigation and prevention of communication disorders.
4. To foster improvement of clinical procedures used in treating disorders of communication.
5. To stimulate exchange of information pertinent to communication and communication disorders.
6. To advocate for individuals with communication disorders.
7. To promote the interests of members of the Association.

ASHA is an organization that is intended to serve the interests of the membership. There are two bodies that govern and establish the policies of the

Association: the Legislative Council and the Executive Board. The Legislative Council establishes the policies of the organization and is composed of elected representatives from every state, and the Executive Board consists of officers who are elected by the ASHA membership, as well as the Executive Director of the Association. Many of the ASHA policies have significant impact on members of the Association, such as defining the scope of practice of the professions, and therefore are of great interest to speech-language pathologists and audiologists. The Executive Board also manages the affairs of the Association and often serves as official representatives of the Association. The committees, task forces, and boards that operate within the ASHA structure provide opportunities for the membership to significantly contribute to the professions.

Certification and Accreditation

Most practitioners in speech-language pathology and audiology in the United States are members of ASHA and have received the Certificate of Clinical Competence (CCC) in either audiology or speech-language pathology, or both, from ASHA. To be eligible to obtain the CCC, ASHA requires the completion of graduate coursework and graduate clinical practicum from a program that is accredited by ASHA (ASHA, 1997b). Academic coursework includes basic sciences and professional coursework that meets the ASHA standards. Clinical observation and supervised practicum must be completed across a range of ages and disorders as specified by the ASHA standards (ASHA, 1997c). Following the completion of the graduate degree, the CCC applicant must spend a Clinical Fellowship Year (CFY) working in an approved clinical setting, under the direct supervision of a clinically certified clinician. The applicant also must pass a certification examination. ASHA membership is not required for certification by the organization, but the percentage of nonmembers holding certification is small. Most states require a license to practice, although those requirements are often consistent with the standards set forth by ASHA for the CCC. Evidence of continuing education also may be required for periodic state licensure renewal.

Continuing Education

ASHA is devoted to continuing education and advancement of scientific and clinical knowledge in the professions. The Association publishes several scholarly journals that are available to members and are carried in many libraries: *American Journal of Audiology*; *American Journal of Speech-Language Pathology*; *Journal of Speech and Hearing Research*; and *Language, Speech, and Hearing Services in Schools*. These journals contain research articles that have been reviewed by experts in the professions (a process called peer review) and have been deemed worthy of publication. A biweekly newspaper called *ASHA Leader* helps keep the membership abreast of current events of interest to the profession, and a quarterly *Asha* magazine covers

timely professional issues. Another continuing education opportunity is provided by the annual ASHA Convention. This convention often draws more than 10,000 participants, who have the opportunity to listen to professional presentations, view new books and clinical materials, and meet for a variety of formal and informal gatherings. Although the ASHA Convention is the largest educational event each year, there are many other activities such as workshops, telephone seminars, and videoconferences available throughout the year that are sponsored by ASHA, state and local organizations, academic programs, and private groups.

Ethical Conduct

A primary concern of ASHA is for certified speech-language pathologists and audiologists to practice their professions ethically. Consequently, all certified audiologists or speech-language pathologists (regardless of ASHA membership) must adhere to the Association's Code of Ethics (ASHA, 2002b). The Code of Ethics provides guidelines for professional practice and is a helpful resource when ethical questions arise (Figure 13.1, pp. 328–330). A timely example of the value of the Code of Ethics pertains to the discussion of clinical cases via electronic mail and listserv discussion groups. There are many opportunities for clinicians to solicit the opinions and advice of other professionals regarding the diagnosis or treatment of a particularly difficult or unusual case by internet and electronic mail interactions. When seeking information, common sense would suggest that it would be inappropriate for a clinician to reveal the name or other identifying information about a specific patient in the context of a listserv discussion (Principle I in Figure 13.1). However, it might not be so obvious that it is unethical to conduct evaluation or treatment solely by correspondence, as indicated by Principle I-I (Figure 13.1). That principle should caution clinicians who seek and offer advice about specific patients. Whereas it is appropriate for clinicians to discuss clinical practice in the electronic mail venue, there are potential problems when diagnostic and treatment suggestions are given by someone who has not actually seen the patient. Therefore, advice proffered by mail (electronic or otherwise) should be taken as suggestions rather than prescriptions for treatment. The Code of Ethics can help clarify these issues for the clinician.

Student Membership

There is a student organization, the National Student Speech Language Hearing Association (NSSLHA), that undergraduate and graduate students may join as they pursue preprofessional education in speech-language pathology, audiology, and the associated sciences. Many colleges and universities have NSSLHA chapters. NSSLHA membership offers students the opportunity to receive professional journals, participate in educational activities, and even become involved in association governance activities.

AMERICAN
SPEECH-LANGUAGE-
HEARING
ASSOCIATION

Code of Ethics

Last Revised November 16, 2001

Preamble

The preservation of the highest standards of integrity and ethical principles is vital to the responsible discharge of obligations in the professions of speech-language pathology and audiology. This Code of Ethics sets forth the fundamental principles and rules considered essential to this purpose.

Every individual who is (a) a member of the American Speech-Language-Hearing Association, whether certified or not, (b) a nonmember holding the Certificate of Clinical Competence from the Association, (c) an applicant for membership or certification, or (d) a Clinical Fellow seeking to fulfill standards for certification shall abide by this Code of Ethics.

Any action that violates the spirit and purpose of this Code shall be considered unethical. Failure to specify any particular responsibility or practice in this Code of Ethics shall not be construed as denial of the existence of such responsibilities or practices.

The fundamentals of ethical conduct are described by Principles of Ethics and by Rules of Ethics as they relate to responsibility to persons served, to the public, and to the professions of speech-language pathology and audiology.

Principles of Ethics, aspirational and inspirational in nature, form the underlying moral basis for the Code of Ethics. Individuals shall observe these principles as affirmative obligations under all conditions of professional activity.

Rules of Ethics are specific statements of minimally acceptable professional conduct or of prohibitions and are applicable to all individuals.

Reference this material as: American Speech-Language-Hearing Association. (2001, December 26). Code of ethics (revised). *ASHA Leader*, vol. 6 (23), p. 2.

Index terms: ASHA reference products, ethics (professional practice issues), ethics and related papers

Document type: Ethics and related documents

Principle of Ethics I

Individuals shall honor their responsibility to hold paramount the welfare of persons they serve professionally.

Rules of Ethics

A. Individuals shall provide all services competently.

B. Individuals shall use every resource, including referral when appropriate, to ensure that high-quality service is provided.

C. Individuals shall not discriminate in the delivery of professional services on the basis of race or ethnicity, gender, age, religion, national origin, sexual orientation, or disability.

D. Individuals shall not misrepresent the credentials of assistants, technicians, or support personnel and shall inform those they serve professionally of the name and professional credentials of persons providing services.

E. Individuals who hold the Certificates of Clinical Competence shall not delegate tasks that require the unique skills, knowledge, and judgment that are within the scope of their profession to assistants, technicians, support personnel, or any nonprofessionals over whom they have supervisory responsibility. An individual may delegate support services to assistants, technicians, support personnel, or any other persons only if those services are adequately supervised by an individual who holds the appropriate Certificate of Clinical Competence.

F. Individuals shall fully inform the persons they serve of the nature and possible effects of services rendered and products dispensed.

G. Individuals shall evaluate the effectiveness of services rendered and of products dispensed and shall provide services or dispense products only when benefit can reasonably be expected.

FIGURE 13.1   ASHA Code of Ethics (Used with permission of the American Speech-Language-Hearing Association).

H. Individuals shall not guarantee the results of any treatment or procedure, directly or by implication; however, they may make a reasonable statement of prognosis.

I. Individuals shall not provide clinical services solely by correspondence.

J. Individuals may practice by telecommunication (for example, telehealth/e-health), where not prohibited by law.

K. Individuals shall maintain adequate records of professional services rendered and products dispensed and shall allow access to these records when appropriately authorized.

L. Individuals shall not reveal, without authorization, any professional or personal information about the person served professionally, unless required by law to do so, or unless doing so is necessary to protect the welfare of the person or of the community.

M. Individuals shall not charge for services not rendered, nor shall they misrepresent,[1] in any fashion, services rendered or products dispensed.

N. Individuals shall use persons in research or as subjects of teaching demonstrations only with their informed consent.

O. Individuals whose professional services are adversely affected by substance abuse or other health-related conditions shall seek professional assistance and, where appropriate, withdraw from the affected areas of practice.

Principle of Ethics II

Individuals shall honor their responsibility to achieve and maintain the highest level of professional competence.

Rules of Ethics

A. Individuals shall engage in the provision of clinical services only when they hold the appropriate Certificate of Clinical Competence or when they are in the certification process and are supervised by an individual who holds the appropriate Certificate of Clinical Competence.

B. Individuals shall engage in only those aspects of the professions that are within the scope of their competence, considering their level of education, training, and experience.

---

[1] For purposes of this Code of Ethics, misrepresentation includes any untrue statements or statements that are likely to mislead. Misrepresentation also includes the failure to state any information that is material and that ought, in fairness, to be considered.

C. Individuals shall continue their professional development throughout their careers.

D. Individuals shall delegate the provision of clinical services only to: (1) persons who hold the appropriate Certificate of Clinical Competence; (2) persons in the education or certification process who are appropriately supervised by an individual who holds the appropriate Certificate of Clinical Competence; or (3) assistants, technicians, or support personnel who are adequately supervised by an individual who holds the appropriate Certificate of Clinical Competence.

E. Individuals shall prohibit any of their professional staff from providing services that exceed the staff member's competence, considering the staff member's level of education, training, and experience.

F. Individuals shall ensure that all equipment used in the provision of services is in proper working order and is properly calibrated.

Principle of Ethics III

Individuals shall honor their responsibility to the public by promoting public understanding of the professions, by supporting the development of services designed to fulfill the unmet needs of the public, and by providing accurate information in all communications involving any aspect of the professions.

Rules of Ethics

A. Individuals shall not misrepresent their credentials, competence, education, training, or experience.

B. Individuals shall not participate in professional activities that constitute a conflict of interest.

C. Individuals shall refer those served professionally solely on the basis of the interest of those being referred and not on any personal financial interest.

D. Individuals shall not misrepresent diagnostic information, services rendered, or products dispensed or engage in any scheme or artifice to defraud in connection with obtaining payment or reimbursement for such services or products.

E. Individuals' statements to the public shall provide accurate information about the nature and management of communication disorders, about the professions, and about professional services.

FIGURE 13.1   (continued)

F. Individuals' statements to the public—advertising, announcing, and marketing their professional services, reporting research results, and promoting products—shall adhere to prevailing professional standards and shall not contain misrepresentations.

Principle of Ethics IV

Individuals shall honor their responsibilities to the professions and their relationships with colleagues, students, and members of allied professions. Individuals shall uphold the dignity and autonomy of the professions, maintain harmonious interprofessional and intraprofessional relationships, and accept the professions' self-imposed standards.

Rules of Ethics

A. Individuals shall prohibit anyone under their supervision from engaging in any practice that violates the Code of Ethics.

B. Individuals shall not engage in dishonesty, fraud, deceit, misrepresentation, sexual harrassment, or any other form of conduct that adversely reflects on the professions or on the individual's fitness to serve persons professionally.

C. Individuals shall not engage in sexual activities with clients or students over whom they exercise professional authority.

D. Individuals shall assign credit only to those who have contributed to a publication, presentation, or product. Credit shall be assigned in proportion to the contribution and only with the contributor's consent.

E. Individuals shall reference the source when using other persons' ideas, research, presentations, or products in written, oral, or any other media presentation or summary.

F. Individuals' statements to colleagues about professional services, research results, and products shall adhere to prevailing professional standards and shall contain no misrepresentations.

G. Individuals shall not provide professional services without exercising independent professional judgment, regardless of referral source or prescription.

H. Individuals shall not discriminate in their relationships with colleagues, students, and members of allied professions on the basis of race or ethnicity, gender, age, religion, national origin, sexual orientation, or disability.

I. Individuals who have reason to believe that the Code of Ethics has been violated shall inform the Board of Ethics.

J. Individuals shall comply fully with the policies of the Board of Ethics in its consideration and adjudication of complaints of violations of the Code of Ethics.

FIGURE 13.1 (continued)

Special Interest Divisions

Although members of ASHA are generally trained to manage a broad array of communication disorders, many members have special interests in particular disorders or aspects of the profession. In 1988, special interest divisions were established to allow ASHA members with common interests to identify themselves and affiliate with one another. The divisions have varied objectives but common purposes are to advance the education of their affiliates and to represent their special interests within ASHA. In 2002, there were sixteen special interest divisions, which are listed in Table 13.1. In addition to ASHA members and international affiliates, members of NSSLHA may choose to affiliate with one or more of the divisions, which may provide them with insight into current issues in prospective areas of interest. Affiliation with special interest divisions is optional; affiliate dues may be paid at the same time that ASHA or NSSLHA dues are paid.

TRENDS IN THE PROFESSION

Specialty Recognition

Professional preparation in speech-language pathology and audiology is relatively broad-based so that there are many clinical populations and settings from which to choose. However, many professionals find that over time they tend to specialize in a particular area (or areas) of clinical practice. Until recently, there was no way for professionals to establish or document that they had gained advanced knowledge

TABLE 13.1   Special Interest Divisions of the American Speech-Language-Hearing Association

Division 1:	Language Learning and Education
Division 2:	Neurophysiology and Neurogenic Speech and Language Disorders
Division 3:	Voice and Voice Disorders
Division 4:	Fluency and Fluency Disorders
Division 5:	Speech Science and Orofacial Disorders
Division 6:	Hearing and Hearing Disorders: Research and Diagnostics
Division 7:	Aural Rehabilitation and Its Instrumentation
Division 8:	Hearing Conservation and Occupational Audiology
Division 9:	Hearing and Hearing Disorders in Childhood
Division 10:	Issues in Higher Education
Division 11:	Administration and Supervision
Division 12:	Augmentative and Alternative Communication
Division 13:	Swallowing and Swallowing Disorders (Dysphagia)
Division 14:	Communication Disorders and Sciences in Culturally and Linguistically Diverse Populations
Division 15:	Gerontology
Division 16:	School-Based Issues

and clinical expertise in a particular clinical specialty. In 1994, the Legislative Council of ASHA approved a program for specialty recognition within the professions of speech pathology and audiology. This voluntary program allows practitioners within a given specialty to petition for the establishment of specialty recognition in their area of expertise. The Clinical Specialty Board established by ASHA oversees the application process as groups within the profession take the responsibility to institute specialty recognition. The Clinical Specialty Board does not initiate the establishment of specialty recognition; the initiative comes from a group of practitioners in a given specialty. So in effect, speech-language pathologists and audiologists who have become specialists in a particular area take the responsibility to establish the criteria for such specialization. In some cases, the Special Interest Division may choose to petition for specialty recognition, in other cases, the petitioner may be a related professional organization. The specialty recognition process is in its infancy. Students and new professionals in speech, language, and hearing may be interested in researching the status of specialty recognition as they prepare to enter the profession.

Use of Support Personnel

The use of support personnel is an emerging trend within the professions. These individuals are sometimes referred to as speech-language assistants or aides, audiometric technicians, or audiology assistants. They work in a variety of settings under the supervision of an ASHA-certified speech-language pathologist or audiologist. Unlike the requirements for clinical certification of master's level clinicians, there is no widely accepted training standard for support personnel. However, ASHA has provided guidelines for the training, credentialing, use, and supervision of these individuals in clinical and educational settings (ASHA, 1995, 1998). In addition, the ASHA Code of Ethics provides principles related to work by support personnel. The use of support personnel is intended to occur as an adjunct to and under the supervision of clinically certified personnel. When managed properly, a program that includes both certified personnel and support personnel can be effective. Let's take a look at one such team.

> Kendall, an ASHA certified speech-language pathologist, "inherited" a speech aide when she took a part-time job at a state residential facility for adults with severe developmental disorders. Her aide, Julie, had been working at this center for twenty years, the last six as a speech aide. She has a high school education and received on-the-job training for her current position. They have been working together for three years.
>   Kendall is responsible for initial assessments of the center's residents. She interviews the center staff concerning the residents' level of functioning and develops programs designed to increase their functional communication. She discusses a new program with Julie to get her insights on how it might be integrated into the daily activities at the center. It is Julie who is at the center on a daily basis, who oversees the implementation of those programs. She works with the center staff to explain the communication goals and provides them with materials for training

those communication behaviors during the day. She also collects and compiles data on the frequency with which goals were addressed by the staff and how effective the program has been for a resident.

Julie's duties are fairly typical of support personnel. These duties may include clerical work, making materials for intervention programs, and implementing the programs planned by the certified clinician (Kimbarow, 1997). Julie's contribution on a daily basis increases frequency of services to the residents beyond what Kendall could provide on her own. Effective use of support personnel may mean that the certified clinician may have to rethink the components of his or her job and how to best carry them out.

"One of the things that has been very important for me in working with my aide was learning to prioritize," said Kendall. "I had to decide which tasks were critical for me to complete, and let Julie do the rest."

As Kendall's experience shows, support personnel can make a positive contribution to the professions. However, the use of support personnel in clinical settings is not without controversy. Some clinicians are concerned that bureaucratic decisions will be made that increase the use of support personnel beyond their training and abilities, eroding the quality of services. Those who have had experience working with support personnel offered guidance for those who might have the opportunity to work with support personnel (Kimbarow, 1997). Their advice includes:

- Establish clear guidelines for use of support personnel.
- Establish minimum competencies for the work setting.
- Learn how to supervise and train support personnel.
- Allow for a training period for developing competencies before working with patients.
- Explain the rationale behind therapy procedures so that they are implemented correctly.
- Do not assign support personnel to work with new clients or with certain types of complex disorders.
- Establish a plan of supervision and feedback.

Employment Outlook

Speech-language pathology and audiology are relatively young professions that continue to grow. In fact, they were ranked among the fastest growing occupations in the country by the U. S. Bureau of Labor Statistics (2002). For the remainder of this decade, the number of positions is expected to increase by 45 percent for audiology and 39 percent for speech-language pathology (Hecker, 2001). Among the job settings that will see the biggest demand are colleges and universities. Data from the Council on Graduate Programs (2001) suggest that job openings for those

with research doctorates will exceed the number of doctoral graduates for much of this decade.

The outlook is good for the professions, given factors such as increased awareness of communication disorders; early detection of hearing, speech, and language disorders in children; the aging of the population and associated increased prevalence of age-related communication impairments; and increased concern over occupationally related hearing disorders (ASHA, 1998). These trends suggest continued growth of the professions well into the future. While work settings and models of service delivery are likely to change over time, the professions will remain devoted to increased understanding of the nature and treatment of communication disorders.

REFERENCES

American Speech-Language-Hearing Association (ASHA). (2002). Code of ethics. www.asha.org

American Speech-Language-Hearing Association (ASHA). (1995). Position statement for the training, credentialing, use, and supervision of support personnel in speech-language pathology. *Asha, 37* (Suppl. 14), 21.

American Speech-Language-Hearing Association (ASHA). (1997a). Bylaws and policies associated with the bylaws of the American Speech-Language-Hearing Association. *ASHA desk reference*, Vol. 1. Rockville, MD: Author.

American Speech-Language-Hearing Association (ASHA). (1997b). Standards for accreditation of educational programs in speech-language pathology and audiology. *ASHA desk reference*, Vol. 1 (pp. 113–144). Rockville, MD: Author.

American Speech-Language-Hearing Association (ASHA). (1997c). *Membership certification handbook*. Rockville, MD: Author.

American Speech-Language-Hearing Association (ASHA). (1998). Position statement and guidelines on support personnel in audiology. *Asha, 40* (Spring Suppl. 18).

American Speech-Language-Hearing Association (ASHA). (2002). *Annual counts of the ASHA membership and affiliation*. Retrieved December 23, 2002, from http://www.professional.ASHA.org/resources/factsheets/index.cfm#counts

Cherry, R., & Giolas, T. G. (1997). Preface to aural rehabilitation with adults. *Seminars in hearing, 18*, 75.

Council on Graduate Programs in Communication Sciences and Disorders. (2002). *Demographic survey of undergraduate and graduate programs in communication sciences and disorders*. Minneapolis, MN: Author.

Frattali, C. M. (1998). Outcomes assessment in speech-language pathology. In A. F. Johnson & B. H. Jacobson (Eds.), *Medical speech-language pathology: A practitioner's guide*. New York: Thieme.

Golper, L. C. (1992). *Sourcebook for medical speech pathology*. San Diego: Singular.

Hecker, D. E. (2001). Occupational employment projections to 2010. *Monthly Labor Review, 124*, 58–84.

Johnson, A. F., & Jacobson, B. H. (1998). *Medical speech-language pathology: A practitioner's guide*. New York: Thieme.

Kimbarow, M. L. (1997). Ahead of the curve: Improving services with speech-language pathology assistants. *Asha, 39*, 41–44

Lubinski, R., & Frattali, C. (1994). *Professional issues in speech-language pathology and audiology: A textbook*. San Diego: Singular.

Paden, E. (1970). *A history of the American Speech and Hearing Association, 1925–1958*. Bethesda, MD: American Speech and Hearing Association.

U.S. Bureau of Labor Statistics. (2002). *Occupational outlook handbook, 2002–03 edition*. Washington, DC: Author.

GLOSSARY

acoustic neuroma   A nonmalignant tumor that involves the myelin sheath of the VIIIth nerve.

addition error   A type of speech articulation error characterized by adding a sound to the target phoneme or word; for example, for the word, *blue*, a child pronounces it *bolu*.

affricate   A consonant that begins with a plosive phoneme and ends with a fricative, such as *ch*, written phonetically as /tʃ/.

agraphia   An acquired impairment of writing caused by brain damage.

air-conduction audiometry   Testing hearing by introducing the tone into the ear canal, with the sound waves then traveling to the drum membrane at the end of the canal (as opposed to bone conduction).

alexia   An acquired impairment of reading caused by brain damage.

alerting devices   Devices to warn a hearing-impaired person to sounds in the environment (e.g., a telephone ringing, a doorbell, a baby's cry, or an emergency alarm) through vibration, a light signal, or a combination.

alexia with agraphia   An acquired impairment of reading and writing due to brain damage without other language impairments.

alexia without agraphia   An acquired impairment of reading that is not accompanied by a writing impairment; also called pure alexia.

allophone   One of the variant forms of a phoneme that is still recognized by the listener as the target phoneme.

alveolar ridge   The ridge of bone just behind the upper front teeth.

Alzheimer's disease   The most common form of dementing illness; a chronic, progressive disease that results in intellectual decline affecting language, memory, and cognition.

anarthria   A severe impairment of motor control for speech resulting in complete lack of articulate speech.

anomia   The inability to name objects or retrieve desired words.

anomic aphasia   A fluent aphasia that is characterized by relatively good verbal expression and auditory comprehension, but notable difficulty coming up with the names of things.

APGAR   A five-point evaluation system for identifying the status of newborns.

aphasia   An acquired impairment of language due to damage to the language-dominant hemisphere, typically the left. See fluent aphasia and nonfluent aphasia.

aphonia   Attempts to produce a voice result in a whisper-like sound. This usually occurs with voice disorders that prevent the vocal folds from vibrating to produce sound.

apraxia of speech   An impairment of motor planning for the movements for speech so that voluntary control for speech is disrupted.

arcuate fasciculus   A bundle of nerve fibers (white matter) that originate in cell bodies in the superior temporal gyrus and project anteriorly to the frontal lobe.

articulation   Production of speech sounds.

articulation index   A theoretical construct that attempts to quantify the contribution of different frequency bands to the intelligibility of speech.

arytenoid cartilage   The paired, pyramid-shaped cartilages that sit on the signet portion of the cricoid cartilage and aid in abduction and adduction of vocal folds.

aspiration   Inhalation of fluids or other matter into the airway.

assimilation   A speech phenomenon in which the sounds that precede or follow a particular sound influence the production of that sound.

assistive listening device (ALD)   Any device designed to reduce the effects of distance, background noise, and reverberation on the perception of speech.

ataxia   A motor disorder characterized by marked loss of coordination, often associated with cerebellar disease.

athetosis   A form of cerebral palsy characterized by twisting and flailing of the extremities, neck, and trunk.

audibility index   *See* articulation index.

audiogram   A graphic representation of the results of a hearing test with axes for hearing level and frequency.

audiologist   A professional who is concerned with the prevention, evaluation, and rehabilitation of auditory, balance, and related disorders.

audiology   The study of normal and disordered hearing.

audiometer   An electronic instrument used to evaluate the auditory system.

auditory brainstem response   An electrophysiological response to sounds that results in five to seven peaks that appear within 10 ms after the presentation of a signal (usually a click).

auditory training   The training of a hearing-impaired individual to make use of residual hearing abilities.

auricle   The external ear, also known as pinna.

basal ganglia   A collection of subcortical gray matter structures, including the putamen, globus pallidus, and caudate, that contribute to control of motor behavior.

basilar membrane   A thin tissue layer found within the cochlea on which the organ of Corti rests.

bolus   Refers to a cohesive mass of some substance such as food.

bone-conduction audiometry   In hearing testing, introducing the sound waves directly into the cochlea via the bones of the skull.

brainstem   The brain structures at the base of the brain excluding the hemispheres above, the cerebellum, and the spinal cord below.

Broca's aphasia   A nonfluent aphasia with relatively preserved auditory comprehension, associated with damage to the inferior portions of the left frontal lobe.

canonical babbling   Consonant-vowel or consonant-vowel-consonant-vowel combinations produced by babies.

carcinoma   A cancer or malignancy.

central auditory processing disorder   Difficulties understanding speech as a result of structural changes in the central auditory nervous system. The difficulties are most pronounced in background noise and other difficult listening situations (e.g., reverberation).

central nervous system   The brain and spinal cord, exclusive of the cranial and peripheral nerves.

cerebrovascular accident   *See* stroke.

cerebellum   A brain structure that sits below the cerebral hemispheres and above the pons, playing an important role in muscular coordination.

cerebral localization   A theory of brain function that associates particular functions and behaviors to particular sites of the brain.

cerebral palsy   A developmental motor disorder related to brain injury; the most common forms are spasticity, athetosis, and ataxia.

cerebrum   The largest division of the brain, containing the cerebral hemispheres and corpus callosum.

cerumen   A waxy substance produced by glands that lie within the skin of the ear canal.

chromosome   A structure containing genes that transmit genetic information.

cilia   Hairlike structures that extend from the surface of a cell.

circumlocution   Talking with an excess number of words; or talking around the topic rather than being direct because of a failure to retrieve desired words, as in anomia.

cleft lip and cleft palate   A congenital fissure or absence of tissue of the lip, premaxilla, hard palate, and/or velum.

closed caption decoder   An electronic device that decodes the captioned signals that are often broadcast with television programs. It enables captions to appear on the television screen and helps hearing-impaired individuals to understand the dialogue of television programs and movies.

cluttering   A disorder of fluency characterized by rapid speech, breaks in fluency, and faulty articulation.

coarticulation   The simultaneous production of two or more consonants or vowels in normal speech production of a word, such as the word *tram*—the first three phones (/t/ /r/ /æ/) might overlap in production.

cochlea   The snail-shaped part of the inner ear containing the sensory organs of hearing.

cochlear implant   A coil and electrodes surgically placed in the inner ear and connected to an external transmitter/signal processor. It is intended to produce sensations of sound for those with profound hearing impairments.

code switching   Shifting by speakers among one or more dialects or languages to accommodate social rules or situational demands.

cognate   A pair of sounds, such as /p/ and /b/, produced similarly except that one (/p/) is unvoiced and one (/b/) voiced.

communication   An interaction or exchange of one's feelings, ideas, thoughts, and wants among two or more people by such modes as speech, writing, facial expression, gesture, or touch.

conduction aphasia   A fluent aphasia characterized by relatively good auditory comprehension and poor verbal repetition.

conductive hearing loss   A loss of hearing related to obstruction or disease in the outer or middle ear in which sound transmission fails to reach the cochlea in the inner ear.

congenital   Present at birth.

consanguineous   Between blood relatives.

content   The elements of language that carry meaning; also called semantics.

continuant   A speech sound that can be continued or prolonged, such as /m/ or /s/.

corpus callosum   A large band of fibers that joins the two hemispheres of the brain.

cortex   The surface layer of the brain that contains the bodies of neurons.

cranial nerves   Twelve paired peripheral nerves that derive from or come into the cranial cavity, such as cranial nerves I, olfactory, or II, optic.

cricoid cartilage   The ring of cartilage that forms the base of the larynx.

criterion-referenced test   A type of measure that is used to compare a child's performance against a standard, or criterion, for behavior.

decibel (dB)   A logarithmic unit of measurement of sound intensity.

dementia   A behavioral syndrome of generalized intellectual deficit that results from a number of diseases.

denasality   Insufficient nasal resonance; hyponasality.

developmental language disorder   A condition involving poor language skills that appears during childhood.

diadochokinesis   The rapid, alternating movements of a body part, such as in the lips and tongue rapidly saying *pataka*.

diagnosogenic theory of stuttering   Theory that posits stuttering begins when normal disfluencies are labeled as stuttering.

diaphragm   The muscular-tendonous partition that separates the thorax from the abdomen, serving as the primary muscle of respiration.

diphthong   A blending together of two vowels in the same syllable, such as heard as /aɪ/ in the word *right*.

diplophonia   This describes a voice that has two pitches occurring at the same time.

disfluency   A breakdown in the prosodic flow or fluency of speech.

distinctive features   Particular elements that are characteristic of a phoneme such as its duration and voicing elements.

distortion error   The production of a target phoneme utilizing a sound that is not in the language, such as in a lateral lisp.

dyadic communication   Two people communicating with each other.

dysarthria   An impairment of motor control for speech caused by weakness, paralysis, slowness, incoordination, or sensory loss in the muscle groups responsible for speech.

dyslexia   An impairment of reading to developmental brain damage or dysfunction.

dysphagia   An impairment of the ability to swallow.

dysphonia   A disorder of voice, such as hoarseness, breathiness, or harshness.

effusion   Fluid that has exuded into the middle ear space.

electrolarynx   An electronic device that creates sound that can be used as a substitute for the voice (usually because the larynx has been surgically removed).

endogenous   Caused by genetic factors

epiglottis   An oblong cartilage that sits at the top of the larynx and covers its opening during swallowing.

eustachian tube   The air tube that connects the middle ear with the nasopharynx.

exogenous   Acquired or caused by factors outside the genes.

external ear canal   The external opening into the ear.

fluency   The rhythm and flow of spoken (or signed) language.

fluent aphasia   An aphasia profile that is characterized by spoken output of relatively normal utterance length, ease of production, and prosodic variation.

FM system   A device that uses a transmitter to send the desired signal to a receiver using a radio wave. The receiver is coupled to the listener via earphones or a hearing aid.

form   The phonological, syntactic, and morphological elements of language.

four kilohertz (4k Hz) notch   An increase in hearing impairment in the 3000 to 6000 Hz region with recovery of hearing at 8000 Hz. This pattern is associated with noise-induced hearing impairment.

frequency   The number of cycles per second of a sound wave; perceived as pitch.

fricative   A speech sound produced by the airstream passing between or through a constricted opening, such as /f/ and /v/.

frontal lobe   The anterior part of each cerebral hemisphere, from the Rolandic fissure forward.

global aphasia   A nonfluent aphasia characterized by marked impairment of verbal expression and auditory comprehension, typically caused by large lesions to the perisylvian region of the left hemisphere.

glossectomy   The surgical removal of the tongue.

glottis   The opening between the vocal folds.

habitual pitch   The modal or most frequently occurring voice pitch.

habituation   Gradual decrease in responsiveness following repeated exposure to a stimulus.

handicap   A disadvantage resulting from an impairment or disability that limits the fulfillment of a role that is normal for an individual.

hearing   The perception of sound.

hearing disability   The restrictions in daily activities that result from a hearing impairment.

hearing impairment   Any loss or abnormality of structure or function of the auditory system.

hearing loss   *See* hearing impairment.

hemiparesis   Weakness of one side of the body.

hemisphere   Literally, half circle. In reference to brain anatomy, hemisphere indicates the half of the cerebrum or cerebellum to each side of midline.

Hertz   Unit of measure that reflects cycles per second.

hypernasality   Excessive nasal resonance.

immittance audiometry   Air-pressure and air-volume differences measured in the external and middle ear as a method of detecting conductive hearing loss.

incidence   The number of new cases that appear in a population over a set period of time.

incus   An anvil-shaped bone found in the middle ear.

intensity   A measure of the magnitude or pressure of a sound wave; perceived as loudness.

involuntary repetitions   A form of stuttering characterized by unexpected syllable or word repetitions.

jargon aphasia   An acquired impairment of language characterized by meaningless utterances.

language   The coding of meaning into a system of arbitrary symbols that are recognized by members of the community. Language may be spoken, written, or manual (signed).

laryngectomy   Surgical removal of the larynx (usually because of cancer).

learning disability   Educational difficulties in reading, writing, listening, speaking, or arithmetic, believed to be related to some kind of central brain dysfunction.

left neglect   Reduced awareness or responsiveness to sensory input from the left side of the body (intrapersonal space) or left half of the environment (extrapersonal space) that cannot be attributed to sensory or motor defects.

lesion   Damage to the nervous system.

lexicon   The terms and words of one's vocabulary.

malleus   A hammer-shaped bone attached to the tympanic membrane within the middle ear.

mandible   The lower jaw.

Ménière's disease   A disease of the inner ear thought to be associated with an overproduction of endolymph. Symptoms include tinnitus, vertigo, and hearing loss.

mental retardation   Reduced cognitive abilities, confirmed by measured intelligence quotients of 70 or below and poor adaptive abilities.

middle ear   The air-filled space located in the temporal bone containing the three small middle-ear bones, incus, malleus, and stapes.

misarticulations   Speech-articulation errors of omission, addition, substitution, or distortion.

mixed hearing loss   A hearing loss caused by both conductive and sensorineural problems.

morpheme Words or the smallest unit of a word that has meaning. For example, the word *cat* is one morpheme; in the plural form *cats*, the *s* is an added morpheme.

morphology The study of words and word forms; the study of morphemes.

multi-infarct dementia A form of dementia related to many small strokes (or infarcts).

myofunctional therapy Muscle training of the tongue to reduce tongue pressures on dentition, that is, therapy for reverse swallow and tongue thrust.

nasoendoscope A scope used during a videoendoscopy examination of the larynx. This scope is shaped like a long thin tube that is flexible. It is placed through the nose to view the soft palate and can also be positioned in the pharynx to view the larynx.

neologism A nonword, or literally "new word," produced by an individual with aphasia.

neuron Cell within the brain that supports activity through the conduction of chemical-electrical signals.

nonfluent aphasia An aphasia profile that is characterized by effortful speech production, reduced grammatical complexity, and short utterance length.

normative sample A representative sample of individuals whose performance on a test or measure serves as a reference against which a single individual's performance can be compared.

norm-referenced test Test designed to allow comparisons between an individual's performance and a group of individuals of similar age.

occipital lobe The posterior part of each cerebral hemisphere.

omission error One of the four types of articulatory errors, in which the sound is totally omitted.

oral-peripheral examination An examination of the structure and function of the face, mouth, and oral cavity, intended to assess the integrity of the articulatory mechanisms of speech.

organ of Corti Area within the cochlea containing the tectorial membrane and hair cells.

organogenesis The development of organs, which in humans occurs during the fetal period.

ossicles The three small bones (incus, malleus, stapes) that form the ossicular chain in the middle ear.

otitis media Inflammation of the middle ear.

otoacoustic emissions Sounds produced by the inner ear.

otosclerosis A disorder of the ear that is characterized by increased vascularity and bone resorption of the stapes It results in a progressive, conductive hearing loss when it interferes with the movement of the stapes.

otoscope A lighted device with a speculum on the end used to visualize the tympanic membrane and ear canals.

ototoxicity Sensory damage to the cochlear or vestibular systems from exposure to a chemical.

oval window A membrane-covered opening of the vestibule of the cochlea that is attached to the footplate of the stapes. Vibration of the stapes footplate sets the oval window in vibration.

palate The roof of the mouth. Anteriorly, the hard palate is bone, covered with a membrane; posteriorly, the soft palate (velum) is muscle covered with a membrane. The palate separates the oral and nasal cavities.

papilloma A wartlike tumor that can grow in the airway and larynx of primarily young children, possibly causing airway obstruction and severe dysphonia.

paraphasia An erroneous word or a nonword that reflects disorders of word choice (e.g., *man* for *woman*) or sound substitution errors (e.g., *tike* for *bike*).

parietal lobe One of the four lobes of the cerebral hemisphere, extending posteriorly from the Rolandic fissure to the occipital lobe.

perinatal The period surrounding birth; between the twenty-ninth week of gestation to one to four weeks after birth.

peripheral nervous system The nervous system that extends beyond the brain and the spinal cord, including peripheral sensory nerves that send impulses to the central nervous system and motor nerves that carry effector impulses to peripheral structures.

peristaltic contractions In the esophagus, this term describes how the muscles squeeze together starting at the top and moving downward. Each neighboring segment squeezes together to push food toward the stomach.

perisylvian region The region of the brain that surrounds the Sylvian fissure, which is the primary horizontal fissure for each cerebral hemisphere.

permanent threshold shift (PTS) Permanent sensorineural hearing loss due to damage that occurs after prolonged exposure to noise or after exposure to very high sound levels.

perseveration   Involuntary repetition of a word, phrase, sentence, or idea.

phone   A speech sound.

phoneme   The smallest sound unit of speech represented by a symbol of the International Phonetic Alphabet.

phonemic regression   Poor auditory comprehension often associated with advanced age.

phonological decoding   The process of sounding out a word from its letters during reading.

phonological process   The systematic simplification by children of the production of adult-modeled articulation, such as deleting the final consonant of words or deleting a syllable within a word.

phonology   The study of the sounds of spoken language, including the rules of phoneme use, phonemes, phonetic production, and voicing characteristics of prosody and suprasegmentals.

Pick's disease   A dementing disease that is associated with atrophy of the frontal and temporal lobes.

pinna   The visible outer ear, also known as the auricle.

pitch   The perceptual correlate of the frequency of a sound as heard by the ear.

plosive   A speech sound produced by impounding air behind an articulator and suddenly releasing it, as in /p/ or /b/.

postnatal   Occurring after birth.

prelingual   Before the development of speech.

prenatal   Preceding birth.

presbycusis   Hearing impairment associated with the aging process.

prevalence   The total number of cases present in a population in a given period of time.

progressive aphasia   An acquired impairment of language that follows a slowly progressive, rather than abrupt, onset and is not associated with dementia.

prolongation   A form of disfluency often observed in stuttering, when a speech sound or syllable has increased in duration.

prosody   The melody, flow, and rhythm of a spoken language; melodic changes in syllable stress, pitch, loudness, and duration.

protoword   Early form of an actual word that usually contains some of the sounds of the target word.

pure tone   A periodic sound wave of a particular frequency that is generated in the audiometric testing of hearing.

reflux   Refers to backward movement of food during swallowing. Often, reflux refers to acid from the stomach spilling upward into the throat, causing irritation to the tissues.

reliability   Quality of providing consistent information.

Rolandic fissure   The central fissue that divides the posterior frontal lobe from the anterior parietal lobe.

rollover   A phenomenon in which word recognition scores decrease as the presentation level of the stimuli increases.

round window   An opening in the vestibule of the cochlea beneath the oval window on the cochlea, permitting the displacement or movement of fluid within the cochlea.

screening   The detection of individuals at risk for a condition (e.g., hearing loss, language disorder).

seizures   The convulsions of an epileptic attack; epilepsy.

semantics   The study of the history and meaning of words.

sensorineural hearing loss   A hearing loss caused by disease of the inner ear or eighth cranial nerve.

sequelae   Conditions that follow or occur as a consequence of another condition (e.g., illness) or event (e.g., trauma).

sight word vocabulary   Words that a reader knows by sight without having to "sound out."

spasticity   A paralysis characterized by extreme tension and hypercontraction of muscles with hyperactive tendon reflexes.

specific language impairment   A diagnosis of a child who demonstrates impairment in understanding spoken language, speaking, reading, and writing with no other demonstrable impairment.

spectrogram   A visual display of the sound frequencies of a spoken utterance.

speech   Sound production via changes in the vocal mechanism and oral structures to form words and sentences in auditory-oral communication.

speech-language pathologist   A professional who specializes in the diagnosis and treatment of communication and swallowing disorders.

speech-language pathology   A profession that specializes in the diagnosis and treatment of communication disorders related to problems of hearing, articulation, language, voice, fluency, and swallowing.

speechreading The use of visual cues from a talker's face to identify this or her speech.

speech-reception threshold The amplification level or threshold at which the subject is able to repeat correctly after the examiner 50 percent of the words presented on a spondee list.

spinal cord The lower portion of the central nervous system, originating at the medulla and extending down within the spinal vertebra.

spinal nerves Thirty-one pairs of nerves that enter or exit the spinal cord.

spondaic words Two-syllable words pronounced with equal stress on each syllable.

stapedectomy An operation in which the stapes is removed and replaced with a prosthesis in an attempt to improve a hearing impairment that was caused by otosclerosis.

stapes A stirrup-shaped bone within the middle ear that attaches to the round window of the inner ear.

stimulability testing In testing articulation, a determination of how well the client can produce the target sound when the sound has been repeatedly presented (visually and auditorially).

STORCH Acronym for syphillis, toxoplasmosis, other, rubella, cytomegalovirus, and herpes simplex infections.

stroke Sudden onset of disturbed neurological functioning caused by disruption of blood flow. Also called a cerebrovascular accident (CVA), usually one of three types: thrombosis, embolus, or hemorrhage.

stuttering The involuntary repetition, interruption, and prolongation of speech sounds and syllables, which the individual struggles to end.

subglottal air pressure The air pressure within the airway below the vocal folds; outgoing air moves between the vocal folds when pressure below the folds is greater than air pressure above them.

substitution error A type of articulation error characterized by an incorrect phoneme used in place of a target phoneme, such as /w/ said for /r/.

Sylvian fissure The horizontal fissure that divides the inferior border of the frontal and parietal lobes from the superior temporal lobe.

syndrome A collection of physical features that co-occur and characterize a disorder or condition.

syntax The grammatical structure and word order of a language.

target sound The correct model; the phoneme selected for articulation therapy.

telecommunication device for the deaf (TDD) A keyboard that attaches to a telephone to allow typewritten communication with other TDDs. It enables individuals with hearing difficulties to communicate using the telephone.

telegraphic speech Spoken communication that consists primarily of content words and is lacking functor words, such as pronouns, auxilary verbs, and articles.

temporal lobe One of the four lobes of a cerebral hemisphere, lying below the Sylvian fissure.

temporary threshold shift Temporary sensorineural hearing loss due to noise exposure; hearing recovers after being away from the noise exposure.

thalamus A large gray mass of sensory nuclei deep within the hemisphere, bordering the third ventricle.

thyroid cartilage The shield-shaped outer cartilage protecting the larynx; popularly called the Adam's apple.

tinnitus Noises in the ear(s) usually described as ringing, hissing, or roaring.

tongue thrust Abnormal tongue positioning, particularly during swallowing, that may have an adverse effect on the anterior dental bite.

tracheostoma A permanent opening in the neck that is surgically created. This is usually done because the larynx has been surgically removed or is not able to open enough to allow breathing, such as with bilateral vocal fold paralysis or injury to the larynx.

tracheosotomy Surgical procedure that creates an opening into the trachea through which a patient can breathe.

transformer A device or mechanism that changes the nature or properties of a signal or substance.

traumatic laryngitis A dysphonia related to excessive use of harmful voicing behaviors such as yelling and screaming.

tympanic membrane The round membrane between the ear canal and middle ear, also known as the eardrum.

use The rules for communicative interactions, including the social-interactive aspects of language, sometimes called pragmatics.

validity The quality of providing accurate or true information.

velum The soft palate.

videoendoscopy This procedure uses special fiberoptic equipment to obtain views of the internal structure of the larynx.

videofluorography A motion picture x-ray that can be recorded on videotape.

video otoscopy A system that provides enlarged images that can be viewed on a monitor, stored on disk, or printed. Applications include visualization of the outer ear, tympanic membrane, and middle ear and counseling regarding hearing instrument insertion, operation, and hygiene.

vocalization Voicing or phonation.

vocal nodules Benign growths on the vocal folds, usually bilateral, which are typically the result of laryngeal abuse and voice misuse.

vocal polyps Benign growths on the vocal folds that usually occur unilaterally and are soft and compliant fluid-filled bags. These occur as a result of excessive use of harmful vocal habits such as yelling and screaming.

voice The production of sound by vibration of the vocal folds.

waveform The graph of the oscillations corresponding to the frequency of a sound.

Wernicke's aphasia A fluent aphasia characterized by poor auditory comprehension and paraphasic utterances.

AUTHOR INDEX

SUBJECT INDEX

A

Abductor spasmodic dysphonia, 136–137
Academic/clinical training programs, 320
Acoustic aspects of sound, 40–45
    complex sounds, 43–45
    frequency, 40–42
    intensity, 42
Acoustic neuroma, 299–301
Acoustic reflex, 240
Acquired language disorders, 8
Adaptive model theory of stuttering, 111
Additions, articulation errors, 63, 64
Adductor spasmodic dysphonia, 136–137
Affricate consonants, 49
Agraphia, 224
Air conduction audiometry, 254
Alerting devices, 310–311
Alexia, 224
    with agraphia, 224
    without agraphia, 224
Allophone, 47
Alveolar ridge, 69
Alzheimer's disease (AD), 227
American Educational Research Association (AERA), 196
American Psychological Association (APA), 196
American Sign Language (ASL), 3
American Speech-Language-Hearing-Association (ASHA), 10, 11, 186, 277, 304, 307, 325–331
    certification and accreditation, 326
    code of ethics, 328–330
    continuing education, 326–327
    ethical conduct, 327
    history and purpose of, 325–326
    laws of, 325
    special interest divisions, 331
    student membership, 327
Americans with Disabilities Act (ADA), 313

Anomia, 209
Anomic aphasia, 218
APGAR scoring system, 263
Aphasia, 8, 208–225
    acquired reading and writing impairments, 224–225
    assessment, 219–220
    auditory comprehension, 213
    causes of, 218–219
    characteristics of, 209–210
    fluent *vs.* nonfluent, 210–213
    repetition, 213–214
    summary of neuroanatomical principles, 214–215
    treatment, 220–223
    types, 215–218
Aphonia, 130
Approach-avoidance theory, 108
Apraxia, 72–74, 89
    of speech, 89
Arcuate fasciculus, 214
Articulation, 9, 290
Articulation disorders, 61–93
    in adults, 87–89
    articulation errors, 62–64
    childhood articulation disorders, evaluation of, 76–83
    in children, 64–76
Articulation evaluation, 77–83
    articulation inventory, 79–80
    audiometric testing, 77
    distinctive feature analysis, 81
    language testing, 83
    oral peripheral evaluation, 77–78
    phonological process analysis, 80–81
    severity estimation, 81–82
    stimulability testing, 82
Articulation inventory, 79–90
Articulation screening, 76–77
Articulation therapy for children, 83–87
    acquisition training, 83–86
    generalization, 86–87
Articulatory mechanism(s), 28–30
    mandible, 29
    palate, 29

teeth, 29–30
tongue, 28–29
Arytenoid cartilage, 25
Asphyxia, 263
Aspiration, 23
Assimilation, 50
Assistive listening devices (ALDs), 309–311
Ataxia, cerebral palsy, 75
Athetosis, cerebral palsy, 75
Attention Deficit Disorder (ADD), 186–187
Audibility index, 290
Audiogram, 254
Audiological evaluation, 304–306
    hearing assessment, 304–306
    hearing screenings, 304
Audiological testing, 271–278
    auditory brainstem response testing, 275
    behavioral testing, 271–275
    Behavioral Observation Audiometry (BOA), 272
    Conditioned Play Audiometry (CPA), 275
    Visual Reinforcement Audiometry (VRA), 273–275
Audiologists, 10
Audiology, 10
Audiology and speech–language pathology, introduction to the professions of, 1–18
    careers in communication disorders, 10–17
    clinical, 11–14
    research, 14–17
    communication disorders, classification of, 7–10
    communication impairment, six individuals with, 4–7
Audiometer, 254
Audiometric testing, 77
Auditory brainstem response (ABR), 275, 299
    testing, 275
Auditory comprehension, 213